Coffee and Caffeine Consumption for Human Health

Coffee and Caffeine Consumption for Human Health

Editor

Raquel Abalo

MDPI • Basel • Beijing • Wuhan • Barcelona • Belgrade • Manchester • Tokyo • Cluj • Tianjin

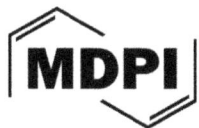

Editor
Raquel Abalo
Universidad Rey Juan Carlos
(URJC)
Spain

Editorial Office
MDPI
St. Alban-Anlage 66
4052 Basel, Switzerland

This is a reprint of articles from the Special Issue published online in the open access journal *Nutrients* (ISSN 2072-6643) (available at: https://www.mdpi.com/journal/nutrients/special_issues/Coffee_Health).

For citation purposes, cite each article independently as indicated on the article page online and as indicated below:

LastName, A.A.; LastName, B.B.; LastName, C.C. Article Title. *Journal Name* **Year**, *Volume Number*, Page Range.

ISBN 978-3-0365-5499-0 (Hbk)
ISBN 978-3-0365-5500-3 (PDF)

© 2022 by the authors. Articles in this book are Open Access and distributed under the Creative Commons Attribution (CC BY) license, which allows users to download, copy and build upon published articles, as long as the author and publisher are properly credited, which ensures maximum dissemination and a wider impact of our publications.
The book as a whole is distributed by MDPI under the terms and conditions of the Creative Commons license CC BY-NC-ND.

Contents

About the Editor ix

Raquel Abalo
Coffee and Caffeine Consumption for Human Health
Reprinted from: *Nutrients* **2021**, *13*, 2918, doi:10.3390/nu13092918 1

Christèle Rochat, Chin B. Eap, Murielle Bochud and Angeline Chatelan
Caffeine Consumption in Switzerland: Results from the First National Nutrition Survey MenuCH
Reprinted from: *Nutrients* **2020**, *12*, 28, doi:10.3390/nu12010028 7

Guilherme Falcão Mendes, Caio Eduardo Gonçalves Reis, Eduardo Yoshio Nakano, Teresa Helena Macedo da Costa, Bryan Saunders and Renata Puppin Zandonadi
Translation and Validation of the Caffeine Expectancy Questionnaire in Brazil (CaffEQ-BR)
Reprinted from: *Nutrients* **2020**, *12*, 2248, doi:10.3390/nu12082248 21

Lluis Rodas, Aina Riera-Sampol, Antoni Aguilo, Sonia Martínez and Pedro Tauler
Effects of Habitual Caffeine Intake, Physical Activity Levels, and Sedentary Behavior on the Inflammatory Status in a Healthy Population
Reprinted from: *Nutrients* **2020**, *12*, 2325, doi:10.3390/nu12082325 41

Saskia Antwerpes, Camelia Protopopescu, Philippe Morlat, Fabienne Marcellin, Linda Wittkop, Vincent Di Beo, Dominique Salmon-Céron, Philippe Sogni, Laurent Michel, Maria Patrizia Carrieri and the ANRS CO13 HEPAVIH Study Group
Coffee Intake and Neurocognitive Performance in HIV/HCV Coinfected Patients (ANRS CO13 HEPAVIH)
Reprinted from: *Nutrients* **2020**, *12*, 2532, doi:10.3390/nu12092532 55

Lena Herden and Robert Weissert
The Effect of Coffee and Caffeine Consumption on Patients with Multiple Sclerosis-Related Fatigue
Reprinted from: *Nutrients* **2020**, *12*, 2262, doi:10.3390/nu12082262 69

Chien Tai Hong, Lung Chan and Chyi-Huey Bai
The Effect of Caffeine on the Risk and Progression of Parkinson's Disease: A Meta-Analysis
Reprinted from: *Nutrients* **2020**, *12*, 1860, doi:10.3390/nu12061860 83

Hye Jin Jee, Sang Goo Lee, Katrina Joy Bormate and Yi-Sook Jung
Effect of Caffeine Consumption on the Risk for Neurological and Psychiatric Disorders: Sex Differences in Human
Reprinted from: *Nutrients* **2020**, *12*, 3080, doi:10.3390/nu12103080 95

Magdalena Nowaczewska, Michał Wiciński and Wojciech Kaźmierczak
The Ambiguous Role of Caffeine in Migraine Headache: From Trigger to Treatment
Reprinted from: *Nutrients* **2020**, *12*, 2259, doi:10.3390/nu12082259 115

Taiyue Jin, Jiyoung Youn, An Na Kim, Moonil Kang, Kyunga Kim, Joohon Sung and Jung Eun Lee
Interactions of Habitual Coffee Consumption by Genetic Polymorphisms with the Risk of Prediabetes and Type 2 Diabetes Combined
Reprinted from: *Nutrients* **2020**, *12*, 2228, doi:10.3390/nu12082228 131

Jihee Han, Jinyoung Shon, Ji-Yun Hwang and Yoon Jung Park
Effects of Coffee Intake on Dyslipidemia Risk According to Genetic Variants in the *ADORA* Gene Family among Korean Adults
Reprinted from: *Nutrients* **2020**, *12*, 493, doi:10.3390/nu12020493 147

Yin-Tso Liu, Disline Manli Tantoh, Lee Wang, Oswald Ndi Nfor, Shu-Yi Hsu, Chien-Chang Ho, Chia-Chi Lung, Horng-Rong Chang and Yung-Po Liaw
Interaction between Coffee Drinking and TRIB1 rs17321515 Single Nucleotide Polymorphism on Coronary Heart Disease in a Taiwanese Population
Reprinted from: *Nutrients* **2020**, *12*, 1301, doi:10.3390/nu12051301 159

Elizabeth D. Moua, Chenxiao Hu, Nicole Day, Norman G. Hord and Yumie Takata
Coffee Consumption and C-Reactive Protein Levels: A Systematic Review and Meta-Analysis
Reprinted from: *Nutrients* **2020**, *12*, 1349, doi:10.3390/nu12051349 171

Shou En Wu and Wei-Liang Chen
Exploring the Association between Urine Caffeine Metabolites and Urine Flow Rate: A Cross-Sectional Study
Reprinted from: *Nutrients* **2020**, *12*, 2803, doi:10.3390/nu12092803 187

Daniel T. Fuller, Matthew Lee Smith and Ali Boolani
Trait Energy and Fatigue Modify the Effects of Caffeine on Mood, Cognitive and Fine-Motor Task Performance: A Post-Hoc Study
Reprinted from: *Nutrients* **2021**, *13*, 412, doi:10.3390/nu13020412 203

Michal Wilk, Aleksandra Filip, Michal Krzysztofik, Mariola Gepfert, Adam Zajac and Juan Del Coso
Acute Caffeine Intake Enhances Mean Power Output and Bar Velocity during the Bench Press Throw in Athletes Habituated to Caffeine
Reprinted from: *Nutrients* **2020**, *12*, 406, doi:10.3390/nu12020406 219

Norzahirah Ahmad, Bee Ping Teh, Siti Zaleha Halim, Nor Azlina Zolkifli, Nurulfariza Ramli and Hussin Muhammad
Eurycoma longifolia—Infused Coffee—An Oral Toxicity Study
Reprinted from: *Nutrients* **2020**, *12*, 3125, doi:10.3390/nu12103125 233

Ana Magdalena Velázquez, Núria Roglans, Roger Bentanachs, Maria Gené, Aleix Sala-Vila, Iolanda Lázaro, Jose Rodríguez-Morató, Rosa María Sánchez, Juan Carlos Laguna and Marta Alegret
Effects of a Low Dose of Caffeine Alone or as Part of a Green Coffee Extract, in a Rat Dietary Model of Lean Non-Alcoholic Fatty Liver Disease without Inflammation
Reprinted from: *Nutrients* **2020**, *12*, 3240, doi:10.3390/nu12113240 251

Benedikt Treml, Elisabeth Schöpf, Ralf Geiger, Christian Niederwanger, Alexander Löckinger, Axel Kleinsasser and Mirjam Bachler
Red Bull Increases Heart Rate at Near Sea Level and Pulmonary Shunt Fraction at High Altitude in a Porcine Model
Reprinted from: *Nutrients* **2020**, *12*, 1738, doi:10.3390/nu12061738 271

Lavinia Liliana Ruta and Ileana Cornelia Farcasanu
Saccharomyces cerevisiae and Caffeine Implications on the Eukaryotic Cell
Reprinted from: *Nutrients* **2020**, *12*, 2440, doi:10.3390/nu12082440 283

Hubert Kolb, Kerstin Kempf and Stephan Martin
Health Effects of Coffee: Mechanism Unraveled?
Reprinted from: *Nutrients* **2020**, *12*, 1842, doi:10.3390/nu12061842 305

Amaia Iriondo-DeHond, José Antonio Uranga, Maria Dolores del Castillo and Raquel Abalo
Effects of Coffee and Its Components on the Gastrointestinal Tract and the Brain–Gut Axis
Reprinted from: *Nutrients* **2021**, *13*, 88, doi:10.3390/nu13010088 . . . . **319**

About the Editor

Raquel Abalo

Raquel Abalo is a Full Professor of Pharmacology, Functional Coordinator of the Department of Basic Health Sciences, and Coordinator of the PhD Program in Health Sciences at Universidad Rey Juan Carlos (URJC). As Head of the High-Performance Research Group in Physiopathology and Pharmacology of the Digestive System (NeuGut-URJC), her research is focused on the gastrointestinal tract and the brain–gut axis. Distinct from other labs, radiographic methods, developed in-house, are used for the non-invasive evaluation of gastrointestinal motor function in preclinical models. Her group is currently working on several lines of research: (1) influence of sex on the brain–gut axis functions, disorders, and responses to treatments; (2) involvement of the endocannabinoid system in the side effects of antitumoral drugs on the brain–gut axis; (2) short- and long-term consequences of the cytokine storm and sepsis on the brain–gut axis; (3) effects of coffee and coffee byproducts on the brain–gut axis. All these projects are developed in a highly national and international collaborative environment, within a lively lab full of motivated multidisciplinary students.

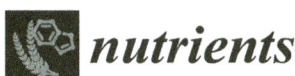

Editorial

Coffee and Caffeine Consumption for Human Health

Raquel Abalo [1,2,3,4]

1. Department of Basic Health Sciences, Faculty of Health Sciences, University Rey Juan Carlos (URJC), 28922 Alcorcón, Spain; raquel.abalo@urjc.es; Tel.: +34-91-488-8854
2. High Performance Research Group in Physiopathology and Pharmacology of the Digestive System (NeuGut-URJC), URJC, 28922 Alcorcón, Spain
3. Associated I+D+i Unit to the Institute of Medicinal Chemistry (IQM), Scientific Research Superior Council (CSIC), 28006 Madrid, Spain
4. Working Group of Basic Sciences in Pain and Analgesia of the Spanish Pain Society (Grupo de Trabajo de Ciencias Básicas en Dolor y Analgesia de la Sociedad Española del Dolor), 28046 Madrid, Spain

Coffee is one of the most popular and consumed beverages worldwide, and caffeine is its best-known component, present also in many other beverages (tea, soft drinks, energy drinks), foodstuffs (cocoa, chocolate, guarana), sport supplements and even medicines. Besides caffeine, many other components, either beneficial for health (chlorogenic acids, polyphenols, diterpenes, micronutrients, melanoidins, fiber) or not (lipids in unfiltered coffee, or acrylamide resulting from coffee bean roasting), are present in coffee. Just to illustrate the scientific interest of coffee and caffeine, when these terms are combined in PubMed (as "coffee OR caffeine"), almost 50,000 papers can be retrieved (as of 10 August 2021). Furthermore, from 2000 to 2020, the number of manuscripts published per year has more than doubled (from 972 to 2601). Within this context of increasing interest in the topic, the Special Issue (SI) on "Coffee and Caffeine Consumption for Human Health" has collected twenty-one manuscripts (five narrative reviews and sixteen original articles, including two meta-analyses).

Most of the original reports obtained information on coffee or caffeine consumption in humans through dietary surveys or interviews. These studies have the limitation of recall bias. In addition, caffeine content needs to be estimated for most foods from packaging, databases, scientific literature or extrapolated from similar foods, although in some cases it was directly measured from samples of coffee or soft drinks. Rochat et al. found that, in agreement with reports from other high-income countries, coffee is the main source of caffeine consumption in Switzerland, mostly consumed early in the morning (6–9 am), although some differences were found across age groups, smoking status, and linguistic regions [1]. Cultural differences in coffee/caffeine consumption are important and may contribute to the health effects observed in different geographic regions. Furthermore, coffee/caffeine consumption may be likewise modulated by expectation (placebo) effects and vice versa. Mendes et al. translated, adapted, and validated the Caffeine Expectancy Questionnaire (CaffEQ), originally designed for the American population [2], to the Brazilian culture (CaffEQ-BR), and confirmed that coffee is the main source of daily caffeine intake in Brazil [3], the largest coffee producer and exporter in the world market.

Most studies tried to determine whether there is an association between coffee/caffeine intake and different health outcomes. Rodas et al. specifically evaluated the effect of caffeine intake, physical activity levels, and sedentary behavior on the inflammatory status in healthy staff and students at the University of the Balearic Islands (Mallorca, Spain). In this sample, sedentary behavior and body fat accumulation had clear pro-inflammatory effects, whereas regular but relatively low caffeine consumption (whose main source was also coffee) could not be demonstrated to exert robust anti-inflammatory effects [4]. Antwerpes et al., analyzed the relationship between regular coffee intake and neurocognitive performance in patients coinfected with human immunodeficiency virus and hepatitis C

Citation: Abalo, R. Coffee and Caffeine Consumption for Human Health. *Nutrients* **2021**, *13*, 2918. https://doi.org/10.3390/nu13092918

Received: 15 August 2021
Accepted: 23 August 2021
Published: 24 August 2021

Publisher's Note: MDPI stays neutral with regard to jurisdictional claims in published maps and institutional affiliations.

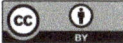

Copyright: © 2021 by the author. Licensee MDPI, Basel, Switzerland. This article is an open access article distributed under the terms and conditions of the Creative Commons Attribution (CC BY) license (https://creativecommons.org/licenses/by/4.0/).

virus, who experience an accelerated aging process and cognitive impairment. The authors showed a positive association between elevated coffee intake (three or more cups per day) and neurocognitive functioning parameters, even after adjusting for liver disease correlates, suggesting that coffee intake may be neuroprotective in these patients [5]. Likewise, Herden and Weissert studied the effect of coffee and caffeine consumption on patients with multiple sclerosis (MS)-related fatigue. Importantly, the authors showed that coffee intake did not cause severe side effects in MS patients and identified a specific set of patients who might benefit from coffee consumption [6]. One meta-analysis evaluated the effect of caffeine consumption on the risk and progression of Parkinson's disease (PD). Individuals consuming caffeine on a regular basis had a significantly lower risk of developing PD during follow-up evaluation, and those that already had the disease and consumed caffeine showed a significantly decelerated PD progression. However, Hong et al. could not determine the optimal daily dosage or food source of caffeine [7]. According to the review by Jee et al., coffee/caffeine neuroprotective effects seem to be broader and sex- and age-specific. Indeed, they concluded that caffeine consumption reduces the risk of stroke, dementia, and depression in women and that of PD in men. Nevertheless, it may increase sleep disorders and anxiety disorders in adolescence in both men and women. They suggested that caffeine use should be individualized according to sex (and age) in the context of neurologic and psychiatric diseases [8]. Nowaczewska et al., on the other hand, reviewed the ambiguous role of caffeine in migraine headache. They did not find any scientific evidence showing that a single dose of caffeine may trigger migraine, although it may influence migraines (i.e., through its vasoconstrictor actions during the premonitory symptoms). Chronic caffeine overuse may lead to migraine chronification and sudden caffeine cessation may trigger migraine attacks. Thus, as recommended by the authors, migraine sufferers should avoid caffeine withdrawal headache by keeping a consistent daily intake, not exceeding 200 mg [9].

Three studies evaluated the relationship of coffee consumption with the risk of metabolic, endocrine, or cardiovascular diseases according to genetic polymorphisms. Using data from the Korean Genome and Epidemiology Study (KGES), Jin et al. identified five single nucleotide polymorphisms (SNPs) related with habitual coffee consumption in this Korean population and showed the lowest risk of prediabetes and type 2 diabetes among black-coffee consumers with minor alleles of these SNPs compared with those with major alleles [10]. Using data from KGES too, Han et al. found that subsets of genetic variants in the adenosine receptors (involved in caffeine signaling) gene family modulate the effect of coffee intake on dyslipidemia risk in a sex-dependent manner [11]. In the third study, Liu et al. found that consumption of coffee was significantly associated with a decreased risk of coronary heart disease among Taiwanese adults carrying the GG genotype of TRIB1 (tribbles pseudokinase 1, a gene involved in cholesterol metabolism and atherosclerosis process) [12]. These three examples of genetic studies strongly suggest that dietary guidelines for coffee intake in the prevention and management of metabolic, endocrine, and cardiovascular disorders should consider the influence of genetic polymorphisms.

The main problem with the survey/interview-based studies is the lack of accurate information regarding type (roasting) or brand of coffee, caffeine content (caffeinated, decaffeinated), methods of preparation (boiled, filtered, brewed), and consumption of other caffeine sources. Thus, quantification of daily consumption of caffeine (and other compounds) is a real challenge in this kind of studies. Moua et al. tried to overcome this limitation by using volume of coffee consumed (not number of cups) in a dose-response meta-analysis of the association between coffee consumption and c-reactive protein, a general biomarker of chronic inflammation. Unfortunately, heterogeneity of study populations (differences in sample size; cultural differences in coffee composition; relevant individual confounders such as age, sex, body mass index, smoking, alcohol intake, diet, activity, comorbidities, etc.) produced inconsistent associations [13]. Thus, in addition to collecting detailed information on coffee type and preparation method, measuring biomarkers of coffee consumption such as urinary metabolites may be helpful to more precisely determine the amounts of bioactive compounds consumed and their effects. In this sense, Wu and Chen explored the association between urine caffeine metabolites and urine flow rate, using data from the US National Health and Nutrition Examination Survey (NHANES) and metabolomics for urine analyses. The association was positive, with more metabolites showing certain flow-dependency in males compared to females and in young compared to elderly participants [14]. This factor is important to correctly interpret urinary data regarding caffeine.

Intervention studies allow to establish more robust cause-effect associations. In this SI, two original studies used a double-blind, placebo-controlled crossover design to evaluate the ergogenic effects of caffeine. In 13 males and 17 females, Fuller et al. examined the effects of trait (long-standing pre-disposition) mental and physical energy and fatigue to changes in moods, cognitive and fine-motor task performance. The results suggest that evaluating trait may be a practical, low-cost method to control for interindividual differences in the ergogenic neurocognitive effects of caffeine, without the need for genetic testing [15]. On the other hand, Wilk et al. demonstrated that a single moderate dose of caffeine (3–6 mg/kg b.m.) increased mean power output and mean bar velocity during an explosive bench press throw in 12 male athletes habituated to caffeine ingestion, meaning that caffeine enhances performance in this context, although the long-term training effects with caffeine need to be determined [16].

This SI includes three original studies showing new data in animal models using different beverages for different purposes, somehow representative of those also addressed in humans. Ahmad et al. performed a classical toxicity study in rats of the beverage Tongkat ali, widely used in Malaysia, made of coffee infused with the additive *Eurycoma longifolia*. This study demonstrated a good safety profile for this beverage in male and female rats [17]. The other rat study, by Velázquez et al., investigated the effects of caffeine alone or as part of a green coffee extract (GCE) in lean female rats with diet-induced hepatic steatosis, as a preclinical model of non-alcoholic fatty liver disease, a highly prevalent condition nowadays, without specific pharmacological treatment. Using different techniques, including lipidomics on liver tissue, the GCE, but not caffeine alone, was found to reduce liver triglyceride levels, through a combination of different molecular mechanisms of action [18]. Whether longer treatment duration and/or higher doses might be even more effective is unknown. In the last preclinical study, a controlled laboratory trial performed in piglets, Treml et al. showed that a high dose of Red Bull, a popular energy drink among athletes containing caffeine, taurine and glucose among other compounds, increased heart rate at near sea level. However, a high dose of this beverage did not worsen tachycardia during acute short-term hypoxia (simulating high altitude conditions). The authors demonstrated that this beverage significantly increased pulmonary shunt fraction without changing distribution of pulmonary blood flow during hypoxia [19]. The specific contributions of the different components of this beverage remain to be identified.

Ruta and Farcasanu reviewed the studies evaluating the molecular mechanisms of action of caffeine in *Saccharomyces cerevisiae* as a simple model of eukaryotic cell. In addition to its three well-known mechanisms, namely intracellular mobilization of calcium, inhibition of phosphodiesterases and antagonism of adenosine receptors, the studies performed in this yeast model have confirmed that the pleiotropic effects of caffeine involve also key molecular mechanisms related with DNA repair mechanisms, cancer, and aging [20]. In contrast, Kolb et al. reviewed the mechanisms that might contribute to explain the beneficial effects of habitual coffee consumption on health. The authors excluded caffeine content as well as radical scavenging properties, anti-inflammatory activity, and genetic polymorphisms as major contributors to coffee healthy effects. Instead, they propose that the mechanisms involve a combination of factors promoting cell protection, namely upregulation of proteins with antioxidant, detoxifying and repair functions through coffee phenolic phytochemicals, as well as modulation of the gut-microbiota, through the non-digestible components of coffee (prebiotics), although this has been scarcely explored [21]. Since the gastrointestinal tract is the first body system that gets in contact with ingested coffee, Iriondo-DeHond et al. reviewed the effects produced by coffee and its components on the different constituents of the gut wall (mucosa, muscle layers, enteric nervous system), the different gastrointestinal organs, the gastrointestinal tract as a whole and the brain-gut axis, only to find that the effects of coffee and its derivatives on the health of this axis (that affect not only gastrointestinal motility, permeability and sensitivity but also a complete spectrum of central nervous functions and disorders, from emotions to neurodegeneration) have not been deeply investigated yet [22].

Altogether, the current view is that coffee/caffeine intake exerts multiple health benefits in humans, at least in specific populations (with a particular genetic profile or suffering from specific diseases), but the specific effects in the different organs and systems, as well as the mechanisms involved are far from clear. Furthermore, within the current context aiming to sustainable development, the coffee plant *Coffee* sp. and its so-far relatively neglected by-products are expected to become soon a source of ingredients for new functional foods whose properties will need to be precisely determined. We hope the readers of this SI will find inspiration for new studies on the topic.

Funding: This research received no external funding.

Acknowledgments: The author research is funded by the following projects: "Novel Coffee by-Product Beverages for an Optimal Health of the Brain–Gut Axis (COFFEE4BGA)", by the Ministerio de Ciencia e Innovación (PID2019-111510RB-I00); "N-acetilcisteína frente a la COVID-19 grave y sus secuelas: estudio en un modelo preclínico de pseudoinfección y sepsis (NACfightsCOVID-19)", funded by URJC-Banco de Santander (2020 call). The author is grateful to all the researchers that submitted their interesting reports to this SI.

Conflicts of Interest: The author declares no conflict of interest.

References

1. Rochat, C.; Eap, C.B.; Bochud, M.; Chatelan, A. Caffeine Consumption in Switzerland: Results from the First National Nutrition Survey MenuCH. *Nutrients* **2019**, *12*, 28. [CrossRef]
2. Huntley, E.D.; Juliano, L.M. Caffeine Expectancy Questionnaire (CaffEQ): Construction, psychometric properties, and associations with caffeine use, caffeine dependence, and other related variables. *Psychol. Assess.* **2012**, *24*, 592–607. [CrossRef] [PubMed]
3. Mendes, G.F.; Reis, C.E.G.; Nakano, E.Y.; Da Costa, T.H.M.; Saunders, B.; Zandonadi, R.P. Translation and Validation of the Caffeine Expectancy Questionnaire in Brazil (CaffEQ-BR). *Nutrients* **2020**, *12*, 2248. [CrossRef] [PubMed]
4. Rodas, L.; Riera-Sampol, A.; Aguilo, A.; Martínez, S.; Tauler, P. Effects of Habitual Caffeine Intake, Physical Activity Levels, and Sedentary Behavior on the Inflammatory Status in a Healthy Population. *Nutrients* **2020**, *12*, 2325. [CrossRef] [PubMed]
5. Antwerpes, S.; Protopopescu, C.; Morlat, P.; Marcellin, F.; Wittkop, L.; Di Beo, V.; Salmon-Céron, D.; Sogni, P.; Michel, L.; Carrieri, M.P.; et al. Coffee Intake and Neurocognitive Performance in HIV/HCV Coinfected Patients (ANRS CO13 HEPAVIH). *Nutrients* **2020**, *12*, 2532. [CrossRef] [PubMed]
6. Herden, L.; Weissert, R. The Effect of Coffee and Caffeine Consumption on Patients with Multiple Sclerosis-Related Fatigue. *Nutrients* **2020**, *12*, 2262. [CrossRef]
7. Hong, C.T.; Chan, L.; Bai, C.-H. The Effect of Caffeine on the Risk and Progression of Parkinson's Disease: A Meta-Analysis. *Nutrients* **2020**, *12*, 1860. [CrossRef]
8. Jee, H.J.; Lee, S.G.; Bormate, K.J.; Jung, Y.-S. Effect of Caffeine Consumption on the Risk for Neurological and Psychiatric Disorders: Sex Differences in Human. *Nutrients* **2020**, *12*, 3080. [CrossRef]
9. Nowaczewska, M.; Wiciński, M.; Kaźmierczak, W. The Ambiguous Role of Caffeine in Migraine Headache: From Trigger to Treatment. *Nutrients* **2020**, *12*, 2259. [CrossRef]
10. Jin, T.; Youn, J.; Na Kim, A.; Kang, M.; Kim, K.; Sung, J.; Lee, J.E. Interactions of Habitual Coffee Consumption by Genetic Polymorphisms with the Risk of Prediabetes and Type 2 Diabetes Combined. *Nutrients* **2020**, *12*, 2228. [CrossRef]
11. Han, J.; Shon, J.; Hwang, J.-Y.; Park, Y.J. Effects of Coffee Intake on Dyslipidemia Risk According to Genetic Variants in the ADORA Gene Family among Korean Adults. *Nutrients* **2020**, *12*, 493. [CrossRef]
12. Liu, Y.-T.; Tantoh, D.M.; Wang, L.; Nfor, O.N.; Hsu, S.-Y.; Ho, C.-C.; Lung, C.-C.; Chang, H.-R.; Liaw, Y.-P. Interaction between Coffee Drinking and TRIB1 rs17321515 Single Nucleotide Polymorphism on Coronary Heart Disease in a Taiwanese Population. *Nutrients* **2020**, *12*, 1301. [CrossRef]
13. Moua, E.D.; Hu, C.; Day, N.; Hord, N.G.; Takata, Y. Coffee Consumption and C-Reactive Protein Levels: A Systematic Review and Meta-Analysis. *Nutrients* **2020**, *12*, 1349. [CrossRef] [PubMed]
14. Wu, S.E.; Chen, W.-L. Exploring the Association between Urine Caffeine Metabolites and Urine Flow Rate: A Cross-Sectional Study. *Nutrients* **2020**, *12*, 2803. [CrossRef] [PubMed]

15. Fuller, D.; Smith, M.; Boolani, A. Trait Energy and Fatigue Modify the Effects of Caffeine on Mood, Cognitive and Fine-Motor Task Performance: A Post-Hoc Study. *Nutrients* **2021**, *13*, 412. [CrossRef] [PubMed]
16. Wilk, M.; Filip, A.; Krzysztofik, M.; Gepfert, M.; Zajac, A.; Del Coso, J. Acute Caffeine Intake Enhances Mean Power Output and Bar Velocity during the Bench Press Throw in Athletes Habituated to Caffeine. *Nutrients* **2020**, *12*, 406. [CrossRef] [PubMed]
17. Ahmad, N.; Teh, B.P.; Halim, S.Z.; Zolkifli, N.A.; Ramli, N.; Muhammad, H. Eurycoma longifolia—Infused Coffee—An Oral Toxicity Study. *Nutrients* **2020**, *12*, 3125. [CrossRef] [PubMed]
18. Velázquez, A.M.; Roglans, N.; Bentanachs, R.; Gené, M.; Sala-Vila, A.; Lázaro, I.; Rodríguez-Morató, J.; Sánchez, R.M.; Laguna, J.C.; Alegret, M. Effects of a low dose of caffeine alone or as part of a green coffee extract, in a rat dietary model of lean non-alcoholic fatty liver disease without inflammation. *Nutrients* **2020**, *12*, 3240. [CrossRef] [PubMed]
19. Treml, B.; Schöpf, E.; Geiger, R.; Niederwanger, C.; Löckinger, A.; Kleinsasser, A.; Bachler, M. Red Bull Increases Heart Rate at Near Sea Level and Pulmonary Shunt Fraction at High Altitude in a Porcine Model. *Nutrients* **2020**, *12*, 1738. [CrossRef]
20. Ruta, L.L.; Farcasanu, I.C. Saccharomyces cerevisiae and Caffeine Implications on the Eukaryotic Cell. *Nutrients* **2020**, *12*, 2440. [CrossRef]
21. Kolb, H.; Kempf, K.; Martin, S. Health Effects of Coffee: Mechanism Unraveled? *Nutrients* **2020**, *12*, 1842. [CrossRef] [PubMed]
22. Iriondo-DeHond, A.; Uranga, J.A.; Del Castillo, M.D.; Abalo, R. Effects of coffee and its components on the gastrointestinal tract and the brain–Gut axis. *Nutrients* **2020**, *13*, 88. [CrossRef] [PubMed]

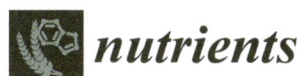

Article

Caffeine Consumption in Switzerland: Results from the First National Nutrition Survey MenuCH

Christèle Rochat [1], Chin B. Eap [2,3], Murielle Bochud [1,*] and Angeline Chatelan [1]

[1] Center of Primary Care and Public Health (Unisanté), University of Lausanne, Route de la Corniche 10, 1010 Lausanne, Switzerland; christele.rochat@unil.ch (C.R.); angeline.chatelan@unisante.ch (A.C.)
[2] Unit of Pharmacogenetics and Clinical Psychopharmacology, Centre for Psychiatric Neuroscience, Department of Psychiatry, Lausanne University Hospital, University of Lausanne, 1008 Prilly-Lausanne, Switzerland; chin.eap@chuv.ch
[3] Institute of Pharmaceutical Sciences of Western Switzerland, 1205 Geneva, Switzerland
* Correspondence: murielle.bochud@unisante.ch; Tel.: +41-21-314-0899

Received: 2 December 2019; Accepted: 17 December 2019; Published: 20 December 2019

Abstract: Caffeine is a natural psychostimulant with a potentially positive impact on health when consumed in moderation and a negative impact at high dose (>400 mg/day). So far, no study has examined self-reported caffeine consumption in Switzerland. Our objectives were to determine (1) the caffeine consumption per adult, (2) the main sources of caffeine intake in the Swiss diet, and (3) the timing of caffeine consumption during the day. We used data from the 2014–2015 national nutrition survey menuCH (adults aged 18 to 75 years old, $n = 2057$, weighted $n = 4{,}627{,}878$), consisting of two 24-h dietary recalls. Caffeine content in consumed foods was systematically assessed using laboratory analyses in samples of Swiss caffeinated beverages, information from food composition databases, and estimations from standard recipes. Mean (±SD) daily caffeine consumption per person and percentile 95 were 191 mg/day (±129) and 426 mg/day, respectively. We observed differences in mean caffeine consumption across age groups (18–34 y: 140 mg/day; 50–64 y: 228 mg/day), linguistic regions (German-speaking: 204 mg/day; French-speaking: 170 mg/day, Italian-speaking: 136 mg/day), and smoking status (never smokers: 171 mg/day; current smokers: 228 mg/day). The three main sources of caffeine intake were 1) coffee (83% of total caffeine intake), 2) tea (9%) and 3) soft drinks (4%). Caffeine consumption was highest between 06:00 and 09:00 (29%) and the circadian rhythm slightly differed across linguistic regions and age groups. The mean caffeine consumption in the Swiss adult population was similar to that reported in neighbouring countries.

Keywords: caffeine intake; Switzerland; national nutrition survey; coffee; tea; soft drinks

---

1. Introduction

Caffeine is a psychostimulant naturally present in coffee and cocoa beans, tea leaves, mate, kola nuts and guarana berries [1–3]. Short-term effects of caffeine on health are well documented: stimulation of the central nervous system [2,4], increased metabolism [4], acute elevation of blood pressure [2,4–6], and diuresis [4]. Caffeine is particularly known and sought for its effects on alertness [7] and cognitive performance [7]. However, in some individuals, it can have a negative impact on sleep in a dose-dependent manner if consumed late in the day [2,7,8]. Longer-term effects of caffeine intake on health are more debated. A meta-analysis of randomized controlled trials indicated that caffeine may increase systolic blood pressure after several weeks of moderate to high caffeine intake [5,9]. On the other hand, the umbrella review by Grosso et al. [5] showed that, based on data from observational studies (i.e., cohorts and case-controls studies), caffeine probably decreases the risk of Parkinson's disease and type 2 diabetes, and possibly decreases the risk of cognitive disorders. In pregnant women, observational and experimental studies have warned about a potential increased risk of pregnancy loss and of infants having a low birth weight [5]. In this context, the European Food Safety Authority (EFSA) [2] and other authors [1,6,10] recommend a caffeine consumption of a maximum 400 mg per day in healthy adults, and 200–300 mg during pregnancy.

Data from the 2007–2012 National Health and Nutrition Examination Survey (NHANES) informed that consumption of caffeine in U.S. adults was on average of 169 mg/day [7] and had been relatively stable for at least 10 years [7,11,12]. In Western Europe, the average daily intake of caffeine is similar as in the U.S [2,7]. In Europe, the most important sources of caffeine are: (1) coffee, (2) cola-based soft drinks and 3) tea [13]. Currently, little is known on the timing of caffeine consumption throughout the day [14]. One study in the U.S., based on the 2007–2012 NHANES data, showed that caffeine is mainly consumed before noon (70% of total daily intake) with a peak between 06:00 and 09:00 (40%) [7].

In Switzerland—a wealthy country whose population exhibits one of the highest life expectancies worldwide [15] and where dietary habits highly vary between the three main linguistic regions (German, French and Italian) [16]—information on caffeine consumption is lacking, although some data on 24-h urinary caffeine and methylxanthine excretion in the general adult population have been recently published [17]. Therefore, we quantified caffeine consumption in the Swiss population aged 18 to 75 using data from the first national nutrition survey, menuCH. We calculated the average consumption of caffeine per person, as well as the main sources of caffeine in the Swiss diet and the timing of caffeine consumption during the day.

2. Methods

2.1. Study Design and Population

This study uses cross-sectional data from the first national population-based nutrition survey in Switzerland, menuCH, conducted between January 2014 and February 2015 [16]. A stratified random sample covering the three main linguistic regions and five categories of predefined age between 18 and 75 years was taken from the national sampling frame for surveys of persons and households by the Federal Statistical Office [18]. Out of the 5496 eligible people invited and reachable by phone, 2086 took part in the survey (response rate: 38%) [19]. Among them, 2057 participants had two complete 24-h dietary recalls (24 HDR). This survey was conducted in accordance with the guidelines of the Helsinki Declaration and all participants signed a written informed consent. The survey was registered in the primary clinical trial registry (ID number: ISRCTN16778734). Further information about menuCH is available in these references [16,19,20].

2.2. Dietary Assessment

Details on dietary assessment methods were described in a previous article [20]. In brief, dietary intake was assessed by dietitians through two non-consecutive 24 HDR, spread across all days of the week and all seasons. The 24 HDRs were multiple-pass automated using the GloboDiet®software (International Agency for Research on Cancer, Lyon, France), which had been adapted to the Swiss food market. To support survey participants in food intake quantification, dietitians used a set of about 60 actual household measures (e.g., cups, glasses, spoons, plates) and a picture book with 119 series of six graduated portion-sizes and with the household measures [21]. The picture book was particularly useful for the second 24 HDR conducted by phone. Detailed descriptions of all consumed foods, beverages, and ingredients of recipes, including flavours and brand names, were collected. For coffee-based beverages, information about caffeine content (i.e., decaffeinated vs. caffeinated coffee) and the preparation method (i.e., prepared from instant powder vs. not) were available. We had, however, no information regarding the brewing methods, such as made from branded capsules, coffee maker brand, moka pot, etc. All foods were grouped into five groups: (1) beverages made of coffee and/or coffee substitutes (e.g., chicory coffee), (2) tea and mate (e.g., white, green and black tea, jasmine tea), (3) soft and energy drinks (e.g., Coca Cola®, iced teas, Red Bull®), (4) pure chocolate and chocolate-based confectionary (e.g., chocolate bars, chocolate spread, chocolate powder,

Easter Bunny) and (5) all other foods (e.g., mocha yogurt). These groups came from the pre-defined GloboDiet®classification (18 food groups and 85 subgroups) and were selected based on the published literature [2,12,13,22].

2.3. Estimated Caffeine Content (Most Foods)

We estimated the caffeine content for most foods reported by survey participants following a systematic approach, described in Supplementary Figure S1: (1) contain caffeine (e.g., coffee), (2) may contain caffeine depending on flavour, brand, etc. (e.g., soft drinks), (3) do not contain caffeine (e.g., vegetables). Since the Swiss Food Composition Database [23] does not include caffeine, the caffeine level reported on the packaging, when present, and the American (ndb.nal.usda.gov) and Canadian (food-nutrition.canada.ca) food composition databases, were the main references to assign caffeine value in consumed foods (see values in Supplementary Table S1). For some specific Swiss or European foods or recipes manufactured locally (e.g., branded chocolate bars), we estimated caffeine content based on the quantity of ingredients containing caffeine from standard recipes/compositions: e.g., cocoa or chocolate powder, milk and dark chocolate. If no information was found in these references, we used values published in a scientific article (e.g., white tea [24]). Finally, we relied on www.caffeineinformer.com for Jasmin tea (reported 22 times out of a total of 121,047 reported foods) and mate (8×), and www.frc.ch/yaourt-a-la-cafeine for mocha yogurt (122×) to estimate caffeine content. For foods having "coffee extract" in their ingredient list (22×), we extrapolated their caffeine content from similar foods because we could not find this item in food composition databases nor the literature. When caffeine concentrations were estimated to be less than 1 mg/100 g of product (70×, e.g., rocket ice cream with coated chocolate on the top), we assigned these foods a caffeine content equal to zero for simplification.

2.4. Measured Caffeine Content (Coffee and Soft Drinks)

For coffee and a few soft drinks, we measured the caffeine content in Swiss samples. Several reasons justify this decision: (1) coffees and soft drinks are the main providers of caffeine in Western Europe [13], (2) we found large differences regarding their caffeine content in food composition databases and literature, and (3) coffee preparation and soft drink recipes/compositions may vary from country to country [25]. In total, we collected 8 samples of soft drinks and 42 samples of coffees for laboratory analyses (Supplementary Table S2). For soft drinks, we measured caffeine in five branded cola-based soft drinks (i.e., Coca Cola®and Pepsi®) and three branded iced teas. As for coffee, we measured caffeine content in ristrettos (about 35 mL, according to menuCH data), espressos (about 64 mL), and lungos (about 144 mL). In this study, we focused only on caffeinated coffees. Decaffeinated coffees were assigned a caffeine concentration of 2 mg/100 mL based on previous analyses conducted in the same Swiss laboratory (unpublished data). In addition, this value corresponded to information found in the literature [26]. Ristrettos were divided into two categories: "self-made" (one Nespresso®capsule) and "take-away/restaurant/vending machine" (four different places). Espressos and lungos were each divided into three categories: "powder-based" (one Nescafé®instant powder), "self-made" (three different Nespresso®capsules), and "take-away/restaurant/vending machine" (four different places). For each type of coffee, two samples were collected, one directly after the other and both results were averaged. Levels of caffeine, paraxanthine, theophylline and theobromine were quantified by ultra-high-performance liquid chromatography (Waters ACQUITY UPLC system, Waters Corporation, Milford, USA) coupled to a tandem quadrupole mass spectrometer (Waters TQD) with electrospray ionization. The limit of quantification for all analytes was 5 ng/mL. The method was validated according to international guidelines using a stable isotope-labelled internal standard for each analyte (detailed method available on request). Because we only had information on whether the coffee was prepared from instant powder or not (no information on brewing method), and because there were important variations regarding caffeine content measured in "self-made" coffee (capsules) and coffee prepared in "take-away/restaurant/vending machine", we calculated an average caffeine concentration in ristrettos (265 mg/100 mL), espressos (119 mg/100 mL) and lungos (67 mg/100 mL) by hypothesizing that 2/3 of coffees were "self-made" using branded capsules and 1/3 were bought in "take-away/restaurant/vending machine" [27]. The contents of caffeine in coffee-based beverages (e.g., cappuccino, latte macchiato) were then calculated from these data using standard recipes/compositions. For details on the estimated and measured caffeine content in the different foods, see Supplementary Table S1.

2.5. Anthropometry and Other Parameters

Following the World Health Organization's MONICA Manual [28], dietitians measured body weight and height to the nearest 0.1 kg/cm with a calibrated Seca 701 scale, equipped with a Seca 220 telescopic measuring rod (Seca GmbH, Hamburg, Germany) [20]. For pregnant and lactating women, or where measurements were impossible (e.g., disability, refusal), self-reported weight and/or height were used ($n = 34$) [16,28]. Body mass index (BMI) was then calculated and categorised as follows: normal weight (BMI < 25 kg/m^2), overweight (25 ≤ BMI < 30 kg/m^2), and obesity (BMI ≥ 30 kg/m^2). A standardized questionnaire was used to assess: (1) sex [men, women], (2) age [age groups: 18–34 years, 35–49 years, 50–64 years, 65–75 years], (3) the language region based on home address (German-, French-, Italian-speaking parts of Switzerland), (4) nationality [Swiss, not Swiss], (5) education [lower (max. 1–2 years after compulsory school), middle (3–4 years after compulsory school), higher (>5 years after compulsory school)], (6) household income [lower (<5999 CHF), middle (6000–8999 CHF), higher (>9000 CHF)] and (7) smoking status [never smokers (<100 cigarettes in life), ex-smokers (used to smoke, >100 cigarettes in life), current smokers (occasional or daily smokers)].

2.6. Statistical Analyses

Usual daily consumption of caffeine intake was modelled out of the two 24 HDR ($n = 2057$) using the Multiple Source Method (MSM, https://nugo.dife.de/msm) [29]. MSM has been developed to predict typical consumption based on short-term measurements, such as 24 HDR, accounting for day-to-day variations (within-person variations). In MSM, we assumed that all survey participants were potential consumers of caffeine. We calculated the percentage of people with consumption of caffeine potentially harmful for health based on thresholds defined by EFSA: i.e., 400 mg/day and 5.7 mg/kg/day [2]. The contribution of main food group sources of caffeine was estimated using the mean intake of the two recorded days (no use of MSM). The timing of caffeine consumption was assessed only in the first 24 HDR, as was the case in Lieberman et al. [7]. We estimated caffeine intake per 3-hour period [7] and per hour [11], assuming that the time of meal/snack start reported by survey participants was the time of consumption. Findings are presented by sex, age groups, linguistic regions, and when appropriate, nationality, educational level, income, smoking status, and weight status. All results were weighted for age, sex, marital status, administrative regions of Switzerland, nationality and household size to take into account sampling design and non-response. Results were also weighted to correct for the slightly uneven distribution of 24 HDR over seasons and weekdays. The weighing strategy intends to provide results that are more representative of the Swiss population aged 18 to 75 years old and of any day in the year. A detailed documentation about the weighting strategy is available at https://menuch.iumsp.ch/index.php/home. All statistical analyses were carried out using STATA version 13 (Stata Corp., College Station, TX, USA).

3. Results

Table 1 describes the daily caffeine consumption across selected strata. Mean (± SD) of caffeine for the entire Swiss population aged 18 to 75 years was 191 mg/day (± 129) with a P95 estimated at 426 mg/day. Mean caffeine intake was higher in men than in women, with 210 (± 138) and 172 mg/day (± 117), respectively. Pregnant women ($n = 14$) had a much lower caffeine intake, with a mean intake of 74 mg/day (± 49) (data not shown). P95 for men and women were 445 and 388 mg/day, respectively. The daily consumption of caffeine tended to increase with age with a peak in people aged

50–64 years, then decreased in those aged 65 to 75 years. People aged 18–34 years had a mean intake of 140 mg/day (± 111), 35–49 years of 202 mg/day (± 134), 50–64 years of 228 mg/day (± 135) and 65–75 years of 202 mg/day (± 111). We also found differences across linguistic regions: German-, French- and Italian-speaking had a mean caffeine intake of 204 (± 136), 170 (± 112), 136 mg/day (± 85) and P95 of 445, 399 and 270 mg/day, respectively. Smokers (228 mg/day ± 152) appeared to be larger caffeine consumers than ex-smokers (197 mg/day ± 115), who themselves consumed more caffeine than never smokers (171 mg/day ± 121). Table 1 also highlights that P95 was above 500 mg/day in three groups of the Swiss population: smokers, people with lower education, and obese people. No major differences were found with respect to nationality and income.

Supplementary Table S3 describes the daily caffeine consumption per kilo of body weight. Mean (± SD) caffeine consumption in the entire population was 2.66 mg/kg/day (± 1.78), with equivalent values in men and women. Table 1 and Supplementary Table S3 also highlight that 6.6% and 5.6% of the Swiss population consumed more than 400 mg/day or 5.7 mg/kg per day of caffeine. None of the 14 pregnant women had a caffeine intake above 200 mg/day (data not shown).

Figure 1 and Supplementary Figure S2 show the main food group sources of caffeine, in relative values (percentage of total intake) and absolute values (mg/day), respectively. The three main sources of caffeine intake at the population level were (1) coffee (83% of total caffeine intake), (2) tea (9%) and (3) soft drinks (4%). Men consumed more caffeine from coffee and soft drinks than women: i.e., 86% (184 mg/day) and 6% (12 mg/day) in men, compared to 81% (139 mg/day) and 3% (5 mg/day) in women. In contrast, women consumed more caffeine from tea: 12% of total daily caffeine intake (21 mg/day) compared to men with 6% (13 mg/day). Coffee was the main caffeine provider in diet among all age groups, and relative values increased with age, from 73% to 87% of total caffeine intake. Respectively, people aged 18–34 years consumed 73% (101 mg/day) of caffeine from coffee, 35–49 years 85% (174 mg/day), 50–64 years 87% (203 mg/day) and 65–75 years 87% (173 mg/day). The absolute intake of caffeine from tea increased with age, with 16 mg/day in the youngest group (18–34 years) to 20 mg/day in the oldest group (65–75 years). Both absolute and relative values of caffeine intake from soft drinks decreased with age, from 11% (15 mg/day) in 18–34 year olds to 1% (1 mg/day) in 65–75 year olds. Individuals residing in the German-speaking, French-speaking and Italian-speaking regions, respectively, consumed caffeine mainly from coffee at 85%, 79% and 85%, and from tea at 7%, 14% and 9%.

Table 2 shows the distribution of caffeine consumption during the day by sex, age group and language region. Caffeine intake in the entire Swiss population was the highest between 06:00 and 09:00 (29%), then decreased gradually during the day: 26% (09:00–12:00), 16% (12:00–15:00), 14% (15:00–18:00), 9% (18:00–21:00) and 3% (21:00–00:00). More than half of the caffeine (58%) was consumed in the morning between 03:00 and 12:00. No major differences were found between men (57%) and women (59%). The largest differences in caffeine consumption regarding age were observed between 06:00 and 12:00. From 06:00 to 09:00, caffeine intake was higher in older people: 22% in people aged 18–34 years and 37% in 65–75 year olds. The trend reversed in the second half of the morning (09:00 to 12:00) with the largest caffeine consumption among people aged 18–34 years (33% of total daily intake) compared to those aged 65–75 years (19%). The German-speaking and French-speaking regions had similar caffeine consumption trends over the day. However, the Italian-speaking region consumed more caffeine in the early morning (40% from 06:00 to 09:00) compared to the other two regions: 28% and 31% for German- and French-speaking, respectively. For more information on hourly caffeine consumption, see Supplementary Figure S3.

Table 1. Daily caffeine consumption in the Swiss population (mg/day) and percentage (%) of the population exceeding the recommendation of 400 mg.

Population Characteristics		n	Weighted n	Weighted %	Weighted Mean	SD	Weighted P5	Weighted P25	Weighted Median	Weighted P75	Weighted P95	>400 mg %
All	Entire population	2057	4,627,878	100%	191	129	29	96	169	260	426	6.6%
Sex	Men	933	2,305,141	50%	210	138	32	108	189	284	445	8.8%
	Women	1124	2,322,737	50%	172	117	27	86	155	229	388	4.5%
Age group	18–34 years	563	1,306,178	28%	140	111	20	58	113	186	359	2.4%
	35–49 years	602	1,421,756	31%	202	134	30	104	175	272	468	8.8%
	50–64 years	554	1,250,918	27%	228	135	62	134	207	294	451	9.4%
	65–75 years	338	649,026	14%	202	111	43	125	193	262	406	5.2%
Language region	German-speaking	1341	3,183,216	69%	204	136	30	104	182	277	445	7.9%
	French-speaking	502	1,187,738	26%	170	112	29	86	148	232	399	4.8%
	Italian-speaking	214	256,925	6%	136	85	22	71	126	193	270	0.3%
Nationality	Swiss	1789	3,470,404	75%	191	128	28	102	172	257	416	6.0%
	Not Swiss	265	1,145,199	25%	192	133	31	84	164	266	445	8.6%
Education	Lower	286	620,712	13%	208	156	31	107	175	261	527	8.7%
	Middle	771	1,589,873	34%	177	120	28	86	160	243	406	5.3%
	Higher	997	2,405,018	52%	196	128	29	101	176	267	426	7.0%
Income	Lower	486	1,128,723	24%	190	133	27	93	167	249	451	6.8%
	Middle	516	1,095,517	24%	188	123	36	100	168	245	401	5.1%
	Higher	802	1,831,768	40%	195	126	28	101	174	266	415	6.2%
	No answer	250	559,595	12%	188	144	15	70	161	262	449	10.9%
Smoking status	Never smokers	1072	2,307,169	50%	171	121	22	74	154	240	400	5.0%
	Ex-smokers	530	1,271,513	27%	197	115	38	111	176	268	415	6.4%
	Smokers	451	1,034,578	22%	228	152	49	131	199	285	519	10.5%
Weight status	Normal weight	1166	2,625,518	57%	179	125	25	85	160	243	413	5.6%
	Overweight	629	1,422,231	31%	204	124	43	112	186	269	423	6.7%
	Obesity	262	580,130	13%	217	154	32	101	195	296	506	11.2%

n: number. SD: standard deviation. p: percentile.

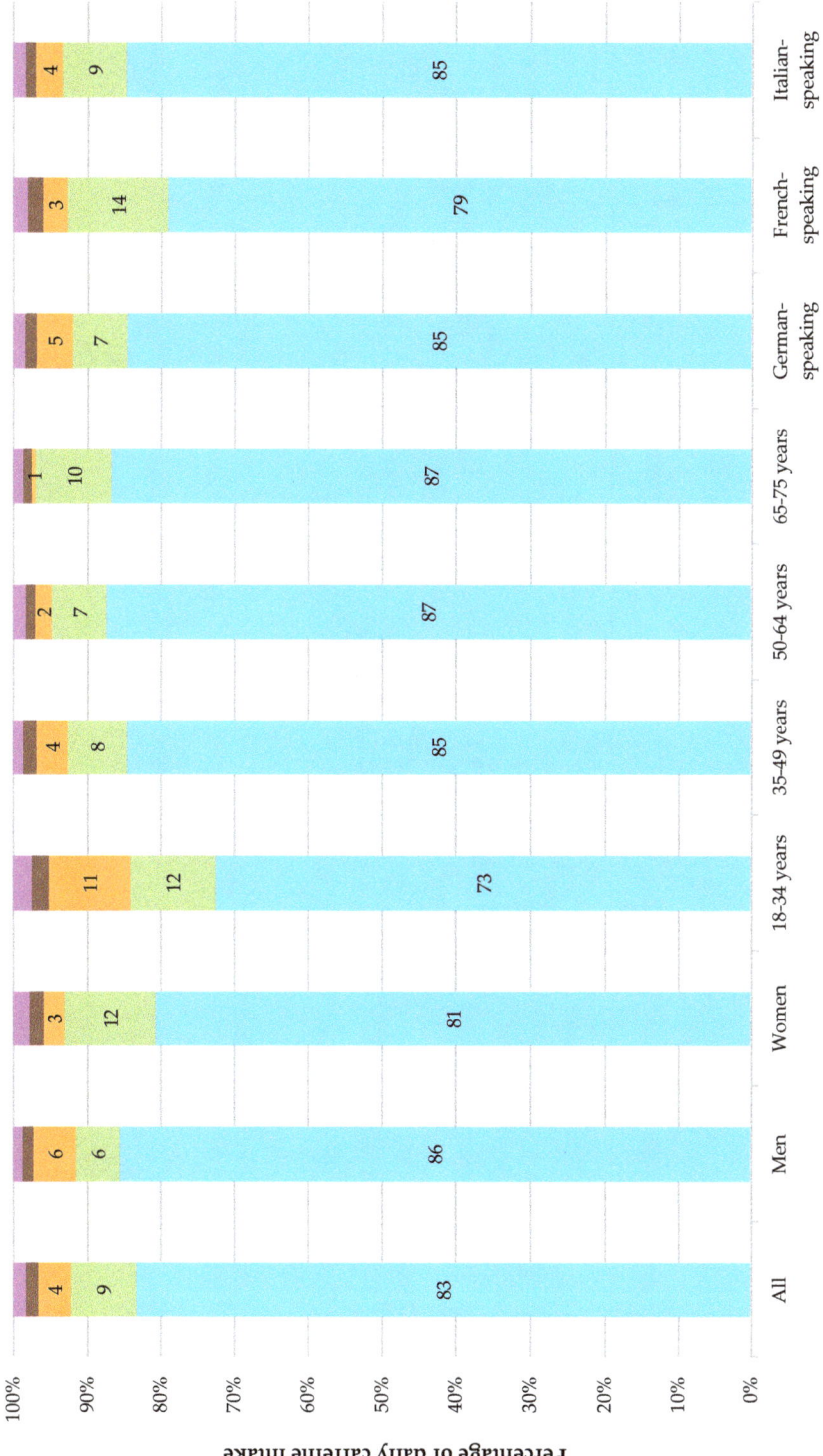

Figure 1. Main food groups sources of caffeine (percentage/day). Labels on bars represent percentage for the specific food group.

Table 2. Distribution of caffeine consumption per 3-hour period during the day (percentage/day).

Population	n	Weighted n	12:00–03:00	03:00–06:00	06:00–09:00	09:00–12:00	12:00–15:00	03:00–06:00	06:00–09:00	9 p.m.–12 a.m.
All	2057	4,627,878	0.2	2.9	29.0	26.2	15.9	13.7	8.9	3.2
Men	933	2,305,141	0.2	3.5	26.9	26.8	15.5	14.3	9.3	3.4
Women	1124	2,322,737	0.1	2.3	31.6	25.5	16.3	12.8	8.4	2.9
18–34 years	563	1,306,178	0.3	3.1	21.7	32.8	13.9	15.0	8.7	4.5
35–49 years	602	1,421,756	0.1	3.6	28.5	26.4	15.8	14.0	8.6	3.0
50–64 years	554	1,250,918	0.2	3.2	30.8	24.7	16.4	13.1	9.0	2.7
65–75 years	338	649,026	0.0	0.6	37.2	19.5	17.8	12.3	9.7	2.9
German-speaking	1341	3,183,216	0.2	3.2	27.9	27.0	15.4	14.0	9.2	3.1
French-speaking	502	1,187,738	0.2	2.1	31.1	24.1	17.6	12.8	8.3	3.7
Italian-speaking	214	256,925	0.0	2.8	39.8	22.0	14.5	12.2	7.2	1.4

n: number.

4. Discussion

The mean caffeine intake of the Swiss adult population was 191 mg/day, with higher intake in the age group 50–64 years (228 mg/day), the German-speaking region (204 mg/day), smokers (228 mg/day), and obese people (217 mg/day). In the Swiss population, the three main sources of caffeine consumption were (1) coffee (83%), (2) tea (9%) and (3) soft drinks (4%). Caffeine was mostly consumed between 06:00 and 09:00, then its intake decreased during the day. The circadian rhythm of caffeine intake slightly differed across linguistic regions and age groups.

4.1. Total Daily Caffeine Intake

Overall, the mean caffeine intake in the entire Swiss population (191 mg/day), was similar to that in other Western European countries [2] and the U.S. (169 mg/day, NHANES data). Because Switzerland has different food and caffeine consumption patterns across linguistic regions, we need to compare our results found in the three different regions. Specifically, our results for the population aged 18–64 years (202, 170, and 133 mg/day for the German-, French- and Italian-speaking regions, respectively, Supplementary Table S4) are very similar to values published in the corresponding neighbouring countries for the same age group: i.e., 238 mg/day in Germany, 155 in France, and 139 in Italy [2]. According to our study, 6.6% of the Swiss population consumed more than 400 mg/day of caffeine, the threshold below which it has been shown that caffeine consumption does not raise health issues in healthy adults [1,2,6]. In this regard, we also found differences between the linguistic regions. However, our observed percentages were lower than in the neighbouring countries (18–64 years old, Supplementary Table S4): 8.5% for the German- (14.6% in Germany), 4.9% in the French- (5.8% in France) and 0.3% for Italian-speaking part of Switzerland (2.1% in Italy) [2]. The comparison between countries should, however, be done with caution because methods used in the different national nutrition surveys were slightly different in terms of data collection years, dietary assessment methods, and sampling design [2].

4.2. Differences Across Population Subgroups

Previous studies have shown similar results as our study with greater consumption of total caffeine in men than in women [7,12,22,30,31]. However, this difference between sexes seemed to be due to confounding factors, such as body weight, as shown in our study. Indeed, Mitchell et al. also demonstrated that, when consumption is adjusted to the body weight, women consumed slightly more caffeine than men [22]. Another study in the U.S. found no significant difference between sex after adjusting for working hours or employment status [7]. The curvilinear association between caffeine consumption and age observed in our study was also already documented in the literature [7,12,22,31]. Consumption increases with age, reaching a peak at around 51–70 years old and declines among older people. Although our results suggest that people with lower education consumed more caffeine, studies in the U.S. did not find a systematic association between caffeine consumption and education [7,31], nor income [31]. Finally, as expected from the literature [32], our study found higher caffeine consumption among smokers. This association might have several explanations: (1) smoking causes the induction of cytochrome P450 1 A2 (CYP1A2), causing an acceleration of the elimination of caffeine, which may lead to a better tolerance to caffeine [33], (2) genetic factors [34] and (3) behavioural and environmental factors [35].

4.3. Main Sources of Caffeine

The large proportion of caffeine brought by coffee in Switzerland (83% of total daily intake) is comparable to proportions in the U.S. [12,22] and European countries [2], with the exception of Ireland, the United Kingdom and Latvia, for which a major source of caffeine was tea (between 52% and 60%) [2]. The main food sources of caffeine seemed to be specific to each culture, as the proportions found in the three linguistic regions of Switzerland are, again, very similar to those published in their neighbouring countries [2]. In addition, we found that younger adults (18–34 years) consumed more caffeine from soft drinks (including energy drinks) than older people. An Austrian study of young adults showed similar results with a decreasing consumption of caffeine from soft and energy drinks with age: 94 mg/day in 18–25 year olds vs. 74 mg/day in 26–39 year olds [36]. Mitchell et al. also found a higher consumption of caffeine from energy drinks in younger than older U.S. adults [22]. This difference may be due to a preference for soft and energy drinks rather than coffee among young people [37].

4.4. Timing of Caffeine Consumption

Our study showed a maximum consumption of caffeine in the morning (58%), with a decreasing consumption throughout the day, as already demonstrated in several North-American studies [7,11,14]. For instance, Martyn et al. showed that 61% of caffeine was consumed in the morning, defined as from before breakfast until lunch (not included), 21% between lunch and dinner (not included) and 18% in the evening (i.e., during and after dinner) [14]. Lieberman et al. found a much higher caffeine consumption peak in the morning, with about 70% of caffeine consumed between 03:00 and 12:00 (58% in our study) and 40% just between 06:00 and 09:00 (29% in our study) [7]. Our results have also shown that caffeine intake in the younger population is slightly delayed in the morning (09:00–12:00 instead of 06:00–09:00), afternoon (03:00–06:00 instead of 12:00–15:00), and evening (21:00–00:00 instead of 06:00–21:00), compared to the older population. However, it seems there are no major differences in caffeine consumption among the four age groups, when grouping periods by two: i.e., 55%–57% of caffeine consumed in the morning (06:00–12:00), 29%–30% in the afternoon (12:00–18:00) and 12%–13% in the evening (18:00–00:00) (Table 2). In the U.S., Martyn et al. found a positive association between age and caffeine intake in the morning: 18–24 year olds consumed 50% of their daily caffeine intake in the morning, whereas those aged 65 consumed over 66% (and 23% vs. 16% in the evening, respectively) [14]. To our knowledge, no study has yet investigated the timing of caffeine consumption in Western Europe.

4.5. Strengths and Limitations of the Study

The strengths of our study were that we used data from a representative sample of the Swiss population, we took into account all the different sources of caffeine, not only beverages, and we used MSM to predict the usual consumption. However, since a menuCH project was not planned to assess caffeine intake, we did not have a detailed description of the different types of coffee with their brand, place of purchase and/or brewing method, even though this information highly influences caffeine concentration in coffee, as shown in literature [38,39] and our measurements (Supplementary Table S2). In this context, we lack precision in the assignment of caffeine concentration in different types of coffees, and had to rely on averages.

5. Conclusions

To the best of our knowledge, this is the first study looking at self-reported caffeine intake in Switzerland. The average consumption in the entire adult population was 191 mg/d, which was consistent with data from other high-income countries, particularly neighbouring countries. Only a small proportion of the Swiss adult population (6.6%) consumes above the maximum intake of 400 mg/day recommended by EFSA. Differences in caffeine consumption were observed across age groups, linguistic regions and smoking status, but in all population subgroups, coffee was the main source of caffeine intake, and caffeine was mostly consumed in the morning.

Supplementary Materials: The following are available online at http://www.mdpi.com/2072-6643/12/1/28/s1, Figure S1: Decision tree regarding food groups with or without caffeine, Table S1: Overview of caffeine concentration in foods, by food groups, Table S2: Measurements of caffeine concentration in coffee and soft drinks, Table S3: Daily caffeine consumption per kg of body weight (mg/kg/day), Figure S2: Main food groups sources of caffeine (mg/day), Figure S3: Distribution of caffeine consumption per hour during the day (percentage/day), Table S4: Daily caffeine consumption in the population aged 18–64 years old (mg/day).

Author Contributions: C.R. and M.B. wrote the study protocol. C.R. and A.C. assigned values for caffeine to all consumed foods reported by survey participants. A.C. conducted the statistical analyses. A.C., M.B. and C.R. contributed to the concept and the design of the manuscript. C.R. collected coffee and soft drinks samples. C.B.E. supervised laboratory analyses. C.R. and A.C. wrote the manuscript. All the authors have revised the writing of the manuscript. All authors have read and agreed to the published version of the manuscript.

Funding: The national nutrition survey menuCH was co-funded by the Swiss Federal Food Safety and Veterinary Office and the Federal Office of Public Health. The work related to this project, which was part of a master thesis, received no funding.

Acknowledgments: The authors thank the Swiss Federal Food Safety and Veterinary Office, www.blv.admin.ch, for providing menuCH data.

Conflicts of Interest: The authors declare no conflict of interest.

References

1. Nawrot, P.; Jordan, S.; Eastwood, J.; Rotstein, J.; Hugenholtz, A.; Feeley, M. Effects of caffeine on human health. *Food Addit. Contam.* **2003**, *20*, 1–30. [CrossRef] [PubMed]
2. EFSA Panel on Dietetic Products. Nutrition and Allergies (NDA) Scientific Opinion on the safety of caffeine. *EFSA J.* **2015**, *13*, 4120.
3. Heckman, M.A.; Weil, J.; De Mejia, E.G. Caffeine (1, 3, 7-trimethylxanthine) in Foods: A Comprehensive Review on Consumption, Functionality, Safety, and Regulatory Matters. *J. Food Sci.* **2010**, *75*, R77–R87. [CrossRef]
4. Higdon, J.V.; Frei, B. Coffee and Health: A Review of Recent Human Research. *Crit. Rev. Food Sci. Nutr.* **2006**, *46*, 101–123. [CrossRef] [PubMed]
5. Grosso, G.; Godos, J.; Galvano, F.; Giovannucci, E.L. Coffee, Caffeine and Health Outcomes: An Umbrella Review. *Annu. Rev. Nutr.* **2017**, *37*, 131–156. [CrossRef]
6. Wikoff, D.; Welsh, B.T.; Henderson, R.; Brorby, G.P.; Britt, J.; Myers, E.; Goldberger, J.; Lieberman, H.R.; O'Brien, C.; Peck, J.; et al. Systematic review of the potential adverse effects of caffeine consumption in healthy adults, pregnant women, adolescents, and children. *Food Chem. Toxicol.* **2017**, *109*, 585–648. [CrossRef]
7. Lieberman, H.R.; Agarwal, S.; Fulgoni, V.L. Daily Patterns of Caffeine Intake and the Association of Intake with Multiple Sociodemographic and Lifestyle Factors in US Adults Based on the NHANES 2007–2012 Surveys. *J. Acad. Nutr. Diet.* **2019**, *119*, 106–114. [CrossRef]
8. O'Callaghan, F.; Muurlink, O.; Reid, N. Effects of caffeine on sleep quality and daytime functioning. *Risk Manag. Healthc. Policy* **2018**, *11*, 263–271. [CrossRef]
9. Noordzij, M.; Uiterwaal, C.S.; Arends, L.R.; Kok, F.J.; Grobbee, D.E.; Geleijnse, J.M. Blood pressure response to chronic intake of coffee and caffeine: A meta-analysis of randomized controlled trials. *J. Hypertens.* **2005**, *23*, 921–928. [CrossRef]
10. Turnbull, D.; Rodricks, J.V.; Mariano, G.F.; Chowdhury, F. Caffeine and cardiovascular health. *Regul. Toxicol. Pharmacol.* **2017**, *89*, 165–185. [CrossRef]
11. Benson, S.M.; Unice, K.M.; Glynn, M.E. Hourly and daily intake patterns among U.S. caffeinated beverage consumers based on the National Health and Nutrition Examination Survey (NHANES, 2013–2016). *Food Chem. Toxicol.* **2019**, *125*, 271–278. [CrossRef] [PubMed]
12. Fulgoni, V.L.; Keast, D.R.; Lieberman, H.R. Trends in intake and sources of caffeine in the diets of US adults: 2001–2010. *Am. J. Clin. Nutr.* **2015**, *101*, 1081–1087. [CrossRef] [PubMed]
13. Verster, J.C.; Koenig, J. Caffeine intake and its sources: A review of national representative studies. *Crit. Rev. Food Sci. Nutr.* **2018**, *58*, 1250–1259. [CrossRef] [PubMed]
14. Martyn, D.; Lau, A.; Richardson, P.; Roberts, A. Temporal patterns of caffeine intake in the United States. *Food Chem. Toxicol.* **2018**, *111*, 71–83. [CrossRef] [PubMed]
15. Kontis, V.; Bennett, J.E.; Mathers, C.D.; Li, G.; Foreman, K.; Ezzati, M. Future life expectancy in 35 industrialised countries: Projections with a Bayesian model ensemble. *Lancet* **2017**, *389*, 1323–1335. [CrossRef]
16. Chatelan, A.; Beer-Borst, S.; Randriamiharisoa, A.; Pasquier, J.; Blanco, J.; Siegenthaler, S.; Paccaud, F.; Slimani, N.; Nicolas, G.; Camenzind-Frey, E.; et al. Major Differences in Diet across Three Linguistic Regions of Switzerland: Results from the First National Nutrition Survey menuCH. *Nutrients* **2017**, *9*, 1163. [CrossRef]

17. Petrovic, D.; Estoppey Younes, S.; Pruijm, M.; Ponte, B.; Ackermann, D.; Ehret, G.; Ansermot, N.; Mohaupt, M.; Paccaud, F.; Vogt, B.; et al. Relation of 24-h urinary caffeine and caffeine metabolite excretions with self-reported consumption of coffee and other caffeinated beverages in the general population. *Nutr. Metab.* **2016**, *13*, 81. [CrossRef]
18. Federal Statistical Office. Stichprobenrahmen für Personen- und Haushaltserhebungen (Swiss persons and households registry). Available online: https://www.bfs.admin.ch/bfs/de/home/grundlagen/volkszaehlung/volkszaehlung-teil-gesamtsystem/stichprobenrahmen.html (accessed on 16 October 2019).
19. Chatelan, A.; Gaillard, P.; Kruseman, M.; Keller, A. Total, Added, and Free Sugar Consumption and Adherence to Guidelines in Switzerland: Results from the First National Nutrition Survey menuCH. *Nutrients* **2019**, *11*, 1117. [CrossRef]
20. Chatelan, A.; Marques-Vidal, P.; Bucher, S.; Siegenthaler, S.; Metzger, N.; Zuberbühler, C.A.; Camenzind-Frey, E.; Reggli, A.; Bochud, M.; Beer-Borst, S. Lessons Learnt About Conducting a Multilingual Nutrition Survey in Switzerland: Results from menuCH Pilot Survey. *Int. J. Vitam. Nutr. Res.* **2017**, *87*, 25–36. [CrossRef]
21. Camenzind-Frey, E.; Zuberbuehler, C.A. *menuCH-Schweizerisches Fotobuch/Livre Photo Suisse/Manuale Fotografico Svizzero (menuCH Picture Book)*; Federal Office of Public Health & Federal Food Safety and Veterinary Office: Berne, Switzerland, 2014.
22. Mitchell, D.C.; Knight, C.A.; Hockenberry, J.; Teplansky, R.; Hartman, T.J. Beverage caffeine intakes in the U.S. *Food Chem. Toxicol.* **2014**, *63*, 136–142. [CrossRef]
23. Federal Food Safety and Veterinary Office. Swiss food composition database. Available online: https://www.naehrwertdaten.ch/en/ (accessed on 6 June 2019).
24. Sereshti, H.; Samadi, S. A rapid and simple determination of caffeine in teas, coffees and eight beverages. *Food Chem.* **2014**, *158*, 8–13. [CrossRef] [PubMed]
25. Vin, K.; Beziat, J.; Seper, K.; Wolf, A.; Sidor, A.; Chereches, R.; Luc Volatier, J.; Ménard, C. Nutritional composition of the food supply: A comparison of soft drinks and breakfast cereals between three European countries based on labels. *Eur. J. Clin. Nutr.* **2019**, *1*. [CrossRef] [PubMed]
26. McCusker, R.R.; Fuehrlein, B.; Goldberger, B.A.; Gold, M.S.; Cone, E.J. Caffeine Content of Decaffeinated Coffee. *J. Anal. Toxicol.* **2006**, *30*, 611–613. [CrossRef] [PubMed]
27. Center for the Promotion of Imports, Ministry of Foreign Affairs. Through what channels can you get coffee onto the European market? Available online: https://www.cbi.eu/market-information/coffee/channels-segments (accessed on 6 June 2019).
28. World Health Organization MONICA Manual, Part III: Population Survey. Section 1: Population Survey Data Component. 4.6 Height, Weight, Waist and Hip Measurement. Available online: http://www.thl.fi/publications/monica/manual/part3/iii-1.htm#s4-6 (accessed on 1 July 2017).
29. Harttig, U.; Haubrock, J.; Knuppel, S.; Boeing, H.; Consortium, E. The MSM program: Web-based statistics package for estimating usual dietary intake using the Multiple Source Method. *Eur. J. Clin. Nutr.* **2011**, *65*, S87–S91. [CrossRef]
30. Fitt, E.; Pell, D.; Cole, D. Assessing caffeine intake in the United Kingdom diet. *Food Chem.* **2013**, *140*, 421–426. [CrossRef]
31. Drewnowski, A.; Rehm Colin, D. Sources of Caffeine in Diets of US Children and Adults: Trends by Beverage Type and Purchase Location. *Nutrients* **2016**, *8*, 154. [CrossRef]
32. Treur, J.L.; Taylor, A.E.; Ware, J.J.; McMahon, G.; Hottenga, J.-J.; Baselmans, B.M.L.; Willemsen, G.; Boomsma, D.I.; Munafò, M.R.; Vink, J.M. Associations between smoking and caffeine consumption in two European cohorts: Smoking and caffeine consumption. *Addiction* **2016**, *111*, 1059–1068. [CrossRef]
33. Grela, A.; Kulza, M.; Piekoszewsi, W.; Senczuk-Przybylowska, M.; Gomolka, E.; Florek, E. The effects of tobacco smoke exposure on caffeine metabolism. *Ital. J. Food Sci.* **2013**, *25*, 76–82.
34. Treur, J.L.; Taylor, A.E.; Ware, J.J.; Nivard, M.G.; Neale, M.C.; McMahon, G.; Hottenga, J.-J.; Baselmans, B.M.L.; Boomsma, D.I.; Munafò, M.R.; et al. Smoking and caffeine consumption: A genetic analysis of their association: Smoking and caffeine. *Addict. Biol.* **2017**, *22*, 1090–1102. [CrossRef]
35. Hettema, J.M.; Corey, L.A.; Kendler, K.S. A multivariate genetic analysis of the use of tobacco, alcohol, and caffeine in a population based sample of male and female twins. *Drug Alcohol Depend.* **1999**, *57*, 69–78. [CrossRef]

36. Rudolph, E.; Faerbinger, A.; Koenig, J. Caffeine intake from all sources in adolescents and young adults in Austria. *Eur. J. Clin. Nutr.* **2014**, *68*, 793–798. [CrossRef] [PubMed]
37. Bleich, S.N.; Vercammen, K.A.; Koma, J.W.; Li, Z. Trends in Beverage Consumption Among Children and Adults, 2003-2014: Trends in Beverage Consumption. *Obesity* **2018**, *26*, 432–441. [CrossRef]
38. Hečimović, I.; Belščak-Cvitanović, A.; Horžić, D.; Komes, D. Comparative study of polyphenols and caffeine in different coffee varieties affected by the degree of roasting. *Food Chem.* **2011**, *129*, 991–1000. [CrossRef] [PubMed]
39. McCusker, R.R.; Goldberger, B.A.; Cone, E.J. Caffeine Content of Specialty Coffees. *J. Anal. Toxicol.* **2003**, *27*, 520–522. [CrossRef] [PubMed]

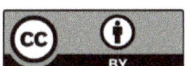

© 2019 by the authors. Licensee MDPI, Basel, Switzerland. This article is an open access article distributed under the terms and conditions of the Creative Commons Attribution (CC BY) license (http://creativecommons.org/licenses/by/4.0/).

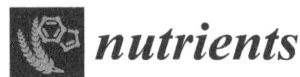

Article

Translation and Validation of the Caffeine Expectancy Questionnaire in Brazil (CaffEQ-BR)

Guilherme Falcão Mendes [1,*], Caio Eduardo Gonçalves Reis [1], Eduardo Yoshio Nakano [2], Teresa Helena Macedo da Costa [1], Bryan Saunders [3,4] and Renata Puppin Zandonadi [1,*]

- [1] Department of Nutrition, School of Health Sciences, University of Brasilia (UnB), Campus Darcy Ribeiro, Asa Norte, Brasilia DF 70910-900, Brazil; caioedureis@gmail.com (C.E.G.R.); thmdacosta@gmail.com (T.H.M.d.C.)
- [2] Department of Statistics, Central Institute of Sciences, University of Brasilia (UnB), Campus Darcy Ribeiro, Asa Norte, Brasilia DF 70910-900, Brazil; eynakano@gmail.com
- [3] Applied Physiology and Nutrition Research Group, School of Physical Education and Sport; Rheumatology Division; Faculdade de Medicina FMUSP, University of São Paulo, Sao Paulo 01246-903, Brazil; drbryansaunders@outlook.com
- [4] Institute of Orthopaedics and Traumatology, Faculty of Medicine FMUSP, University of São Paulo, Sao Paulo 01246-903, Brazil
- * Correspondence: guilherme.falcao@aluno.unb.br (G.F.M.); renatapz@unb.br (R.P.Z.); Tel.: +55-(61)3107-1782 (G.F.M. & R.P.Z.)

Received: 4 June 2020; Accepted: 22 July 2020; Published: 28 July 2020

Abstract: Caffeine is the world's most commonly used stimulant of the central nervous system. Caffeine is present in coffee and other beverages such as tea, soft drinks, and cocoa-based foods. The caffeine expectancy questionnaire was developed to investigate the effects of caffeine expectations and thus contribute to knowledge about its usage and subjective effects (response expectancies). This study aimed to evaluate caffeine expectation psychometrically in a sample of the Brazilian population. The original version of the "Caffeine Expectancy Questionnaire (CaffEQ)" was translated and validated into Brazilian-Portuguese and adapted to Brazilian culture to be used in the Brazilian adult (19–59 y) population. After the translation and back-translation processes of the original CaffEQ questionnaire, the content and semantic validation were performed by a group of experts. The Brazilian-Portuguese version of the questionnaire consists of 47 items, in seven factors, which assess subjective perceptions about the effects of caffeine. Interobserver reproducibility and internal consistency of the questionnaire were tested with a convenience sample ($n = 50$) of Brazilian adult consumers of caffeine sources, who completed the Brazilian CaffEQ (CaffEQ-BR) on two occasions separated by 24 h. All of the 47 questions were adequate regarding reliability, clarity, and comprehension. Psychometric properties could be replicated consistently. Appropriate internal consistency and validation were confirmed by Cronbach's alpha (α) 0.948, and an intraclass correlation coefficient of 0.976 was observed. The CaffEQ-BR was applied using a web-based platform to a convenience sample of Brazilian adults from all 27 Brazilian states ($n = 4202$ participants), along with measures of sociodemographic and caffeine consumption data. Factor validity was verified by confirmatory factor analysis. The seven factors presented a good fit for Root Mean Square Error of Approximation—RMSEA = 0.0332 (95% CI: 0.0290–0.0375). By confirming the validity and reliability of CaffEQ-BR, a useful tool is now available to assess caffeine expectations in the Brazilian adult population.

Keywords: caffeine; subjective; expectancy; instrument; validation; Brazilian; Portuguese

1. Introduction

Caffeine (1,3,7-trimethylxanthine) is the most widely consumed psychoactive substance in the world [1,2] with several guidelines addressing the form of use, dosage, and limits for safe consumption [3–5]. Worldwide, and in Brazil, caffeine intake occurs primarily through coffee consumption [1]. The estimation of the Brazilian population's average daily coffee intake is 163 mL [6], being the most consumed non-alcoholic drink in Brazil [7,8]. In addition, caffeine is also widely consumed in other foods and beverages such as cola, cocoa, chocolate, guarana, and in matte, black, and green teas [9]. Furthermore, a range of energy drinks and sports supplements also contain caffeine in their composition [5]. The differences in biological individuality and cultural factors can influence the habits of caffeine consumption [10,11]. Therefore, the ingestion of products that contain caffeine is not only associated with their sensorial characteristics and eating habits but also with caffeine effect expectations [12].

It is well established that placebo effects are associated with caffeine supplementation, likely due to an expectancy surrounding its effects. Double-blind studies have shown that participants receiving a placebo treatment perceived to be caffeine improved exercise performance to a similar extent when compared with caffeine ingestion [13,14]. Positive expectation associated with caffeine ingestion appeared to drive this effect since individuals correctly believing that they had ingested caffeine improved to a greater extent than the average effect of caffeine [13,15]. However, these results were not observed in physiological variables, such as heart rate and blood pressure [16], further reinforcing the notion that the expected effect of caffeine plays a subjective role in the belief around its consumption [16,17]. Regarding expectancy, factors such as motivation and belief can influence the ergogenic response of caffeine in adults [17]. Therefore, expectancies associated with caffeine use/outcome may play an important role in the development, maintenance, and reinforcement of its consumption patterns [12,18,19]. Studies have attempted to associate habitual caffeine consumption with changes in mood, appetite, sleep/alertness, exercise performance, and other factors [19–21]. Based on these observations, standardized questionnaires were constructed using psychometric techniques [22] to assess expectancy about caffeine consumption [19–21], or to evaluate the motives for caffeine consumption [12].

In this regard, Heinz et al. (2009) [18] proposed a questionnaire with 37 items to examine caffeine expectancy comprising four factors: 'withdrawal symptoms', 'positive effects', 'acute negative effects', and 'mood effects'. Subsequently, Huntley and Juliano (2012) [20] proposed the Caffeine Expectancy Questionnaire (CaffEQ), a structured questionnaire based on a detailed review of the literature and a series of preliminary studies for construction of the items. The final version of the CaffEQ (originally in English, designed for the United States of America) includes 47 items, evaluated using a six-point Likert scale, distributed across seven factors: 'withdrawal/dependence', 'energy/work enhancement', 'appetite suppression', 'social/mood enhancement', 'physical performance enhancement', 'anxiety/negative physical effects' and 'sleep disturbance'. Besides its use in the English language, the CaffEQ was also translated and validated for German-speaking countries (Germany, Switzerland, and Austria) by the authors Schott et al. (2016) [21].

However, since the validation and standardization of the CaffEQ questionnaire were performed only for English and German speaking populations [19–21], there are currently no studies with Latin American countries using the CaffEQ due to linguistic barriers and cultural differences that cause difficulties in using the original questionnaire. In this sense, there has been no study proposed to evaluate caffeine expectations in the Brazilian population due to the lack of a valid questionnaire in the Brazilian-Portuguese language. Therefore, this study aimed to translate, culturally adapt, and validate the CaffEQ to the Brazilian population (CaffEQ-BR), and also to evaluate caffeine expectations in Brazilian adult participants. We expect that this study can provide a questionnaire with internal and external validity to characterize caffeine expectations in the Brazilian adult population and be an easy questionnaire to incorporate into research and clinical contexts.

2. Materials and Methods

The present study used the original CaffEQ and translated it from the English version to Brazilian-Portuguese [20]. The CaffEQ is composed of 47 items, evaluated using a six-point Likert scale. In order to create the CaffEQ for the Brazilian population (CaffEQ-BR), our study was conducted in four stages: (1) Translation, Cultural Adaptation, and Semantic Evaluation; (2) Internal Consistency and Reproducibility of CaffEQ-BR; (3) Brazilian nationwide CaffEQ-BR application; (4) Statistical analysis. The study was approved by the Ethics Committee of the University Católica of Brasília (Brasília, Brazil) (number: 23019319.3.0000.0029) and followed the guidelines established by the Declaration of Helsinki. The volunteers were informed about the study protocol and provided web-based consent.

In the present study, the survey was carried out using Google Forms™ web-based platform [23]. The online form maintained the original CaffEQ version layout and content [20]. The expert panel suggested inserting an explanation about the meaning of the word caffeine (as well as about its main sources) in the questionnaire heading for a better understanding of the questionnaire by the general public, since the term "caffeine" is not common to the Brazilian population.

2.1. Translation, Cultural Adaptation, and Semantic Assessment

The translation and cultural adaptation of the questionnaire was performed according to World Health Organization (WHO) recommendations [24]. A bilingual researcher native in Portuguese (T.H.M.d.C.) translated the original version (in English) of the CaffEQ into the Brazilian-Portuguese language. Subsequently, another bilingual researcher, a native English speaker (resident in Brazil for eight years) (B.S.), with no knowledge of the original work, back-translated the Brazilian-Portuguese version (made by T.H.M.d.C.) into English. After that, three collaborators (G.F.M.; C.E.G.R.; R.P.Z.) compared the back-translated version (in English, made by B.S.) with the original questionnaire and analyzed the Brazilian-Portuguese translation version to make adjustments in case of non-conformities. The final version was agreed upon by the bilingual translators (T.H.M.d.C. and B.S.) as a final step in the translation process.

The questionnaire was subsequently analyzed and revised by a panel of health professional experts ($n = 20$) distributed across the following academic degrees: Master's ($n = 7$; 35%), Doctorate ($n = 9$; 45%) and Post-doctorate ($n = 4$; 20%), all associated with universities and all residents in Brasília Federal District [22]. The experts individually analyzed the cultural adaptation and semantic assessment using parameters of the 'importance' and 'clarity' of each question ($n = 47$) on a Likert scale of 1 to 5, where 1 indicates "I totally disagree with the item"; 2—"I partially disagree with the item"; 3—"I neither agree nor disagree with the item"; 4—"I partially agree with the item"; and 5—"I fully agree with the item". The objective was to achieve more than 80% agreement among the experts (mean > 3) for each question [25,26]. Pending items were adjusted according to the experts' observations and sent back to them for compliance analysis. This process occurred until all items achieved at least 80% agreement (mean > 3). The degree of agreement among experts in the evaluation of the 'importance' and 'clarity' of the questions was performed by the Kendall correlation coefficient (W) ranging from 0 to 1. A W-value ≥ 0.66 indicates that the experts applied the same evaluation standards, and W-values < 0.66 suggest disagreement between experts. To approve an item, it was deemed necessary that at least 80% agreement was achieved among the experts (W values ≥ 0.8) [26].

2.2. Internal Consistency and Reproducibility of CaffEQ-BR

The reproducibility of the translated and adapted instrument CaffEQ-BR was analyzed before nationwide application since, before application in a large sample, it is important to test the reproducibility (reliability) and internal consistency with a small sample size [27]. Internal consistency refers to the variation in measurements made under changing conditions and reproducibility evaluates the agreement between any two measurements made on the same subject [27].

For this purpose, the questionnaire was applied using the Google Forms™ platform to a convenience sample ($n = 50$) of Brazilian adults (>19–59 y) who were regular consumers of caffeine from various sources. Participants were invited through pilot advertising on social media (for example, Facebook™, Instagram™, and WhatsApp™). The questionnaire was answered twice (test-retest) by each person. The second questionnaire was sent within 24 h and returned within the next 24 h. The test-retest questionnaires evaluated reproducibility. It is important to note that the participants did not previously know that they would have to answer the questionnaire a second time. The test-retest reliability (reproducibility) analysis was performed using the intraclass correlation coefficient (ICC), and the internal consistency of the factors was verified using Cronbach's alpha (α). The number of individuals used in this step was considered sufficient once the results were statistically significant ($p < 0.05$) and the effect size was significant (alpha > 0.9 and ICC > 0.6) [28,29].

2.3. Brazilian Nationwide Application of CaffEQ-BR

In order to validate the CaffEQ-BR in Brazil and also to evaluate the Brazilian adult population, we used a questionnaire composed of three parts: (i) sociodemographic and health-related questions; (ii) evaluation of caffeine consumption; and (iii) the CaffEQ-BR. According to Hair et al. (2010) [30], the process of validating a questionnaire requires 20 respondents per item (20:1). In this sense, the minimum sample size was estimated as 940 participants to validate this questionnaire composed of 47 items. In addition, as this is a nationally external validation study, the sample size adopted for calculation was in accordance with the last Brazilian national census [26], with adequacy greater than or equal to 70% of the sample distribution, according to the various states of Brazil. In the example of the state of Rio de Janeiro, the population of 17,264,943, represents 8.22% of the population of Brazil. Therefore, the CaffEQ-BR sample, to obtain 100% adequacy, must have 8.22% of its total sample composed of participants from the state of Rio de Janeiro. In this way, we balanced the sample among the states of Brazil.

The questionnaire was applied using the Google Forms™ platform to a convenience sample of Brazilian adults from all 27 Brazilian states. Participants were recruited by advertising on social media (e.g., Facebook™, Instagram™, and WhatsApp™) [21]. The data collection period occurred from December 2019 to April 2020.

The initial page of the online survey presented the informed consent form with details of the inclusion criteria: (i) adults (>19–59 y) [31,32]) living in Brazil; (ii) regular consumer of caffeine sources (at least three times per week [33]), later confirmed by the caffeine consumption questionnaire. Those who did not agree to participate were directed to a page thanking them for their time, while those who agreed were directed to the first page of the questionnaire with sociodemographic and health-related questions, then caffeine consumption assessment and the 47-item CaffEQ-BR.

2.3.1. Sociodemographic and Health Data

Sociodemographic variables were gender; self-identification of ethnicity; state of the federation of current residence; education level; and average monthly income (BRL/month/person or family). The variables concerning health aspects were height (m) and weight (kg) (self-reported); ≥150 min weekly physical exercise; and previous diagnosis of self-reported chronic diseases with current medication.

2.3.2. Caffeine Consumption

The caffeine consumption questionnaire [33,34] was used to assess the caffeine consumed over the past two weeks prior to the completion of the questionnaire. Participants were asked to indicate the number of servings of coffee, tea, soft drinks, energy drinks, and other caffeine-containing products consumed. The questionnaire also includes a list categorized into eight groups of caffeine sources: 1. Filtered or espresso, hot or iced coffee; 2. Tea sources of caffeine like mate, green and black tea; 3. Pure chocolate with 50% cocoa; 4. Chocolate beverages with 50% cocoa; 5. Cola or guarana based soft drinks; 6. Caffeinated drugs; 7. Commercial drink sources of anhydrous caffeine or guarana extract beverage; 8. Sports supplements sources of anhydrous caffeine. Standardized doses of coffee, in homemade measures, were adopted according to the national reference study [35]. The typical serving size and caffeine values were based on the products' manufacturer information and the food composition table [36].

2.4. Statistical Analysis

A confirmatory factor analysis verified the factor validity. The factor validity was evaluated by the Root Mean Square Error of Approximation (RMSEA). The RMSEA ranges from 0 to 1, where the value 0 indicates a perfect model fit. A value of 0.05 or less is indicative of an acceptable model fit. Caffeine intake was expressed as a mean ± standard deviation (SD). Shapiro-Wilk test was used to evaluate the normality of distribution. The independent samples t-test was used to compare means between gender. All tests were conducted considering a significance level of 5%. The statistical packages IBM SPSS (Statistical Package for Social Sciences) version 22 (IBM SPSS Statistics for Windows, IBM Corp, Armonk, NY, USA) and IBM SPSS AMOS (Analysis of Moment Structures) version 22 (Amos, IBM SPSS, Chicago, IL, USA) were used for the analyses.

3. Results

3.1. Translation, Cultural Adaptation, Semantic Evaluation, and Content Validation

The CaffEQ-BR (available in Brazilian-Portuguese in Appendix A) was constructed considering the translation/back-translation process and the suggestions made by the expert panel. Following the translation/back-translation phase, the first stage of semantic evaluation and content validation was carried out by the panel of 20 experts who decided to keep 47 items with cultural and semantic adaptations, since we chose to follow the original CaffEQ questionnaire [20]. Throughout three rounds of assessment, with modifications in the items regarding cultural and semantic aspects, the experts reached agreement (≥80%) on the evaluation of the 47 items in the questionnaire. After that, with a convenience sample of 50 Brazilian adults (60% female, 36.4 ± 12.4 y, 62.2% self-identification as white), the internal consistency and reproducibility of CaffEQ-BR were verified. A summary of the translation, cultural adaptation, semantic evaluation, and content validation processes for CaffEQ-BR is shown in Figure 1.

3.2. Reproducibility and Internal Consistency of the CaffEQ-BR

All seven factors of the CaffEQ-BR showed no significant difference (ICC > 0.9) in the responses from the same individual (n = 50) (Table 1). As shown in Table 1, all seven factors indicated good internal consistency ($\alpha \geq 0.8$) [29,37].

Table 1. Reproducibility and internal consistency of the instrument and factors of the Caffeine Expectancy Questionnaire in Brazil (CaffEQ-BR) *.

Factors	N. Items	Internal Consistency Cronbach Alpha (95% CI)	Reproducibility Intraclass Correlation Coefficient (95% CI)
Withdrawal/dependence	12	0.948 (0.923–0.968)	0.983 (0.969–0.991)
Energy/work enhancement	8	0.926 (0.888–0.923)	0.953 (0.912–0.975)
Appetite suppression	5	0.872 (0.802–0.923)	0.951 (0.903–0.974)
Social/mood enhancement	6	0.889 (0.829–0.932)	0.949 (0.900–0.973)
Physical performance enhancement	3	0.924 (0.875–0.956)	0.965 (0.936–0.981)
Anxiety/negative physical effects	9	0.872 (0.807–0.921)	0.953 (0.907–0.976)
Sleep disturbance	4	0.941 (0.907–0.965)	0.970 (0.945–0.983)
Overall	**47**	**0.948 (0.923–0.967)**	**0.976 (0.935–0.989)**

* For reproducibility and internal consistency of items and factors of the CaffEQ-BR, conducted with a convenience sample of 50 Brazilian adults: 60% female, 36.4 ± 12.4 y, 62.2% of self- identification as white.

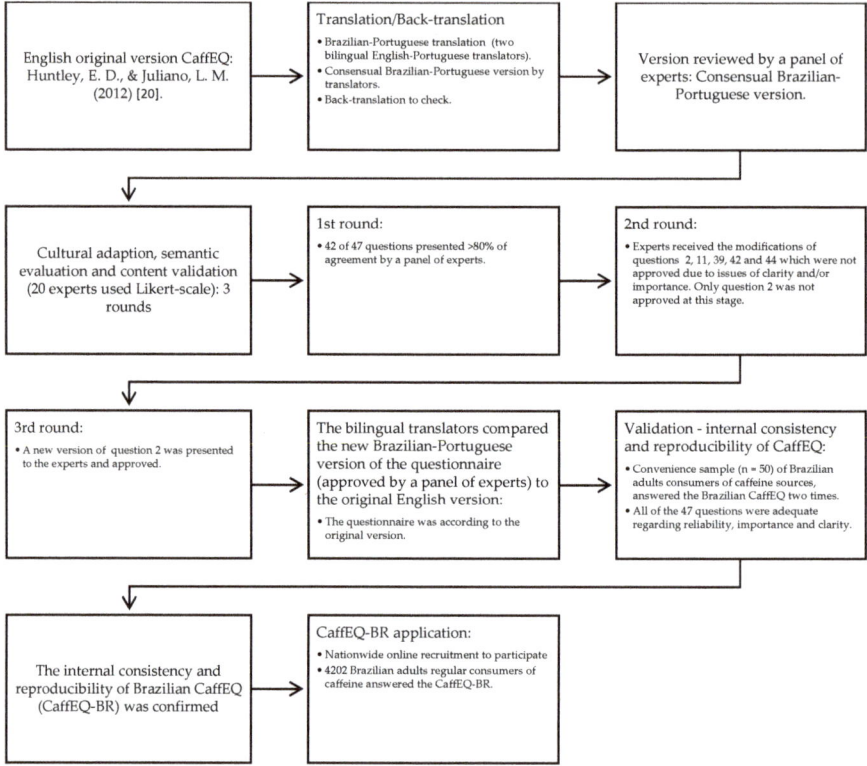

Figure 1. Flowchart of translation, cultural adaptation, semantic evaluation, content validation processes and application of the Caffeine Expectancy Questionnaire in Brazil (CaffEQ-BR).

3.3. Brazilian Nationwide Application of the CaffEQ-BR

3.3.1. Participants

From 4339 individuals who responded to the online CaffEQ-BR questionnaire, the final sample was composed of 4202 participants, since some participants ($n = 137$) did not provide all the data necessary for their inclusion in the survey. The nationwide distribution of the participants among the Brazilian states is presented in Figure 2. Participants were mostly from the Southeast Brazilian region ($n = 1390$; 33.08%), followed by the Northeast ($n = 1175$; 27.96%), Midwest ($n = 716$; 17.04%), South ($n = 566$; 13.47%) and North ($n = 355$; 8.45%). The state with the highest participation was São Paulo-Southeast region ($n = 683$; 16.25%), and the lowest was Acre-North region ($n = 18$; 0.43%). Figure 2 shows the methodological rigor of adequacy of 70% or more in the sample representation, according to the last national census [38], since all Brazilian states achieved this goal. Figure 2 also displays the mean of participants' caffeine and coffee consumption by each Brazilian state.

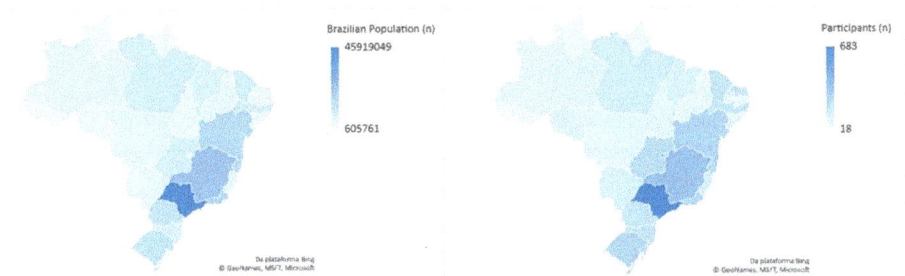

Brazil states	Brazilian population		Participants		Adequacy ≥ 70%*	Caffeine ** (mg/day)	
	(n)	(%)	(n)	(%)		Mean	SD
São Paulo	45,919,049	21.85%	683	16.25%	74%	265.2	150.9
Minas Gerais	21,168,791	10.07%	328	7.81%	77%	274.8	165.3
Rio de Janeiro	17,264,943	8.22%	250	5.95%	72%	272.2	178.5
Bahia	14,873,064	7.08%	249	5.93%	84%	264.3	150.3
Paraná	11,433,957	5.44%	161	3.83%	70%	271.1	169.4
Rio Grande do Sul	11,377,239	5.41%	229	5.45%	101%	263.3	158.5
Pernambuco	9,557,071	4.55%	195	4.64%	102%	252.8	141.5
Ceará	9,132,078	4.35%	180	4.28%	99%	260.0	172.3
Pará	8,602,865	4.09%	135	3.21%	78%	221.5	125.3
Santa Catarina	7,164,788	3.41%	176	4.19%	123%	292.9	167.9
Maranhão	7,075,181	3.37%	112	2.67%	79%	269.6	166.6
Goiás	7,018,354	3.34%	188	4.47%	134%	289.4	164.9
Amazonas	4,144,597	1.97%	70	1.67%	84%	293.6	163.1
Espírito Santo	4,018,650	1.91%	129	3.07%	161%	254.3	133.9
Paraíba	4,018,127	1.91%	73	1.74%	91%	288.4	196.4
Rio Grande do Norte	3,506,853	1.67%	179	4.26%	255%	251.4	142.5
Mato Grosso	3,484,466	1.66%	64	1.52%	92%	303.1	200.8
Alagoas	3,337,357	1.59%	60	1.43%	90%	287.5	165.4
Piauí	3,273,227	1.56%	57	1.36%	87%	236.0	158.6
Distrito Federal	3,015,268	1.43%	298	7.09%	494%	234.6	149.7
Mato Grosso do Sul	2,778,986	1.32%	109	2.59%	196%	288.1	148.4
Sergipe	2,298,696	1.09%	70	1.67%	152%	276.4	157.1
Rondônia	1,777,225	0.85%	86	2.05%	242%	266.9	157.7
Tocantins	1,572,866	0.75%	57	1.36%	181%	289.5	171.6
Acre	881,935	0.42%	18	0.43%	102%	280.6	139.5
Amapá	845,731	0.40%	25	0.59%	148%	248.0	157.1
Roraima	605,761	0.29%	21	0.50%	173%	247.6	189.4
OVERALL	210,147,125	100%	4,202	100%	All in accordance	265.9	159.0

Figure 2. National distribution of participants and average caffeine consumption. * As this is an external validation study of national scope, the sample calculation was performed according to the last Brazilian national census [38], with adequacy greater than or equal to 70% of the sample distribution according to the states of Brazil; ** caffeine in general sources. Northeast Region-Alagoas, Bahia, Ceará, Maranhão, Paraíba, Pernambuco, Piauí, Rio Grande do Norte, Sergipe; North Region-Acre, Amazonas, Amapá, Pará, Rondônia, Roraima, Tocantins; Midwest Region-Distrito Federal, Goiás, Mato Grosso, Mato Grosso do Sul; South Region-Paraná, Santa Catarina, Rio Grande do Sul; Southeast Region-Espírito Santo, Minas Gerais, Rio de Janeiro, São Paulo.

Table 2 shows the balanced distribution of participants by gender, with the highest frequency of participants aged between 31 and 59 y (n = 2625; 62.5%) and the majority of people of normal weight (classified by BMI between 18.5–24.9 kg/m^2 [31]). More than half of the sample (n = 2328; 55.4%) was white, as well as physically active (n = 2278; 54.2%). Graduates and postgraduates were the most frequent educational level (n = 2477; 59%). A monthly income between 3000.01 and 5000.00 (BRL) was the most frequent (n = 865; 20.6%). A large part of the sample did not report having any chronic disease (n = 3397; 80.8%). More information on sociodemographic aspects is shown in Table 2.

Table 2. Sociodemographic data, sample profile of the CaffEQ-BR study (2019–2020).

	Categories	Total (n = 4202)	
		n	%
Gender	Male	2063	49.1
	Female	2139	50.9
Age	19–24	822	19.5
	25–30	755	18.0
	31–40	1331	31.7
	41–59	1294	30.8
Body Mass Index * (kg/m^2)	<18.5	106	2.5
	18.5–24.9	1751	41.7
	25–29.9	1498	35.6
	≥30	847	20.2
Self-Identified ethnicity	Asia descendants	114	2.7
	White	2328	55.4
	Indigenous	41	1.0
	Pardo	1330	31.6
	Black	309	7.4
	Without description	80	1.9
Physical Exercises ≥ 150 min/week	No	1924	45.8
	Yes	2278	54.2
Educational Level	No schooling	3	0.1
	Incomplete elementary school	17	0.4
	Completed elementary school	37	0.9
	Incomplete high school	101	2.4
	Completed high school	596	14.2
	Incomplete higher education	955	22.7
	Higher education graduate	1162	27.6
	Postgraduate studies	1315	31.3
	Without description	16	0.4
Monthly Income (BRL) **	1000.00	407	9.7
	1000.01 to 2000.00	769	18.3
	2000.01 to 3000.00	669	15.9
	3000.01 to 5000.00	865	20.6
	5000.01 to 10,000.00	796	18.9
	Above 10,000.00	575	13.7
	Without description	121	2.9
Self-Reported Chronic Diseases	No	3397	80.8
	Yes	805	19.2

* Body mass index (BMI) followed the criteria adopted by the World Health Organization (WHO) [39] underweight (BMI < 18.5 kg/m^2), adequate (BMI between 18.5 and 24.9 kg/m^2), overweight (BMI between 25 and 29.9 kg/m^2) and obesity (BMI ≥ 30 kg/m^2). ** 5.55 BRL = 1.00 USD on the last day of data collection, April 2020.

3.3.2. Caffeine Consumption

Based on weekly consumption of caffeine sources, the average daily intake observed was 265 ± 159 mg (minimum 49 mg; maximum 1200 mg). The total caffeine intake for males (274 ± 162 mg/day) and for females (256 ± 155 mg/day) was statistically different (t = 3703; df = 4200; p < 0.001). Figure 2 shows descriptive data of average caffeine consumption by Brazilian states. A very similar pattern of consumption was observed between states. The average consumption by regions was as follows: North (n = 355; caffeine consumption: 253 ± 150 mg/day); Northeast (n = 1175; caffeine consumption: 262 ± 157 mg/day); Midwest (n = 716; caffeine consumption: 267 ± 162 mg/day); Southeast (n = 1390; caffeine consumption: 267 ± 158 mg/day); South (n = 566; caffeine consumption: 274 ± 164 mg/day). Thus, the highest absolute consumption of caffeine was in the southern region. Table 3 shows the distribution of consumption of caffeine sources and the time of the day that these were consumed.

Table 3. Distribution frequency of regular consumption of sources of caffeine per week (n = 4202).

Caffeine Sources [1]		Coffee [2]		Tea [3]		Chocolate [4]		Chocolate Beverages [5]		Soft Drinks [6]		Medication [7]		Energy Drinks [8]		Sports Supplements [9]	
		N	(%)	N	(%)	N	(%)	N	(%)	N	(%)	N	(%)	N	(%)	N	(%)
Time of the Day	Early morning (00:00–06:00)	202	4.8%	79	1.9%	153	3.6%	70	1.7%	149	3.5%	115	2.7%	109	2.6%	19	0.5%
	Morning (06:00–12:00)	3853	91.7%	503	12.0%	644	15.3%	653	15.5%	362	8.6%	505	12.0%	188	4.5%	333	7.9%
	Afternoon (12:00–18:00)	2829	67.3%	686	16.3%	1594	37.9%	523	12.4%	1361	32.4%	396	9.4%	324	7.7%	206	4.9%
	Evening (18:00–24:00)	1508	35.9%	878	20.9%	1291	30.7%	563	13.4%	1058	25.2%	699	16.6%	348	8.3%	122	2.9%
N° of Servings Per Day	1	971	23.1%	1178	28.0%	1647	39.2%	908	21.6%	985	23.4%	824	19.6%	530	12.6%	463	11.0%
	2	1958	46.6%	322	7.7%	537	12.8%	273	6.5%	543	12.9%	209	5.0%	141	3.4%	78	1.9%
	3	983	23.4%	92	2.2%	235	5.6%	89	2.1%	209	5.0%	111	2.6%	43	1.0%	19	0.5%
	4	139	3.3%	12	0.3%	64	1.5%	22	0.5%	58	1.4%	35	0.8%	7	0.2%	1	0.0%
Total Recorded		4051	96.4%	1604	38.2%	2483	59.1%	1292	30.7%	1795	42.7%	1179	28.1%	721	17.2%	561	13.4%

[1] Standardization of the portions in the consumption frequency table was adopted based on the dose of 50 mg of caffeine/portion. The percentages exceed 100% because consumption can occur in two or more periods. [2] Filtered or espresso, hot or iced coffee. [3] Tea sources of caffeine like mate, green and black tea. [4] Pure chocolate with ≥ 50% cocoa. [5] Chocolate beverages with ≥ 50% cocoa. [6] Cola nut or guarana based soft drinks. [7] Caffeinated medications. [8] Commercial drink sources of anhydrous caffeine or guarana extract beverage. [9] Sports supplements sources of anhydrous caffeine.

The participants' main source of caffeine was coffee, mostly consumed in the morning. In the afternoon, soft drinks and chocolates were the primary sources of caffeine. In the evening, the consumption of coffee, teas, chocolate, soft drinks, caffeine medications, and energy drinks was more frequent. Chocolate beverages showed no difference in consumption during the day. Caffeine-based sports supplements were most frequent in the morning. Coffee was the only source of caffeine with a predominance (73.3%) of consumption of two or more servings daily.

3.3.3. Confirmatory Factor Analysis and Associations of the CaffEQ-BR

Based on the national sample ($n = 4202$), the external factor validity of CaffEQ-BR was verified by confirmatory factor analysis. The seven factors presented RMSEA = 0.0332 (95% CI: 0.0290–0.0375), which shows satisfactory external validity.

Table 4 shows the results of the Pearson correlation coefficient between the CaffEQ-BR scores, divided between the seven factors, and the consumption of caffeine. All correlation between caffeine consumption and CaffEQ-BR factors (F1 to F6) were positive weak ($r < 0.4$) and significant ($p < 0.001$), except for F7 (-0.074; $p < 0.001$). Therefore, the higher the consumption, the higher the score. Despite the weak correlation ($r < 0.4$), the association between caffeine consumption and the CaffEQ-BR scores were all significant ($p < 0.001$), due to the large sample size ($n = 4202$).

Table 4. Correlations Between Caffeine Expectancy Questionnaire in Brazil (CaffEQ-BR) Factors and Caffeine-Related Variables ($n = 4202$).

Sources	Factors of the CaffEQ-BR *						
	F1	F2	F3	F4	F5	F6	F7
Caffeine ** (mg/day)	0.085 ***	0.102 ***	0.081 ***	0.141 ***	0.097 ***	0.095 ***	−0.074 ***

* Factors of the CaffEQ-BR: F1 Withdrawal/dependence; F2 Energy/work enhancement; F3 Appetite suppression; F4 Social/mood enhancement; F5 Physical performance enhancement; F6 Anxiety/negative physical effects; F7 Sleep disturbance; ** Caffeine in general sources (Tea, coffee, chocolate above 50% cocoa, chocolate beverages, cola nut or guarana based soft drinks, caffeinated drugs, commercial drinks and sports supplements sources of anhydrous caffeine or guarana extract beverage); Pearson correlation *** $p < 0.001$.

In Table 5, the region of Brazil with the highest average for F1 factor (withdrawal/dependence) was the southeast. The F2 (energy/work) enhancement factor resulted in the highest average score among all factors and was similar between regions in Brazil. The F3 factor (appetite suppression) was below 3 on the six-point Likert scale for all regions of Brazil. The factors F4 (social/mood enhancement) and F5 (physical performance enhancement) were above 3 on the Likert scale, with emphasis on the upper average for F4 in the north region, and the lower average for F5 in the south region of Brazil. The F6 factor (anxiety/negative physical effects) resulted in the lowest average score among all factors, with a similarity between regions. The F7 factor (sleep disturbance) was also below 3 on the Likert scale, with the lowest average for the south region of Brazil.

Table 5. Mean and Standard Deviation (SD) of the scores on a six-point Likert scale of the seven factors of the CaffEine Expectancy Questionnaire in Brazil (CaffEQ-BR) by regions of Brazil ($n = 4202$).

Regions **	Factors of the CaffEQ-BR * Mean (SD)						
	F1	F2	F3	F4	F5	F6	F7
North	3.48 (1.49)	4.16 (1.37)	2.21 (1.15)	3.56 (1.45)	3.49 (1.55)	1.78 (0.69)	2.51 (1.60)
Northeast	3.44 (1.41)	4.15 (1.31)	2.24 (1.14)	3.44 (1.38)	3.55 (1.53)	1.81 (0.77)	2.45 (1.58)
Midwest	3.34 (1.39)	4.08 (1.32)	2.13 (1.14)	3.25 (1.34)	3.50 (1.53)	1.85 (0.82)	2.62 (1.69)
Southeast	3.60 (1.45)	4.17 (1.33)	2.26 (1.18)	3.41 (1.38)	3.47 (1.49)	1.75 (0.75)	2.44 (1.62)
South	3.47 (1.43)	4.08 (1.30)	2.36 (1.24)	3.42 (1.34)	3.24 (1.48)	1.74 (0.75)	2.36 (1.57)
Brazil	3.48 (1.43)	4.14 (1.32)	2.24 (1.17)	3.41 (1.38)	3.47 (1.51)	1.78 (0.77)	2.47 (1.62)

* Factors of the CaffEQ-BR, range: 1.00–6.00: F1 Withdrawal/dependence; F2 Energy/work enhancement; F3 Appetite suppression; F4 Social/mood enhancement; F5 Physical performance enhancement; F6 Anxiety/negative physical effects; F7 Sleep disturbance. ** Regions of Brazil: North Region-Acre, Amazonas, Amapá, Pará, Rondônia, Roraima, Tocantins; Northeast Region-Alagoas, Bahia, Ceará, Maranhão, Paraíba, Pernambuco, Piauí, Rio Grande do Norte, Sergipe; Midwest Region-Distrito Federal, Goiás, Mato Grosso, Mato Grosso do Sul; South Region-Paraná, Santa Catarina, Rio Grande do Sul; Southeast Region-Espírito Santo, Minas Gerais, Rio de Janeiro, São Paulo.

4. Discussion

In this original study, we developed and validated the Brazilian version of the CaffEQ. Until now, there has been no adaptation of CaffEQ to Brazilian-Portuguese in the cultural context of Brazil, or in Latin American countries. Its application may assist in observational studies for clinical trials that assess caffeine consumption in Brazil. The selected questionnaire also allowed us to make comparisons with data available from other countries that used the same questionnaire [19–21]. The CaffEQ-BR is a questionnaire designed to identify the expectations that Brazilian individuals have about the subjective effects of caffeine on the biopsychosocial aspects involved in its consumption [19–21].

In order to create the CaffEQ-BR, the translation and back-translation process (linguistic validation of the instrument) was necessary, since the original questionnaire was developed in another language and there was no translated and validated version in the target language [24]. Therefore, the first step of this study was to translate/retranslate the original version of CaffEQ from English to Brazilian-Portuguese to English following the scientific guidelines proposed by the WHO [12,24]. After this, the questionnaire was sent to experts for evaluation, since semantic evaluation is necessary to ensure its clarity and comprehension [40,41]. In this sense, CaffEQ-BR presented cultural and semantic adequacy according to the consensus of the experts (at least 80% of agreement). After this stage, the test-retest with 50 individuals was used to assess the reliability of the CaffEQ-BR, which analyzes the questionnaire's ability to reproduce consistent results [29,41]. The internal consistency of CaffEQ-BR was measured by Cronbach's alpha coefficient ($\alpha = 0.94$), considered acceptable when ≥ 0.8 [28,37]. This result was similar to the findings of Huntley and Juliano (2012) [20] ($n = 1046$; $\alpha = 0.96$), and Schott et al. [21] ($n = 352$; $\alpha = 0.98$) for the same questionnaire in English and German, respectively. In addition, the CaffEQ-BR presented excellent measures of reproducibility (ICC = 0.97). This result confirms that the questionnaire is able to consistently measure the subjective effects of caffeine perceived by the interviewed user. Every scale used to measure health results needs this reliability performed by exploratory and confirmatory factor analysis [37].

After internal validation of the CaffEQ-BR, we conducted a national study in Brazil, using a sample of all 27 Brazilian states (Figure 2) with uniform distribution of age and sex (Table 2), similar to the last available national census (Brazil-IBGE (Instituto Brasileiro de Geografia e Estatística) 2010) [42]. The national census is usually held every decade, and the 2020 edition is in progress. The first five most populous Brazilian states (Figure 2) had two or more rounds of dissemination of the survey on social networks, to achieve the established interview number goal. The Federal District had the highest representation in percentage points because the research group is based in Brasília, Federal District. Naturally, in a convenience sample, there was greater participation in our hometown.

The sociodemographic data of the CaffEQ-BR participants are closer to the measures of the adult Brazilian population on gender and age than the sample of the original study (CaffEQ) [20], which had a predominance of young female students. Although the CaffEQ-BR sample is representative of the population distribution parameters in the Brazilian states [38], there is a selection bias in relation to the respondents' education and socioeconomic level, which was above the national average family income (1439 BRL per month in 2019) [43] directly influencing educational status [44]. Another factor was the use of social networks to disseminate the research questionnaire. Other nationwide surveys in Brazil from our institution/research groups, released through web-base, also observed greater access by higher economic classes compared to the national average [45,46]. Therefore, it is not possible to extrapolate our results to the entire Brazilian adult population. This is not a national census or national sample representation.

Regarding the self-reported categories for BMI ≥ 25 and chronic disease being treated, our sample data showed a lower incidence of these two variables (55.8%; 19.2%, respectively) compared to the results of the Brazilian national study "Surveillance of risk and protective factors for chronic diseases by telephone research" (VIGITEL 2019) (75.7%; 31.9%, respectively). However, our sample showed a higher frequency of people who self-reported being physically active: 54.2%, compared to the last VIGITEL (2019) which showed 39.5% [47]. The VIGITEL study used a representative random sample only from the state capitals of Brazil, through phone interviews. Our survey did not cover capitals only, with a convenience sample by invitation on social networks with predominant access via mobiles. There was an inclination towards greater sample composition of middle-aged adults, with a higher level of education and income for the CaffEQ-BR. There are studies that indicate a greater preference, especially for coffee, in individuals with this sociodemographic profile [6–8]. The VIGITEL study in different periods of time (2006 to 2019) showed that that part of the population that has more years of schooling (≥12 years) is less overweight, sedentary, and chronically ill. The reverse context, low income and education level and high morbidity rate, are also observed [48]. The self-reported ethnicity comparison between the National Household Sample Survey (2018/2019) [43] and that obtained in the CaffEQ-BR was: 45.2–55.4% of Brazilians that declared themselves as white, 45.0–31.6% as pardo, 8.8–8% as black, 0.47–2.7% as Asian descendants and 0.38–1.0% as indigenous.

The average caffeine intake in our sample (265 ± 159 mg/day) is above the published standards for Brazil (115 ± 96 mg/day) [49]. According to Sartori et al., the survey on caffeine consumption in Brazil was based on food sources, extracted from data from the national survey of 2008 and 2009 [49]. In addition to the difference in the observation periods (2008/09 vs. 2019/20), our survey included other sources of caffeine as supplements and medications. This fact is relevant according to Arrais et al. (2016) [50], as self-medication is a recurrent practice in Brazil, including among young adults, mainly associated with the use of non-prescription medications, such as analgesics and muscle relaxants. In the national market, these drugs take in their composition, on average, 30 to 50 mg of caffeine per serving. Our study also focused on individuals who are regular consumers of caffeine (from different sources); therefore, we expect that the participants' average usual intake could be higher than the general Brazilian population. These values were similar to those found by Schott et al. (from Germany, Switzerland, and Austria: 236 ± 235 mg/day) [21] but considerably below the consumption found by Huntley and Juliano (from U.S.: 323 ± 297 mg/day), which was based on the consumption of a younger population, containing many college/university students [20]. Another point is that the volume of coffee consumed in Brazil is not a standard variable to be compared with a North American or European study, since Brazilians and inhabitants of other Latin American countries usually drink small portions of stronger coffee (approx. 50 mL of small cups) compared to the American culture of large cups (approx. 250 mL) of lighter coffee, a fact observed by De Paula and Farah (2019) [51]. Total caffeine intake in males (274 ± 162 mg/day) was higher than in females (256 ± 155 mg/day), similar to the results observed by other studies [8,49,52]. Probably these gender differences are related to cultural and behavioral factors in males as well as to the gender differences in physiological responses to caffeine [53–56]. A study showed that males differ in cardiovascular responses to caffeine, while females did not differ in their responses as a function of typical caffeine use [55]. Males also presented greater decreases in heart rate in response to caffeine than did females, probably related to changes in circulating steroid hormone, in which increased circulating estradiol increases the physiological and subjective effects associated with caffeine, influencing the high consumption of caffeine on males [53].

Across previous CaffEQ studies, caffeine was consumed mainly in coffee, a habit also observed in Brazil [6–8]. Globally, habitual coffee consumption ranges from about 1 to more than 5 cups per day, which indicates that the daily dose is defined by several reasons, like lifestyle, gender, expectance of caffeine effects, culture, genetics, health effects, among others [2,36,57]. Most of our sample (69%) are used to consuming 2 or 3 portions of coffee daily (Table 3). The culture of coffee in Brazil has a historical origin in its production capacity, as it is the largest coffee exporter in the world market [58]. Brazil accounts for one-third of the world's coffee production, making it the world's largest producer, a position it has occupied for more than 150 years. In Brazil, at the beginning of the 19th century, coffee was already treated as an investment. With the expansion of plantations in the country, there was also an expansion of investment favoring urbanization, such as the construction of railroads responsible for the national distribution and export of coffee, in addition to the arrival of immigrants. Thus, in Brazil, coffee is considered one of those products responsible for the modernization, urbanization and development of some cities [59], and it is still widely consumed and appreciated throughout the country. Annual per capita Brazilian consumption is 6.02 kg, which represents 13% of world demand [60]. Easy access to coffee naturally influences the consumption culture of Brazilians [8]. Coffee is the main drink consumed, with an average of 163 mL per day, and is also the second most consumed food [6,7].

In Brazil, coffee consumption is widespread [6]. This reflects a very similar average consumption between regions [6], as observed in the CaffEQ-BR survey. The differences are greater when other eating habits are associated with the daily use of coffee. For example, the habit of consuming a hot mate called "Chimarrão" in the south region, a cold mate called "Terere" in the Midwest region [61] and guarana extract in the northern region of Brazil [62]. The fact that the Northeast region is the largest consumer of coffee was also confirmed by the study of Sousa and Da Costa [6]. We also emphasize that coffee and other caffeine sources are also sources of other bioactive compounds, including polyphenols and chlorogenic acids [63]. However, the main substance with psychoactive properties is caffeine, confirmed by several meta-analyses [4]. The construction of the original CaffEQ [20] takes into account the estimated average consumption of caffeine in general (from all sources), without the intention of associating it with other compounds present in food sources of caffeine.

The statistical correlations ($r < 0.4$) shown between CaffEQ factors, scores and caffeine consumption were also observed in previous studies that used the original CaffEQ in the United States [20] and the translated and validated version in German-speaking countries [21].

When observing the descriptive results of the CaffEQ-BR scores divided into seven factors using the original questionnaire [20], it is possible to observe similarity in the factors Withdrawal/dependence 3.48 (1.43)–3.22 (1.45), Energy/work enhancement 4.14 (1.32)–3.92 (1.17), Appetite suppression 2.24 (1.17)–2.70 (1.20), Social/mood enhancement 3.41 (1.38)–2.98 (1.21), respectively. However, there was a difference of approximately one point for the factors Physical performance enhancement 3.47 (1.51)–2.41 (1.07), Anxiety/negative physical effects 1.78 (0.77)–2.68 (1.04) and Sleep disturbance 2.47 (1.62)–3.20 (1.45). Differences in mean scores in the seven factors were also observed in the other cultures where CaffEQ was studied [20,21].

Data from the latest survey published by the Brazilian Institute of Geography and Statistics showed that three out of four Brazilians in metropolitan capitals (Belém (Pará), Fortaleza (Ceará), Recife (Pernambuco), Salvador (Bahia), Belo Horizonte (Minas Gerais), Rio (Rio de Janeiro), São Paulo (São Paulo), Curitiba (Paraná) and Porto Alegre (Rio Grande do Sul)) have access to the Internet, and the number of households with landlines dropped from 33.6 % to 31.5%, while ownership of devices with mobile internet increased from 92.6% to 93.2% [64]. The smartphone was also the main tool used to access the internet. Therefore, although web-based research may be limited because it is not possible to reach every portion of the population, it can still be considered a viable strategy since our web search could be answered on any device with internet. There is also the limitation of memory and intake bias, which is intrinsically related to frequency questionnaires [65].

There is no other scientifically validated Brazilian research questionnaire that evaluates consumption related to caffeine. Therefore, there are no parameters for comparison except with the original version of the CaffEQ [20] and the German version [21]. Another important factor is the heterogeneity of the Brazilian-Portuguese language in the national territory. Certainly, there are aspects of regionality, but despite these limitations, due to the construction process in several stages and the wide statistical confirmation, the Brazilian version of CaffEQ represents a reliable and valid questionnaire to assess expectations of caffeine intake. Analytical item analysis confirms the quality of the translated items. Overall, the CaffEQ's translation and validation for Portuguese and Brazilian culture were successful.

5. Conclusions

The full version of the Caffeine Expectancy Questionnaire in Brazil (CaffEQ-BR) is available for Brazilian adults, translated into Portuguese and adapted to Brazilian culture. This study confirmed the validity and reliability of the CaffEQ-BR. Its internal and external consistency allows its use throughout the national territory, if the sampling conditions are similar. The CaffEQ-BR observed the pattern of consumption of caffeine sources by Brazilian adults, confirming the national preference for coffee as the main source of daily caffeine. Future studies may validate the CaffEQ-BR in children, adolescents and the elderly, since caffeine is widely consumed across the lifespan. The present study contributes to a better understanding of the expectations of the most used psychoactive substance in Brazil, systematizing several expectations in seven factors that can be explored and categorized. Thus, the CaffEQ-BR can be used to facilitate our understanding of the use of caffeine. Other studies may also replicate our results, pointing out the temporal stability of the CaffEQ-BR, monitoring changes in expectations in longitudinal exposure to caffeine.

Author Contributions: Conceptualization, G.F.M., C.E.G.R. and R.P.Z.; methodology, G.F.M., C.E.G.R. and R.P.Z.; software, G.F.M. and E.Y.N.; validation, G.F.M., C.E.G.R., E.Y.N., T.H.M.d.C., B.S. and R.P.Z.; formal analysis, E.Y.N.; investigation, G.F.M.; resources, C.E.G.R. and R.P.Z.; data curation, G.F.M. and E.Y.N.; writing—original draft preparation, G.F.M.; writing—review and editing, G.F.M., C.E.G.R., E.Y.N., T.H.M.d.C., B.S. and R.P.Z.; visualization, G.F.M., and R.P.Z.; supervision, R.P.Z.; project administration, G.F.M. and C.E.G.R.; funding acquisition, C.E.G.R. and R.P.Z. All authors have read and agreed to the published version of the manuscript.

Funding: This research received no external funding.

Acknowledgments: The authors acknowledge DPG/DPI/UnB, PPGNH/UnB, Capes for the support, the expert panel of judges, social communicator Luciana Nogueira for support with social networks, and all participants who completed the CaffEQ-BR. Bryan Saunders acknowledges a personal research grant (2016/50438-0) from Fundação de Amparo à Pesquisa do Estado de Sao Paulo. Teresa H M da Costa acknowledges a personal research grant (308630-2017-3) from CNPq (Conselho Nacional de Desenvolvimento Científico e Tecnológico—National Council for Scientific and Technological Development).

Conflicts of Interest: The authors declare no conflict of interest.

Appendix A

Questionário de Expectativa de efeitos da Cafeína/café, versão brasileira (CaffEQ-BR)

Instruções: Estamos interessados em suas crenças sobre os efeitos que a cafeína tem sobre você. Abaixo há uma lista de possíveis efeitos da cafeína presentes nos produtos listados na tabela acima preenchida. Usando a escala como guia, avalie cada afirmação em termos de quanto é PROVÁVEL ou IMPROVÁVEL para esses efeitos como consequências do consumo da cafeína. As possibilidades de respostas são: 1 = Muito improvável; 2 = Improvável; 3 = Um pouco improvável; 4 = Um pouco provável; 5 = Provável; 6 = Muito provável. Baseie suas respostas no produto com cafeína que escolheu. Se você usa muitos tipos de produtos com cafeína, escolha o mais usual para basear suas respostas, ou você pode optar por basear suas respostas em "cafeína/café".

Itens	Muito Improvável	Improvável	Um Pouco Improvável	Um Pouco Provável	Provável	Muito Provável
1. Cafeína/café me dá ânimo quando estou cansado	☐	☐	☐	☐	☐	☐
2. Eu fico extrovertido quando tomo cafeína/café	☐	☐	☐	☐	☐	☐
3. Cafeína/café me ajuda a não comer mais do que deveria	☐	☐	☐	☐	☐	☐
4. Fico facilmente estressado depois de tomar cafeína/café	☐	☐	☐	☐	☐	☐
5. Cafeína/café melhora meu desempenho físico	☐	☐	☐	☐	☐	☐
6. Fico menos cansado depois de tomar cafeína	☐	☐	☐	☐	☐	☐
7. A cafeína/café tira minha fome	☐	☐	☐	☐	☐	☐
8. Fico triste quando não tomo cafeína/café	☐	☐	☐	☐	☐	☐
9. Cafeína/café melhora meu humor	☐	☐	☐	☐	☐	☐
10. Eu fico ansioso quando não tomo cafeína/café	☐	☐	☐	☐	☐	☐
11. Eu me sinto angustiado quando tomo cafeína/café	☐	☐	☐	☐	☐	☐
12. Eu me exercito melhor depois de tomar cafeína/café	☐	☐	☐	☐	☐	☐
13. Eu sinto muita falta de cafeína/café quando não tomo	☐	☐	☐	☐	☐	☐
14. Eu não gosto do jeito que eu me sinto após tomar cafeína/café	☐	☐	☐	☐	☐	☐
15. Eu me sinto mal se ficar sem cafeína/café	☐	☐	☐	☐	☐	☐
16. Cafeína/café aumenta minha motivação para trabalhar	☐	☐	☐	☐	☐	☐
17. Eu me sinto mais confiante depois de tomar cafeína/café	☐	☐	☐	☐	☐	☐
18. Tomar cafeína/café a qualquer hora do dia atrapalha o meu sono	☐	☐	☐	☐	☐	☐
19. Quando tomo cafeína/café fico nervoso(a)	☐	☐	☐	☐	☐	☐
20. Quando tomo cafeína/café fico mais alerta	☐	☐	☐	☐	☐	☐
21. Mesmo quando tomo uma pequena quantidade de cafeína/café fico ansioso	☐	☐	☐	☐	☐	☐
22. Cafeína/café melhora minha concentração	☐	☐	☐	☐	☐	☐
23. Quando tomo cafeína/café fico mais amigável	☐	☐	☐	☐	☐	☐
24. Eu tenho que tomar cafeína/café todos os dias	☐	☐	☐	☐	☐	☐
25. Cafeína/café me faz suar	☐	☐	☐	☐	☐	☐
26. Cafeína/café me faz pular refeições	☐	☐	☐	☐	☐	☐
27. Tenho muita vontade de tomar cafeína/café se não tiver tomado a quantidade de sempre	☐	☐	☐	☐	☐	☐
28. Tomar cafeína/café na hora de dormir atrapalha meu sono	☐	☐	☐	☐	☐	☐
29. Cafeína/café me deixa irritado	☐	☐	☐	☐	☐	☐
30. Eu desejo cafeína/café o tempo todo	☐	☐	☐	☐	☐	☐

Itens	Muito Improvável	Improvável	Um Pouco Improvável	Um Pouco Provável	Provável	Muito Provável
31. Cafeína/café me ajuda a trabalhar por mais tempo	☐	☐	☐	☐	☐	☐
32. Cafeína/café me faz sentir feliz	☐	☐	☐	☐	☐	☐
33. Eu não funciono sem tomar cafeína/café	☐	☐	☐	☐	☐	☐
34. Quando tomo cafeína/café meu coração acelera	☐	☐	☐	☐	☐	☐
35. Eu tenho dificuldade em começar o dia sem tomar cafeína/café	☐	☐	☐	☐	☐	☐
36. Sinto dor de estômago quando tomo cafeína/café	☐	☐	☐	☐	☐	☐
37. Eu não conseguiria parar de tomar cafeína/café	☐	☐	☐	☐	☐	☐
38. Tomar cafeína/café no final da tarde atrapalha o meu sono	☐	☐	☐	☐	☐	☐
39. Cafeína/café me ajuda a regular o peso	☐	☐	☐	☐	☐	☐
40. Quanto não tomo cafeína/café sinto dor de cabeça	☐	☐	☐	☐	☐	☐
41. Cafeína/café melhora minha atenção	☐	☐	☐	☐	☐	☐
42. Eu fico mais extrovertido(a) quando tomo cafeína/café	☐	☐	☐	☐	☐	☐
43. Cafeína/café me ajuda a me exercitar por mais tempo	☐	☐	☐	☐	☐	☐
44. Sinto-me mais disposto quando tomo cafeína/café	☐	☐	☐	☐	☐	☐
45. Cafeína/café me faz sentir com mais energia	☐	☐	☐	☐	☐	☐
46. Cafeína/café diminui o meu apetite	☐	☐	☐	☐	☐	☐
47. Tomar cafeína/café no final do dia não me deixa dormir	☐	☐	☐	☐	☐	☐

References

1. Reyes, C.M.; Cornelis, M.C. Caffeine in the diet: Country-level consumption and guidelines. *Nutrients* **2018**, *10*, 1772. [CrossRef] [PubMed]
2. Boolani, A.; Fuller, D.T.; Mondal, S.; Wilkinson, T.; Darie, C.C.; Gumpricht, E. Caffeine-Containing, Adaptogenic-Rich Drink Modulates the Effects of Caffeine on Mental Performance and Cognitive Parameters: A Double-Blinded, Placebo-Controlled, Randomized Trial. *Nutrients* **2020**, *12*, 1922. [CrossRef] [PubMed]
3. Wikoff, D.; Welsh, B.T.; Henderson, R.; Brorby, G.P.; Britt, J.; Myers, E.; Goldberger, J.; Lieberman, H.R.; O'Brien, C.; Peck, J.; et al. Systematic review of the potential adverse effects of caffeine consumption in healthy adults, pregnant women, adolescents, and children. *Food Chem. Toxicol.* **2017**, *109*, 585–648. [CrossRef] [PubMed]
4. Poole, R.; Kennedy, O.J.; Roderick, P.; Fallowfield, J.A.; Hayes, P.C.; Parkes, J. Coffee consumption and health: Umbrella review of meta-analyses of multiple health outcomes. *BMJ* **2017**. [CrossRef]
5. Maughan, R.J.; Burke, L.M.; Dvorak, J.; Larson-Meyer, D.E.; Peeling, P.; Phillips, S.M.; Rawson, E.S.; Walsh, N.P.; Garthe, I.; Geyer, H.; et al. IOC consensus statement: Dietary supplements and the high-performance athlete. *Br. J. Sports Med.* **2018**, *28*, 104–105.
6. Sousa, A.G.; Da Costa, T.H.M. Usual coffee intake in Brazil: Results from the National Dietary Survey 2008-9. *Br. J. Nutr.* **2015**, *113*, 1615–1620. [CrossRef]
7. Pereira, R.A.; Souza, A.M.; Duffey, K.J.; Sichieri, R.; Popkin, B.M. Beverage consumption in Brazil: Results from the first National Dietary Survey. *Public Health Nutr.* **2015**, *18*, 1164–1172. [CrossRef]
8. Souza, A.D.M.; Pereira, R.A.; Yokoo, E.M.; Levy, R.B.; Sichieri, R. Most consumed foods in Brazil: National dietary survey 2008–2009. *Rev. Saude Publica* **2014**, *18*, 1164–1172. [CrossRef]

9. Heckman, M.A.; Weil, J.; de Mejia, E.G. Caffeine (1, 3, 7-trimethylxanthine) in foods: A comprehensive review on consumption, functionality, safety, and regulatory matters. *J. Food Sci.* **2010**, *75*, R77–R87. [CrossRef]
10. Mahoney, C.R.; Giles, G.E.; Marriott, B.P.; Judelson, D.A.; Glickman, E.L.; Geiselman, P.J.; Lieberman, H.R. Intake of caffeine from all sources and reasons for use by college students. *Clin. Nutr.* **2019**, *38*, 668–675. [CrossRef]
11. Fulton, J.L.; Dinas, P.C.; Carrillo, A.E.; Edsall, J.R.; Ryan, E.J.; Ryan, E.J. Impact of genetic variability on physiological responses to caffeine in humans: A systematic review. *Nutrients* **2018**, *10*, 1373. [CrossRef] [PubMed]
12. Ágoston, C.; Urbán, R.; Király, O.; Griffiths, M.D.; Rogers, P.J.; Demetrovics, Z. Why Do You Drink Caffeine? The Development of the Motives for Caffeine Consumption Questionnaire (MCCQ) and Its Relationship with Gender, Age and the Types of Caffeinated Beverages. *Int. J. Ment. Health Addict.* **2017**, *16*, 981–999. [CrossRef] [PubMed]
13. Saunders, B.; de Oliveira, L.F.; da Silva, R.P.; de Salles Painelli, V.; Gonçalves, L.S.; Yamaguchi, G.; Mutti, T.; Maciel, E.; Roschel, H.; Artioli, G.G.; et al. Placebo in sports nutrition: A proof-of-principle study involving caffeine supplementation. *Scand. J. Med. Sci. Sport.* **2016**, *27*, 1240–1247. [CrossRef] [PubMed]
14. Beedie, C.J.; Stuart, E.M.; Coleman, D.A.; Foad, A.J. Placebo effects of caffeine on cycling performance. *Med. Sci. Sports Exerc.* **2006**, *38*, 2159–2164. [CrossRef]
15. Saunders, B.; Saito, T.; Klosterhoff, R.; de Oliveira, L.F.; Barreto, G.; Perim, P.; Pinto, A.J.; Lima, F.; de Sá Pinto, A.L.; Gualano, B. "I put it in my head that the supplement would help me": Open-placebo improves exercise performance in female cyclists. *PLoS ONE* **2019**, *14*, e0222982. [CrossRef]
16. Dömötör, Z.; Szemerszky, R.; Köteles, F. Subjective and objective effects of coffee consumption—Caffeine or expectations? *Acta Physiol. Hung.* **2015**, *102*, 77–85. [CrossRef]
17. Shabir, A.; Hooton, A.; Tallis, J.; Higgins, M.F. The influence of caffeine expectancies on sport, exercise, and cognitive performance. *Nutrients* **2018**, *10*, 1528. [CrossRef]
18. Heinz, A.J.; Kassel, J.D.; Smith, E.V. Caffeine Expectancy: Instrument Development in the Rasch Measurement Framework. *Psychol. Addict. Behav.* **2009**, *23*, 500–511. [CrossRef]
19. Kearns, N.T.; Blumenthal, H.; Natesan, P.; Zamboanga, B.L.; Ham, L.S.; Cloutier, R.M. Development and initial psychometric validation of the brief-caffeine expectancy questionnaire (B-CaffEQ). *Psychol. Assess.* **2018**, *30*, 1597–1611. [CrossRef]
20. Huntley, E.D.; Juliano, L.M. Caffeine Expectancy Questionnaire (CaffEQ): Construction, psychometric properties, and associations with caffeine use, caffeine dependence, and other related variables. *Psychol. Assess.* **2012**, *24*, 592–607. [CrossRef]
21. Schott, M.; Beiglböck, W.; Neuendorff, R. Translation and Validation of the Caffeine Expectancy Questionnaire (CaffEQ). *Int. J. Ment. Health Addict.* **2016**, *14*, 514–525. [CrossRef]
22. Pasquali, L. Psicometria. *Rev. Esc. Enferm. USP* **2009**, *43*, 992–999. [CrossRef]
23. Knapp, H.; Kirk, S.A. Using pencil and paper, Internet and touch-tone phones for self-administered surveys: Does methodology matter? *Comput. Human Behav.* **2003**, *19*, 117–134. [CrossRef]
24. World Health Organization. Process of Translation and Adaptation of Instruments. Available online: https://www.who.int/substance_abuse/research_tools/translation/en/ (accessed on 26 May 2020).
25. Meijering, J.V.; Kampen, J.K.; Tobi, H. Quantifying the development of agreement among experts in Delphi studies. *Technol. Forecast. Soc. Chang.* **2013**, *80*, 1607–1614. [CrossRef]
26. Watson, P.F.; Petrie, A. Method agreement analysis: A review of correct methodology. *Theriogenology* **2010**, *73*, 1167–1179. [CrossRef]
27. Bartlett, J.W.; Chris, F. Reliability, repeatability and reproducibility: Analysis of measurement errors in continuous variables. *Ultrasound Obstet. Gynecol.* **2008**, *31*, 466–475. [CrossRef]
28. Streiner, D.L.; Norman, G.R. *Health Measurement Scales: A Practical Guide to Their Development and Use*; Oxford University Press: Oxford, UK, 2008; ISBN 9780191724015.
29. Streiner, D.L.; Streiner, D.L. Starting at the Beginning: An Introduction to Coefficient Alpha and Internal Consistency. *J. Pers. Assess.* **2003**, *80*, 99–103. [CrossRef]
30. Hair, J.F.; Black, W.C.; Babin, B.J.; Anderson, R.E. *Multivariate Data Analysis*; Pearson new international edition; Essex, Pearson Education Limited: London, UK, 2014. [CrossRef]
31. World Health Organization. *WHO Guideline: Sugars Intake for Adults and Children*; WHO: Geneva, Switzerland, 2015; ISBN 9789241549028.

32. Institute of Medicine (IOM). *DRI Dietary Reference Intakes: Applications in Dietary Assessment*; National Academies Press: Washington, DC, USA, 2000; ISBN 9780309502543.
33. Shohet, K.L.; Landrum, R.E. Caffeine consumption questionnaire: A standardized measure for caffeine consumption in undergraduate students. *Psychol. Rep.* **2001**, *89*, 521–526. [CrossRef]
34. Irons, J.G.; Bassett, D.T.; Prendergast, C.O.; Landrum, R.E.; Heinz, A.J. Development and Initial Validation of the Caffeine Consumption Questionnaire-Revised. *J. Caffeine Res.* **2016**, *6*, 20–25. [CrossRef]
35. IBGE—Instituto Brasileiro de Geografia e Estatística. Pesquisa de Orçamentos Familiares: 2008–2009. Antropometria e Estado Nutricional de Crianças, Adolescentes e Adultos no Brasil. ISBN 978-85-240-4131-0. Available online: https://biblioteca.ibge.gov.br/visualizacao/livros/liv50000.pdf (accessed on 7 July 2020).
36. Dharmasena, S.; Capps, O.; Clauson, A. Ascertaining the Impact of the 2000 USDA Dietary Guidelines for Americans on the Intake of Calories, Caffeine, Calcium, and Vitamin C from At-Home Consumption of Nonalcoholic Beverages. *J. Agric. Appl. Econ.* **2011**, *43*, 13–27. [CrossRef]
37. Vogelzang, J.L. Health Measurement Scales: A Practical Guide to Their Development and Use. *J. Nutr. Educ. Behav.* **2015**, *47*, 484.e1. [CrossRef]
38. IBGE—Instituto Brasileiro de Geografia e Estatística. IBGE Divulga As Estimativas da População dos Municípios para 2019. Estatísticas Sociais 2019. Available online: https://agenciadenoticias.ibge.gov.br/media/com_mediaibge/arquivos/7d410669a4ae85faf4e8c3a0a0c649c7.pdf (accessed on 26 May 2020).
39. World Health Organization (WHO). Mean Body Mass Index (BMI). WHO 2017. Available online: https://www.who.int/gho/ncd/risk_factors/bmi_text/en/ (accessed on 26 May 2020).
40. Baeza, F.L.C.; Caldieraro, M.A.K.; Pinheiro, D.O.; Fleck, M.P. Translation and cross-cultural adaptation into Brazilian Portuguese of the Measure of Parental Style (MOPS)—A self-reported scale—According to the International Society for Pharmacoeconomics and Outcomes Research (ISPOR) recommendations. *Rev. Bras. Psiquiatr.* **2010**, *32*, 159–163. [CrossRef]
41. Santo, R.M.; Ribeiro-Ferreira, F.; Alves, M.R.; Epstein, J.; Novaes, P. Enhancing the cross-cultural adaptation and validation process: Linguistic and psychometric testing of the Brazilian-Portuguese version of a self-report measure for dry eye. *J. Clin. Epidemiol.* **2015**, *68*, 370–378. [CrossRef]
42. IBGE—Instituto Brasileiro de Geografia e Estatística. Censo Demográfico 2010. Características da População e dos Domicílios. 2010. Available online: https://biblioteca.ibge.gov.br/visualizacao/periodicos/93/cd_2010_caracteristicas_populacao_domicilios.pdf (accessed on 26 May 2020).
43. IBGE—Instituto Brasileiro de Geografia e Estatística. Características Gerais dos Domicílios e dos Moradores: 2018. Available online: https://biblioteca.ibge.gov.br/index.php/biblioteca-catalogo?view=detalhes&id=2101654 (accessed on 26 May 2020).
44. Gori-Maia, A. Relative Income, Inequality and Subjective Wellbeing: Evidence for Brazil. *Soc. Indic. Res.* **2013**, *113*, 1193–1204. [CrossRef]
45. Pratesi, C.P.; Häuser, W.; Uenishi, R.H.; Selleski, N.; Nakano, E.Y.; Gandolfi, L.; Pratesi, R.; Zandonadi, R.P. Quality of life of celiac patients in Brazil: Questionnaire translation, cultural adaptation and validation. *Nutrients* **2018**, *10*, 1167. [CrossRef] [PubMed]
46. Hargreaves, S.M.; Araújo, W.M.C.; Nakano, E.Y.; Zandonadi, R.P. Brazilian vegetarians diet quality markers and comparison with the general population: A nationwide cross-sectional study. *PLoS ONE* **2020**, *15*, e0232954. [CrossRef]
47. Ministério da Saúde, Secretaria de Vigilância em Saúde, Departamento de Análise em Saúde e Vigilância de Doenças Não Transmissíveis. Vigitel Brasil 2019: Surveillance of Risk and Protective Factors for Chronic Diseases by Telephone Survey: Estimates of Frequency and Sociodemographic Distribution of Risk and Protective Factors for Chronic Diseases in the Capitals of the 26 Brasilian States. Available online: http://www.crn1.org.br/wp-content/uploads/2020/04/vigitel-brasil-2019-vigilancia-fatores-risco.pdf?x53725 (accessed on 26 May 2020).
48. Sommer, I.; Griebler, U.; Mahlknecht, P.; Thaler, K.; Bouskill, K.; Gartlehner, G.; Mendis, S. Socioeconomic inequalities in non-communicable diseases and their risk factors: An overview of systematic reviews. *BMC Public Health* **2015**, *15*, 914. [CrossRef] [PubMed]
49. Giovanini de Oliveira Sartori, A.; Vieira da Silva, M. Caffeine in Brazil: Intake, socioeconomic and demographic determinants, and major dietary sources. *Nutrire* **2016**, *41*, 147. [CrossRef]

50. Dourado, P.; Porto, M.; Dal Pizzol, T.; Ramos, L.; Serrate, S.; Luiza, V.; Leão, N.; Rocha, M.; Oliveira, M.; Dâmaso, A.; et al. Prevalência da automedicação no Brasil e fatores associados. *Rev. Saúde Pública* **2016**, *50*. [CrossRef]
51. dePaula, J.; Farah, A. Caffeine Consumption through Coffee: Content in the Beverage, Metabolism, Health Benefits and Risks. *Beverages* **2019**, *5*, 37. [CrossRef]
52. Choi, J. Motivations Influencing Caffeine Consumption Behaviors among College Students in Korea: Associations with Sleep Quality. *Nutrients* **2020**, *14*, 953. [CrossRef] [PubMed]
53. Temple, J.L.; Ziegler, A.M. Gender Differences in Subjective and Physiological Responses to Caffeine and the Role of Steroid Hormones. *J. Caffeine Res.* **2011**, *1*, 41–48. [CrossRef] [PubMed]
54. Temple, J.L.; Bulkley, A.M.; Briatico, L.; Dewey, A.M. Sex differences in reinforcing value of caffeinated beverages in adolescents. *Behav. Pharmacol.* **2009**, *20*, 731–741. [CrossRef] [PubMed]
55. Temple, J.L.; Dewey, A.M.; Briatico, L.N. Effects of Acute Caffeine Administration on Adolescents. *Exp. Clin. Psychopharmacol.* **2010**, *18*, 510–520. [CrossRef]
56. Dillon, P.; Kelpin, S.; Kendler, K.; Thacker, L.; Dick, D.; Svikis, D. Gender Differences in Any-Source Caffeine and Energy Drink Use and Associated Adverse Health Behaviors. *J. Caffeine Adenosine Res.* **2019**, *9*, 12–19. [CrossRef]
57. Kolb, H.; Kempf, K.; Martin, S. Health Effects of Coffee: Mechanism Unraveled? *Nutrients* **2020**, *12*, 1842. [CrossRef]
58. International Coffee Organization. *Trade Statistics*; International Coffee Organization (ICO), 2019. Available online: http://www.ico.org/trade_statistics.asp (accessed on 26 May 2020).
59. Toledo, R.A. O ciclo do café e o processo de urbanização do Estado de São Paulo. *Historien* **2012**, *6*, 76–89. [CrossRef]
60. Associação Brasileira de Industria do Café—ABIC. Consórcio Pesquisa Café Brasil. Available online: http://www.consorciopesquisacafe.com.br/index.php/publicacoes/637 (accessed on 26 May 2020).
61. Gebara, K.S.; Gasparotto-Junior, A.; Santiago, P.G.; Cardoso, C.A.L.; De Souza, L.M.; Morand, C.; Costa, T.A.; Cardozo-Junior, E.L. Daily Intake of Chlorogenic Acids from Consumption of Maté (Ilex paraguariensis A.St.-Hil.) Traditional Beverages. *J. Agric. Food Chem.* **2017**, *65*, 10093–10110. [CrossRef] [PubMed]
62. Schimpl, F.C.; Da Silva, J.F.; Gonçalves, J.F.D.C.; Mazzafera, P. Guarana: Revisiting a highly caffeinated plant from the Amazon. *J. Ethnopharmacol.* **2013**, *150*, 14–31. [CrossRef]
63. Liang, N.; Kitts, D.D. Role of chlorogenic acids in controlling oxidative and inflammatory stress conditions. *Nutrients* **2016**, *8*, 16. [CrossRef]
64. IBGE—Instituto Brasileiro de Geografia e Estatística. Acesso à Internet e à Televisão e Posse de Telefone Móvel. Available online: https://biblioteca.ibge.gov.br/index.php/biblioteca-catalogo?view=detalhes&id=2101543 (accessed on 26 May 2020).
65. Schatzkin, A.; Kipnis, V.; Carroll, R.J.; Midthune, D.; Subar, A.F.; Bingham, S.; Schoeller, D.A.; Troiano, R.P.; Freedman, L.S. A comparison of a food frequency questionnaire with a 24-hour recall for use in an epidemiological cohort study: Results from the biomarker-based Observing Protein and Energy Nutrition (OPEN) study. *Int. J. Epidemiol.* **2003**, *32*, 1054–1062. [CrossRef] [PubMed]

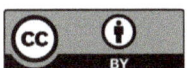

© 2020 by the authors. Licensee MDPI, Basel, Switzerland. This article is an open access article distributed under the terms and conditions of the Creative Commons Attribution (CC BY) license (http://creativecommons.org/licenses/by/4.0/).

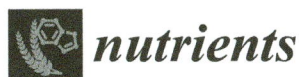

Article

Effects of Habitual Caffeine Intake, Physical Activity Levels, and Sedentary Behavior on the Inflammatory Status in a Healthy Population

Lluis Rodas [1], Aina Riera-Sampol [2], Antoni Aguilo [3], Sonia Martínez [3,*] and Pedro Tauler [4,*]

[1] Research Group on Evidence, Lifestyles and Health, University of the Balearic Islands, 07122 Palma, Spain; lluisrodas@hotmail.com
[2] Research Group on Evidence, Lifestyles and Health, Department of Nursing and Physiotherapy, University of the Balearic Islands, 07122 Palma, Spain; ana.riera@uib.es
[3] Research Group on Evidence, Lifestyles and Health, Department of Nursing and Physiotherapy, Health Research Institute of the Balearic Islands (IdISBa), University of the Balearic Islands, 07122 Palma, Spain; aaguilo@uib.es
[4] Research Group on Evidence, Lifestyles and Health, Department of Fundamental Biology and Health Sciences, Health Research Institute of the Balearic Islands (IdISBa), University of the Balearic Islands, 07122 Palma, Spain
* Correspondence: sonia.martinez@uib.es (S.M.); pedro.tauler@uib.es (P.T.); Tel.: +34-971-172-867 (S.M.); +34-971-259-960 (P.T.)

Received: 24 June 2020; Accepted: 2 August 2020; Published: 3 August 2020

Abstract: Low-grade chronic inflammation is associated with many chronic diseases and pathological conditions. The aim of the present study was to determine the effect of regular caffeine intake, physical activity levels, and sedentary behavior on the inflammatory status in healthy participants. In total, 112 men and 132 women aged 18 to 55 years and belonging to the staff and student population of the University of the Balearic Islands volunteered to participate in this descriptive cross-sectional study. Plasma concentrations of pro-inflammatory and anti-inflammatory markers were measured. Weight, height, and body composition (bioelectrical impedance) were determined. Caffeine intake, physical activity levels and sitting time, and diet quality were determined using questionnaires. Statistical regression analysis showed that caffeine intake was a negative predictor of C-reactive protein (CRP) ($p = 0.001$). Body fat percentage was positively associated with CRP ($p < 0.001$) and inversely associated with adiponectin ($p = 0.032$) and interleukin (IL)-10 levels ($p = 0.001$). Visceral fat was the main predictor for IL-6 ($p < 0.001$) and tumor necrosis factor (TNF)-α ($p < 0.001$). Sitting time was found to be the main, inverse, predictor for IL-10 ($p < 0.001$), and a positive predictor for TNF-α ($p < 0.001$). In conclusion, regular caffeine consumption induced very limited anti-inflammatory effects. Sedentary behavior and body fat accumulation induced significant pro-inflammatory effects.

Keywords: caffeine; coffee; physical activity; siting time; inflammation; body fat

1. Introduction

Low-grade chronic inflammation is characterized by chronically (two to three-fold) increased concentrations of several cytokines such as interleukin (IL)-6 and tumor necrosis factor (TNF)-α, as well as other pro-inflammatory substances such as C-reactive protein (CRP) [1]. Fat accumulation has been suggested to be the main reason for increased levels of these pro-inflammatory markers [2,3]. Many chronic diseases such as arthritis, type-2 diabetes or cancer, and pathological conditions such as insulin resistance or atherosclerosis have been found to be associated with low-grade systemic inflammation [2–4].

Physical inactivity has also been linked to low-grade systemic inflammation and subsequent increased risk for the development of chronic diseases [5]. On the other hand, regular exercise has been associated with an anti-inflammatory status, characterized by higher levels of anti-inflammatory markers such as IL-10 and adiponectin, and lower levels of pro-inflammatory cytokines, including IL-6, TNF-α, and IL-1β [2,4]. It has been pointed out that exercise-induced anti-inflammatory effects could be produced by reduced fat accumulation [2]. Interestingly, sedentary behavior, commonly defined as any sitting activity with a low energy expenditure, has been also linked to low-grade inflammation, independently of physical activity levels or adiposity [6–9].

Caffeine, due to its widespread presence in foods such as coffee, tea, and chocolate, and its stimulant effects, is highly consumed around the world. In vitro studies have suggested an anti-inflammatory role for caffeine, mainly inhibiting TNF-α production [10]. Regarding in vivo studies, only a few have addressed the effects of caffeine supplementation on blood inflammatory markers in humans [11]. These studies used a single dose of caffeine or used coffee as supplement when longer interventions were tested, reporting slight anti-inflammatory effects from the supplementation [12,13]. However, when coffee is used, many more components than caffeine alone are included in the supplement, as coffee is rich in bioactive compounds with antioxidant and anti-inflammatory properties, mainly chlorogenic acids [14,15]. In a similar way, when effects of habitual caffeine intake are analyzed it is impossible not to consider coffee consumption and the contribution of other coffee components, because in most countries, including Spain, coffee has been reported to be the main dietary source of caffeine [16]. In this regard, it has been shown that regular coffee intake is associated with reduced risk of type 2 diabetes [17,18] and metabolic syndrome [19] among other clinical conditions where low-grade inflammation and oxidative stress is involved in their development [11]. Furthermore, studies have shown anti-inflammatory effects of regular coffee consumption [20–23].

To our knowledge the effect of habitual caffeine intake on the inflammatory status of people performing different levels of physical activity, while taking into consideration the amount of sitting time, in a healthy young population has not yet been determined. Therefore, the aim of the present study was to determine the effect of regular caffeine intake, physical activity levels and sedentary behavior on the inflammatory status in healthy participants. Because physical activity and also caffeine, or coffee, have been suggested to induce anti-inflammatory effects, it could be expected that physically active participants consuming caffeine could present a more anti-inflammatory profile.

2. Materials and Methods

2.1. Study Design and Participants

Two hundred and forty-four participants (112 men and 132 women) volunteered to participate in this descriptive cross-sectional study. Participants were recruited among healthy students, workers, researchers and lecturers from the University of the Balearic Islands. All the participants were informed of the purpose and demands of the study before giving their written consent to participate. The protocol was in accordance with the Declaration of Helsinki for research of human participants and was approved by the Balearic Islands Clinical Investigation Ethics Committee (IB 2399/14 PI).

Participants were enrolled after fulfilling all inclusion criteria and presenting none of the exclusion criteria. Participants could be included if they were currently healthy, aged between 18 and 55 years and to have maintained constant physical activity levels (regardless of how high or low the level of activity) and sedentary behavior within the previous two months. Exclusion criteria were: smokers, professional, elite and those athletes with a habitual participation in endurance and ultra-endurance events, significant body weight fluctuations within the previous two months (±2 kg), regular alcohol or drugs consumption, and habitual consumption, or consumption within the 2 weeks preceding the study, of anti-inflammatory medication. Two hundred and forty-eight participants were recruited, but blood samples could not be obtained from four, leading to the final number of participants indicated above.

2.2. Laboratory Visit

Participants arrived at the laboratory between 08:00 and 10:00 h following an overnight fast of approximately 12 h. They had been previously informed about the study demands and about the inclusion and exclusion criteria. They had also been instructed to abstain from any moderate-vigorous intensity exercise during the 24 h before coming to the laboratory. Information about the study was given again to the participants, they completed an inclusion/exclusion criteria questionnaire and they then signed an informed consent form. Each participant was asked to empty their bladder before body mass, height and body composition were recorded. Participants then sat quietly for 10 min and completed questionnaires to determine physical activity levels, caffeine intake and adherence to the Mediterranean diet, before a blood sample was taken. The women were also asked about the date of their last menstruation. Seated venous blood samples were collected in suitable vacutainers with ethylenediaminetetraacetic acid (EDTA). Plasma was obtained from the blood samples within 30 min after blood collection by centrifugation (15 min, 1000× g, 4 °C). Plasma aliquots were stored at −70 °C until measurements were performed.

2.3. Anthropometrical Measurements

Height was measured to the nearest 0.5 cm using a stadiometer (Seca 220 (CM) Telescopic Height Rod for Column Scales, Seca gmbh, Hamburg). Body weight, percentage of body fat mass, and rating of visceral fat were measured using a Body Composition Analyzer (Bioelectrical Impedance Analysis, TANITA MC-780MA, TANITA Europe BV, Amsterdam, The Netherlands). Body weight was measured to the nearest 0.1 kg. The visceral fat measurement using this methodology provides a rating from 1 to 59, with values from 1 to 12 considered healthy (arbitrary units and information provided by the manufacturer, https://tanita.eu/help-guides/products-manuals/). Body mass index (BMI) was calculated as weight (kg) divided by height (m) squared (kg·m^{-2}).

2.4. Questionnaires

Physical activity levels were determined using the standard short form of the validated International Physical Activity Questionnaire (IPAQ), thus providing quantitative information on physical activity levels in metabolic equivalents (MET)-h·week^{-1}. Total weekly physical activity time and daily sitting time were also determined.

Diet quality was measured as the Adherence to the Mediterranean diet using a simplified assessment of adherence to the Mediterranean Diet (14-item questionnaire), previously developed and validated for the Spanish population [24]. Each item was scored as 0 or 1. A global score of 9 or higher indicates a good adherence to the Mediterranean Diet.

Habitual caffeine intake was measured using a self-reported questionnaire previously developed and used by our group [25,26]. The frequency intake of common products containing caffeine was ascertained, and caffeine daily consumption determined by using the caffeine content of each product [16]. Products included in the questionnaire were coffee preparations, including decaffeinated coffee, instant coffee (as cups or spoons), tea, chocolate, cola drinks, energy or stimulant beverages, and pharmaceutical caffeine supplements. Coffee intake was estimated from the intake of each coffee preparation contained in the questionnaire. The most common preparations in Spain were considered: espresso, "cortado" (espresso coffee, one serving, with a shot of milk), and "café con leche" (white coffee, or espresso coffee, one serving, with the remaining half of a cup filled with milk or steamed milk). Because a dose-response plasma appearance of the chlorogenic and phenolic acids contained in coffee has been shown after instant coffee ingestion [27], and because of its caffeine content, instant coffee was also considered as a coffee preparation. When applicable, the number of instant coffee servings was determined considering the number of spoons indicated by participants and that each serving contained 3.4 g of instant coffee [27]. Therefore, the total coffee intake, in number of servings, was determined considering all preparations indicated above.

2.5. Measurement of Inflammatory Markers

Plasma IL-10, IL-6, IL-1β, TNF-α, adiponectin, and CRP concentrations were determined to describe the inflammatory status of participants. These inflammatory markers were measured using commercially available solid-phase sandwich enzyme-linked immunosorbent assays and performed according to the manufacturers' instructions. Concentrations of IL-10, IL-6, and TNF-α were measured using Invitrogen high sensitivity kits (ThermoFisher SCIENTIFIC, Waltham, MA, USA). IL-10 was measured using the "IL-10 Human ELISA Kit, High Sensitivity" (BMS215HS); IL-6 was measured using the "IL-6 Human ELISA Kit, High Sensitivity" (BMS213HS); and TNF-α was measured using the "TNF alpha Human ELISA Kit, High Sensitivity" (BMS223HS). IL-1β, adiponectin and CRP were measured using RayBio® kits (RayBiotech, Norcross, GA, USA). IL-1β was measured using the "Human IL-1 beta ELISA" (ELH-IL1b); Adiponectin was measured using the "Human Adiponectin (Acrp30) ELISA" (ELH-Adiponectin); and CRP was measured using the "Human CRP ELISA" (ELH-CRP). All kits were exclusive for human samples (plasma, serum, and culture supernatants), and micro-plates were supplied with wells pre-coated with the specific antibody. For all assays, the absorbance was measured spectrophotometrically on a microplate reader (PowerWavei; BioTek, Winooski, VT, USA), and the concentration of each cytokine was calculated by comparison with a calculation curve established in the same measurement.

2.6. Statistical Analysis

Statistical analysis was carried out using IBM SPSS Statistics 22.0 software (SPSS/IBM, Chicago, IL, USA). All the data were tested for their normal distribution (Kolmogorov–Smirnov test). The results are expressed as means and standard deviations (SD), or median and interquartile ranges as specified. Percentages were also used when required. Student's t-test for unpaired data or the Mann-Whitney U test were used to evaluate differences between sexes. Kruskal-Wallis one-way ANOVA was used to determine the effect of the menstrual cycle on cytokine, adiponectin and CRP concentrations in women. Because no effect of menstrual cycle was observed (results not shown), this variable was not included in the following main analysis. The existence of significant bivariate correlations between the main variables was ascertained by determining Pearson correlation coefficients. These correlations were determined for the whole sample and for male and female participants separately. Multiple linear regression analysis, using the stepwise procedure, was applied to determine the relation between each dependent variable (logarithmic transformed IL-10, IL-6, IL-1β, TNF-α, adiponectin, and CRP concentrations) and independent and control variables. Habitual caffeine intake, IPAQ score and sitting time were included in the analysis as independent variables. Sex, body fat percentage, visceral fat rating, and diet quality, measured as the Adherence to the Mediterranean diet, were included in the analysis as control variables. Kruskal-Wallis one-way ANOVA was used to analyze IL-10 and TNF-α values depending on sitting time categorized in tertiles. A post-hoc power analysis calculation was performed (G*Power 3.1.9.4. Universität Kiel, Germany) for the regression analysis ($n = 244$, eight predictors, $\alpha = 0.05$). The power statistical calculation reported values higher than 90% for all significant regression reported. Statistical significance was accepted at $p < 0.05$.

3. Results

3.1. General Characteristics of Participants in the Study

Table 1 shows the general characteristics of participants in the study stratified per sex. The study population was, on average, young, with a BMI value within the normal weight range, a Mediterranean diet score slightly under the threshold for a good adherence, and with a higher number of women. Regarding anthropometrical characteristics, 20.5% of participants were overweight (BMI between 25 and 30 kg·m^{-2}), and 3.7% were obese (BMI higher than 30 kg·m^{-2}). On the other hand, 2.2% of participants showed an unhealthy visceral fat rating. Regarding caffeine intake, 4.9% of participants did not take caffeine, and 17% of participants took more than 400 mg per day (which is considered the higher-end value for a throughout the day, not in a single dose, safe consumption in healthy people [16]). Regarding coffee intake, 22.1% of participants reported no coffee intake, and 7% of participants reported an intake greater than 3 servings. Men reported non-significantly higher physical activity levels, both when expressed in METs and in hours. No significant differences between sexes were observed in the sitting time.

Table 1. General characteristics of participants in the study.

	All (n = 244)	Men (n = 112)	Women (n = 132)	p Value
Age (years)	32.1 ± 10.8	33.4 ± 10.8	31.1 ± 10.8	0.098
Weight (kg)	66.9 ± 13.3	76.3 ± 11.4	58.9 ± 8.7	**<0.001 ***
Height (cm)	170.0 ± 9.0	177.0 ± 6.5	164.0 ± 6.0	**<0.001 ***
BMI (kg·m^{-2})	23.0 ± 3.4	24.3 ± 3.3	22.0 ± 3.2	**<0.001 ***
Fat mass (%)	23.3 ± 7.9	18.3 ± 6.3	27.6 ± 6.5	**<0.001 ***
Visceral fat rating	4.01 ± 3.30	5.66 ± 3.68	2.63 ± 2.12	**<0.001 ***
Mediterranean diet score	8.18 ± 1.91	8.22 ± 1.93	8.15 ± 1.91	0.771
Caffeine intake (mg·day^{-1})	164.3 ± 143.4	174.7 ± 152.4	155.5 ± 135.3	0.298
Caffeine intake (mg·kg body weight^{-1}·day^{-1})	2.48 ± 2.18	2.33 ± 2.18	2.60 ± 2.18	0.346
Coffee intake (servings·day^{-1})	1.32 ± 1.35	1.41 ± 1.47	1.24 ± 1.25	0.311
Physical activity levels (METs-hour·week^{-1})	43.8 ± 36.1	48.7 ± 33.7	39.7 ± 37.5	0.054
Physical activity (hours·week^{-1})	9.18 ± 8.50	9.90 ± 7.36	8.57 ± 9.35	0.224
Sitting time (hours·day^{-1})	6.96 ± 2.77	7.20 ± 3.09	6.77 ± 2.46	0.235

Values are expressed as means ± standard deviations. * indicates significant differences between sexes (with p significant values also in bold) ($p < 0.05$), Student's t-test for unpaired data. BMI: body mass index.

3.2. Sources of Caffeine Consumption

Among caffeine consumers, coffee was the main caffeine source for participants in the study (Table 2). No significant differences were found between male and female participants.

Table 2. Sources of caffeine intake among those participants consuming caffeine.

Source	All (n = 228)	Men (n = 105)	Women (n = 123)	p Value
Coffee (%)	67.5 ± 37.1	69.6 ± 37.4	66.0 ± 36.9	0.538
Tea (%)	10.1 ± 19.8	8.9 ± 19.4	11.0 ± 20.1	0.425
Cola drinks (%)	12.8 ± 24.7	14.0 ± 26.8	11.8 ± 22.9	0.506
Chocolate (%)	7.9 ± 20.4	5.2 ± 14.1	10.2 ± 24.2	0.054
Energetic drinks (%)	1.6 ± 7.6	2.2 ± 9.0	1.0 ± 6.1	0.241
Sport products (%)	0.1 ± 0.7	0.1 ± 1.0	n.d.	0.175

Values are expressed as means ± standard deviations and represent the caffeine contribution in percentage of each source with respect to total caffeine intake. No differences between men and women were found, Student's t-test for unpaired data. n.d.: non detected (no consumption reported).

3.3. Concentration of Inflammatory Markers

Table 3 shows cytokine concentrations of all participants and categorized by sex. Significant differences were observed for IL-6, TNF-α, CRP, and adiponectin, with higher values in men for IL-6 ($p = 0.003$) and TNF-α ($p = 0.005$), and higher values in women for CRP ($p < 0.001$) and adiponectin ($p < 0.001$).

3.4. Bivariate Correlations between Dependent and Independent Variables

Table 4 shows bivariate correlations between all dependent and independent (continuous) variables. Positive correlations were found for IL-6 ($p = 0.001$) and TNF-α ($p = 0.014$) with age. However, IL-10 was inversely correlated with age ($p = 0.032$). Caffeine intake was inversely correlated with CRP levels ($p = 0.044$). Physical activity levels were correlated with IL-10 ($p = 0.002$). Sitting time showed a positive correlation with TNF-α ($p < 0.001$) and an inverse correlation with IL-10 levels ($p < 0.001$).

Percentage of body fat was correlated with CRP ($p < 0.001$), while it was inversely correlated with IL-10 ($p = 0.001$) and adiponectin ($p < 0.001$). An inverse correlation was found between visceral fat rating and IL-10 ($p = 0.013$). However, visceral fat showed positive correlations with IL-6 ($p < 0.001$) and TNF-α ($p < 0.001$). IL-1β levels were correlated with the adherence to the Mediterranean diet ($p = 0.039$).

Table 3. Cytokine concentrations of participants in the study.

Inflammatory Marker	All ($n = 244$)	Men ($n = 112$)	Women ($n = 132$)	p Value
IL-10 ($\mu g \cdot mL^{-1}$)	0.65 (0.54, 0.77)	0.65 (0.55, 0.83)	0.66 (0.54, 0.74)	0.333
IL-6 ($\mu g \cdot mL^{-1}$)	2.17 (1.44, 3.04)	2.38 (1.84, 3.12)	1.89 (1.14, 2.99)	**0.003 ***
IL-1β ($pg \cdot mL^{-1}$)	3.84 (2.66, 6.29)	4.02 (2.88, 6.40)	3.58 (2.43, 6.00)	0.205
TNF-α ($pg \cdot mL^{-1}$)	1.98 (1.52, 2.68)	2.11 (1.64, 3.04)	1.76 (1.49, 2.51)	**0.005 ***
CRP ($\mu g \cdot mL^{-1}$)	3.50 (1.81, 5.67)	2.46 (1.58, 4.28)	4.26 (2.42, 6.34)	**<0.001 ***
Adiponectin ($\mu g \cdot mL^{-1}$)	5.78 (3.62, 7.96)	4.59 (3.12, 6.22)	6.72 (4.77, 8,78)	**<0.001 ***

Values are expressed as median (25th, 75th percentile). * indicates significant differences between men and women (with p values in bold) ($p < 0.05$), Mann Whitney U test. IL: interleukin; TNF: tumor necrosis factor; CRP: C-reactive protein.

Table 4. Bivariate correlations between dependent and independent variables (all participants).

	Age	%Fat	Vis Fat	MD	Caffeine	PA	Sit
IL-10	−0.138 (**0.032 ***)	−0.219 (**0.001 ***)	−0.159 (**0.013 ***)	−0.083 (0.197)	−0.094 (0.142)	0.195 (**0.002 ***)	−0.325 (**<0.001***)
IL-6	0.205 (**0.001 ***)	0.063 (0.329)	0.290 (**<0.001 ***)	−0.032 (0.615)	0.089 (0.164)	−0.037 (0.561)	0.003 (0.957)
IL-1β	0.006 (0.932)	0.071 (0.267)	0.052 (0.417)	0.132 (**0.039 ***)	−0.006 (0.930)	−0.009 (0.889)	−0.030 (0.639)
TNF-α	0.157 (**0.014 ***)	0.086 (0.180)	0.335 (**<0.001 ***)	−0.023 (0.717)	0.067 (0.299)	−0.081 (0.208)	0.249 (**<0.001 ***)
CRP	0.009 (0.889)	0.427 (**<0.001 ***)	0.115 (0.074)	−0.109 (0.088)	−0.129 (**0.044 ***)	−0.037 (0.563)	−0.039 (0.549)
Adiponectin	−0.107 (0.095)	−0.222 (**<0.001 ***)	−0.117 (0.072)	−0.012 (0.429)	−0.087 (0.182)	−0.041 (0.520)	−0.003 (0.963)

Pearson correlation coefficient and (p value) is shown ($n = 244$). * indicates significant correlations (with p values in bold) ($p < 0.05$). % Fat: percentage of total body fat; Vis fat: visceral fat rating; MD: adherence to the Mediterranean diet; Caffeine: caffeine intake; PA: physical activity levels. Sit: sitting daily time. Logarithmic transformations of dependent variables were used. IL: interleukin; CRP: C-reactive protein; TNF: tumor necrosis factor.

Table 5 shows bivariate correlations between all dependent and independent variables in female participants. An inverse correlation was found between IL-10 and age ($p = 0.020$). However, a positive correlation was found for IL-6 with age ($p = 0.023$). Physical activity levels were correlated with IL-10 ($p = 0.033$). Sitting time showed a positive correlation with TNF-α ($p = 0.001$) and an inverse correlation with IL-10 levels ($p = 0.001$). Percentage of body fat showed a positive correlation with CRP ($p < 0.001$). Positive correlations were found for IL-6 ($p = 0.037$) and TNF-α ($p = 0.049$) with visceral fat. No correlation was found for adherence to the Mediterranean diet or caffeine intake with any of the dependent variables.

Table 6 shows bivariate correlation between all dependent and independent variables in male participants. A positive correlation was found between TNF-α and age ($p = 0.042$). Physical activity levels were positively correlated with IL-10 ($p = 0.010$) and inversely correlated with TNF-α ($p = 0.005$). Sitting time showed a positive correlation with TNF-α ($p = 0.047$) and an inverse correlation with IL-10 levels ($p < 0.001$). Percentage of body fat was correlated with IL-6 ($p = 0.001$), TNF-α ($p < 0.001$), and CRP ($p < 0.001$), while it was inversely correlated with adiponectin ($p < 0.001$) and IL-10 ($p = 0.002$). Visceral fat was correlated with IL-6 ($p = 0.002$), TNF-α ($p < 0.001$), and CRP ($p < 0.001$), and it was inversely correlated with IL-10 ($p = 0.008$). No correlation was found for adherence to the Mediterranean diet or caffeine intake with any of the dependent variables.

Table 5. Bivariate correlations between dependent and independent variables in females.

	Age	%Fat	Vis Fat	MD	Caffeine	PA	Sit
IL-10	−0.203 (**0.020** *)	−0.133 (0.128)	−0.170 (0.052)	−0.045 (0.605)	−0.098 (0.265)	0.185 (**0.033** *)	−0.281 (**0.001** *)
IL-6	0.198 (**0.023** *)	0.162 (0.064)	0.182 (**0.037** *)	−0.046 (0.597)	0.054 (0.539)	−0.100 (0.254)	0.017 (0.844)
IL-1β	−0.005 (0.959)	−0.011 (0.902)	0.048 (0.588)	0.157 (0.072)	−0.016 (0.854)	−0.028 (0.754)	−0.091 (0.300)
TNF-α	0.096 (0.274)	0.164 (0.060)	0.172 (**0.049** *)	−0.062 (0.479)	−0.034 (0.699)	−0.016 (0.856)	0.297 (**0.001** *)
CRP	−0.066 (0.455)	0.330 (**<0.001** *)	0.158 (0.070)	−0.097 (0.267)	−0.155 (0.077)	0.030 (0.729)	0.048 (0.582)
Adiponectin	−0.111 (0.243)	0.063 (0.510)	−0.053 (0.579)	0.152 (0.109)	−0.027 (0.773)	−0.106 (0.268)	−0.062 (0.513)

Pearson correlation coefficient and (p value) is shown ($n = 132$). * indicates significant correlations (with p values in bold) ($p < 0.05$). % Fat: percentage of total body fat; Vis fat: visceral fat rating; MD: adherence to the Mediterranean diet; Caffeine: caffeine intake; PA: physical activity levels. Sit: sitting daily time. Logarithmic transformations of dependent variables were used. IL: interleukin; CRP: C-reactive protein; TNF: tumor necrosis factor.

Table 6. Bivariate correlations between dependent and independent variables in males.

	Age	%Fat	Vis Fat	MD	Caffeine	PA	Sit
IL-10	−0.100 (0.296)	−0.295 (**0.002** *)	−0.249 (**0.008** *)	−0.120 (0.207)	−0.102 (0.286)	0.242 (**0.010** *)	−0.369 (**<0.001** *)
IL-6	0.180 (0.058)	0.300 (**0.001** *)	0.293 (**0.002** *)	−0.024 (0.803)	0.130 (0.164)	−0.023 (0.806)	−0.042 (0.662)
IL-1β	−0.002 (0.980)	−0.054 (0.577)	−0.011 (0.913)	0.094 (0.323)	−0.006 (0.953)	0.004 (0.953)	0.026 (0.784)
TNF-α	0.193 (**0.042** *)	0.353 (**<0.001** *)	0.378 (**<0.001** *)	0.115 (0.226)	0.148 (0.118)	−0.262 (**0.005** *)	0.188 (**0.047** *)
CRP	0.166 (0.079)	0.366 (**<0.001** *)	0.381 (**<0.001** *)	−0.122 (0.200)	−0.074 (0.440)	−0.051 (0.594)	0.076 (0.424)
Adiponectin	−0.107 (0.095)	−0.222 (**<0.001** *)	−0.117 (0.072)	−0.012 (0.429)	−0.087 (0.182)	−0.041 (0.520)	−0.003 (0.963)

Pearson correlation coefficient and (p value) is shown ($n = 112$). * indicates significant correlations (with p values in bold) ($p < 0.05$). % Fat: percentage of total body fat; Vis fat: visceral fat rating; MD: adherence to the Mediterranean diet; Caffeine: caffeine intake; PA: physical activity levels. Sit: sitting daily time. Logarithmic transformations of dependent variables were used. IL: interleukin; CRP: C-reactive protein; TNF: tumor necrosis factor.

3.5. Multivariable Linear Regression Analysis

Table 7 shows the results of the regression analysis for IL-10. Regression analysis revealed that sitting time ($p < 0.001$) and the percentage of fat ($p = 0.001$) were negative predictors for IL-10 levels, while physical activity was a positive predictor ($p = 0.028$). Sitting time was found to be the main predictor (change in R^2 0.106 vs. 0.040 for fat mass and 0.017 for physical activity).

Table 8 shows de-regression analysis results for adiponectin. Sex was revealed as the main predictor for adiponectin (change in R^2 0.097, $p < 0.001$), with higher values for females, as has been indicated above. Percentage of fat mass was inversely associated with adiponectin (change in R^2 0.017, $p = 0.032$).

Table 7. Multiple linear regression for IL-10.

Variable	B	95% CI	β	t	p Value
Age	−0.002	(−0.006, 0.002)	−0.104	−1.706	0.089
Sex	0.010	(−0.060, 0.080)	0.042	0568	0.570
Fat mass	−0.003	(−0.005, −0.001)	−0.189	−3.171	**0.002 ***
Visceral fat rating	−0.002	(−0.014, 0.010)	−0.066	−1.346	0.180
Adherence to MD	−0.005	(−0.013, 0.003)	−0.078	−1.324	0.187
Caffeine intake	0.000	(−0.001, 0.000)	−0.080	−1.336	0.183
Physical activity	0.000	(0.000, 0.001)	0.136	2.218	**0.028 ***
Sitting time	−0.012	(−0.017, −0.007)	−0.281	−4.607	**<0.001 ***

Model: R: 0.405; R^2 0.164; Adjusted R^2 0.153; $p < 0.001$; * indicates significant predictors (with p values in bold) ($p < 0.05$). IL: interleukin; MD: Mediterranean diet; CI: confidence intervals.

Table 8. Multiple linear regression for adiponectin.

Variable	B	95% CI	β	t	p Value
Age	0.000	(−0.004, 0.004)	−0.019	−0.285	0.776
Sex	0.194	(0.124–0.265)	0.407	5.426	**<0.001 ***
Fat mass	−0.005	(−0.009, −0.001)	−0.162	−2.156	**0.032 ***
Visceral fat rating	0.004	(−0.004–0.012)	0.050	0.443	0.658
Adherence to MD	0.008	(−0.006, 0.022)	0.065	1.075	0.283
Caffeine intake	0.000	(−0.001, 0.000)	−0.068	−1.092	0.276
Physical activity	0.000	(−0.001, 0.000)	−0.012	0.010	0.846
Sitting time	0.003	(−0.007, 0.013)	0.039	0.637	0.585

Model: R^2 0.115; Adjusted R^2 0.107; $p < 0.001$; * indicates significant predictors (with p values in bold) ($p < 0.05$). MD: Mediterranean diet; CI: confidence intervals.

Table 9 shows the results of the regression analysis for IL-6. Visceral fat was revealed as the only significant predictor for IL-6 ($p < 0.001$), with a positive association.

Table 9. Regression analysis for IL-6.

Variable	B	95% CI	β	t	p Value
Age	0.001	(−0.003, 0.005)	0.013	0.151	0.880
Sex	−0.035	(−0.075, 0.005)	−0.073	−1.055	0.292
Fat mass	−0.001	(−0.003, 0.001)	−0.028	−0.439	0.661
Visceral fat rating	0.021	(0.012, 0.030)	0.290	4.701	**<0.001 ***
Adherence to MD	−0.005	(−0.017, 0.007)	−0.044	−0.706	0.481
Caffeine intake	0.000	(0.000, 0.001)	0.039	0.579	0.563
Physical activity	−0.001	(−0.002, 0.001)	−0.059	−0.948	0.344
Sitting time	−0.003	(−0.011, 0.005)	−0.033	−0.532	0.595

Model: R^2 0.084; Adjusted R^2 0.080; $p < 0.001$; * indicates significant predictors (with p values in bold) ($p < 0.05$). IL: interleukin; MD: Mediterranean diet; CI: confidence intervals.

Sitting time (change in R^2 0.044, $p < 0.001$,) and visceral fat rating (change in R^2 0.112, $p < 0.001$) were found as positive predictors for TNF-α concentrations, with visceral fat as the main predictor (Table 10).

Table 11 shows the results of the regression analysis for CRP. Percentage of fat mass was found as the main predictor for CRP (change in R^2 0.182, $p < 0.001$), showing a positive association. Caffeine intake was shown to be a negative predictor for CRP (change in R^2 0.037, $p = 0.001$). The regression analysis did not report any significant predictor for IL-1β.

Table 10. Multiple linear regression for tumor necrosis factor (TNF) -α.

Variable	B	95% CI	β	t	p Value
Age	−0.002	(−0.005, 0.001)	−0.108	−1.327	0.186
Sex	−0.014	(−0.128, 0.100)	−0.041	−0.608	0.544
Fat mass	−0.001	(−0.011, 0.010)	−0.023	−0.367	0.714
Visceral fat rating	0.016	(0.010, 0.022)	0.309	5.166	**<0.001 ***
Adherence to MD	0.001	(−0.009, 0.012)	0.007	0.119	0.905
Caffeine intake	0.000	(−0.001, 0.000)	−0.060	−0.936	0.350
Physical activity	0.000	(−0.001, 0.000)	−0.025	−0.984	0.326
Sitting time	0.013	(0.004, 0.019)	0.211	3.538	**<0.001 ***

Model: R^2 0.156; Adjusted R^2 0.149; $p < 0.001$; * indicates significant predictors (with p values in bold) ($p < 0.05$). TNF: tumor necrosis factor; MD: Mediterranean diet; CI: confidence intervals.

Table 11. Multiple linear regression for C-reactive protein (CRP).

Variable	B	95% CI	β	t	p Value
Age	−0.002	(−0.010, 0.006)	−0.039	−0.601	0.549
Sex	−0.016	(−0.082, 0.050)	−0.021	−0.288	0.774
Fat mass	0.018	(0.013, 0.022)	0.454	7.885	**<0.001 ***
Visceral fat rating	0.006	(−0.022, 0.034)	0.063	0.980	0.328
Adherence to MD	−0.011	(−0.029, 0.007)	−0.070	−1.219	0.224
Caffeine intake	−0.002	(−0.003, −0.001)	−0.195	−3.379	**0.001 ***
Physical activity	0.000	(−0.004, 0.004)	0.023	0.407	0.684
Sitting time	0.000	(−0.013, 0.013)	0.011	0.187	0.852

Model: R^2 0.219; Adjusted R^2 0.213; $p < 0.001$; * indicates significant predictors (with p values in bold) ($p < 0.05$). CRP: C-reactive protein; MD: Mediterranean diet; CI: confidence intervals.

3.6. Effects of Sitting Time on IL-10 and Tumor Necrosis Factor (TNF) -α Concentrations

Figure 1 shows values of IL-10 (a) and TNF-α (b) categorized by sitting time tertiles. A significant effect of sitting time was found for both IL-10 ($p = 0.001$) and TNF-α ($p < 0.001$). IL-10 values in the third tertile (longer sitting time, 9 to 15 h) were significantly lower ($p = 0.001$) than in the first tertile (shortest sitting time, 1 to 5 h). TNF-α values in the third tertile were significantly higher than in the second tertile ($p = 0.004$) and in the first tertile ($p < 0.001$).

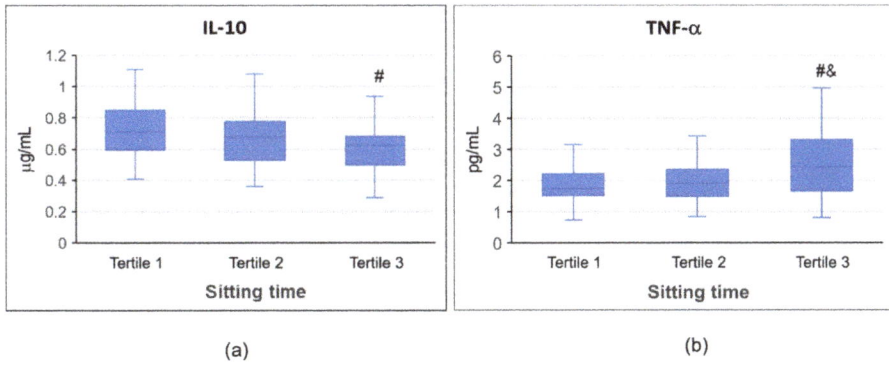

Figure 1. IL-10 (**a**) and TNF-α (**b**) plasma concentrations categorized by sitting time tertiles. Median, 25th, 75th percentile, and lowest and highest values are shown for IL-10 and TNF-α values. # indicates significant differences to first tertile. & indicates significant differences to second tertile. IL: interleukin; TNF: tumor necrosis factor.

4. Discussion

The main finding of the present study was that in a healthy population, low caffeine intake could exert a slight anti-inflammatory effect characterized by lower CRP plasma levels. Body fat, both total and visceral, and sedentary behavior have been shown to be important and independent inflammatory predictors, inducing higher levels of pro-inflammatory markers, but also decreased levels of anti-inflammatory markers.

Participants in the study population were, on average, young and with a higher number of women. These characteristics reflect properly the university population, with higher figures for young female students. Caffeine intake observed in the present study was similar to previous studies in Spain, and similar, or slightly lower to the average value, when participants of a similar age from most occidental countries were considered [16,28–30]. Concerning this consumption, coffee remains the main source for caffeine intake, a common finding in most European countries, except for the UK and Ireland [16]. As coffee preparations in Spain are quite different from the ones in other countries, it becomes difficult to compare coffee intake observed in the present study with the habitual intake of other countries. For these reasons, caffeine intake, rather than coffee intake, has been used as the main variable for the analysis, and also as an indicator of coffee consumption.

Previous studies, both observational and clinical trials, have reported that coffee intake increases adiponectin levels [13,20]. The mechanism involved seems to be the stimulatory effect of caffeine on the expression of the peroxisome proliferator activated receptor γ (PPARγ), which positively elevates the adiponectin concentration [31]. In fact, a previous study reported increased levels of adiponectin after a supplementation with caffeinated coffee but no effect with decaffeinated coffee [13]. However, a higher daily intake of coffee (four cups, or more than 600 mg of caffeine) than that observed in the present study, seems to be required to increase adiponectin levels [20]. Therefore, and as suggested, low amounts of coffee or caffeine consumption may be the reason for not observing a significant effect of caffeine intake on adiponectin [32] but also on IL-10, TNF-α, and IL-6 concentrations in the present study. It should also be considered that some studies reporting positive effects of regular coffee consumption on adiponectin levels were performed in overweight participants [13], while in the present study only ~24% of participants were overweight or obese; or in older populations [20]. Therefore, it is possible that the protective effect of coffee was emphasized in such conditions.

The association between CRP, which is considered an appropriate marker for low grade systemic inflammation [33], and coffee intake has been recently reviewed [34]. Despite this review suggesting that on average, coffee consumption is not associated with CRP levels, some studies have reported a protective healthy effect because decreased levels of CRP have been observed in participants ingesting at least a daily cup of coffee [20–23]. Results of the present study are in agreement with this observation as it was observed that caffeine consumption is inversely associated with CRP levels. Therefore, it seems that in contrast with the other inflammatory markers analyzed, low regular coffee intake could be enough to prevent higher CRP levels. It is worth noting however, that decaffeinated coffee seems to also be effective in decreasing CRP levels, therefore other components of coffee rather than caffeine itself, could contribute to this effect [22]. It has been suggested that chlorogenic acid, the main phenolic acid in coffee with antioxidant and anti-inflammatory properties [14], can play an important role in the reduction of inflammatory factors such as CRP [35]. The low, on average, BMI of participants in the present study could have been an important factor that influenced the inverse association between coffee intake and CRP, as all studies reporting the protective anti-inflammatory effect of coffee consumption were performed in populations with low BMIs [20–23]. In fact, it has been suggested that the different BMI of populations considered in previous studies could be a key factor for the inconsistent results found regarding this association [34]. Interestingly, in the present study, and in agreement with previous reports [36,37], a positive association was found between body fat mass and CRP. Therefore, our data indicates that, in the context of an average low BMI, caffeine consumption, probably as a coffee consumption marker, presents an inverse association with CRP, inducing the opposite effect of body fat mass accumulation.

Inverse associations were found between percentage of body fat and anti-inflammatory markers such as adiponectin and IL-10. Adiponectin is an anti-inflammatory adipokine secreted almost exclusively from adipose tissue [38], and low adiponectin levels have been associated with body fat accumulation and obesity, leading to increased risk of inflammation [3]. It is striking that in the present study this potential negative effect was observed in young and healthy participants, with an incidence of obesity as low as 3.7%. In addition, and despite the fact women present a relatively greater percentage body fat, adiponectin levels were found to be higher in women, which is in agreement with previous results, mainly when lean populations have been considered [39].

The anti-inflammatory IL-10 has not been commonly measured when associations between fat mass and inflammation have been investigated. In the present study, and in the same line of results indicated above, IL-10 was inversely associated with body fat mass. It has been reported that fat accumulation is accompanied by adipose tissue infiltration by pro-inflammatory immune cells (T2), increased release of pro-inflammatory markers such as TNF-α, decreased production of anti-inflammatory markers, such as IL-10, and the development of the low-grade systemic inflammatory state described above [3]. Within this picture, and regarding adipose tissue, visceral fat has been suggested to play an important role [2]. In the present study positive associations were found between visceral fat and TNF-α and also between visceral fat and IL-6. Previous studies, using different approaches to measure visceral fat, have shown similar associations [40–42]. Whether TNF-α and IL-6 levels are more dependent on total body fat or visceral fat remains to be elucidated, because some studies have reported associations with both parameters [37,42,43]. However, taken together, the opposite associations found for IL-10 and, on the other hand, TNF-α and IL-6 with regard to fat content, total or visceral, could reflect the predominant anti-inflammatory production when fat content is low as well as the predominant pro-inflammatory release when fat is accumulated.

In the present study only a small effect of physical activity levels on the IL-10 concentrations were observed. However, more strong associations were found for sedentary time: a positive association with TNF-α and an inverse association with IL-10, which, together, define a pro-inflammatory picture induced by sedentary behavior and independent of physical activity levels. It is possible that the average moderate levels reported could limit the effects of physical activity. However, previous studies showed that sedentary behavior was linked to low-grade inflammation, independently of physical activity levels or adiposity [6–9]. This observation is in agreement with results obtained in the present study and suggests an independent link between sitting time and low-grade inflammation [7]. To our knowledge, the association between sedentary time and IL-10 has not been reported, as previous studies focused on the pro-inflammatory markers. This novel result could indicate that sedentary behavior, independent of fat mass and physical activity, influences levels of both pro-inflammatory and anti-inflammatory compounds.

This study presents some limitations that should be acknowledged. In addition to the limitations due to the observational nature, the current study was limited to cross-sectional data from a single university population. However, the patterns of physical activity and sedentary behavior observed in the present study could be applied to other populations, even outside the university. Both sedentary time and physical activity levels, two of the main variables of the study, were self-reported. However, the IPAQ, which is a widely used and validated questionnaire, was utilized to collect these data, as has been done in previous studies using the same or similar questionnaires [6,9]. Regarding sedentary time, an important limitation was that the number, duration, and frequency of sedentary breaks were not recorded. In this regard, it has been reported that these breaks could modify to some extent associations between sedentary time and inflammatory markers [8], at least when sitting time is not too long [7]. Furthermore, methodology used to determine both percentage of fat mass and visceral fat rating has been reported to present some limitations [44]. Finally, despite the statistical power analysis revealed high power for most of the associations found, these associations could be considered weak. However, there is a concordance between most of them, highlighting the pro-inflammatory role of sedentary behavior and fat mass accumulation.

5. Conclusions

The limited effects of caffeine or coffee intake observed in the present study could be explained by relatively low caffeine and coffee intakes. However, this relatively low caffeine or coffee consumption could slightly prevent CRP increases induced by increased fat mass. Sedentary behavior and body fat accumulation, even within the young, healthy and, on average, normal weight participants in the present study induced pro-inflammatory effects. However, only slight effects of physical activity levels were observed. Interestingly, both sedentary behavior and fat accumulation induced lower levels of the essential anti-inflammatory cytokine IL-10. Future studies should be performed to determine coffee intake needed to observe greater health effects and, also, to determine the mechanism linking sedentary behavior to inflammation.

Author Contributions: Conceptualization, P.T. and S.M.; Methodology, P.T., S.M., A.R.-S. and L.R.; Formal Analysis, P.T. and A.A.; Investigation, L.R., S.M., A.R.-S., A.A. and P.T.; Writing-Original Draft Preparation, L.R.; Writing-Review and Editing, P.T., A.R.-S., A.A. and S.M.; Visualization, L.R.; Supervision, P.T. and S.M.; Project Administration, P.T. and S.M.; Funding Acquisition, P.T. All authors have read and agreed to the published version of the manuscript.

Funding: This research was funded by the Ministerio de Economía, Industria y Competitividad (MINECO), the Agencia Estatal de Investigación (AEI) and the European Regional Development Funds (ERDF), project DEP2013-45966-P (MINECO/AEI/ERDF, EU).

Acknowledgments: The authors would like to thank all the participants in the study.

Conflicts of Interest: The authors declare no conflict of interest. The funders had no role in the design of the study; in the collection, analyses, or interpretation of data; in the writing of the manuscript, or in the decision to publish the results.

References

1. Ross, R. Atherosclerosis—An inflammatory disease. *N. Engl. J. Med.* **1999**, *340*, 115–126. [CrossRef] [PubMed]
2. Gleeson, M.; Bishop, N.C.; Stensel, D.J.; Lindley, M.R.; Mastana, S.S.; Nimmo, M.A. The anti-inflammatory effects of exercise: Mechanisms and implications for the prevention and treatment of disease. *Nat. Rev. Immunol.* **2011**, *11*, 607–615. [CrossRef] [PubMed]
3. Ouchi, N.; Parker, J.L.; Lugus, J.J.; Walsh, K. Adipokines in inflammation and metabolic disease. *Nat. Rev. Immunol.* **2011**, *11*, 85–97. [CrossRef] [PubMed]
4. Petersen, A.M.W.; Pedersen, B.K. The anti-inflammatory effect of exercise. *J. Appl. Physiol.* **2005**, *98*, 1154–1162. [CrossRef] [PubMed]
5. Pedersen, B.K. Health Benefits Related to Chronic Low-Grade Exercise in Patients with Systemic Inflammation. *Am. J. Lifestyle Med.* **2007**, *1*, 289–298. [CrossRef]
6. Allison, M.A.; Jensky, N.E.; Marshall, S.J.; Bertoni, A.G.; Cushman, M. Sedentary behavior and adiposity-associated inflammation: The multi-ethnic study of atherosclerosis. *Am. J. Prev. Med.* **2012**, *42*, 8–13. [CrossRef]
7. Henson, J.; Yates, T.; Edwardson, C.L.; Khunti, K.; Talbot, D.; Gray, L.J.; Leigh, T.M.; Carter, P.; Davies, M.J. Sedentary time and markers of chronic low-grade inflammation in a high risk population. *PLoS ONE* **2013**, *8*, 4–9. [CrossRef]
8. Healy, G.N.; Matthews, C.E.; Dunstan, D.W.; Winkler, E.A.H.; Owen, N. Sedentary time and cardio-metabolic biomarkers in US adults: NHANES 200306. *Eur. Heart J.* **2011**, *32*, 590–597. [CrossRef]
9. Yates, T.; Khunti, K.; Wilmot, E.G.; Brady, E.; Webb, D.; Srinivasan, B.; Henson, J.; Talbot, D.; Davies, M.J. Self-reported sitting time and markers of inflammation, insulin resistance, and adiposity. *Am. J. Prev. Med.* **2012**, *42*, 1–7. [CrossRef]
10. Horrigan, L.A.; Kelly, J.P.; Connor, T.J. Caffeine suppresses TNF-alpha production via activation of the cyclic AMP/protein kinase A pathway. *Int. Immunopharmacol.* **2004**, *4*, 1409–1417. [CrossRef]
11. Paiva, C.L.R.S.; Beserra, B.T.S.; Reis, C.E.G.; Dorea, J.G.; Da Costa, T.H.M.; Amato, A.A. Consumption of coffee or caffeine and serum concentration of inflammatory markers: A systematic review. *Crit. Rev. Food Sci. Nutr.* **2019**, *59*, 652–663. [CrossRef] [PubMed]

12. Kempf, K.; Herder, C.; Erlund, I.; Kolb, H.; Martin, S.; Carstensen, M.; Koenig, W.; Sundvall, J.; Bidel, S.; Kuha, S.; et al. Effects of coffee consumption on subclinical inflammation and other risk factors for type 2 diabetes: A clinical trial. *Am. J. Clin. Nutr.* **2010**, *91*, 950–957. [CrossRef] [PubMed]
13. Wedick, N.M.; Brennan, A.M.; Sun, Q.; Hu, F.B.; Mantzoros, C.S.; Van Dam, R.M. Effects of caffeinated and decaffeinated coffee on biological risk factors for type 2 diabetes: A randomized controlled trial. *Nutr. J.* **2011**, *10*, 93. [CrossRef] [PubMed]
14. Naveed, M.; Hejazi, V.; Abbas, M.; Kamboh, A.A.; Khan, G.J.; Shumzaid, M.; Ahmad, F.; Babazadeh, D.; FangFang, X.; Modarresi-Ghazani, F.; et al. Chlorogenic acid (CGA): A pharmacological review and call for further research. *Biomed. Pharmacother.* **2018**, *97*, 67–74. [CrossRef]
15. Gómez-Ruiz, J.Á.; Leake, D.S.; Ames, J.M. In vitro antioxidant activity of coffee compounds and their metabolites. *J. Agric. Food Chem.* **2007**, *55*, 6962–6969. [CrossRef]
16. EFSA NDA Panel (EFSA Panel on Dietetic Products, Nutrition and Allergies). Scientific Opinion on the safety of caffeine. *EFSA J.* **2015**, *13*, 4102.
17. Akash, M.S.H.; Rehman, K.; Chen, S. Effects of coffee on type 2 diabetes mellitus. *Nutrition* **2014**, *30*, 755–763. [CrossRef]
18. Ding, M.; Bhupathiraju, S.N.; Chen, M.; van Dam, R.M.; Hu, F.B. Caffeinated and decaffeinated coffee consumption and risk of type 2 diabetes: A systematic review and a dose-response meta-analysis. *Diabetes Care* **2014**, *37*, 569–586. [CrossRef]
19. Shang, F.; Li, X.; Jiang, X. Coffee consumption and risk of the metabolic syndrome: A meta-analysis. *Diabetes Metab.* **2016**, *42*, 80–87. [CrossRef]
20. Williams, C.J.; Fargnoli, J.L.; Hwang, J.J.; Van Dam, R.M.; Blackburn, G.L.; Hu, F.B.; Mantzoros, C.S. Coffee consumption is associated with higher plasma adiponectin concentrations in women with or without type 2 diabetes a prospective cohort study. *Diabetes Care* **2008**, *31*, 1434–1437. [CrossRef]
21. Kotani, K.; Tsuzaki, K.; Sano, Y.; Maekawa, M.; Fujiwara, S.; Hamada, T.; Sakane, N. The relationship between usual coffee consumption and serum C-reactive protein level in a Japanese female population. *Clin. Chem. Lab. Med.* **2008**, *46*, 1434–1437. [CrossRef] [PubMed]
22. Lopez-Garcia, E.; Van Dam, R.M.; Qi, L.; Hu, F.B. Coffee consumption and markers of inflammation and endothelial dysfunction in healthy and diabetic women. *Am. J. Clin. Nutr.* **2006**, *84*, 888–893. [CrossRef] [PubMed]
23. Maki, T.; Pham, N.M.; Yoshida, D.; Yin, G.; Ohnaka, K.; Takayanagi, R.; Kono, S. The relationship of coffee and green tea consumption with high-sensitivity C-reactive protein in Japanese men and women. *Clin. Chem. Lab. Med.* **2010**, *48*, 849–854. [CrossRef] [PubMed]
24. Martínez-González, M.A.; Fernández-Jarne, E.; Serrano-Martínez, M.; Wright, M.; Gomez-Gracia, E. Development of a short dietary intake questionnaire for the quantitative estimation of adherence to a cardioprotective Mediterranean diet. *Eur. J. Clin. Nutr.* **2004**, *58*, 1550–1552. [CrossRef] [PubMed]
25. Tauler, P.; Martinez, S.; Moreno, C.; Monjo, M.; Martinez, P.; Aguilo, A. Effects of caffeine on the inflammatory response induced by a 15-km run competition. *Med. Sci. Sports Exerc.* **2013**, *45*, 1269–1276. [CrossRef] [PubMed]
26. Tauler, P.; Martinez, S.; Martinez, P.; Lozano, L.; Moreno, C.; Aguiló, A. Effects of caffeine supplementation on plasma and blood mononuclear cell IL-10 levels after exercise. *Int. J. Sport Nutr. Exerc. Metab.* **2016**, *26*, 8–16. [CrossRef]
27. Renouf, M.; Marmet, C.; Giuffrida, F.; Lepage, M.; Barron, D.; Beaumont, M.; Williamson, G.; Dionisi, F. Dose-response plasma appearance of coffee chlorogenic and phenolic acids in adults. *Mol. Nutr. Food Res.* **2014**, *58*, 301–309. [CrossRef]
28. Fitt, E.; Pell, D.; Cole, D. Assessing caffeine intake in the United Kingdom diet. *Food Chem.* **2013**, *140*, 421–426. [CrossRef]
29. Rochat, C.; Eap, C.B.; Bochud, M.; Chatelan, A. Caffeine consumption in switzerland: Results from the first national nutrition survey menuCH. *Nutrients* **2020**, *12*, 28. [CrossRef]
30. Sousa, A.G.; da Costa, T.H.M. Usual coffee intake in Brazil: Results from the National Dietary Survey 2008–9. *Br. J. Nutr.* **2015**, *113*, 1615–1620. [CrossRef]
31. Gressner, O.A.; Lahme, B.; Rehbein, K.; Siluschek, M.; Weiskirchen, R.; Gressner, A.M. Pharmacological application of caffeine inhibits TGF-β-stimulated connective tissue growth factor expression in hepatocytes via PPARγ and SMAD2/3-dependent pathways. *J. Hepatol.* **2008**, *49*, 758–767. [CrossRef] [PubMed]

32. Rebello, S.A.; Chen, C.H.; Naidoo, N.; Xu, W.; Lee, J.; Chia, K.S.; Tai, E.S.; Van Dam, R.M. Coffee and tea consumption in relation to inflammation and basal glucose metabolism in a multi-ethnic Asian population: A cross-sectional study. *Nutr. J.* **2011**, *10*, 61. [CrossRef] [PubMed]
33. Pearson, T.A.; Mensah, G.A.; Alexander, R.W.; Anderson, J.L.; Cannon, R.O.; Criqui, M.; Fadl, Y.Y.; Fortmann, S.P.; Hong, Y.; Myers, G.L.; et al. Markers of inflammation and cardiovascular disease: Application to clinical and public health practice: A statement for healthcare professionals from the centers for disease control and prevention and the American Heart Association. *Circulation* **2003**, *107*, 499–511. [CrossRef] [PubMed]
34. Moua, E.D.; Hu, C.; Day, N.; Hord, N.G.; Takata, Y. Coffee consumption and c-reactive protein levels: A systematic review and meta-analysis. *Nutrients* **2020**, *12*, 1349. [CrossRef]
35. Izadi, V.; Larijani, B.; Azadbakht1, L. Is coffee and green tea consumption related to serum levels of adiponectin and leptin? *Int. J. Prev. Med.* **2018**, *9*, 106. [CrossRef]
36. Visser, M.; Bouter, L.M.; McQuillan, G.M.; Wener, M.H.; Harris, T.B. Elevated C-reactive protein levels in overweight and obese adults. *J. Am. Med. Assoc.* **1999**, *282*, 2131–2135. [CrossRef]
37. Pou, K.M.; Massaro, J.M.; Hoffmann, U.; Vasan, R.S.; Maurovich-Horvat, P.; Larson, M.G.; Keaney, J.F.; Meigs, J.B.; Lipinska, I.; Kathiresan, S.; et al. Visceral and subcutaneous adipose tissue volumes are cross-sectionally related to markers of inflammation and oxidative stress: The Framingham Heart Study. *Circulation* **2007**, *116*, 1234–1241. [CrossRef]
38. Scherer, P.E.; Williams, S.; Fogliano, M.; Baldini, G.; Lodish, H.F. A novel serum protein similar to C1q, produced exclusively in adipocytes. *J. Biol. Chem.* **1995**, *270*, 26746–26749. [CrossRef]
39. Kern, P.A.; Di Gregorio, G.B.; Lu, T.; Rassouli, N.; Ranganathan, G. Adiponectin expression from human adipose tissue: Relation to obesity, insulin resistance, and tumor necrosis factor-α expression. *Diabetes* **2003**, *52*, 1779–1785. [CrossRef]
40. Thorand, B.; Baumert, J.; Döring, A.; Herder, C.; Kolb, H.; Rathmann, W.; Giani, G.; Koenig, W.; Wichmann, H.E.; Löwel, H.; et al. Sex differences in the relation of body composition to markers of inflammation. *Atherosclerosis* **2006**, *184*, 216–224. [CrossRef]
41. Panagiotakos, D.B.; Pitsavos, C.; Yannakoulia, M.; Chrysohoou, C.; Stefanadis, C. The implication of obesity and central fat on markers of chronic inflammation: The ATTICA study. *Atherosclerosis* **2005**, *183*, 308–315. [CrossRef] [PubMed]
42. Park, H.S.; Park, J.Y.; Yu, R. Relationship of obesity and visceral adiposity with serum concentrations of CRP, TNF-α and IL-6. *Diabetes Res. Clin. Pract.* **2005**, *69*, 29–35. [CrossRef] [PubMed]
43. Rexrode, K.M.; Pradhan, A.; Manson, J.E.; Buring, J.E.; Ridker, P.M. Relationship of total and abdominal adiposity with CRP and IL-6 in women. *Ann. Epidemiol.* **2003**, *13*, 674–682. [CrossRef]
44. Day, K.; Kwok, A.; Evans, A.; Mata, F.; Verdejo-garcia, A.; Hart, K.; Ward, L.C.; Truby, H. Comparison of a Bioelectrical Impedance Device against the Reference Method Dual Energy X-Ray Absorptiometry and Anthropometry for the Evaluation of Body Composition in Adults. *Nutrients* **2018**, *10*, 1469. [CrossRef] [PubMed]

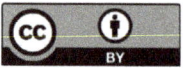

© 2020 by the authors. Licensee MDPI, Basel, Switzerland. This article is an open access article distributed under the terms and conditions of the Creative Commons Attribution (CC BY) license (http://creativecommons.org/licenses/by/4.0/).

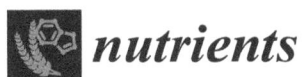

Article

Coffee Intake and Neurocognitive Performance in HIV/HCV Coinfected Patients (ANRS CO13 HEPAVIH)

Saskia Antwerpes [1], Camelia Protopopescu [1,2,*], Philippe Morlat [3], Fabienne Marcellin [1,2], Linda Wittkop [4,5], Vincent Di Beo [1,2], Dominique Salmon-Céron [6,7], Philippe Sogni [6,8], Laurent Michel [9,10], Maria Patrizia Carrieri [1,2] and the ANRS CO13 HEPAVIH Study Group [†]

1. Aix Marseille Univ, INSERM, IRD, SESSTIM, Sciences Économiques & Sociales de la Santé & Traitement de l'Information Médicale, 13385 Marseille, France; saskia.antwerpes@univ-amu.fr (S.A.); fabienne.marcellin@inserm.fr (F.M.); vincent.di-beo@inserm.fr (V.D.B.); maria-patrizia.carrieri@inserm.fr (M.P.C.)
2. ORS PACA, Observatoire Régional de la Santé Provence-Alpes-Côte d'Azur, 13385 Marseille, France
3. Service de Médecine Interne et Maladies Infectieuses, CHU de Bordeaux, Université de Bordeaux, 33000 Bordeaux, France; philippe.morlat@chu-bordeaux.fr
4. ISPED, Inserm, Bordeaux Population Health Research Center, Team MORPH3EUS, UMR 1219, CIC-EC 1401, University of Bordeaux, F-33000 Bordeaux, France; linda.wittkop@u-bordeaux.fr
5. CHU de Bordeaux, Pole de Sante Publique, F-33000 Bordeaux, France
6. Université Paris Descartes, 75006 Paris, France; dominique.salmon@aphp.fr (D.S.-C.); philippe.sogni@aphp.fr (P.S.)
7. Service Maladies Infectieuses et Tropicales, AP-HP, Groupe Hospitalier Cochin Hôtel Dieu, 75014 Paris, France
8. Service d'Hépatologie, Groupe Hospitalier Cochin Hôtel Dieu, Assistance Publique-Hôpitaux de Paris, 75014 Paris, France
9. UMRS 1018, Paris-Saclay University, 94807 Villejuif, France; laurent.michel@croix-rouge.fr
10. Centre Pierre Nicole, French Red Cross, 75005 Paris, France
* Correspondence: camelia.protopopescu@inserm.fr; Tel.: +33-4137-32290
† Membership of the ANRS CO13 HEPAVIH Study Group is provided in the Acknowledgments.

Received: 9 July 2020; Accepted: 12 August 2020; Published: 21 August 2020

Abstract: Coffee is one of the most consumed beverages worldwide. Previous research has demonstrated its neuroprotective effects in the elderly. People coinfected with human immunodeficiency virus (HIV) and hepatitis C virus (HCV) experience an accelerated aging process and cognitive impairment, which significantly impair quality of life and may affect disease-related dimensions such as treatment adherence. This study aimed to analyse the relationship between regular coffee intake and neurocognitive performance (NCP) in HIV-HCV coinfected people. We used data from 139 coinfected patients who participated in both the ANRS CO13 HEPAVIH cohort and the HEPAVIH-Psy cross-sectional survey. Linear regression models adjusting for potential sociodemographic (age, gender, educational level), clinical (liver disease status, ongoing HCV treatment, HIV viral load, major depressive disorder) and socio-behavioural (cannabis use) correlates of NCP were used. Our results showed significant, positive associations between elevated coffee intake (ECI) (three or more cups of coffee per day) and NCP in verbal fluency, psychomotor speed (coding) and executive functioning. ECI might therefore preserve neurocognitive functioning in people living with HIV and HCV.

Keywords: coffee; hepatitis C; HIV; neurocognitive disorders

1. Introduction

Coffee is one of the most widely consumed drinks in the world, especially in high-resource settings [1]. It is associated with better overall health and a reduced risk of both mortality [2] and cancer [3] in the general population.

In people infected with hepatitis C virus (HCV), coffee consumption is associated with lower liver stiffness [4] and with decreased rates of liver disease progression and severity [5]. Specifically, an in vitro study showed that coffee extract and caffeic acid inhibit HCV viral propagation [6]. Elevated coffee intake (ECI) (three or more cups per day) is an independent predictor of improved virological response to peginterferon plus ribavirin therapy in patients with chronic HCV infection [7] and is associated with improved treatment tolerance.

In people living with HIV and HCV, previous research has shown that ECI can reduce the risk of mortality by 50% [8]. With regard to liver function, Yaya et al. pointed out that ECI is associated with a significantly reduced risk of advanced liver fibrosis in HIV-HCV coinfected patients, even in those with unhealthy alcohol use [9]. Furthermore, reduced levels of liver enzymes have been highlighted in patients with ECI by Morisco et al. [5] and Carrieri et al. [10]. Other beneficial effects of ECI in this population are its positive effects on insulin resistance [10], perceived toxicity and fatigue [11].

Apart from its beneficial effects on liver disease, coffee intake also significantly impacts cognition because of its stimulating effects on the central nervous system (CNS). In a study performed in 1875 healthy adults, habitual caffeine consumption was significantly related to better long-term memory performance and faster locomotor speed. No relationships were found between habitual caffeine consumption and short-term memory, information processing, planning and attention [12]. A meta-analysis showed a J-shaped association between coffee intake and incident cognitive disorders, with the lowest risk of incident cognitive disorders observed for a daily consumption level of 1–2 cups of coffee [13]. In the elderly, Haller et al. (2018) demonstrated an association between moderate caffeine consumption (from one to two cups of coffee/day) and better neurocognitive performance (NCP) and between moderate to ECI and better white matter preservation and cerebral blood flow [14]. ECI has also been associated with a reduced risk of Alzheimer's disease [15]. Furthermore, people living with HIV and HCV experience an accelerated aging process [16] and suffer from neurocognitive aging.

Cognitive impairment is prevalent in HIV-HCV coinfected people, with rates ranging from 40% to 63% [17]. Compared with HIV mono-infected patients, coinfected patients have higher levels of cognitive impairment, particularly in information processing speed [18]. Vivithanaporn et al. showed that the presence of HCV coinfection in HIV-infected individuals is likely to increase the neurologic disease burden and risk of death [19]. With regard to the underlying mechanisms, an HCV-encoded protein, named Core, has been found to cause neuroinflammation and neuronal death by potentiating HIV-associated neurotoxicity [20].

No study, to date, has examined the association between coffee consumption and neurocognitive functioning in HIV-HCV coinfected patients. The present study aimed to analyse the relationship between coffee consumption and neurocognitive performance (NCP) in a sample of HIV-HCV coinfected patients, characterized by a high rate of HIV viral suppression.

2. Materials and Methods

We used data from 139 HIV-HCV coinfected patients who participated in both the ANRS CO13 HEPAVIH cohort [21] and the HEPAVIH-Psy cross-sectional survey [22]. The latter was nested in the former and was designed to estimate the prevalence of mental health and substance use disorders in HIV-HCV coinfected patients recruited in 10 French HIV services between 2012 and 2014. Exclusion criteria for HEPAVIH-Psy were diagnosis of a current psychotic episode and neurological or medical disorders that may affect NCP, such as cerebrovascular disease or head trauma.

HEPAVIH-Psy provided data about current major depressive disorder (MDD) and NCP, the latter being assessed by measuring the following functions (with associated test/scale in brackets): visuospatial abilities and visual memory (Rey–Osterrieth complex figure test (ROCF) [23], vocabulary size or lexical access speed (verbal fluency task) [24], processing speed (coding task, a subtest of the fourth version of the Wechsler Adult Intelligence Scale (WAIS-IV)) [25] and executive functioning (Trail Making Test (TMT) part B minus A) [26]. The TMT B-A score was calculated as the difference between TMT-A and TMT-B times and is considered a measure of cognitive flexibility relatively independent of manual dexterity [27]. These cognitive functions, which have been shown to be sensitive enough to detect a possible neurocognitive impairment in HIV-infected individuals [28], were considered outcomes in our study. We tested coffee consumption in the previous six months and other factors, including age, gender, educational level, liver disease status (presence of cirrhosis), ongoing HCV treatment, HIV viral load and MDD, as potential correlates of neurocognitive performance. All of these variables were included in the HEPAVIH cohort and measured at the closest visit to the date of the HEPAVIH-Psy survey, except for MDD, which was documented in the HEPAVIH-Psy survey itself.

Our study outcomes were the five raw test scores measuring NCP (ROCF—direct copy and delayed reproduction, verbal fluency, coding, TMT B-A), with higher scores indicating better results for all tests/scales except TMT. Results for TMT are reported as the logarithm of the number of seconds required to complete the given task. Therefore, higher scores reflect greater impairment. Distributions of raw test scores are illustrated in Section 3.2. We used linear regression models to study the association between coffee intake during the previous six months (≥3 cups per day (ECI), ≤2 cups per day, no consumption) and each of the five outcomes. First, we selected all variables associated with the outcomes using a liberal p-value < 0.20 in the univariable analysis. We then built the five multivariable models. Only variables associated with at least one out of the five outcomes in univariable and multivariable analyses (using a p-value < 0.05) were included in order to have comparable multivariable models. Educational level was forced into all models, as it is an important cofactor of NCP.

3. Results

3.1. Study Population

Study patients were mostly men (66.9%), median (IQR) age was 50 (48–53) years, and 40.3% of patients had an educational level above or equal to the French high school diploma. A total of 91.3% of patients had an undetectable HIV viral load and 23.7% had cirrhosis. A total 28.8% reported ECI in the previous six months (Table 1).

Table 1. Characteristics of HIV-HCV coinfected patients in the study population, the ANRS CO13 HEPAVIH cohort and the HEPAVIH-Psy cross-sectional survey (N = 139).

	N (%)
Age, years Median (IQR)	50 (48–53)
Gender	
Male	93 (66.9)
Female	46 (33.1)
High school certificate *	
No	83 (59.7)
Yes	56 (40.3)
Current MDD (N = 137)	
No	107 (78.1)
Yes	30 (21.9)
HIV-related characteristics:	
CD4 count, cells/mm^3 (N = 138)	
Median (IQR)	522 (346–726)

Table 1. *Cont.*

	N (%)
Detectable HIV viral load (N = 138)	
No	126 (91.3)
Yes	12 (8.7)
HCV-related characteristics:	
Ongoing HCV-treatment	
No	116 (83.5)
Yes	23 (16.6)
Presence of cirrhosis	
No	106 (76.3)
Yes	33 (23.7)
Cannabis use	
No	81 (58.3)
Yes	58 (41.7)
Coffee intake	
≥3 cups/day	40 (28.8)
≤2 cups/day	81 (58.3)
No consumption	18 (13.0)

* Educational level above or equal to the French Baccalaureate. Abbreviations: IQR—interquartile range; MDD—major depressive disorder; HIV—human immunodeficiency virus; HCV—hepatitis C virus.

3.2. Outcomes

The distributions of the five raw test scores measuring NCP (ROCF—direct copy and delayed reproduction, verbal fluency, coding, TMT B-A) are presented as boxplots. We stratified by coffee consumption, comparing the distributions of test scores in the three groups: no consumption, ≤ 2 cups/day and ≥ 3 cups/day (Figure 1).

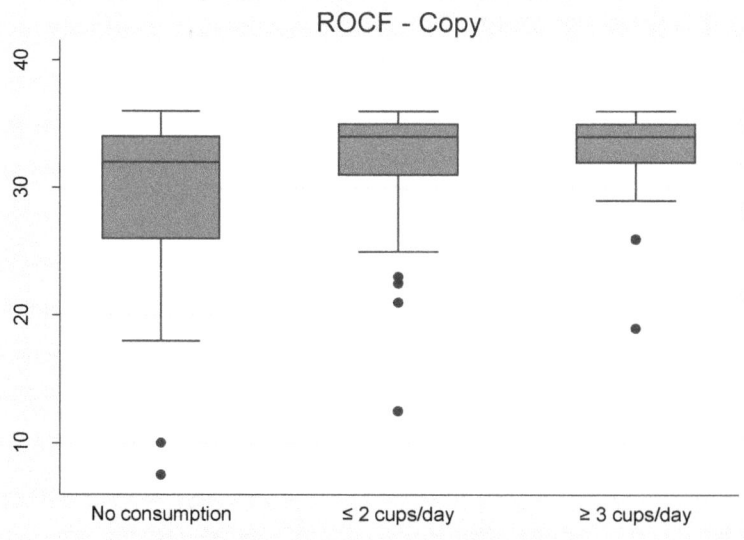

Figure 1. *Cont.*

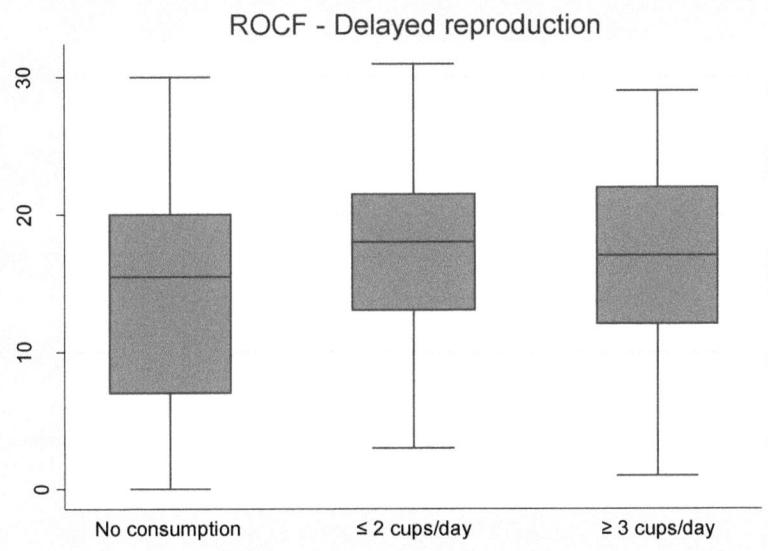

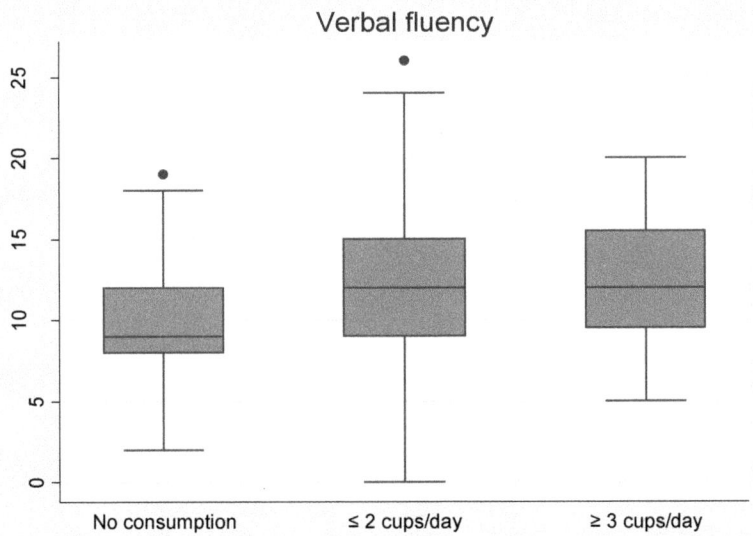

Figure 1. *Cont.*

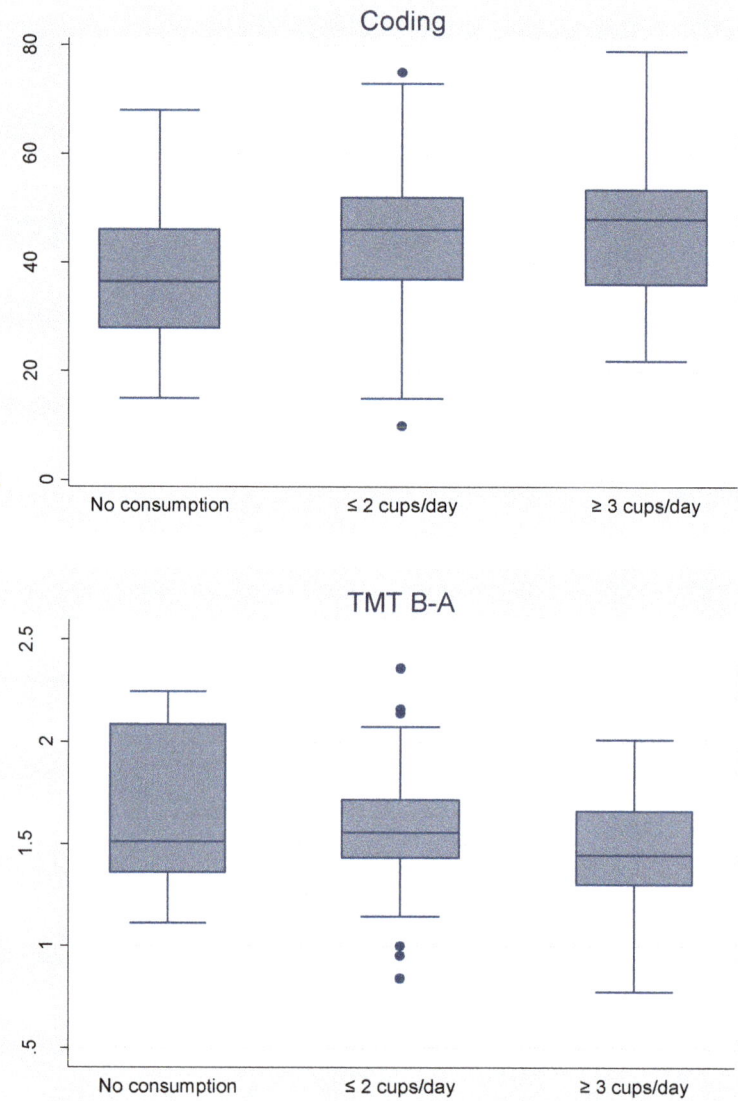

Figure 1. Distribution of raw test scores of HIV-HCV coinfected patients in the study population, the ANRS CO13 HEPAVIH cohort and the HEPAVIH-Psy cross-sectional survey (N = 139). Abbreviations: ROCF: Rey-Osterrieth complex figure; TMT B-A: Trail Making Test part B minus A.

3.3. Coffee Consumption Associated with Neurocognitive Performance in HIV-HCV Coinfected People

Interestingly, we found that ECI was positively associated with four of the five outcomes, as follows: ROCF (copy score only), verbal fluency, coding and TMT B-A. This result was confirmed after adjusting for clinical (presence of cirrhosis, ongoing HCV treatment, detectable HIV viral load, MDD), sociodemographic (age, gender, educational level) and socio-behavioural (cannabis use) correlates of the outcomes (Table 2).

Table 2. Factors associated with neurocognitive performance in HIV-HCV coinfected patients, multivariable linear regression models, the ANRS CO13 HEPAVIH cohort and the HEPAVIH-Psy cross-sectional survey (N = 139).

	ROCF				Verbal Fluency (N = 134)		Coding (N = 135)		TMT B-A [1] (N = 132)	
	Copy (N = 134)		Delayed Reproduction (N = 131) [2]							
	Coefficient (95% CI)	p-Value	Coefficient (95% CI)	p-Value	Coefficient (95% CI)	p-Value	Coefficient (95% CI)	p-Value	Coefficient (95% CI)	p-Value
Coffee intake										
≤2 cups/day	3.35 (−0.28 to 6.99)	0.070	3.05 (−0.78 to 6.87)	0.117	2.32 (−0.33 to 4.97)	0.085	7.58 (0.18 to 14.97)	0.045	−0.11 (−0.28 to 0.07)	0.226
≥3 cups/day	4.63 (0.88 to 8.39)	**0.016**	2.70 (−1.44 to 6.84)	0.199	3.08 (0.18 to 5.97)	**0.037**	9.24 (1.26 to 17.36)	**0.024**	−0.27 (−0.47 to −0.07)	**0.009**
Age	0.10 (−0.04 to 0.25)	0.165	−0.09 (−0.26 to 0.09)	0.333	0.03 (−0.12 to 0.16)	0.701	−0.82 (−1.18 to −0.46)	**0.000**	0.00 (−0.01 to 0.01)	0.608
Educational level [3]	−1.19 (−2.79 to 0.41)	0.145	2.06 (−0.08 to 4.20)	0.059	0.59 (−1.25 to 2.42)	0.527	1.03 (−2.93 to 5.00)	0.607	−0.06 (−0.17 to 0.05)	0.302
Current MDD	−1.88 (−4.61 to 0.85)	0.176	−2.81 (−5.23 to −0.38)	**0.024**	−0.73 (−2.74 to 1.29)	0.477	−6.75 (−11.50 to −2.00)	**0.006**	0.05 (−0.11 to 0.22)	0.529
Presence of cirrhosis	−2.28 (−4.49 to −0.07)	**0.043**	−1.12 (−3.60 to 1.38)	0.380	−1.07 (−3.04 to 0.89)	0.282	−4.38 (−9.23 to 0.47)	0.076	0.07 (−0.06 to 0.19)	0.288
Ongoing HCV treatment	0.26 (−1.67 to 2.18)	0.792	0.13 (−3.15 to 3.40)	0.939	−2.43 (−4.72 to −0.13)	**0.039**	−9.01 (−14.14 to −3.88)	**0.001**	0.00 (−0.14 to 0.15)	0.988
Detectable HIV viral load	0.13 (−1.83 to 2.09)	0.896	−0.71 (−3.56 to 2.14)	0.623	−1.73 (−4.41 to 0.96)	0.205	−10.97 (−17.38 to −4.55)	**0.001**	0.21 (0.05 to 0.38)	**0.013**
Cannabis use	−0.89 (−2.65 to 0.87)	0.320	−0.46 (−2.70 to 1.78)	0.685	−1.77 (−3.61 to 0.06)	0.058	−4.91 (−8.98 to −0.84)	**0.019**	0.09 (−0.03 to 0.20)	0.149

[1] TMT B-A was log10-transformed so results must be interpreted as 10^Est. [2] Adjusted for quality of the copy and for reproduction time (log10 transformed). [3] Educational level above or equal to the French Baccalaureate. Abbreviations: ROCF: Rey-Osterrieth complex figure; MDD: major depressive disorder; HCV: hepatitis C virus; TMT B-A: trail making test part B minus A.

4. Discussion

This is the first study to explore the relationship between coffee intake and neurocognitive performance in people coinfected with HIV and HCV. We showed that elevated coffee intake (ECI) (i.e., three cups or more per day) was associated with better NCP, as measured by the ROCF (direct copy only), verbal fluency, coding and TMT B-A tests. These results are clinically relevant given that the HIV-HCV coinfected population is doubly affected by their vulnerability to cognitive impairments and the burden of their diseases [17,19]. A meta-analysis comparing cognitive performance between HIV-HCV coinfected and HIV and HCV mono-infected patients showed significantly poorer information processing speed in the coinfected group [18]. Our results showed significant, positive associations between information processing speed (measured by the coding task test) and ECI.

Our findings are in line with previous research in people living with HIV [29], showing the protective effects of moderate coffee intake on cognitive function. For example, Bragança and colleagues showed that regularly drinking espresso was associated with better Global Deficit Scores (GDS) and improved cognitive performance in five out of eight cognitive tests. They also found daily espresso consumption to be a positive predictor for performance in attention, working memory, executive functions and GDS.

Interestingly, our results remained valid after adjustment for known correlates of neurocognitive impairment. We presume that this observed effect is not "acute" but attributable to prolonged exposure to ECI.

In particular, the positive relationship between ECI and NCP persisted even after adjusting for known liver disease correlates (cirrhosis and ongoing HCV treatment), which suggests that the beneficial influence of coffee intake on NCP may occur irrespective of liver disease related factors. Accordingly, our results might be explained by a direct effect of caffeine on the CNS [30]. Caffeine targets specific brain regions involved in executive and verbal working memory functions [31], explaining the positive associations with NCP in verbal fluency observed in our study. In addition, caffeine enhances information processing speed and attention, which are two cognitive functions mobilised during the coding test [32].

With regard to the underlying mechanisms, our results may be explained, at least in part, by the antioxidant properties of coffee [33], which are able to counter the harmful effects of HCV- and HIV-induced neuro-inflammation. More specifically, chlorogenic acid, an important polyphenol found in coffee, has been shown to improve the oxidative system [34] and, therefore, may counter the inflammatory effects of HCV and HIV on the CNS. This is particularly relevant since HCV is characterized by high oxidative stress, which is shown to promote liver fibrosis, cirrhosis and cancer, as well as metabolic dysfunction [35]. This study's strengths include rigorous control for several clinical (HIV viral load, presence of cirrhosis, treatment status) and socio-behavioural (age, gender, educational level) confounding factors. Moreover, MDD in the study population was diagnosed by psychiatrists and taken into account in our analysis.

Our study also has limitations. First, because it was cross-sectional, we were not able to infer causality for the associations found. Furthermore, we used raw scores as outcomes instead of a global deficit score, which is frequently used in other studies [18,29]. However, not aggregating our results into a single score enabled us to distinguish the cognitive functions assessed by the different tests and to provide more detailed results. Furthermore, we did not have information about the type of coffee consumed (caffeinated or decaffeinated, green or roasted), and we did not consider other caffeine sources, such as energy drinks, tea, chocolate or cocoa, which are likely to affect cognitive functioning [36]. Future research using consistent and comprehensive neuropsychological assessment batteries is needed in order to clarify the effects of coffee intake (including the cumulative effect of prolonged coffee consumption) on cognitive function and the mechanisms underlying these effects. It may also be useful to disentangle the effects of the numerous coffee compounds and their potential antioxidant activity on NCP and inflammation indicators in HIV-HCV coinfected patients to further explore these effects in certain categories of patients (such as patients with metabolic syndrome) and to assess the potential dose–response pattern of coffee intake on neurocognitive functioning in this population.

5. Conclusions

The strong relationship we found between coffee intake and NCP underlines the multiple benefits of coffee consumption in HIV-HCV coinfected people, ranging from reduced inflammation and risk of liver disease to reduced morbidity and mortality risk. Because cognitive deficits can have significant functional consequences for patients' everyday lives—such as difficulties in remembering important information, reduced quality of life, and poor adherence to treatments—our results may have important implications for the planning of effective clinical management of these diseases. The effect of coffee and other functional food on HIV-HCV-related outcomes should also be included in the clinical and public health research agenda.

Author Contributions: Conceptualization, S.A., L.M. and M.P.C.; methodology, S.A., M.P.C., F.M. and C.P.; software, V.D.B., C.P. and S.A.; validation, S.A. and C.P.; formal analysis, S.A., L.M. and C.P.; investigation, P.S, D.S.-C. and P.M.; resources, S.A., L.M., F.M. and M.P.C.; data curation, V.D.B. and C.P.; writing—original draft preparation, S.A.; writing—review and editing, S.A., C.P., P.M., F.M., L.W., D.S.-C., P.S., L.M. and M.P.C.; visualization, S.A.; supervision, M.P.C.; project administration, L.M. and M.P.C.; funding acquisition, F.M., M.P.C. and L.M. All authors have read and agreed to the published version of the manuscript.

Funding: This project was funded by AbbVie and the French National Agency for Research on Aids and Viral Hepatitis (ANRS). The funding sources were not involved in the study design, data analysis, or in the writing and submission of the manuscript.

Acknowledgments: This project was funded by AbbVie and the French National Agency for Research on Aids and Viral Hepatitis (ANRS). We thank all the members of the ANRS CO13-HEPAVIH Study Group and staff members from the HEPAVIH-Psy centers (Appendix A). We especially thank all physicians and nurses involved in the follow-up of the HEPAVIH cohort and all patients who took part in both studies. Finally, our thanks to Jude Sweeney for the English revision and editing of the manuscript.

Conflicts of Interest: The authors declare no conflict of interest.

Appendix A

The ANRS CO13 HEPAVIH Study Group: *Scientific Committee:* D.Salmon (co-Principal investigator), L.Wittkop (co-Principal Investigator & Methodologist), P.Sogni (co-Principal Investigator), L. Esterle (project manager), P.Trimoulet, J.Izopet, L.Serfaty, V.Paradis, B.Spire, P.Carrieri, M.A.Valantin, G.Pialoux, J.Chas, I.Poizot-Martin, K.Barange, A.Naqvi, E.Rosenthal, A.Bicart-See, O.Bouchaud, A.Gervais, C.Lascoux-Combe, C.Goujard, K.Lacombe, C.Duvivier, D.Neau, P.Morlat, F.Bani-Sadr, L.Meyer, F.Boufassa, B.Autran, A.M.Roque, C.Solas, H.Fontaine, D.Costagliola, L.Piroth, A.Simon, D.Zucman, F.Boué, P.Miailhes, E.Billaud, H.Aumaître, D.Rey, G.Peytavin, V.Petrov-Sanchez, D.Lebrasseur-Longuet. *Clinical Centres* (ward/participating physicians): APHP, Hôpitaux Universitaires Paris Centre, Paris (Médecine Interne et Maladies Infectieuses: D. Salmon, R.Usubillaga; Hépato-gastro-entérologie: P.Sogni; Anatomo-pathologie: B.Terris; Virologie: P.Tremeaux); APHP Pitié-Salpétrière, Paris (Maladies Infectieuses et Tropicales: C.Katlama, M.A.Valantin, H.Stitou; Médecine Interne: A.Simon, P.Cacoub, S.Nafissa; Hépato-gastro-entérologie: Y.Benhamou; Anatomo-pathologie: F.Charlotte; Virologie: S.Fourati; APHM Sainte-Marguerite, Marseille (Service d'Immuno-Hématologie Clinique: I.Poizot-Martin, O.Zaegel, H.Laroche; Virologie: C.Tamalet); APHP Tenon, Paris (Maladies Infectieuses et Tropicales: G.Pialoux, J.Chas; Anatomo-pathologie: P.Callard, F.Bendjaballah; Virologie: C.Amiel, C.Le Pendeven); CHU Purpan, Toulouse (Maladies Infectieuses et Tropicales: B. Marchou; Médecine interne: L.Alric; Hépato-gastro-entérologie: K.Barange, S.Metivier; Anatomo-pathologie: J.Selves; Virologie: F.Larroquette); CHU Archet, Nice (Médecine Interne: E.Rosenthal; Infectiologie: A.Naqvi, V.Rio; Anatomo-pathologie: J.Haudebourg, M.C.Saint-Paul; Virologie: A. De Monte, V.Giordanengo, C.Partouche); APHP Avicenne, Bobigny (Médecine Interne – Unité VIH: O.Bouchaud; Anatomo-pathologie: A.Martin, M.Ziol; Virologie: Y.Baazia, V.Iwaka-Bande, A.Gerber); Hôpital Joseph Ducuing, Toulouse (Médecine Interne: M.Uzan, A.Bicart-See, D.Garipuy,

M.J.Ferro-Collados; Anatomo-pathologie: J.Selves; Virologie: F.Nicot); APHP Bichat – Claude-Bernard, Paris (Maladies Infectieuses: A.Gervais, Y.Yazdanpanah; Anatomo-pathologie: H.Adle-Biassette; Virologie: G.Alexandre, Pharmacologie: G.Peytavin); APHP Saint-Louis, Paris (Maladies infectieuses: C.Lascoux-Combe, J.M.Molina; Anatomo-pathologie: P.Bertheau; Virologie: M.L.Chaix, C. Delaugerre, S. Maylin); APHP Saint-Antoine (Maladies Infectieuses et Tropicales: K. Lacombe, J. Bottero; J. Krause, P.M. Girard, Anatomo-pathologie: D. Wendum, P. Cervera, J. Adam; Virologie: C. Viala); APHP, Hôpitaux Paris Sud, Bicêtre, Paris (Maladies Infectieuses et Tropicales: D. Vittecocq; Médecine Interne: C. Goujard, Y. Quertainmont, E. Teicher; Virologie: C. Pallier); APHP Necker, Paris (Maladies Infectieuses et Tropicales: O. Lortholary, C. Duvivier, C. Rouzaud, J. Lourenco, F. Touam, C. Louisin: Virologie: V. Avettand-Fenoel, E. Gardiennet, A. Mélard); CHU Bordeaux Hôpital Pellegrin, Bordeaux (Maladies Infectieuses et Tropicales: D. Neau, A. Ochoa, E. Blanchard, S. Castet-Lafarie, C. Cazanave, D. Malvy, M. Dupon, H. Dutronc, F. Dauchy, L. Lacaze-Buzy, A. Desclaux; Anatomo-pathologie: P. Bioulac-Sage; Virologie: P. Trimoulet, S. Reigadas; CHU Bordeaux Hôpital Saint-André, Bordeaux (Médecine Interne et Maladies Infectieuses: P. Morlat, D. Lacoste, F. Bonnet, N. Bernard, M. Hessamfar, J, F. Paccalin, C. Martell, M. C. Pertusa, M. Vandenhende, P. Mercié, D. Malvy, T. Pistone, M.C. Receveur, M. Méchain, P. Duffau, C Rivoisy, I. Faure, S. Caldato; Anatomo-pathologie: P. Bioulac-Sage; Virologie: P. Trimoulet, S. Reigadas, P. Bellecave, C. Tumiotto); CHU Bordeaux Hôpital du Haut-Levêque, Bordeaux (Médecine Interne: J.L. Pellegrin, J.F. Viallard, E. Lazzaro, C. Greib; Anatomo-pathologie: P. Bioulac-Sage; Virologie: P. Trimoulet, S. Reigadas); Hôpital FOCH, Suresnes (Médecine Interne: D. Zucman, C. Majerholc; Virologie: M. Brollo, E. Farfour); APHP Antoine Béclère, Clamart (Médecine Interne: F. Boué, J. Polo Devoto, I. Kansau, V. Chambrin, C. Pignon, L. Berroukeche, R. Fior, V. Martinez, S. Abgrall, M. Favier; Virologie: C. Deback); CHU Henri Mondor, Créteil (Immunologie Clinique: Y. Lévy, S. Dominguez, J.D. Lelièvre, A.S. Lascaux, G. Melica); CHU Nantes Hôpital Hôtel Dieu, Nantes (Maladies Infectieuses et Tropicales: E. Billaud, F. Raffi, C. Allavena, V. Reliquet, D. Boutoille, C. Biron; M. Lefebvre, N. Hall, S. Bouchez; Virologie: A. Rodallec, L. Le Guen, C. Hemon); Hôpital de la Croix Rousse, Lyon (Maladies Infectieuses et Tropicales: P. Miailhes, D. Peyramond, C. Chidiac, F. Ader, F. Biron, A. Boibieux, L. Cotte, T. Ferry, T. Perpoint, J. Koffi, F. Zoulim, F. Bailly, P. Lack, M. Maynard, S. Radenne, M. Amiri, F Valour; Hépato-gastro-entérologie: J. Koffi, F. Zoulim, F. Bailly, P. Lack, M. Maynard, S. Radenne, C. Augustin-Normand; Virologie: C. Scholtes, T.T. Le-Thi); CHU Dijon, Dijon (Département d'infectiologie: L. Piroth, P. Chavanet M. Duong Van Huyen, M. Buisson, A. Waldner-Combernoux, S. Mahy, A. Salmon Rousseau, C. Martins); CH Perpignan, Perpignan (Maladies infectieuses et tropicales: H. Aumaître, Virologie: S. Galim); CHU Robert Debré, Reims (Médecine interne, maladies infectieuses et immunologie clinique: F. Bani-Sadr, D. Lambert, Y Nguyen, J.L. Berger, M. Hentzien, Virologie: V. Brodard); CHRU Strasbourg (Le Trait d'Union: D Rey, M Partisani, ML Batard, C Cheneau, M Priester, C Bernard-Henry, E de Mautort, P Fischer, Virologie: P Gantner et S Fafi-Kremer). *Data collection*: F.Roustant, P. Platterier, I. Kmiec, L. Traore, S. Lepuil, S. Parlier, V. Sicart-Payssan, E. Bedel, S. Anriamiandrisoa, C. Pomes, F. Touam, C. Louisin, M. Mole, C. Bolliot, P Catalan, M. Mebarki, A. Adda-Lievin, P. Thilbaut, Y. Ousidhoum, F.Z. Makhoukhi, O. Braik, R. Bayoud, C. Gatey, M.P. Pietri, V. Le Baut, R. Ben Rayana, D. Bornarel, C. Chesnel, D. Beniken, M. Pauchard, S. Akel, S. Caldato, C. Lions, A. Ivanova, A-S. Ritleg, C. Debreux, L. Chalal, J.Zelie, H. Hue, A. Soria, M. Cavellec, S. Breau, A. Joulie, P. Fisher, S. Gohier, D. Croisier-Bertin, S. Ogoudjobi, C. Brochier, V. Thoirain-Galvan, M. Le Cam. *Management, statistical analyses:* P. Carrieri, M. Chalouni, V. Conte, L. Dequae-Merchadou, M. Desvallees, L. Esterle, C. Gilbert, S. Gillet, R. Knight, T. Lemboub, F. Marcellin, L. Michel, M. Mora, C. Protopopescu, P. Roux, B. Spire, S. Tezkratt, T. Barré, M. Baudoin, M. Santos, V. Di Beo, M.Nishimwe, L Wittkop.

HEPAVIH-Psy clinical centres (ward): Centre hospitalo-universitaire (CHU) Cochin (Médecine Interne et Maladies Infectieuses); CHU Pitié-Salpêtrière (Maladies Infectieuses et Tropicales); CHU Sainte-Marguerite, Marseille (Service d'Immuno-Hématologie Clinique/CISIH); CHU Purpan Toulouse (Maladies Infectieuses et Tropicales); CHU Archet, Nice (Médecine Interne); CHU Saint-Louis (Médecine Interne); CHU Saint Antoine (Maladies Infectieuses et Tropicales); CHU Necker (Maladies Infectieuses et Tropicales); ANRS CO3 Aquitaine cohort (Hôpital Saint André and Hôpital Pellegrin).

References

1. Heckman, M.A.; Weil, J.; Mejia, E.G.D. Caffeine (1, 3, 7-trimethylxanthine) in Foods: A Comprehensive Review on Consumption, Functionality, Safety, and Regulatory Matters. *J. Food Sci.* **2010**, *75*, 77–87. [CrossRef] [PubMed]
2. Gunter, M.J.; Murphy, N.; Cross, A.J.; Dossus, L.; Dartois, L.; Fagherazzi, G.; Kaaks, R.; Kühn, T.; Boeing, H.; Aleksandrova, K.; et al. Coffee Drinking and Mortality in 10 European Countries: A Multinational Cohort Study. *Ann. Intern. Med.* **2017**, *167*, 236–247. [CrossRef]
3. Alicandro, G.; Tavani, A.; La Vecchia, C. Coffee and cancer risk: A summary overview. *Eur. J. Cancer Prev.* **2017**, *26*, 424–432. [CrossRef] [PubMed]
4. Hodge, A.; Lim, S.; Goh, E.; Wong, O.; Marsh, P.; Knight, V.; Sievert, W.; De Courten, B. Coffee Intake Is Associated with a Lower Liver Stiffness in Patients with Non-Alcoholic Fatty Liver Disease, Hepatitis C., and Hepatitis B. *Nutrients* **2017**, *9*, 56. [CrossRef]
5. Morisco, F.; Lembo, V.; Mazzone, G.; Camera, S.; Caporaso, N. Coffee and Liver Health. *J. Clin. Gastroenterol.* **2014**, *48*, 87–90. [CrossRef] [PubMed]
6. Tanida, I.; Shirasago, Y.; Suzuki, R.; Abe, R.; Wakita, T.; Hanada, K.; Fukasawa, M. Inhibitory Effects of Caffeic Acid, a Coffee-Related Organic Acid, on the Propagation of Hepatitis C Virus. *Jpn. J. Infect. Dis.* **2015**, *68*, 268–275. [CrossRef] [PubMed]
7. Freedman, N.D.; Curto, T.M.; Lindsay, K.L.; Wright, E.C.; Sinha, R.; Everhart, J.E. Coffee Consumption Is Associated With Response to Peginterferon and Ribavirin Therapy in Patients With Chronic Hepatitis C. *Gastroenterology* **2011**, *140*, 1961–1969. [CrossRef] [PubMed]
8. Carrieri, M.P.; Protopopescu, C.; Marcellin, F.; Rosellini, S.; Wittkop, L.; Esterle, L.; Zucman, D.; Raffi, F.; Rosenthal, E.; Poizot-Martin, I.; et al. Protective effect of coffee consumption on all-cause mortality of French HIV-HCV co-infected patients. *J. Hepatol.* **2017**, *67*, 1157–1167. [CrossRef]
9. Yaya, I.; Marcellin, F.; Costa, M.; Morlat, P.; Protopopescu, C.; Pialoux, G.; Santos, M.E.; Wittkop, L.; Esterle, L.; Gervais, A. Impact of Alcohol and Coffee Intake on the Risk of Advanced Liver Fibrosis: A Longitudinal Analysis in HIV-HCV Coinfected Patients (ANRS CO-13 HEPAVIH Cohort). *Nutrients* **2018**, *10*, 705. [CrossRef]
10. Carrieri, M.P.; Lions, C.; Sogni, P.; Winnock, M.; Roux, P.; Mora, M.; Bonnard, P.; Salmon, D.; Dabis, F.; Spire, B. Association between elevated coffee consumption and daily chocolate intake with normal liver enzymes in HIV-HCV infected individuals: Results from the ANRS CO13 HEPAVIH cohort study. *J. Hepatol.* **2014**, *60*, 46–53. [CrossRef]
11. Carrieri, M.P.; Cohen, J.; Salmon-Ceron, D.; Winnock, M. Coffee consumption and reduced self-reported side effects in HIV-HCV co-infected patients during PEG-IFN and ribavirin treatment: Results from ANRS CO13 HEPAVIH. *J. Hepatol.* **2012**, *56*, 745–747. [CrossRef] [PubMed]
12. Hameleers, P.M.; Van Boxtel, M.J.; Hogervorst, E.; Riedel, W.J.; Houx, P.J.; Buntinx, F.; Jolles, J. Habitual caffeine consumption and its relation to memory, attention, planning capacity and psychomotor performance across multiple age groups. *Hum. Psychopharmacol. Clin. Exp.* **2000**, *15*, 573–581. [CrossRef] [PubMed]
13. Wu, L.; Sun, D.; He, Y. Coffee intake and the incident risk of cognitive disorders: A dose–response meta-analysis of nine prospective cohort studies. *Clin. Nutr.* **2017**, *36*, 730–736. [CrossRef]
14. Haller, S.; Montandon, M.-L.; Rodriguez, C.; Herrmann, F.; Giannakopoulos, P. Impact of Coffee, Wine, and Chocolate Consumption on Cognitive Outcome and MRI Parameters in Old Age. *Nutrients* **2018**, *10*, 1391. [CrossRef]

15. Liu, Q.P.; Wu, Y.F.; Cheng, H.Y.; Xia, T.; Ding, H.; Wang, H.; Wang, Z.M.; Xu, Y. Habitual coffee consumption and risk of cognitive decline/dementia: A systematic review and meta-analysis of prospective cohort studies. *Nutrition* **2016**, *32*, 628–636. [CrossRef]
16. Sheppard, D.P.; Iudicello, J.E.; Morgan, E.E.; Kamat, R.; Clark, L.R.; Avci, G.; Bondi, M.W.; Woods, S.P. Accelerated and Accentuated Neurocognitive Aging in HIV Infection. *J. Neurovirol.* **2017**, *23*, 492–500. [CrossRef]
17. Barokar, J.; McCutchan, A.; Deutsch, R.; Tang, B.; Cherner, M.; Bharti, A.R. Neurocognitive impairment is worse in HIV/HCV-coinfected individuals with liver dysfunction. *J. Neurovirol.* **2019**, *25*, 792–799. [CrossRef]
18. Fialho, R.; Pereira, M.; Bucur, M.; Fisher, M.; Whale, R.; Rusted, J. Cognitive impairment in HIV and HCV co-infected patients: A systematic review and meta-analysis. *AIDS Care* **2016**, *28*, 1481–1494. [CrossRef]
19. Vivithanaporn, P.; Nelles, K.; DeBlock, L.; Newman, S.C.; Gill, M.J.; Power, C. Hepatitis C virus co-infection increases neurocognitive impairment severity and risk of death in treated HIV/AIDS. *J. Neurol. Sci.* **2012**, *312*, 45–51. [CrossRef]
20. Vivithanaporn, P.; Maingat, F.; Lin, L.T.; Na, H.; Richardson, C.D.; Agrawal, B.; Cohen, É.A.; Jhamandas, J.H.; Power, C. Hepatitis C Virus Core Protein Induces Neuroimmune Activation and Potentiates Human Immunodeficiency Virus-1 Neurotoxicity. *PLoS ONE* **2010**, *5*, e12856. [CrossRef]
21. Loko, M.A.; Salmon, D.; Carrieri, P.; Winnock, M.; Mora, M.; Merchadou, L.; Gillet, S.; Pambrun, E.; Delaune, J.; Valantin, M.A. The French national prospective cohort of patients co-infected with HIV and HCV (ANRS CO13 HEPAVIH): Early findings, 2006–2010. *BMC Infect. Dis.* **2010**, *10*, 303. [CrossRef] [PubMed]
22. Michel, L.; Lions, C.; Winnock, M.; Lang, J.P.; Loko, M.A.; Rosenthal, E.; Marchou, B.; Valantin, M.A.; Morlat, P.; Roux, P.; et al. Psychiatric and substance use disorders in HIV/hepatitis C virus (HCV)-coinfected patients: Does HCV clearance matter? [Agence Nationale de Recherche sur le SIDA et les Hépatites Virales (ANRS) HEPAVIH CO13 cohort]. *HIV Med.* **2016**, *17*, 758–765. [CrossRef] [PubMed]
23. Osterrieth, P.A. Le test de copie d'une figure complexe; contribution a l'etude de la perception et de la memoire. *Arch. Psychol.* **1944**, *30*, 205–550.
24. Borkowski, J.G.; Benton, A.L.; Spreen, O. Word fluency and brain damage. *Neuropsychologia* **1967**, *5*, 135–140. [CrossRef]
25. Wechsler, D. Wechsler adult intelligence scale–Fourth Edition (WAIS–IV). *San Antonio TX NCS Pearson* **2008**, *22*, 816–827.
26. Reitan, R.M. Validity of the Trail Making Test as an indicator of organic brain damage. *Percept. Mot. Ski.* **1958**, *8*, 271–276. [CrossRef]
27. Corrigan, J.D.; Hinkeldey, N.S. Relationships between Parts A and B of the Trail Making Test. *J. Clin. Psychol.* **1987**, *43*, 402–409. [CrossRef]
28. Antinori, A.; Arendt, G.; Becker, J.T.; Brew, B.J.; Byrd, D.A.; Cherner, M.; Clifford, D.B.; Cinque, P.; Epstein, L.G.; Goodkin, K. Updated research nosology for HIV-associated neurocognitive disorders. *Neurology* **2007**, *69*, 1789–1799. [CrossRef]
29. Bragança, M.; Marinho, M.; Marques, J.; Moreira, R.; Palha, A.; Marques-Teixeira, J.; Esteves, M. The influence of espresso coffee on neurocognitive function in HIV-infected patients. *AIDS Care* **2016**, *28*, 1149–1153. [CrossRef]
30. Nehlig, A.; Daval, J.L.; Debry, G. Caffeine and the central nervous system: Mechanisms of action, biochemical, metabolic and psychostimulant effects. *Brain Res. Rev.* **1992**, *17*, 139–170. [CrossRef]
31. Koppelstaetter, F.; Poeppel, T.D.; Siedentopf, C.M.; Ischebeck, A.; Kolbitsch, C.; Mottaghy, F.M.; Felber, S.R.; Jaschke, W.R.; Krause, B.J. Caffeine and Cognition in Functional Magnetic Resonance Imaging. *J. Alzheimer's Dis.* **2010**, *20*, 71–84. [CrossRef] [PubMed]
32. Cysneiros, R.M.; Farkas, D.; Harmatz, J.S.; von Moltke, L.L.; Greenblatt, D.J. Pharmacokinetic and Pharmacodynamic Interactions Between Zolpidem and Caffeine. *Clin. Pharmacol. Ther.* **2007**, *82*, 54–62. [CrossRef] [PubMed]
33. Gutiérrez-Grobe, Y.; Chávez-Tapia, N.; Sánchez-Valle, V.; Gavilanes-Espinar, J.G.; Ponciano-Rodríguez, G.; Uribe, M.; Méndez-Sánchez, N. High coffee intake is associated with lower grade nonalcoholic fatty liver disease: The role of peripheral antioxidant activity. *Ann. Hepatol.* **2012**, *11*, 350–355. [CrossRef]
34. Liang, N.; Kitts, D.D. Role of Chlorogenic Acids in Controlling Oxidative and Inflammatory Stress Conditions. *Nutrients* **2016**, *8*, 16. [CrossRef]

35. Ivanov, A.V.; Bartosch, B.; Isaguliants, M.G. Oxidative Stress in Infection and Consequent Disease. Available online: https://www.hindawi.com/journals/omcl/2017/3496043/ (accessed on 4 August 2020).
36. Yoshimura, H. The Potential of Caffeine for Functional Modification from Cortical Synapses to Neuron Networks in the Brain. *Curr. Neuropharmacol.* **2005**, *3*, 309–316. [CrossRef]

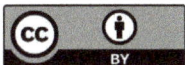
© 2020 by the authors. Licensee MDPI, Basel, Switzerland. This article is an open access article distributed under the terms and conditions of the Creative Commons Attribution (CC BY) license (http://creativecommons.org/licenses/by/4.0/).

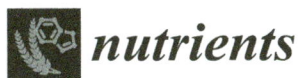

Article

The Effect of Coffee and Caffeine Consumption on Patients with Multiple Sclerosis-Related Fatigue

Lena Herden and Robert Weissert *

Department of Neurology of the University of Regensburg Hospital, D-93053 Regensburg, Germany; lena.herden@stud.uni-regensburg.de
* Correspondence: robert.weissert@ukr.de

Received: 23 June 2020; Accepted: 25 July 2020; Published: 28 July 2020

Abstract: *Background*: Coffee and caffeine are considered to have beneficial effects in patients with multiple sclerosis (MS), an autoimmune disease of the central nervous system (CNS) that can lead to disability and chronic fatigue. *Methods*: In the present study the preference in terms of coffee and caffeine consumption in patients with MS was assessed. In total the opinions of 124 MS patients were explored with a questionnaire, which was developed to investigate the consumption behavior and associated beneficial and harmful effects of coffee and caffeine concerning symptoms of fatigue. *Results*: Our study showed that 37.1% of the included patients experience severe symptoms of fatigue. In our cohort, fatigue was not related to age, type of diagnosis or duration of the disease. The effects of coffee did not differ between MS patients with and without fatigue. Very few side effects linked to coffee consumption were reported, and we could demonstrate that coffee consumption had no negative impact on quality of sleep. A positive effect on everyday life was observed particularly among patients with a mid-level expanded disability status scale (EDSS). The strongest effects of coffee consumption were observed regarding a better ability to concentrate while fulfilling tasks, an expanded attention span and a better structured daily routine. *Conclusions*: Since coffee showed no severe side effects and in the absence of an effective fatigue therapy, coffee consumption might be a therapeutic approach for selected patients with MS-related fatigue.

Keywords: coffee; caffeine; multiple sclerosis; fatigue

1. Introduction

Multiple sclerosis (MS) is considered a chronic inflammatory and degenerating disease of the central nervous system (CNS), which often first manifests in early adulthood. What is known so far is that MS is most likely an autoimmune disease with demyelinating processes, which occur in the white and grey matter of the CNS [1]. These lesions, which are visible on nuclear magnetic resonance (NMR) imaging, lead to reduced nerve conductivity in the course of the disease. It is assumed that auto-reactive, myelin-specific T cells are activated in the periphery due to faulty tolerance development. They enter the brain and trigger an immune response by binding to "their" antigen, which leads to an inflammatory process [2]. MS is not a curable disease, but its course can be very positively influenced by medication. MS can manifest in a variety of disease courses. About 85% of patients first develop relapsing-remitting MS (RRMS), which can evolve into secondary progressive MS (SPMS) over a longer period [3]. The other 15% of patients initially develop primary progressive MS (PPMS). The respective diagnosis is made based on the McDonald Criteria [4]. The variety of possible symptoms of MS differs depending on the location and size of the lesions. Common symptoms include visual disturbances, paresis, bladder dysfunction, gait disturbances, as well as paresthesia and hypoesthesia. Another common symptom of MS is fatigue. Fatigue is an extreme exhaustion that usually occurs very suddenly and cannot be compared to being tired [5]. In 2007, the symptoms of patients with MS-related fatigue were examined in detail and a standardized definition was formulated. They summarized that "fatigue is defined as a reversible motor and cognitive impairment, with reduced motivation and the desire to rest. It either occurs spontaneously, or is triggered by mental or physical stress, infection or after eating. Improvement can be achieved by sleeping or resting without sleep. Fatigue can occur at any time but is usually worse in the afternoon. In MS, fatigue symptoms can occur daily, are usually present for years, and are much more severe compared to fatigue caused by other diseases" [6]. More than 70% of people with MS report symptoms of fatigue [7]. Different studies have shown that 14% of patients perceive fatigue as their worst symptom, 55% of patients report it as one of the symptoms that affects them most [8]. Patients suffering from fatigue often do not manage to get through a whole day without taking breaks. As a result, their ability to work is particularly severely affected [5]. Fatigue is also one of the main causes of unemployment or early retirement in people with MS [9–12]. As therapy, some substances have been tested for their effectiveness. Even a meta-analysis of many pharmacotherapeutic approaches could not define clear therapeutic recommendations [13]. Accordingly, non-drug therapy and comprehensive education about a healthy lifestyle as a therapeutic approach is becoming important, such as the impact of sport and regular physical activity as a preventive measure [13,14]. Therefore, it should be considered whether and to what extent simple therapy approaches, such as coffee or especially caffeine might be an interesting subject for further research. Coffee consists of more than 1000 ingredients, of which caffeine is by far the best studied one. The effect of caffeine is not restricted to a stimulation of the CNS; a short-term improvement of attention, as well as a positive effect on cognition and memory have also been observed [15]. Caffeine reaches its maximum plasma concentration after 20–30 min after intake [16], and caffeine from coffee in particular is absorbed faster as compared to other sources [17]. Due to its hydrophobic structure, caffeine can pass the blood-brain barrier and thus also act on receptors in the brain [16,18]. Its main effect, as a psychostimulant of the CNS, is based on its ability to lower adenosine secretion as an adenosine antagonist on adenosine receptors in certain areas of the brain [19]. Adenosine signals the body that much energy is consumed and causes self-regulation of the body, by having a calming and inhibitory effect via various neurotransmitter-induced pathways [20]. By blocking the adenosine receptors, caffeine prevents adenosine from acting and conversely has a stimulating effect on the CNS. It improves cognitive function, reaction time, concentration, and alertness, as well as motor coordination [21]. The negative reputation of coffee has been reversed in recent years, a coffee consumption of up to four cups per day (a 150 mL, i.e., a total of about 400–500 mg of caffeine) can be considered harmless to human health [22]. Since coffee and caffeine have already shown a positive effect on daytime sleepiness in Parkinson's disease [23], the question is whether this effect can also alleviate the symptoms of fatigue in MS patients. The connection between caffeine and MS-related fatigue has not been investigated yet. The present study intends to evaluate the possible effect of coffee or caffeine on fatigue as well as on the everyday life of the patients. The aim of this work is to better understand the effect of coffee by means of patient interviews and evaluation of further clinical data. Of interest is the possibility of characterizing a specific group of patients for whom consumption of coffee or caffeine could be indicated as a therapeutic approach.

2. Methods

2.1. Participants

Questionnaires were distributed to the patients during the weekly consultation hours for MS patients at the Department of Neurology of the University of Regensburg Hospital between March 2018 and September 2018. Inclusion criteria were a confirmed diagnosis of MS and age of majority (18 years). Patients with initial diagnoses, who presented themselves for the first time, were also included. All patients who presented during this period were properly informed about the study and asked to participate. Those who signed the informed consent form were included in the study. The responsible ethics committee of the University of Regensburg approved this retrospective study by data collection in February 2018 (file number 18-890-101).

2.2. Data Collection

A short, retrospective questionnaire was prepared to provide an overview of coffee consumption habits in patients with MS. A five-page, simply structured questionnaire was designed, asking about the respective preferences of coffee intake. It focuses on fatigue and behavior concerning coffee consumption. To better classify the patients' fatigue, we used the Fatigue Severity Score (FSS) [11], as well as the Epworth sleepiness scale (ESS) [24]. Furthermore, patients were specifically asked about problems falling asleep and/or sleeping through the night. The number of hours awake, as well as the frequency of waking up at night were recorded. In addition, the patients were asked to assess whether they felt fit and well rested in the morning or not. Regarding the behavior of coffee consumption, we focused on the reasons why patients do not drink coffee and the possible associated side effects. They were asked what kind of coffee they prefer or which other caffeinated drinks they consume. This, together with the average number of cups consumed per day, as well as the average time of their coffee consumption should provide a better overview. The times of coffee intake were marked on a timeline. Finally, patients should indicate whether, and if so, what subjective effect of coffee they perceive, on what occasions or for what reasons they primarily consumed coffee and what relevance coffee has in their everyday life. Additionally, all patients were neurologically examined and further clinical data, such as the Expanded Disability Status Score (EDSS) [25] were collected. Data about the course of the disease were supplemented from the files.

2.3. Data Analysis

Data were coded using SPSS version 25.0.0.1, IBM corporation (Armonk, NY, USA), 2019. Descriptive statistics included the calculation, the distribution, the median and the mean with standard deviation. Differences between groups were presented in cross tables and analyzed by the chi-square-test for categorical variables or t-test for all metric variables. A p-value of <0.05 was considered significant. Concerning the presence of fatigue, we decided to set the cut-of score as $\geq$ four points in the FSS, as originally defined by the authors [26].

3. Results

3.1. Characteristics of Patients with MS

126 (84.6%) of the 149 questionnaires distributed in the period from March to September 2018 were completed. Two of the 126 questionnaires were filled out incompletely, resulting in a total of 124 (83.2%) completed questionnaires. There was no significant difference between the groups in terms of age, sex, disease duration, diagnosis, or behavior in coffee consumption (Table 1).

Table 1. Patient characteristics.

		All ($n = 124$)	Fatigue ($n = 46$)	No Fatigue ($n = 78$)	p-Value
Age (y)					
	Median (r)	46 (18–80)	49 (20–80)	45 (18–64)	0.116
Sex					
	Female (%)	79 (63.7)	29 (63.0)	50 (64.1)	0.906
	Male (%)	45 (36.3)	17 (37.0)	28 (35.9)	
Diagnosis					
	RRMS (%)	85 (68.5)	29 (63.0)	56 (71.8)	
	PPMS (%)	12 (9.7)	8 (17.4)	4 (5.1)	
	SPMS (%)	14 (11.3)	6 (13.0)	8 (10.3)	0.177
	Initial diagnosis (%)	6 (4.8)	2 (4.3)	5 (6.4)	
	Unspecified (%)	7 (5.6)	1 (2.2)	5 (6.4)	
Duration of disease					
	Mean (y) ± SD	10.45 ± 9.3	11.28 ± 9.4	10.15 ± 9.6	0.532
EDSS ($n = 120$)					
	Median (r)	2.5 (0–8.5)	2.0 (0–8.5)	3.0 (0–8.5)	0.003
Working status					
	Working (%)	81 (65.3)	20 (43.5)	61 (78.2)	<0.001
	Not Working (%)	43 (34.7)	26 (56.5)	17 (21.8)	
Coffee consumption (cups/day)					
	0 cups (%)	14 (11.3)	7 (15.2)	7 (9.0)	
	<2 cups (%)	48 (38.7)	15 (32.6)	33 (42.3)	0.606
	2 to 4 cups (%)	48 (38.7)	19 (41.3)	29 (37.2)	
	>4 cups (%)	14 (11.3)	5 (10.9)	9 (11.5)	

p, statistical significance; n, number; PPMS, primary progressive multiple sclerosis; r, range; RRMS, relapsing remitting multiple sclerosis; SD, standard deviation; SPMS, secondary progressive multiple sclerosis; y, year.

Nevertheless, the rate of unemployment was significantly higher in patients experiencing fatigue ($p < 0.001$). In total 34.7% ($n = 43$) were not working anymore at the time of filling out the questionnaire. Out of these 43 patients 67.4% ($n = 29$) stated to not be able to work due to their disease. This was accompanied by an increased EDSS value in the group of patients with fatigue (Table 1).

3.2. EDSS

The clinical classification of patients using the standardized EDSS resulted in a median of 2.5 ($n = 124$). For further analysis, we defined three groups based on the EDSS value (Table 2). The EDSS describes the severity of the disease and is correspondingly higher in more severely affected patients. Group-wise a significant difference in mean age could be seen. The duration of the disease since initial diagnosis also showed clear differences in the groups. There was a significant positive correlation between a higher EDSS value and the mean duration of the illness of the patients ($r = 0.493$, $p < 0.001$). Coffee consumption did not differ significantly between the groups.

Table 2. EDSS distribution of patients with MS.

		Frequency, n (%)	Mean Age (y)	Duration of Disease (y)
Groups (n/%)	EDSS = 0	37 (29.8)	34.8 ± 10.2	5.9 ± 6.1
	EDSS < 4	54 (43.6)	44.7 ± 11.6	9.1 ± 7.7
	EDSS ≥ 4	33 (26.6)	53.4 ± 11.5	17.4 ± 11.1
	Total	124 (100.0)	44.1 ± 13.1	10.6 ± 9.5

EDSS, expanded disability status scale, n, number; y, year.

3.3. Fatigue

As previously described, we formed two groups "fatigue" and "no fatigue", based on the FSS-Score. In comparison, a higher mean EDSS score in patients affected by fatigue could be shown. The group "fatigue" contained 39.1% with an EDSS score of at least four, in contrast to group "no fatigue" with 19.2% ($p = 0.003$). As described above (Table 1), the groups presented themselves as homogeneous regarding most characteristics. Based on this assumption, we compared the different effects and side effects of coffee and caffeine consumption. As presented in Table 3, the perceived effects of coffee were remarkably similar regarding fatigue.

Table 3. Effects of coffee consumption of MS patients without and with fatigue.

	No Fatigue ($n = 78$)	Fatigue ($n = 46$)
"I need the coffee to start the day fitter in the morning"		
Yes	36 (46.2%)	22 (47.8%)
No	42 (53.8%)	24 (52.2%)
"I am taking deliberate breaks"		
Yes	37 (47.4%)	19 (41.3%)
No	41 (52.6%)	27 (58.7%)
"I feel more active, so I get a little more exercise in my day"		
Yes	22 (28.2%)	9 (19.6%)
No	56 (71.8%)	37 (80.4%)
"I have more strength to assert myself in difficult situations and feel more competent in everyday life as well"		
Yes	4 (5.1%)	4 (8.7%)
No	74 (94.9%)	42 (91.3%)
"I can concentrate better and thus fulfill my tasks"		
Yes	13 (16.7%)	11 (23.9%)
No	65 (83.3%)	35 (76.1%)
"I can lengthen my attention span and listen more attentively to conversations"		
Yes	10 (12.8%)	7 (15.2%)
No	68 (87.2%)	39 (84.8%)
"I drink coffee from the "custom" of going out for coffee with someone, e.g., to get to know someone or meet a friend again"		
Yes	29 (37.2%)	13 (28.3%)
No	49 (62.8%)	33 (71.7%)
"It stimulates my digestion and I notice that I have to go to the toilet more often and more regularly"		
Yes	22 (28.2%)	11 (23.9%)
No	56 (71.8%)	35 (76.1%)
"I feel my heart beating faster or I'm shaking or sweating afterwards"		
Yes	3 (3.8%)	4 (8.7%)
No	75 (96.2%)	42 (91.3%)
"I get heartburn or stomachache"		
Yes	3 (3.8%)	1 (2.2%)
No	75 (96.2%)	45 (97.8%)
"I feel no effect"		
Yes	21 (26.9%)	11 (23.9%)
No	57 (73.1%)	35 (76.1%)

MS, multiple sclerosis; n, number.

3.4. Sleep Characteristics

In total, 34 of 124 participants (27.4%) stated that they had problems falling asleep. No significant difference in the amount of coffee consumption could be observed in those patients (Table 4).

Table 4. Characteristics of patients with MS regarding sleep.

	All	Problem	No Problem	*p*-Value
Problems with falling asleep	n = 124	n = 34	n = 90	
Lay awake (h)	0.5 ± 0.94	1.86 ± 0.93	0.4 ± 0.17	<0.001
Coffee consumption (mean in cups)	2.67 ± 2.08	2.98 ± 2.13	2.55 ± 2.06	0.316
ESS (median + range)	7 (0–18)	8.5 (0–18)	6 (0–18)	0.013
Problems with sleeping through the night	n = 124	n = 66	n = 58	
Frequency of waking up (median + range)	1 (0–4)	2 (0–4)	0 (0–1)	<0.001
Regular coffee consumption (%)	83.9	80.3	87.9	0.249
Coffee consumption (mean in cups)	2.67 ± 2.08	3.02 ± 2.33	2.28 ± 1.69	0.051

ESS, Epworth sleepiness scale; h, hours; n, number; p, statistical significance.

Furthermore, 66 of the 124 patients (53.2%) surveyed, said that they regularly woke up more than once during the night. Here as well, no significant correlation with regular coffee consumption could be found. More MS patients laid awake at night who had problems with falling asleep ($p < 0.001$) and had a higher ESS ($p = 0.013$). The frequency of waking up at night was higher in MS patients who had problems with sleeping through the night ($p < 0.001$) (Table 4). Patients with fatigue more frequently replied with "sometimes" or "no" when asked whether they felt fit and well rested in the morning (Figure 1). In contrast no impact of coffee consumption was observed (Figure 2).

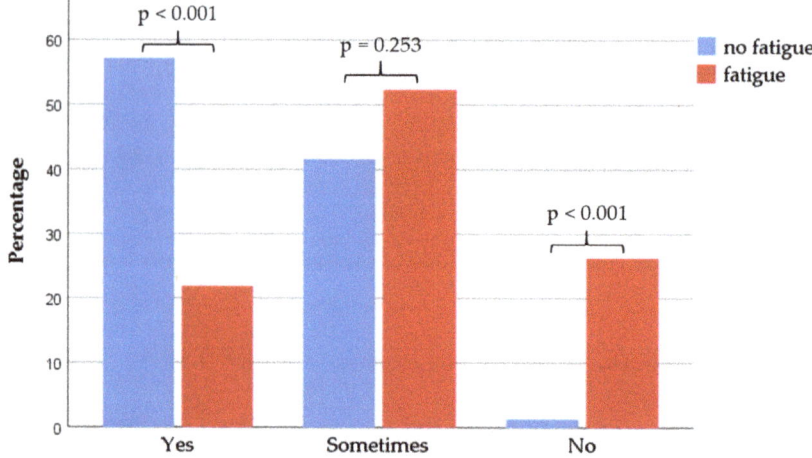

Figure 1. Distribution of sleep quality data in the two groups "fatigue" and "no fatigue". Patients with fatigue ($n = 46$) stated to feel less active and well rested in the morning ($p < 0.001$), whereas patients without fatigue ($n = 78$) felt more fit in the morning ($p < 0.001$; p, statistical significance).

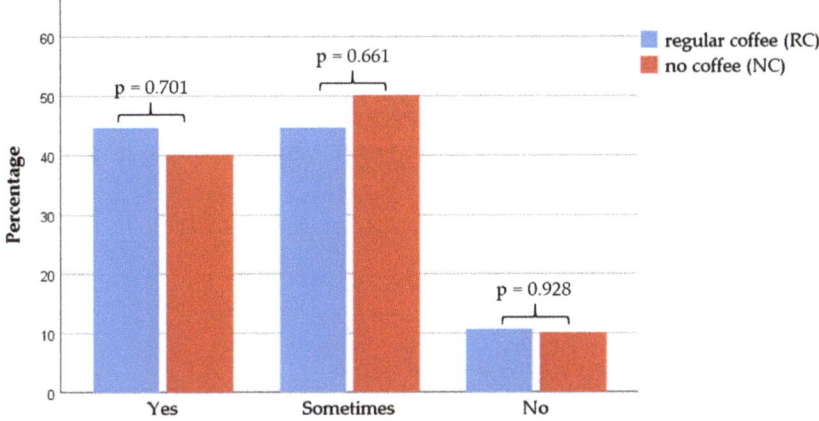

Figure 2. Distribution of sleep quality data in the groups "regular coffee" (RC) and "no coffee" (NC). In the group with RC consumption, patients with an average daily coffee intake of more than 0.5 cups ($n = 104$) are shown. In the group of NC, patients with an average daily coffee intake of lower than 0.5 cups ($n = 20$) are shown. There was no difference in sleep quality regarding coffee consumption (p, statistical significance).

3.5. Coffee Habits

The amount of coffee consumed per day varied from a minimum of one cup to a maximum of 12 cups (mean = 2.67 ± 2.08) among the patients. For further analysis we built four groups, according to their average coffee intake per day (Table 1). Only fourteen patients stated no coffee consumption at all, most of the patients have reported to consume up to four cups per day.

The small group of patients with no regular coffee consumption indicated different reasons for this. By far the most prevalent reason for not drinking coffee was a dislike for the taste of coffee (Figure 3).

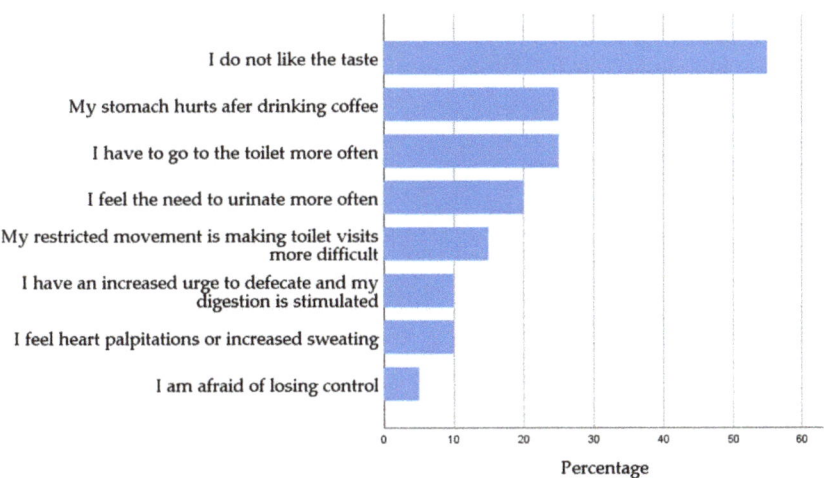

Figure 3. Reasons for patients not to drink coffee indicated in percentages.

We evaluated the average time of coffee intake in all participants (Table 5). In total 79.9% of all patients consume their coffee until 6 p.m. Only 8.1% of patients declared to consume coffee after 6 p.m. (7.3% whole day [in the morning, afternoon, and evening]; 0.8% in the morning and evening [until 12 p.m. and after 6 p.m.]). Patients with late coffee consumption showed a higher mean coffee intake of 6.6 ± 2.94 cups per day, compared to 2.3 ± 1.59 cups per day ($p = 0.001$).

Table 5. Time of coffee consumption.

Time of Coffee Consumption	n	%
In the morning (until 12 p.m.)	24	19.4
In the afternoon (12 p.m. to 6 p.m.)	5	4
In the evening (after 6 p.m.)	0	0
In the morning and afternoon (until 6 p.m.)	70	56.5
In the morning and evening (until 12 p.m. and after 6 p.m.)	1	0.8
Whole day (in the morning, afternoon, and evening)	9	7.3
Never	15	12.0

n, number; p.m., post meridiem (afternoon).

The evaluation of a possible correlation between late coffee consumption and the occurrence of sleep problem, showed no significant effect of coffee intake after 6 p.m. ($p = 0.849$).

In the questionnaire, the patients were asked to state their reasons for drinking coffee and the effects they perceived from it. The most frequently selected answer was "I need coffee in the morning so that I can start the day fitter" 46.8% ($n = 58$). While 25.8% ($n = 32$) said that they did not feel any effect from coffee consumption. The effects and side effects did not differ significantly between the groups with different amount of daily coffee intake. The least common reported effect of coffee was stomach problems, such as heartburn (3.2%, $n = 4$). The effects were examined regarding the duration of the illness, for which none of the statements showed a significant difference. Especially the patients of the group "EDSS between 0 and 4" noticed positive effects regarding concentration and attention span (Table 6).

Table 6. Effects of coffee consumption categorized based on the EDSS value.

	EDSS = 0 (n = 37)	EDSS < 4 (n = 54)	EDSS ≥ 4 (n = 33)	p-Value
"I need the coffee to start the day fitter in the morning"				
Yes	12 (32.4)	31(57.4%)	15 (45.5%)	0.079
No	25 (67.6%)	23 (42.6%)	18 (54.5%)	
"I am taking deliberate breaks"				
Yes	18 (48.6%)	29 (53.7%)	9 (27.3%)	0.049
No	19 (51.4%)	25 (46.3%)	24 (72.7%)	
"I feel more active, so I get a little more exercise in my day."				
Yes	6 (16.2%)	13 (24.1%)	12 (36.4%)	0.151
No	31 (83.8%)	41 (75.9%)	21 (63.6%)	
"I have more strength to assert myself in difficult situations and feel more competent in everyday life as well"				
Yes	2 (5.4%)	3 (5.6%)	3 (9.1%)	0.771
No	35 (94.6%)	51 (94.4%)	30 (90.0%)	
"I can concentrate better and thus fulfill my tasks"				
Yes	2 (5.4%)	18 (33.3%)	4 (12.1%)	0.002
No	35 (94.6%)	36 (66.7%)	29 (87.9%)	
"I can lengthen my attention span and listen more attentive in conversations"				
Yes	3 (8.1%)	13 (24.1%)	1 (3.0%)	0.011
No	34 (91.9%)	41 (75.9%)	32 (97.0%)	
"I drink coffee from the 'custom' of going out for coffee with someone, e.g., to get to know someone or meet a friend again"				
Yes	12 (32.4%)	18 (33.3%)	12 (36.4%)	0.936
No	25 (67.6%)	36 (66.7%)	21 (63.6%)	
"It stimulates my digestion and I notice that I have to go to the toilet more often and more regularly"				
Yes	7 (18.9%)	19 (35.2%)	7 (21.2%)	0.162
No	30 (81.1%)	35 (64.8%)	26 (78.8%)	
"I feel my heart beating faster or I'm shaking or sweating afterwards"				
Yes	3 (8.1%)	3 (5.6%)	1 (3.0%)	0.671
No	34 (91.9%)	51 (94.4%)	32 (97.0%)	
"I get heartburn or stomachache"				
Yes	3 (8.1%)	0(0.0%)	1 (3.0%)	0,101
No	34 (91.9%)	54 (100.0%)	32 (97.0%)	
"I feel no effect"				
Yes	8 (21.6%)	14 (25.9%)	10 (30.3%)	0.661
No	29 (78.4%)	40 (74.1%)	23 (69.7%)	

EDSS, expanded disability status scale; n, number; p, statistical significance.

Comparing the four groups with different daily coffee intake there were no significant differences in the EDSS values, or in ESS and FSS values. No significant correlations to age or gender of the patients could be found. No correlation was observed between the amount of coffee intake per day and the presence of a bladder voiding disorder ($p = 0.514$). The information on the current occupation in all groups was like the distribution of the entire patient collective ($p = 0.205$). Furthermore, no differences could be seen in sleep quality or distribution of difficulties falling asleep.

4. Discussion

The purpose of this study was to determine the characteristics of patients, for whom coffee consumption might have a beneficial effect on fatigue. This retrospective cohort demonstrated that 46 (37.1%) of the included patients experience severe symptoms of fatigue. The results of this study indicated that fatigue is not related to age, type of diagnosis or duration of the disease. This is different from previous studies in which fatigue was more common in progressive MS forms [27]. Fatigue had a significant impact on the patients' ability to work with 56.5% of all patients suffering from fatigue stating that they were currently not able to work. 67.4% of these were no longer working due to their disease. This is consistent with previous studies, which identified fatigue as one of the most relevant causes for unemployment in MS [10,12]. Along with this, a significant correlation between a higher EDSS value and a present fatigue could be found.

Looking at sleep quality 27.4% of all patients reported problems with falling asleep. In comparing these patients with those who state no problems, no difference in the behavior of coffee consumption could be found. Even regular late coffee consumption, after 6 p.m. showed no effect on sleep quality and most importantly on the ability to fall asleep. Analyses of the relationship between the ESS value, i.e., the daytime sleepiness and fatigue, showed a positive correlation Other studies found that prevalence of sleeping disorders in MS patients ranged from 25–54% [28–30]. Better objective sleep was not related to self-reported scores of sleep-disordered breathing and fatigue [31]. We investigated which criteria had an influence on whether patients felt fit in the morning. Interestingly in our cohort, it could not be observed that coffee consumption had any effect. Furthermore, it could be demonstrated that coffee consumption, regardless of the amount consumed had no negative influence on sleep quality. There was no association either with daytime sleepiness (ESS value) or fatigue (FSS value). This was in contradiction to the frequent assumption that coffee consumption has a negative effect on sleep. Patients with a higher FSS value showed significantly more problems with sleeping.

Coffee and especially caffeine have beneficial effects on various neurological diseases as demonstrated in different studies [32]. Caffeine has also been investigated in in vitro experiments, where it showed a significant positive effect on rodents with experimental autoimmune encephalomyelitis (EAE) [33,34]. In previous research, coffee could lead to various beneficial effects regarding cognition. The overall mood of the patients who consumed coffee was better, and they showed lower fatigue levels. Tiredness and headaches also occurred less frequently among these patients [35].

In this study it was not possible to measure the exact amount of caffeine intake of patients, due to the retrospective nature of the data collection. We evaluated the amount of consumed coffee, measured in cups per day. However, while present studies have shown that an average caffeine content of about 30–175 mg caffeine per cup (defined as 150 mL) can be assumed [36], most studies including a prospective study on the effect of espresso in daytime-sleepiness in patients with Parkinson disease [23] indicate an amount of 90–100 mg per 150 mL. Since the average coffee consumption in our cohort amounted two to three cups per day, an estimated amount of 250 to 300 mg caffeine intake can be presumed. Previous studies demonstrated that an intake of caffeine up to 400 mg can be considered safe and harmless regarding side effects on human health [22]. In total, only 20 of the patients (16.1%) stated not to drink coffee regularly, 14 of them never consume coffee. The reason most indicated for not drinking coffee was simply a dislike for the taste of coffee. The possible perceived side effects tended to play a rather minor role. No differences could be found in terms of sleeping behavior in the small group of patients reporting side effects linked to coffee consumption.

In contrast, significant differences in the perceived effects of coffee consumption depending on disease severity were observed. Especially in patients with an EDSS higher than 0, but below 4, positive effects on everyday life could be identified. These beneficial effects included an increased ability to concentrate for performing tasks, a more focused attention, and a better structure in everyday life. It can be hypothesized that these patients are able to benefit from the effects of coffee consumption due to their still preserved cognitive reserves. The important influence of the cognitive reserve in MS has been demonstrated [37–39]. There is also data, which states that this protective role is mostly restricted to memory function and does not refer to the development of the disease in general [40].

Patients with an EDSS score of more than 4 points tended to have a higher quantity of CNS lesions [41,42]. The number of lesions has been shown to be associated with cognitive dysfunction in patients with MS [43]. Lesion load, as defined by conventional NMR imaging techniques, does not correlate with fatigue [44]. However, data show a possible contribution of the gray matter on fatigue development [45]. A recent pilot study demonstrated that patients with MS may link neural resources less efficiently than healthy people, which might result in higher levels of mental fatigue [46]. Even though many studies exist on fatigue and its therapy, treatment options remain extremely limited. The most promising therapy so far has been modafinil. Unfortunately, robust positive effects of modafinil could not be reproducibly shown in every published study [47–49]. On the contrary, it has even been shown that physical activity and a well-executed fatigue management in patients with MS have the same, if not a better effect on fatigue than pharmacological therapy [50]. It must be assumed, that various factors, such as diet, activity, and the pharmacological management of MS play an important role regarding fatigue experience [1,51].

A limitation of this study is the fact that the sample size is quite small. Possibly, similar studies could be performed with larger numbers of patients with multicenter recruitment. It is further not excluded that the effects of coffee drinking are not necessarily only due to the consumption of caffeine. Coffee contains high concentrations of other potentially bioactive natural products such as trigonelline and chlorogenic acids with partly undefined effects on the human body [32]. In addition, some beverages like tea and soft drinks often contain caffeine which could influence the obtained results to some degree [32].

5. Conclusions

The lack of therapeutic options of fatigue in patients with MS is the reason why we initiated this study with the aim to evaluate a simple and maybe helpful approach for fatigue intervention in patients with MS. In our cohort, no negative impact of coffee or caffeine consumption on sleep quality could be found and no serious side effects were observed. Especially MS patients with an EDSS score higher than 0, but lower than 4, noted the strongest effect of coffee consumption on their cognitive abilities, mainly regarding a higher mental capacity and a more structured daily routine.

Author Contributions: L.H. designed the study, acquired, analyzed and interpreted the data, wrote and revised the manuscript and approved the final version of the manuscript. R.W. had the idea, designed and supervised the, analyzed and interpreted the data, wrote and revised the manuscript and approved the final version of the manuscript. L.H. and R.W. agree to be accountable for all aspects of the work in ensuring that questions related to the accuracy or integrity of any part of the work are appropriately investigated and resolved. All authors have read and agreed to the published version of the manuscript.

Funding: This research received no external funding.

Conflicts of Interest: The authors declare no conflict of interest.

References

1. Weissert, R. The immune pathogenesis of multiple sclerosis. *J. Neuroimmune Pharm.* **2013**, *8*, 857–866. [CrossRef] [PubMed]
2. Goverman, J. Autoimmune T cell responses in the central nervous system. *Nat. Rev. Immunol.* **2009**, *9*, 393–407. [CrossRef] [PubMed]
3. Lublin, F.D.; Reingold, S.C. Defining the clinical course of multiple sclerosis. *Neurology* **2014**, *83*, 278–286. [CrossRef]
4. Thompson, A.J.; Banwell, B.L.; Barkhof, F.; Carroll, W.M.; Coetzee, T.; Comi, G.; Correale, J.; Fazekas, F.; Filippi, M.; Freedman, M.S.; et al. Diagnosis of multiple sclerosis: 2017 revisions of the McDonald criteria. *Lancet Neurol.* **2018**, *17*, 162–173. [CrossRef]
5. Popp, R.F.J.; Fierlbeck, A.K.; Knüttel, H.; König, N.; Rupprecht, R.; Weissert, R.; Wetter, T.C. Daytime sleepiness versus fatigue in patients with multiple sclerosis: A systematic review on the Epworth sleepiness scale as an assessment tool. *Sleep Med. Rev.* **2017**, *32*, 95–108. [CrossRef]
6. Mills, R.J.; Young, C.A. A medical definition of fatigue in multiple sclerosis. *QJM* **2008**, *101*, 49–60. [CrossRef]
7. Iriarte, J.; Subirá, M.L.; Castro, P. Modalities of fatigue in multiple sclerosis: Correlation with clinical and biological factors. *Mult. Scler. J.* **2000**, *6*, 124–130. [CrossRef]
8. Fisk, J.D.; Pontefract, A.; Ritvo, P.G.; Archibald, C.J.; Murray, T.J. The Impact of Fatigue on Patients with Multiple Sclerosis. *Can. J. Neurol. Sci.* **1994**, *21*, 9–14. [CrossRef]

9. Hadjimichael, O.; Vollmer, T.; Oleen-Burkey, M. Fatigue characteristics in multiple sclerosis: The North American Research Committee on Multiple Sclerosis (NARCOMS) survey. *Health Qual. Life Outcomes* **2008**, *6*, 100. [CrossRef]
10. Koziarska, D.; Król, J.; Nocoń, D.; Kubaszewski, P.; Rzepa, T.; Nowacki, P. Prevalence and factors leading to unemployment in MS (multiple sclerosis) patients undergoing immunomodulatory treatment in Poland. *PLoS ONE* **2018**, *13*, e0194117. [CrossRef]
11. Krupp, L.B.; LaRocca, N.; Muir-Nash, J.; Steinberg, A. The fatigue severity scale: Application to patients with multiple sclerosis ans systemic lupus erythematosus. *Arch. Neurol.* **1989**, *46*, 1121–1123. [CrossRef] [PubMed]
12. Smith, M.M.; Arnett, P.A. Factors related to employment status changes in individuals with multiple sclerosis. *Mult. Scler.* **2005**, *11*, 602–609. [CrossRef] [PubMed]
13. Veauthier, C.; Paul, F. Therapie der Fatigue bei Multipler Sklerose: Ein Behandlungsalgorithmus. *Nervenarzt* **2016**, *87*, 1310–1321. [CrossRef] [PubMed]
14. Krupp, L.B. Fatigue in multiple sclerosis: Definition, Pathophysiology and Treatment. *CNS Drugs.* **2003**, *17*, 225–234. [CrossRef]
15. Hameleers, P. Habitual caffeine consumption and its relation to memory, attention, planning capacity and psychomotor performance across multiple age groups. *Hum. Psychopharmacol. Clin. Exp.* **2000**, *15*, 573–581. [CrossRef]
16. Bonati, M.; Latini, R.; Galletti, F.; Young, J.F.; Tognoni, G.; Garattini, S. Caffeine disposition after oral doses. *Clin. Pharmacol. Ther.* **1982**, *32*, 98–106. [CrossRef]
17. Marks, V.; Kelly, J.F. Absorption of caffeine from tea, coffee and coca cola. *Lancet* **1973**, *1*, 827. [CrossRef]
18. Blanchard, J.; Sawers, S.J.A. The absolute bioavailability of caffeine in man. *Eur. J. Clin. Pharmacol.* **1983**, *24*, 93–98. [CrossRef]
19. Fisone, G.; Borgkvist, A.; Usiello, A. Caffeine as a psychomotor stimulant: Mechanism of action. *Cell. Mol. Life Sci.* **2004**, *61*, 857–872. [CrossRef]
20. Hauher, W. Adenosin: Ein Purinnukleosid mit neuromodulatorischen Wirkungen. *E-Neuroforum* **2002**, *8*, 228–334. [CrossRef]
21. McLellan, T.M.; Caldwell, J.A.; Lieberman, H.R. A review of caffeine's effects on cognitive, physical and occupational performance. *Neurosci. Biobehav. Rev.* **2016**, *71*, 294–312. [CrossRef] [PubMed]
22. Nieber, K. The Impact of Coffee on Health. *Planta Med.* **2017**, *83*, 1256–1263. [CrossRef] [PubMed]
23. Ferreira, J.J.; Mestre, T.; Guedes, L.C.; Coelho, M.; Rosa, M.M.; Santos, A.T.; Barra, M.; Sampaio, C.; Rascol, O. Espresso Coffee for the Treatment of Somnolence in Parkinson's Disease: Results of n-of-1 Trials. *Front. Neurol.* **2016**, *7*, 455. [CrossRef]
24. Johns, M.W. A new method for measuring daytime sleepiness: The Epworth sleepiness scale. *Sleep* **1991**, *14*, 540–545. [CrossRef] [PubMed]
25. Kurtzke, J.F. Rating neurologic impairment in multiple sclerosis: An expanded disability status scale (EDSS). *Neurology* **1983**, *33*, 1444–1452. [CrossRef] [PubMed]
26. Krupp, L.B.; Coyle, P.K.; Doscher, C.; Miller, A.; Cross, A.H.; Jandorf, L.; Halper, J.; Johnson, B.; Morgante, L.; Grimson, R. Fatigue therapy in multiple sclerosis: Results of a double-blind, randomized, parallel trial of amantadine, pemoline, and placebo. *Neurology* **1995**, *45*, 1956–1961. [CrossRef]
27. Patrick, E.; Christodoulou, C.; Krupp, L.B. Longitudinal correlates of fatigue in multiple sclerosis. *Mult. Scler.* **2009**, *15*, 258–261. [CrossRef]
28. Čarnická, Z.; Kollár, B.; Šiarnik, P.; Krížová, L.; Klobučníková, K.; Turčáni, P. Sleep disorders in patients with multiple sclerosis. *J. Clin. Sleep Med.* **2015**, *11*, 553–557. [CrossRef]
29. Bamer, A.M.; Johnson, K.L.; Amtmann, D.; Kraft, G.H. Prevalence of sleep problems in individuals with multiple sclerosis. *Mult. Scler.* **2008**, *14*, 1127–1130. [CrossRef]
30. Tachibana, N.; Howard, R.S.; Hirsch, N.P.; Miller, D.H.; Moseley, I.F.; Fish, D. Sleep problems in multiple sclerosis. *Eur. Neurol.* **1994**, *34*, 320–323. [CrossRef]
31. Sadeghi Bahmani, D.; Gonzenbach, R.; Motl, R.W.; Bansi, J.; Rothen, O.; Niedermoser, D.; Gerber, M.; Brand, S. Better Objective Sleep Was Associated with Better Subjective Sleep and Physical Activity; Results from an Exploratory Study under Naturalistic Conditions among Persons with Multiple Sclerosis. *Int. J. Environ. Res. Public Health* **2020**, *17*, 3522. [CrossRef] [PubMed]

32. Herden, L.; Weissert, R. The Impact of Coffee and Caffeine on Multiple Sclerosis Compared to Other Neurodegenerative Diseases. *Front. Nutr.* **2018**, *5*, 133. [CrossRef] [PubMed]
33. Chen, G.Q.; Chen, Y.Y.; Wang, X.S.; Wu, S.Z.; Yang, H.M.; Xu, H.Q.; He, J.C.; Wang, X.T.; Chen, J.F.; Zheng, R.Y. Chronic caffeine treatment attenuates experimental autoimmune encephalomyelitis induced by guinea pig spinal cord homogenates in Wistar rats. *Brain Res.* **2010**, *1309*, 116–125. [CrossRef] [PubMed]
34. Wang, T.; Xi, N.-n.; Chen, Y.; Shang, X.-f.; Hu, Q.; Chen, J.-F.; Zheng, R.-y. Chronic caffeine treatment protects against experimental autoimmune encephalomyelitis in mice: Therapeutic window and receptor subtype mechanism. *Neuropharmacology* **2014**, *86*, 203–211. [CrossRef] [PubMed]
35. Haskell-Ramsay, C.F.; Jackson, P.A.; Forster, J.S.; Dodd, F.L.; Bowerbank, S.L.; Kennedy, D.O. The Acute Effects of Caffeinated Black Coffee on Cognition and Mood in Healthy Young and Older Adults. *Nutrients* **2018**, *10*, 1386. [CrossRef] [PubMed]
36. Gilbert, R.M.; Marshman, J.A.; Schwieder, M.; Berg, R. Caffeine content of beverages as consumed. *Can. Med. Assoc. J.* **1976**, *114*, 205–208.
37. Luerding, R.; Gebel, S.; Gebel, E.M.; Schwab-Malek, S.; Weissert, R. Influence of Formal Education on Cognitive Reserve in Patients with Multiple Sclerosis. *Front. Neurol.* **2016**, *7*, 46. [CrossRef]
38. Santangelo, G.; Altieri, M.; Gallo, A.; Trojano, L. Does cognitive reserve play any role in multiple sclerosis? A meta-analytic study. *Mult. Scler. Relat. Disord.* **2019**, *30*, 265–276. [CrossRef]
39. Artemiadis, A.; Bakirtzis, C.; Ifantopoulou, P.; Zis, P.; Bargiotas, P.; Grigoriadis, N.; Hadjigeorgiou, G. The role of cognitive reserve in multiple sclerosis: A cross-sectional study in 526 patients. *Mult. Scler. Relat. Disord.* **2020**, *41*, 102047. [CrossRef]
40. Ifantopoulou, P.; Artemiadis, A.K.; Bakirtzis, C.; Zekiou, K.; Papadopoulos, T.-S.; Diakogiannis, I.; Hadjigeorgiou, G.; Grigoriadis, N.; Orologas, A. Cognitive and brain reserve in multiple sclerosis—A cross-sectional study. *Mult. Scler. Relat. Disord.* **2019**, *35*, 128–134. [CrossRef]
41. Fisniku, L.K.; Brex, P.A.; Altmann, D.R.; Miszkiel, K.A.; Benton, C.E.; Lanyon, R.; Thompson, A.J.; Miller, D.H. Disability and T2 MRI lesions: A 20-year follow-up of patients with relapse onset of multiple sclerosis. *Brain* **2008**, *131*, 808–817. [CrossRef] [PubMed]
42. Luchetti, S.; Fransen, N.L.; van Eden, C.G.; Ramaglia, V.; Mason, M.; Huitinga, I. Progressive multiple sclerosis patients show substantial lesion activity that correlates with clinical disease severity and sex: A retrospective autopsy cohort analysis. *Acta Neuropathol.* **2018**, *135*, 511–528. [CrossRef] [PubMed]
43. Shinoda, K.; Matsushita, T.; Nakamura, Y.; Masaki, K.; Sakai, S.; Nomiyama, H.; Togao, O.; Hiwatashi, A.; Niino, M.; Isobe, N.; et al. Contribution of cortical lesions to cognitive impairment in Japanese patients with multiple sclerosis. *Sci. Rep.* **2020**, *10*, 5228. [CrossRef] [PubMed]
44. Bakshi, R.; Miletich, R.S.; Henschel, K.; Shaikh, Z.A.; Janardhan, V.; Wasay, M.; Stengel, L.M.; Ekes, R.; Kinkel, P.R. Fatigue in multiple sclerosis: Cross-sectional correlation with brain MRI findings in 71 patients. *Neurology* **1999**, *53*, 1151–1153. [CrossRef] [PubMed]
45. Niepel, G.; Tench, C.R.; Morgan, P.S.; Evangelou, N.; Auer, D.P.; Constantinescu, C.S. Deep gray matter and fatigue in MS: A T1 relaxation time study. *J. Neurol.* **2006**, *253*, 896–902. [CrossRef]
46. Chen, M.H.; Wylie, G.R.; Sandroff, B.M.; Dacosta-Aguayo, R.; DeLuca, J.; Genova, H.M. Neural mechanisms underlying state mental fatigue in multiple sclerosis: A pilot study. *J. Neurol.* **2020**, *267*, 2372–2382. [CrossRef]
47. Möller, F.; Poettgen, J.; Broemel, F.; Neuhaus, A.; Daumer, M.; Heesen, C. HAGIL (Hamburg Vigil Study): A randomized placebo-controlled double-blind study with modafinil for treatment of fatigue in patients with multiple sclerosis. *Mult. Scler.* **2011**, *17*, 1002–1009. [CrossRef]
48. Stankoff, B.; Waubant, E.; Confavreux, C.; Edan, G.; Debouverie, M.; Rumbach, L.; Moreau, T.; Pelletier, J.; Lubetzki, C.; Clanet, M. Modafinil for fatigue in MS: A randomized placebo-controlled double-blind study. *Neurology* **2005**, *64*, 1139–1143. [CrossRef] [PubMed]
49. Lange, R.; Volkmer, M.; Heesen, C.; Liepert, J. Modafinil effects in multiple sclerosis patients with fatigue. *J. Neurol.* **2009**, *256*, 645–650. [CrossRef]

50. Asano, M.; Finlayson, M.L. Meta-analysis of three different types of fatigue management interventions for people with multiple sclerosis: Exercise, education, and medication. *Mult. Scler. Int.* **2014**, *2014*, 798285. [CrossRef]
51. Steimer, J.; Weissert, R. Effects of Sport Climbing on Multiple Sclerosis. *Front. Physiol.* **2017**, *8*, 1021. [CrossRef] [PubMed]

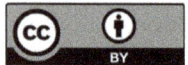

© 2020 by the authors. Licensee MDPI, Basel, Switzerland. This article is an open access article distributed under the terms and conditions of the Creative Commons Attribution (CC BY) license (http://creativecommons.org/licenses/by/4.0/).

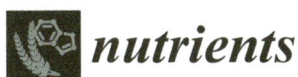 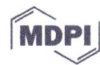

Article

The Effect of Caffeine on the Risk and Progression of Parkinson's Disease: A Meta-Analysis

Chien Tai Hong [1,2], Lung Chan [1,2,*,†] and Chyi-Huey Bai [3,4,5,*,†]

1. Department of Neurology, Shuang-Ho Hospital, Taipei Medical University, New Taipei 23561, Taiwan; ct.hong@tmu.edu.tw
2. Department of Neurology, School of Medicine, College of Medicine, Taipei Medical University, Taipei 11031, Taiwan
3. School of Public Health, College of Public Health, Taipei Medical University, Taipei 11031, Taiwan
4. Department of Public Health, School of Medicine, College of Medicine, Taipei Medical University, Taipei 11031, Taiwan
5. Nutrition Research Center, Taipei Medical University Hospital, Taipei 11031, Taiwan
* Correspondence: 12566@s.tmu.edu.tw (L.C.); baich@tmu.edu.tw (C.-H.B.); Tel.: +886-2-22490088 (ext. 8112) (L.C.); +886-2-2736-1661 (ext. 6510) (C.-H.B.)
† Both authors contributed equally to this study.

Received: 6 May 2020; Accepted: 22 June 2020; Published: 22 June 2020

Abstract: Coffee and caffeine are speculated to be associated with the reduced risk of Parkinson's disease (PD). The present study aimed to investigate the disease-modifying potential of caffeine on PD, either for healthy people or patients, through a meta-analysis. The electronic databases were searched using terms related to PD and coffee and caffeinated food products. Articles were included only upon fulfillment of clear diagnostic criteria for PD and details regarding their caffeine content. Reference lists of relevant articles were reviewed to identify eligible studies not shortlisted using these terms. In total, the present study enrolled 13 studies, nine were categorized into a healthy cohort and the rest into a PD cohort. The individuals in the healthy cohort with regular caffeine consumption had a significantly lower risk of PD during follow-up evaluation (hazard ratio (HR) = 0.797, 95% CI = 0.748–0.849, $p < 0.001$). The outcomes of disease progression in PD cohorts included dyskinesia, motor fluctuation, symptom onset, and levodopa initiation. Individuals consuming caffeine presented a significantly lower rate of PD progression (HR = 0.834, 95% CI = 0.707–0.984, $p = 0.03$). In conclusion, caffeine modified disease risk and progression in PD, among both healthy individuals or those with PD. Potential biological benefits, such as those obtained from adenosine 2A receptor antagonism, may require further investigation for designing new drugs.

Keywords: caffeine; Parkinson's disease; risk; progression; meta-analysis

1. Introduction

Parkinson's disease (PD) is one of the most common neurodegenerative diseases, second only to Alzheimer's disease (AD). Risk factors for PD include genetic mutations, environmental toxins, and lifestyle [1]. An epidemiological study reported some protective factors for PD worldwide, such as female sex, physical activity, and smoking [2]. The consumption of coffee or caffeinated food is associated with the reduction of the risk of PD. Patients with PD are less frequent habitual consumers of caffeinated food [3,4]. The consumption of either tea or coffee exhibited similar effects on the reduction of the risk of PD [5]. In a similar manner, the protective effect of coffee was also noted in dementia and AD [6], whereby caffeine reversed the cognitive impairment and decreased the amyloid burden in transgenic AD mice model [7].

Caffeine is an adenosine A2A receptor antagonist [8]. Different types of adenosine receptors (A1, A2A, A2B, and A3) are widely distributed in the brain. Adenosine A2A receptors are coupled with G-proteins and exclusively expressed in dopaminergic neurons. The activation of adenosine A2A receptors causes an increase in intracellular cAMP levels and the extracellular release of glutamate, resulting in neural excitotoxicity [9]. The neuroprotective effects of caffeine involved the antagonism of the adenosine A2A receptor, down-regulating the down streaming phosphatidylinositol 3-kinase (PI3K)/protein kinase B (AKT) signaling pathway, and avoiding excessive calcium releasing-related neurotoxicity and neuroinflammation [10], which has been experimentally demonstrated in several in vivo models of PD [11–14].

Whether caffeine can reduce the risk and halt the progression of PD remains unclear. In large-scale cohort studies, caffeine consumption was inconsistently associated with a low risk of PD during follow-up [15–18]. However, among patients diagnosed with PD, the administration of caffeine tablets did not modify the disease course [19]. Furthermore, caffeine metabolism varies among patients with PD [20], thus potentially resulting in inconsistent protective effects. This study investigated the association between caffeine and PD progression. Considering disease progression was the primary temporal outcome, only cohort studies rather than case–control studies were included herein, because case–control studies cannot delineate this temporal association.

2. Methods

2.1. Literature Search Strategy

All relevant articles published in English between 1 January 1990, and 31 December 2019 were identified by searching PubMed, BioMed Central, Medline, and Google Scholar. Details regarding search terms are provided in supplementary data. Moreover, the reference lists of relevant articles were reviewed to identify eligible studies not derived using these search terms.

2.2. Inclusion and Exclusion of the Literature

Inclusion criteria were as follows: (1) clear definition of PD diagnosis; (2) clear definition regarding the quantity of caffeine, coffee, or tea consumption; (3) cohort study published as an original article, case series, or letter to the editor; (4) sample size of ≥50 individuals; and (5) published in English. After excluding nonqualified studies, 19 studies were entered the full-article assessment process and another 6 studies were excluded due to the lack of hazard ratio. Finally, 13 studies were included into qualitative synthesis. We further segregated the remaining 13 studies into two categories: the healthy cohort including studies ($n = 9$) that recruited individuals without previous diagnosis of PD, wherein PD diagnosis was performed during follow-up evaluation, and the PD cohort including studies ($n = 4$) on individuals with PD already presenting motor symptoms, wherein PD progression was monitored. The selection process is illustrated in Figure 1.

2.3. Data Extraction

The following data were extracted: name of the first author; year of publication; country and location; study design; the original cohort or clinical trial; the starting time of cohort; diagnostic criteria for PD; the assessment of caffeine consumption; the amount of coffee or caffeine consumption; mean follow-up period of time; the outcome assessment time; and the outcome of the PD progression. All data were independently reviewed by three investigators (BAI CH, Hong CT, and Chan L), and conflicts were resolved through a consensus. Assessing of quality of all studies were done by three investigators (BAI CH, Hong CT, and Chan L) based on the Newcastle–Ottawa Scale. The study was recommended (>7) by at least 2 investigators into this study as candidate. Data from these 13 candidate studies were independently extracted by two investigators (BAI CH and FAN YC).

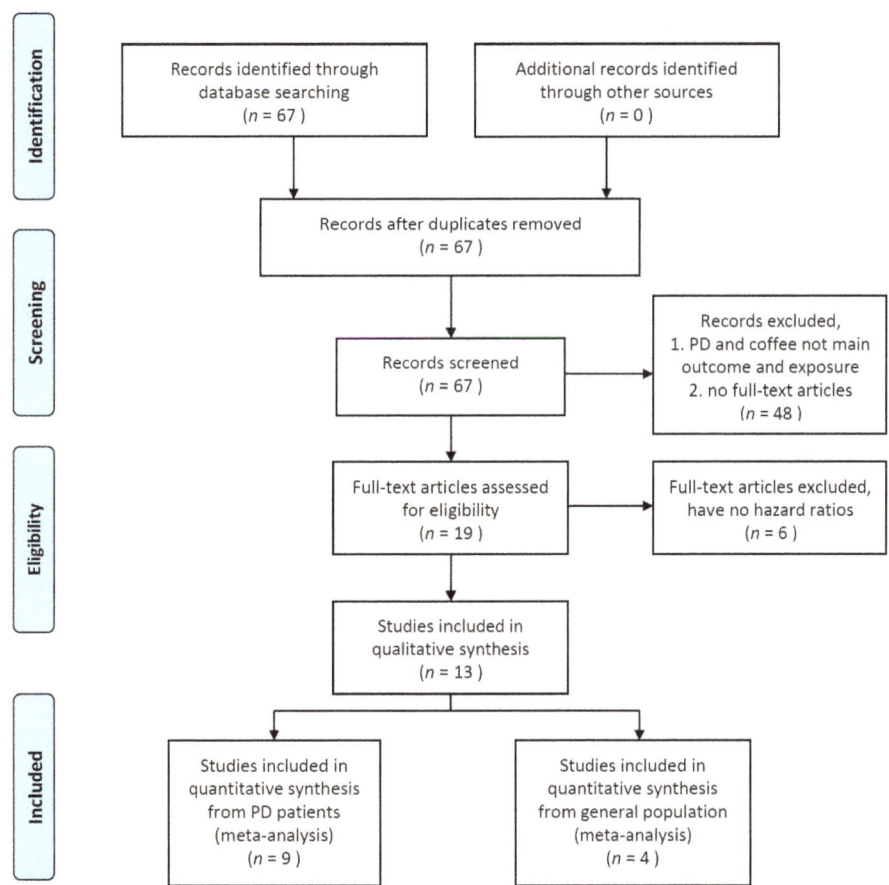

Figure 1. A schematic representation of the literature search.

2.4. Statistical Analysis

The hazard ratio (HR) was determined, and 95% CIs were calculated on the basis of a binomial assumption. I^2 was used to assess heterogeneity across studies. All statistical analyses were performed using SAS software (version 9.3; Statistical Analysis System, SAS.com, USA). All reported probability (p) values were two-sided, with $p < 0.05$ considered statistically significant.

2.5. Data Availability

The present study was a meta-analysis and all the studies enrolled into analysis can be found through the provided searching strategy.

3. Results

Among the nine studies included in the healthy cohort (Table 1) [15–18,21–25], five were conducted in the United States, three in Scandinavia, and one in Singapore. Some studies were large-scale, long-term, population-based epidemiological cohort studies, and the others were specific for individuals with certain characteristics (nurses, healthcare professions, twins, and ancestry of migrants). Caffeine consumption was evaluated using questionnaires, either detailed and comprehensive or simple ones. Five of them investigated overall dietary habits, including coffee, tea, cola, and chocolate consumption, by using the transforming formula. The rest of them only recorded the daily consumption of coffee or tea. PD was diagnosed through either self-report and confirmation of medical records or from the national health care database. Two studies separately reported the results for men and women, and another study reported data only for women.

Most of the included studies categorized caffeine consumption as degree 4–5 based on the amount of caffeine or the number of cups of coffee per day. Only one study simply provided options of "yes" and "no" with regard to regular coffee consumption. Considering the difficulty in transforming the actual caffeine consumption among studies, this study considered results of all individuals consuming coffee at all degrees and considered the no-exposure group as a reference group to determine the HR. Overall, 43 results extracted from nine studies were analyzed herein. Caffeine consumption was significantly associated with a lower risk of developing remarkable symptoms for the diagnosis of PD during the follow-up period of time (HR = 0.797, 95% CI: 0.748–0.849, $p < 0.001$; Figure 2).

This study analyzed the effect of caffeine on patients with PD (Table 2). [26–29] Among the four studies in the PD cohort, three were conducted in European countries and one in the United States. Patients with PD were in the early stage of the disease. Similar to the healthy cohort, levels of caffeine consumption were assessed through either comprehensive questionnaires or simple questions. The four studies set different parameters for PD progression, including the initiation of levodopa, levodopa-induced motor complications, and the transition to Hoehn and Yahr stage III. The average follow-up duration ranged 4 to 10.3 years. Finally, 10 results were extracted from these 4 studies. Caffeine composition among patients at an early stage of PD significantly decelerated PD progression (HR = 0.834, 95% CI = 0.707–0.984, $p = 0.03$; Figure 3).

Table 1. List of the included cohort study.

Study Name	Country	Original Cohort (Established-Last Outcome Assessment)	n	Assessment Caffeine Consumption	Amount of Caffeine Consumption	The Diagnosis of PD
Ascherio et al. [14]	US	Health Professionals' Follow-Up Study and Nurses' Health Study (1976 and 1986/1994)	135,916	semiquantitative food-frequency questionnaire (SFFQ)	caffeine was 137 mg per cup of coffee, 47 mg per cup of tea, 46 mg per can or bottle of cola beverage, and 7 mg per serving of chocolate candy.	Self-report and medical records
Ascherio et al. [19]	US	Nurses' Health Study (1976/1998)	121,700 women	semiquantitative food-frequency questionnaire (SFFQ)	caffeine was 137 mg per cup of coffee, 47 mg per cup of tea, 46 mg per can or bottle of cola beverage, and 7 mg per serving of chocolate candy.	medical records
Grandinetti et al [18]	US	Honolulu Heart Program-Japanese and Okinawan ancestry (1965/1991)	8006 men	Questionnaires	NA	Medical records
Hu et al. [20]	FIN	Four independent cross-sectional population surveys were carried out in five geographic areas of Finland in 1982, 1987, 1992, and 1997 (1982/2002)	29,335	self-administered questionnaire	Cups of coffee	National Social Insurance Institution's Register
Liu et al. [15]	US	NIH-AARP Diet and Health Study (1995/2010)	566,401	Diet History Questionnaire	nutrient calculation: 1994–1996 US Department of Agriculture's Continuing Survey of Food Intakes by Individuals.	Interview and copy of medical records
Palacios et al. [22]	US	CPS II-Nutrition cohort (1992/2007)	184,190	Food Frequency Questionnaire	137 and 47 mg per cup of coffee and tea, respectively, 46 mg per can or bottle of cola; and 7 mg per serving of chocolate.	Interview and copy of medical records
Sääksjärvi et al. [12]	FIN	Finnish Mobile Clinic Health Examination Survey (1973/1994)	7246	self-administered, health questionnaire	Cups of coffee	National Social Insurance Institution's Register
Tan et al. [21]	SG	Singapore Chinese Health Study (1993/2005)	63,257	a validated, semiquantitative food frequency section questionnaire	Singapore Food Composition Table, a food-nutrient database that lists the levels of 96 nutritive/nonnutritive components (including caffeine) per 100 g of cooked food and beverages	Interview and linkage database to medical record
Wirdefeldt et al. [13]	SE	Swedish Twin Registry (1961 and 1973/without clear mentioning)	52,149	questionnaires	Did not provide the formula	Inpatient Discharge Register and Cause of Death Register

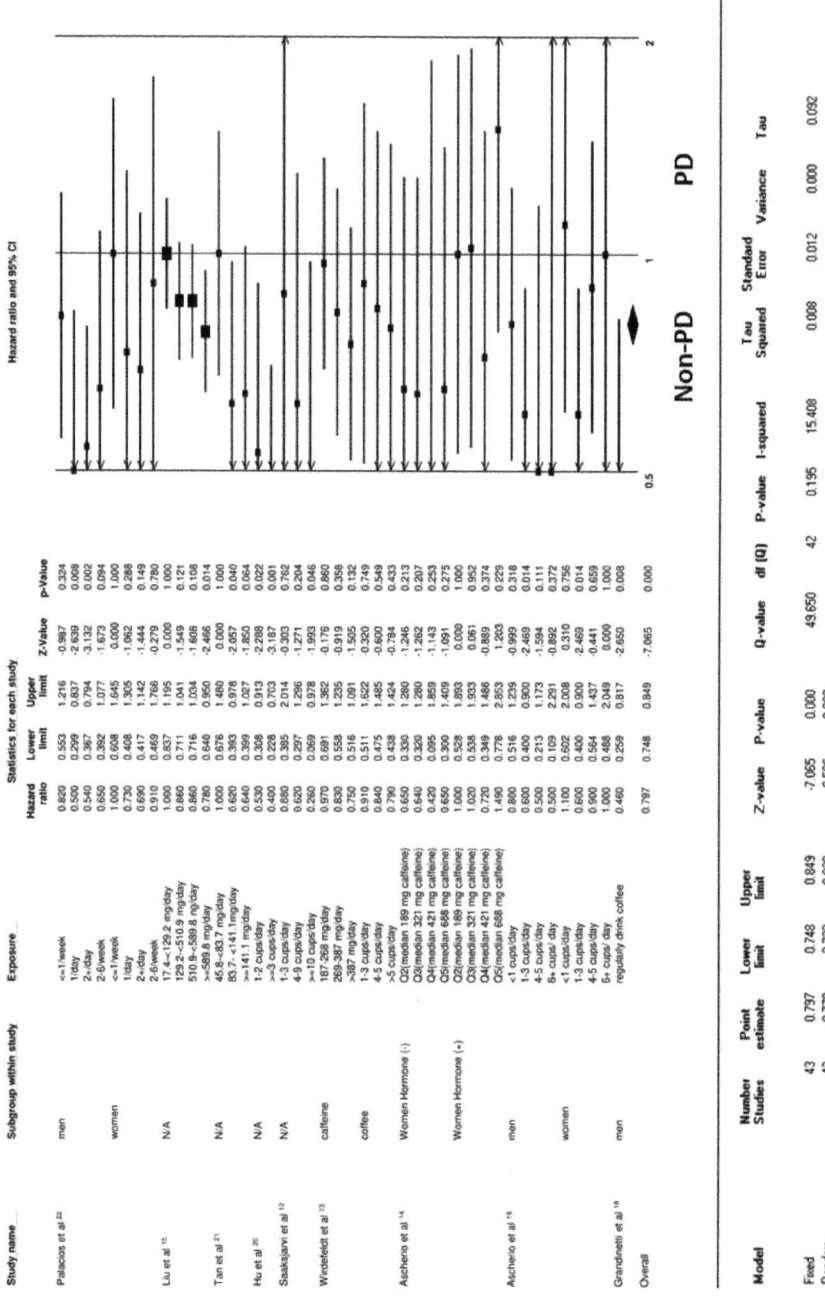

Figure 2. Forest plot illustrating the hazard ratio (HR) of Parkinson's disease (PD) among healthy individuals from cohort studies.

Table 2. List of the included studies on the progression of Parkinson's disease (PD).

Study Name	Country	Number of PD	Stage of PD	Assessment Caffeine Consumption	Amount of Caffeine Consumption	Mean Follow-Up Period of Time	Outcome as the Progression of PD
Kandinov et al. [23]	IL	278	Onset of PD motor symptoms	Interview	the number of cups of coffee per day	10.3 years	Time from onset to Hoehn and Yahr stage 3
Moccia et al. [26]	IL	79	de novo, drug naïve	Caffeine Consumption Questionnaire	i.e., Espresso 1oz = 50 mg caffeine	4 years	Starting L-dopa treatment
Scott et al. [25]	GB	183	Newly diagnosed	Verbal interview about the average level of exposure before baseline	Cups of tea: 47 mg caffeine Cup of coffee: 62 mg caffeine	59 months	1. Motor fluctuation 2. Dyskinesia
Wills et al. [24]	US	228	Early PD	questionnaire assessing both current ("in the past week") and prior ("on average over the past 5 years") caffeine intake	Coffee (85 mg caffeine/5 oz) Tea (36 mg caffeine/5 oz) Soda (45 mg caffeine/12 oz)	5.5 years	Dyskinesia

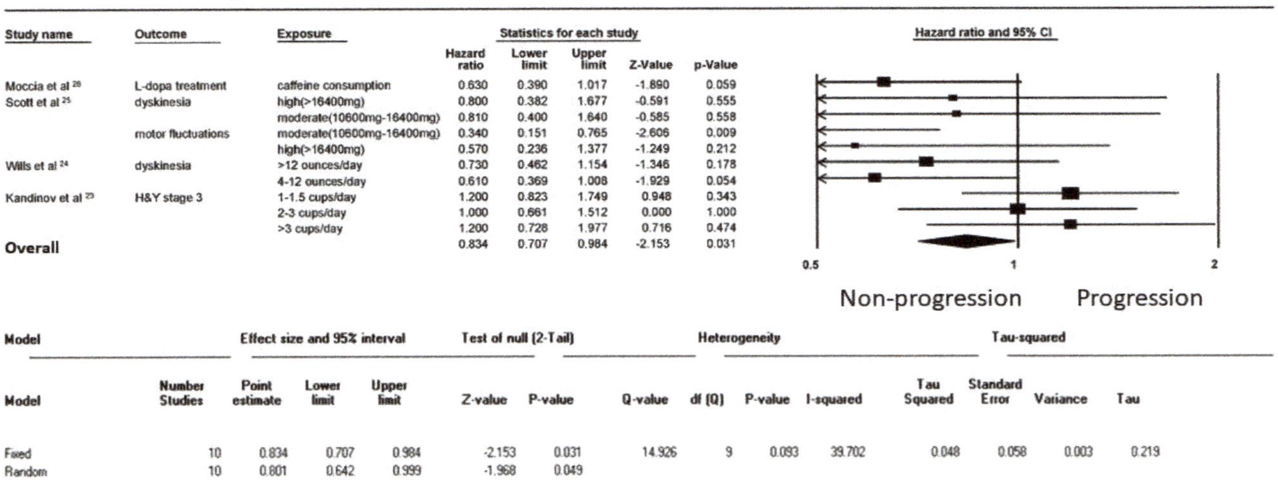

Study name	Outcome	Exposure	Statistics for each study					Test of null (2-Tail)		Hazard ratio and 95% CI
			Hazard ratio	Lower limit	Upper limit	Z-Value	p-Value	Z-value	P-value	
Moccia et al [26]	L-dopa treatment	caffeine consumption	0.630	0.390	1.017	-1.890	0.059			
Scott et al [25]	dyskinesia	high(>16400mg)	0.800	0.382	1.677	-0.591	0.555			
		moderate(10600mg-16400mg)	0.810	0.400	1.640	-0.585	0.558			
	motor fluctuations	moderate(10600mg-16400mg)	0.340	0.151	0.765	-2.606	0.009			
		high(>16400mg)	0.570	0.236	1.377	-1.249	0.212			
Wills et al [24]	dyskinesia	>12 ounces/day	0.730	0.462	1.154	-1.346	0.178			
		4-12 ounces/day	0.610	0.369	1.008	-1.929	0.054			
Kandinov et al [23]	H&Y stage 3	1-1.5 cups/day	1.200	0.823	1.749	0.948	0.343			
		2-3 cups/day	1.000	0.661	1.512	0.000	1.000			
		>3 cups/day	1.200	0.728	1.977	0.716	0.474			
Overall			0.834	0.707	0.984	-2.153	0.031	-2.153	0.031	

Model		Effect size and 95% interval			Test of null (2-Tail)		Heterogeneity				Tau-squared		
Model	Number Studies	Point estimate	Lower limit	Upper limit	Z-value	P-value	Q-value	df (Q)	P-value	I-squared	Tau Squared	Standard Error	Variance	Tau
Fixed	10	0.834	0.707	0.984	-2.153	0.031	14.926	9	0.093	39.702	0.048	0.058	0.003	0.219
Random	10	0.801	0.642	0.999	-1.968	0.049								

Figure 3. Forest plot illustrating the hazard ratio (HR) of progression of Parkinson's disease (PD) among individuals with early-stage PD.

4. Discussion

The results of this study showed that among both healthy individuals and patients with PD, caffeine consumption was significantly associated with a lower HR for the risk or progression of PD, respectively. Considering that steady neurodegeneration in PD precedes the onset of motor symptoms for decades and persists thereafter [30], caffeine was speculated to have disease-modifying potential throughout the course of the disease in this study. Compared with data obtained from case–control studies, data obtained from a combination of multiple cohorts were more likely to demonstrate the beneficial causal relationship between caffeine consumption and the risk of PD.

The potential neuroprotective effect of caffeine consumption against PD was noted on the basis of case–control epidemiological studies. Although another component in coffee, that is, eicosanoyl-5-hydroxytryptamide, is believed to protect against neurodegeneration [31], a similar association found for tea consumption further corroborated the finding that caffeine is the key protective agent in coffee [32]. Instead of psychostimulation, caffeine antagonizes the adenosine A2A receptor. In the central nervous system, the adenosine A2A receptor is exclusively expressed in dopaminergic neurons, and the activation of the adenosine A2A receptor triggers the cAMP-protein kinase A-dependent elevation of intracellular calcium and release of glutamate [33]. Excessive intracellular calcium and glutamate levels are responsible for excitotoxicity in neurodegenerative diseases, including PD [34]. The adenosine A2A receptor is also involved in neuroinflammation-mediated neuronal dysfunction and degeneration [35]. Istradefylline, an FDA-approved adenosine A2A receptor antagonist currently used for treating PD, reduces off time and improves the motor symptoms of patients with PD albeit with complications including the exacerbation of dyskinesia [36]. The neuroprotective effect of istradefylline has been further described in in vivo studies [37–39] but not in clinical.

However, large-scale cohort studies focused on the healthy population, did not consistently demonstrate the risk-reduction effect of caffeine on PD. Studies investigating the effect of caffeine on PD progression among PD patients were also not fruitful. The quantification of daily caffeine consumption is most challenging for studies intending to investigate disease-modifying effects. Except caffeine tablets, the assessment of the daily intake of caffeinated beverages and food products requires a formula for transformation. A structured dietary interview is usually necessary to obtain semi-quantitative data regarding daily caffeine intake. Considering that adults usually adhere to their dietary preferences, the interview would yield reliable data regarding long-term levels of caffeine consumption. However, coffee, tea, cola, and chocolate in different styles, brands, or countries (even areas) have different caffeine contents. Moreover, genetic polymorphism, sex, and heterogeneity in caffeine metabolism also influence the effects of caffeine [20,40,41]. Herein, most studies segregated their participants on the basis of caffeine consumption by relative gradients, thus introducing a slight variation among the enrolled studies. This relative but not absolute grouping deters inter-study comparisons and the obtainment of consistent findings.

Defining PD progression is challenging and problematic. Among healthy individuals, tremors may be visible and can be recognized early. However, the remaining cardinal motor symptoms, including rigidity, bradykinesia, and postural instability, are ambiguous. Most individuals with PD were either misdiagnosed or underwent unnecessary treatment years before reaching a final diagnosis [42]. This delay deters the assessment of disease progression for the cohort study recruiting healthy participants. Regarding disease progression among patients with PD, off-status motor function is the major parameter among clinical trials. However, responses to one-night washout are variable, and the effect of levodopa may last for 2 weeks [43]. Moreover, if the intervention itself causes certain symptomatic effects in conjunction, similar to rasagiline or caffeine, it would be challenging to distinguish between disease modification and symptomatic effect [44]. However, the onset of motor fluctuation and dyskinesia have been considered markers of disease progression among patients with PD. Nevertheless, the degeneration of dopaminergic neurons is not the only underlying factor [45]. The dosage of levodopa, the prescription of dopamine agonists, or amantadine in the early stage of the disease also influences the onset of motor complications [46–48]. One study included herein considered the initiation of levodopa treatment as a marker for disease progression, which was highly influenced by the subjective and objective conditions of patients with PD [49]. Young or old; employed, self-employed, or retired individuals and the self-expectation had an influence on levodopa initiation. These aforementioned issues deter the accurate assessment of disease progression, thus yielding inconsistent disease-modifying effects of caffeine or any other interventions.

The strength of this study is the delineation of the disease-modifying effect of caffeine on PD. The inclusion of exclusive cohort studies was superior to case–control studies owing to the potential temporal association between caffeine and PD, and the prevention of recall bias on the dietary habit. Furthermore, this study pooled all the HR of PD from moderate-to-high levels of caffeine consumption together and determined the lower limit as reference, thus eliminating the ambiguous cut-off level of daily caffeine intake in numerous studies. This blurred "beneficial dosage of caffeine" varied among studies and confounded clinicians and the population. Moreover, no remarkable J-shaped curve was previously obtained for the risk of PD and caffeine consumption, thus yielding an upper limit of permissible caffeine consumption. The present results indicate that caffeine consumption potentially alters the PD risk and progression among both healthy individuals and those with PD, and this concept is easier to pick up by general population and health professions.

This study has some limitations. First, considering the diagnosis of PD heavily relying on the development of the motor symptoms, which may be delayed for decades after the beginning of the neurodegeneration, the utilization of the diagnosis of PD as outcome assessment in the healthy cohorts may bias by either under or overvaluation. Second, variations in the levels of caffeine consumption among studies undoubtedly introduced heterogeneity among studies. Certain studies focused on caffeinated food products, and another study focused only on coffee or tea. The effect of some promising ingredients in coffee, such as eicosanoyl-5-hydroxytryptamide [31] or methylxanthine [50] had not been investigated in the present study due to the lack of standard assessment, such as the dietary questionnaires for the amount of daily intake. None of the studies included in this research focused on the effect of pure caffeine tablets, which would directly demonstrate the effects of caffeine rather than the mixed effects of caffeinated food products. Based on this information provided from the dietary questionnaires, it was not possible to define the optimal daily dosage of caffeine and the food source of caffeine. Third, instead of coffee or caffeine, some factors are known to affect the risk of PD, such as diabetes, pesticide exposure and the well-water drinking [51]. Female is well-known for the lower risk of PD, and the protective role of sex hormone is speculated [52]. However, in the present study, two cohorts separated the results between men and women, which revealed no significant heterogenicity. Meanwhile, one study also sub-grouped female participants based on the hormone replacement therapy, and there was no remarkable heterogenicity either. Moreover, several genetic and environmental factors interact with caffeine, and life style, socioeconomic status, exercise, high-fat diet and alcohol consumption may also be associated with the habitual coffee drinking. There was no clear information about those environmental factors from the included studies for the authors to adjust those possible confounding factors. Lastly, genetic polymorphism may affect the metabolism of caffeine, but to the best of our knowledge, only case-control studies were found to investigate the gene–caffeine interaction in PD [53–55], which did not fit into the inclusion criteria of the present meta-analysis.

In conclusion, this meta-analysis shows that caffeine is associated with a low risk of developing PD in healthy individuals and the deceleration in the progression of motor symptoms in patients with PD. Additional studies are required to investigate not only the optimal daily dosage and food source of caffeine for PD, but also the possible mechanisms underlying the bioprotective effects of caffeine on PD. Among individuals with PD, caffeine intake should be encouraged if adverse effects are tolerable.

Supplementary Materials: The following are available online at http://www.mdpi.com/2072-6643/12/6/1860/s1.

Author Contributions: C.T.H.: study design, article review, quality assessment, draft written. L.C.: study design, article review, quality assessment, manuscript revise. C.-H.B.: study design, article review, quality assessment, data extraction, statistical analysis, manuscript revise. Financial Disclosures of all authors: none to disclose. All authors have read and agreed to the published version of the manuscript.

Funding: The author(s) received no financial support for the research, authorship, and/or publication of this article.

Acknowledgments: We appreciated YC Fan for the help in data extraction and Shennie Tan and Yanie Tan for the proofreading and English editing.

Conflicts of Interest: The authors declare no conflict of interest.

Abbreviations

PD   Parkinson's disease
HR   hazard ratio
CI   confidence interval

References

1. Wirdefeldt, K.; Adami, H.-O.; Cole, P.; Trichopoulos, D.; Mandel, J. Epidemiology and etiology of Parkinson's disease: A review of the evidence. *Eur. J. Epidemiol.* **2011**, *26*, 1. [CrossRef]
2. Kieburtz, K.; Wunderle, K.B. Parkinson's disease: Evidence for environmental risk factors. *Mov. Disord.* **2013**, *28*, 8–13. [CrossRef]
3. Jiméanez-Jiméanez, F.J.; Mateo, D.; Giméanez-Roldan, S. Premorbid smoking, alcohol consumption, and coffee drinking habits in Parkinson's disease: A case-control study. *Mov. Disord.* **1992**, *7*, 339–344. [CrossRef] [PubMed]
4. Hellenbrand, W.; Boeing, H.; Robra, B.-P.; Seidler, A.; Vieregge, P.; Nischan, P.; Joerg, J.; Oertel, W.H.; Schneider, E.; Ulm, G. Diet and Parkinson's disease II, A possible role for the past intake of specific nutrients: Results from a self-administered food-frequency questionnaire in a case-control study. *Neurology* **1996**, *47*, 644–650. [CrossRef]
5. Tan, E.K.; Tan, C.; Fook-Chong, S.M.; Lum, S.Y.; Chai, A.; Chung, H.; Shen, H.; Zhao, Y.; Teoh, M.L.; Yih, Y.; et al. Dose-dependent protective effect of coffee, tea, and smoking in Parkinson's disease: A study in ethnic Chinese. *J. Neurol. Sci.* **2003**, *216*, 163–167. [CrossRef] [PubMed]
6. Eskelinen, M.H.; Kivipelto, M. Caffeine as a protective factor in dementia and Alzheimer's disease. *J. Alzheimers Dis.* **2010**, *20* (Suppl. S1), S167–S174. [CrossRef] [PubMed]
7. Arendash, G.W.; Mori, T.; Cao, C.; Mamcarz, M.; Runfeldt, M.; Dickson, A.; Rezai-Zadeh, K.; Tane, J.; Citron, B.A.; Lin, X.; et al. Caffeine reverses cognitive impairment and decreases brain amyloid-beta levels in aged Alzheimer's disease mice. *J. Alzheimers Dis.* **2009**, *17*, 661–680. [CrossRef] [PubMed]
8. Fredholm, B.B.; Battig, K.; Holmen, J.; Nehlig, A.; Zvartau, E.E. Actions of caffeine in the brain with special reference to factors that contribute to its widespread use. *Pharmacol. Rev.* **1999**, *51*, 83–133.
9. Carpenter, B.; Lebon, G. Human Adenosine A(2A) Receptor: Molecular Mechanism of Ligand Binding and Activation. *Front. Pharmacol.* **2017**, *8*, 898. [CrossRef]
10. Kolahdouzan, M.; Hamadeh, M.J. The neuroprotective effects of caffeine in neurodegenerative diseases. *CNS Neurosci. Ther.* **2017**, *23*, 272–290. [CrossRef]
11. Chen, J.F.; Xu, K.; Petzer, J.P.; Staal, R.; Xu, Y.H.; Beilstein, M.; Sonsalla, P.K.; Castagnoli, K.; Castagnoli, N., Jr.; Schwarzschild, M.A. Neuroprotection by caffeine and A(2A) adenosine receptor inactivation in a model of Parkinson's disease. *J. Neurosci.* **2001**, *21*, RC143. [CrossRef] [PubMed]
12. Bove, J.; Serrats, J.; Mengod, G.; Cortes, R.; Tolosa, E.; Marin, C. Neuroprotection induced by the adenosine A2A antagonist CSC in the 6-OHDA rat model of parkinsonism: Effect on the activity of striatal output pathways. *Exp. Brain Res.* **2005**, *165*, 362–374. [CrossRef] [PubMed]
13. Kelsey, J.E.; Langelier, N.A.; Oriel, B.S.; Reedy, C. The effects of systemic, intrastriatal, and intrapallidal injections of caffeine and systemic injections of A2A and A1 antagonists on forepaw stepping in the unilateral 6-OHDA-lesioned rat. *Psychopharmacology* **2009**, *201*, 529–539. [CrossRef] [PubMed]
14. Reyhani-Rad, S.; Mahmoudi, J. Effect of adenosine A2A receptor antagonists on motor disorders induced by 6-hydroxydopamine in rat. *Acta Cir. Bras.* **2016**, *31*, 133–137. [CrossRef]
15. Saaksjarvi, K.; Knekt, P.; Rissanen, H.; Laaksonen, M.A.; Reunanen, A.; Mannisto, S. Prospective study of coffee consumption and risk of Parkinson's disease. *Eur. J. Clin. Nutr.* **2008**, *62*, 908–915. [CrossRef]
16. Wirdefeldt, K.; Gatz, M.; Pawitan, Y.; Pedersen, N.L. Risk and protective factors for Parkinson's disease: A study in Swedish twins. *Ann. Neurol.* **2005**, *57*, 27–33. [CrossRef]

17. Ascherio, A.; Zhang, S.M.; Hernan, M.A.; Kawachi, I.; Colditz, G.A.; Speizer, F.E.; Willett, W.C. Prospective study of caffeine consumption and risk of Parkinson's disease in men and women. *Ann. Neurol.* **2001**, *50*, 56–63. [CrossRef]
18. Liu, R.; Guo, X.; Park, Y.; Huang, X.; Sinha, R.; Freedman, N.D.; Hollenbeck, A.R.; Blair, A.; Chen, H. Caffeine intake, smoking, and risk of Parkinson disease in men and women. *Am. J. Epidemiol.* **2012**, *175*, 1200–1207. [CrossRef]
19. Postuma, R.B.; Lang, A.E.; Munhoz, R.P.; Charland, K.; Pelletier, A.; Moscovich, M.; Filla, L.; Zanatta, D.; Romenets, S.R.; Altman, R.; et al. Caffeine for treatment of Parkinson disease: A randomized controlled trial. *Neurology* **2012**, *79*, 651–658. [CrossRef]
20. Fujimaki, M.; Saiki, S.; Li, Y.; Kaga, N.; Taka, H.; Hatano, T.; Ishikawa, K.-I.; Oji, Y.; Mori, A.; Okuzumi, A.; et al. Serum caffeine and metabolites are reliable biomarkers of early Parkinson disease. *Neurology* **2018**, *90*, e404–e411. [CrossRef] [PubMed]
21. Grandinetti, A.; Morens, D.M.; Reed, D.; MacEachern, D. Prospective study of cigarette smoking and the risk of developing idiopathic Parkinson's disease. *Am. J. Epidemiol.* **1994**, *139*, 1129–1138. [CrossRef] [PubMed]
22. Ascherio, A.; Chen, H.; Schwarzschild, M.A.; Zhang, S.M.; Colditz, G.A.; Speizer, F.E. Caffeine, postmenopausal estrogen, and risk of Parkinson's disease. *Neurology* **2003**, *60*, 790–795. [CrossRef] [PubMed]
23. Hu, G.; Bidel, S.; Jousilahti, P.; Antikainen, R.; Tuomilehto, J. Coffee and tea consumption and the risk of Parkinson's disease. *Mov. Disord.* **2007**, *22*, 2242–2248. [CrossRef] [PubMed]
24. Tan, L.C.; Koh, W.P.; Yuan, J.M.; Wang, R.; Au, W.L.; Tan, J.H.; Tan, E.K.; Yu, M.C. Differential effects of black versus green tea on risk of Parkinson's disease in the Singapore Chinese Health Study. *Am. J. Epidemiol.* **2008**, *167*, 553–560. [CrossRef]
25. Palacios, N.; Gao, X.; McCullough, M.L.; Schwarzschild, M.A.; Shah, R.; Gapstur, S.; Ascherio, A. Caffeine and risk of Parkinson's disease in a large cohort of men and women. *Mov. Disord.* **2012**, *27*, 1276–1282. [CrossRef]
26. Kandinov, B.; Giladi, N.; Korczyn, A.D. Smoking and tea consumption delay onset of Parkinson's disease. *Parkinsonism Relat. Disord.* **2009**, *15*, 41–46. [CrossRef]
27. Wills, A.-M.A.; Eberly, S.; Tennis, M.; Lang, A.E.; Messing, S.; Togasaki, D.; Tanner, C.M.; Kamp, C.; Chen, J.-F.; Oakes, D.; et al. Study, Caffeine consumption and risk of dyskinesia in CALM-PD. *Mov. Disord. Off. J. Mov. Disord. Soc.* **2013**, *28*, 380–383. [CrossRef]
28. Scott, N.W.; Macleod, A.D.; Counsell, C.E. Motor complications in an incident Parkinson's disease cohort. *Eur. J. Neurol.* **2016**, *23*, 304–312. [CrossRef]
29. Moccia, M.; Erro, R.; Picillo, M.; Vitale, C.; Longo, K.; Amboni, M.; Pellecchia, M.T.; Barone, P. Caffeine consumption and the 4-year progression of de novo Parkinson's disease. *Parkinsonism Relat. Disord.* **2016**, *32*, 116–119. [CrossRef]
30. Vingerhoets, F.J.; Snow, B.J.; Lee, C.S.; Schulzer, M.; Mak, E.; Calne, D.B. Longitudinal fluorodopa positron emission tomographic studies of the evolution of idiopathic parkinsonism. *Ann. Neurol.* **1994**, *36*, 759–764. [CrossRef]
31. Yan, R.; Zhang, J.; Park, H.J.; Park, E.S.; Oh, S.; Zheng, H.; Junn, E.; Voronkov, M.; Stock, J.B.; Mouradian, M.M. Synergistic neuroprotection by coffee components eicosanoyl-5-hydroxytryptamide and caffeine in models of Parkinson's disease and DLB. *Proc. Natl. Acad. Sci. USA* **2018**, *115*, E12053–E12062. [CrossRef] [PubMed]
32. Li, F.-J.; Ji, H.-F.; Shen, L. A meta-analysis of tea drinking and risk of Parkinson's disease. *Sci. World J.* **2012**, *2012*, 923464. [CrossRef] [PubMed]
33. Wei, C.J.; Li, W.; Chen, J.-F. Normal and abnormal functions of adenosine receptors in the central nervous system revealed by genetic knockout studies. *Biochim. Biophys. Acta (BBA) Biomembr.* **2011**, *1808*, 1358–1379. [CrossRef] [PubMed]
34. Ambrosi, G.; Cerri, S.; Blandini, F. A further update on the role of excitotoxicity in the pathogenesis of Parkinson's disease. *J. Neural. Transm.* **2014**, *121*, 849–859. [CrossRef]
35. Machado-Filho, J.A.; Correia, A.O.; Montenegro, A.B.; Nobre, M.E.; Cerqueira, G.S.; Neves, K.R.; Mda, G.N.; Cavalheiro, E.A.; Brito, G.A.; Viana, G.S. Caffeine neuroprotective effects on 6-OHDA-lesioned rats are mediated by several factors, including pro-inflammatory cytokines and histone deacetylase inhibitions. *Behav. Brain Res.* **2014**, *264*, 116–125. [CrossRef]
36. Rascol, O.; Perez-Lloret, S.; Ferreira, J.J. New treatments for levodopa-induced motor complications. *Mov. Disord.* **2015**, *30*, 1451–1460. [CrossRef]

37. Golembiowska, K.; Wardas, J.; Noworyta-Sokolowska, K.; Kaminska, K.; Gorska, A. Effects of adenosine receptor antagonists on the in vivo LPS-induced inflammation model of Parkinson's disease. *Neurotox. Res.* **2013**, *24*, 29–40. [CrossRef] [PubMed]
38. Bibbiani, F.; Oh, J.D.; Petzer, J.P.; Castagnoli, N., Jr.; Chen, J.F.; Schwarzschild, M.A.; Chase, T.N. A2A antagonist prevents dopamine agonist-induced motor complications in animal models of Parkinson's disease. *Exp. Neurol.* **2003**, *184*, 285–294. [CrossRef]
39. Grondin, R.; Bedard, P.J.; Tahar, A.H.; Gregoire, L.; Mori, A.; Kase, H. Antiparkinsonian effect of a new selective adenosine A2A receptor antagonist in MPTP-treated monkeys. *Neurology* **1999**, *52*, 1673–1677. [CrossRef]
40. Arab, L.; Biggs, M.L.; O'Meara, E.S.; Longstreth, W.T.; Crane, P.K.; Fitzpatrick, A.L. Gender differences in tea, coffee, and cognitive decline in the elderly: The Cardiovascular Health Study. *J. Alzheimers Dis.* **2011**, *27*, 553–566. [CrossRef]
41. Yang, A.; Palmer, A.A.; de Wit, H. Genetics of caffeine consumption and responses to caffeine. *Psychopharmacology* **2010**, *211*, 245–257. [CrossRef]
42. Breen, D.P.; Evans, J.R.; Farrell, K.; Brayne, C.; Barker, R.A. Determinants of delayed diagnosis in Parkinson's disease. *J. Neurol.* **2013**, *260*, 1978–1981. [CrossRef] [PubMed]
43. Fahn, S.; Oakes, D.; Shoulson, I.; Kieburtz, K.; Rudolph, A.; Lang, A.; Olanow, C.W.; Tanner, C.; Marek, K. Levodopa and the progression of Parkinson's disease. *N. Engl. J. Med.* **2004**, *351*, 2498–2508. [PubMed]
44. Olanow, C.W.; Rascol, O.; Hauser, R.; Feigin, P.D.; Jankovic, J.; Lang, A.; Langston, W.; Melamed, E.; Poewe, W.; Stocchi, F.; et al. A double-blind, delayed-start trial of rasagiline in Parkinson's disease. *N. Engl. J. Med.* **2009**, *361*, 1268–1278. [CrossRef] [PubMed]
45. Kelly, M.J.; Lawton, M.A.; Baig, F.; Ruffmann, C.; Barber, T.R.; Lo, C.; Klein, J.C.; Ben-Shlomo, Y.; Hu, M.T. Predictors of motor complications in early Parkinson's disease: A prospective cohort study. *Mov. Disord.* **2019**, *34*, 1174–1183. [CrossRef]
46. Wu, T.L.; Wang, C.C.; Lin, F.J.; Wu, R.M. The association between early treatment with amantadine and delayed onset of levodopa-induced dyskinesia in patients with Parkinson's disease. *Parkinsonism Relat. Disord.* **2018**, *46*, e14–e15. [CrossRef]
47. Group, P.S. Pramipexole vs Levodopa as Initial Treatment for Parkinson DiseaseA Randomized Controlled Trial. *JAMA* **2000**, *284*, 1931–1938. [CrossRef]
48. Olanow, C.W.; Kieburtz, K.; Rascol, O.; Poewe, W.; Schapira, A.H.; Emre, M.; Nissinen, H.; Leinonen, M.; Stocchi, F. Factors predictive of the development of Levodopa-induced dyskinesia and wearing-off in Parkinson's disease. *Mov. Disord.* **2013**, *28*, 1064–1071. [CrossRef]
49. Stocchi, F.; Vacca, L.; Radicati, F.G. How to optimize the treatment of early stage Parkinson's disease. *Transl. Neurodegener.* **2015**, *4*, 4. [CrossRef]
50. Oñatibia-Astibia, A.; Franco, R.; Martínez-Pinilla, E. Health benefits of methylxanthines in neurodegenerative diseases. *Mol. Nutr. Food Res.* **2017**, *61*, 1600670. [CrossRef]
51. Martino, R.; Candundo, H.; Lieshout, P.v.; Shin, S.; Crispo, J.A.G.; Barakat-Haddad, C. Onset and progression factors in Parkinson's disease: A systematic review. *NeuroToxicology* **2017**, *61*, 132–141. [CrossRef] [PubMed]
52. Pinares-Garcia, P.; Stratikopoulos, M.; Zagato, A.; Loke, H.; Lee, J. Sex: A Significant Risk Factor for Neurodevelopmental and Neurodegenerative Disorders. *Brain Sci.* **2018**, *8*, 154. [CrossRef] [PubMed]
53. Simon, D.K.; Wu, C.; Tilley, B.C.; Lohmann, K.; Klein, C.; Payami, H.; Wills, A.M.; Aminoff, M.J.; Bainbridge, J.; Dewey, R.; et al. Caffeine, creatine, GRIN2A and Parkinson's disease progression. *J. Neurol. Sci.* **2017**, *375*, 355–359. [CrossRef]
54. Chuang, Y.H.; Lill, C.M.; Lee, P.C.; Hansen, J.; Lassen, C.F.; Bertram, L.; Greene, N.; Sinsheimer, J.S.; Ritz, B. Gene-Environment Interaction in Parkinson's Disease: Coffee, ADORA2A, and CYP1A2. *Neuroepidemiology* **2016**, *47*, 192–200. [CrossRef] [PubMed]
55. Kim, I.Y.; O'Reilly, É, J.; Hughes, K.C.; Gao, X.; Schwarzschild, M.A.; McCullough, M.L.; Hannan, M.T.; Betensky, R.A.; Ascherio, A. Interaction between caffeine and polymorphisms of glutamate ionotropic receptor NMDA type subunit 2A (GRIN2A) and cytochrome P450 1A2 (CYP1A2) on Parkinson's disease risk. *Mov. Disord.* **2018**, *33*, 414–420. [CrossRef]

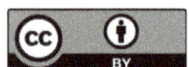

© 2020 by the authors. Licensee MDPI, Basel, Switzerland. This article is an open access article distributed under the terms and conditions of the Creative Commons Attribution (CC BY) license (http://creativecommons.org/licenses/by/4.0/).

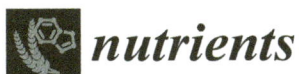

Review

Effect of Caffeine Consumption on the Risk for Neurological and Psychiatric Disorders: Sex Differences in Human

Hye Jin Jee [1,2], Sang Goo Lee [1], Katrina Joy Bormate [1] and Yi-Sook Jung [1,2,*]

1. College of Pharmacy, Ajou University, Suwon 16499, Korea; hjjee@ajou.ac.kr (H.J.J.); cw4646@naver.com (S.G.L.); katbormate96@gmail.com (K.J.B.)
2. Research Institute of Pharmaceutical Sciences and Technology, Ajou University, Suwon 16499, Korea
* Correspondence: yisjung@ajou.ac.kr; Tel.: +82-3-1219-3444

Received: 26 August 2020; Accepted: 4 October 2020; Published: 9 October 2020

Abstract: Caffeine occurs naturally in various foods, such as coffee, tea, and cocoa, and it has been used safely as a mild stimulant for a long time. However, excessive caffeine consumption (1~1.5 g/day) can cause caffeine poisoning (caffeinism), which includes symptoms such as anxiety, agitation, insomnia, and gastrointestinal disorders. Recently, there has been increasing interest in the effect of caffeine consumption as a protective factor or risk factor for neurological and psychiatric disorders. Currently, the importance of personalized medicine is being emphasized, and research on sex/gender differences needs to be conducted. Our review focuses on the effect of caffeine consumption on several neurological and psychiatric disorders with respect to sex differences to provide a better understanding of caffeine use as a risk or protective factor for those disorders. The findings may help establish new strategies for developing sex-specific caffeine therapies.

Keywords: caffeine; neurological and psychiatric disorders; sleep disorder; stroke; dementia; depression; sex differences

1. Introduction

Caffeine (1,3,7-trimethylxanthine), a type of methylxanthine series alkaloid [1], is commonly found in coffee, tea, and soft drinks, and also exists in cocoa, chocolate, and a number of dietary supplements [2]. Caffeine is commonly taken orally in the form of coffee or tea, and 99% of it is absorbed into the bloodstream from the gastrointestinal tract, reaching peak concentrations 30–60 min after ingestion and circulation throughout the body [3]. In the USA, adults consume an average of 179 mg of caffeine daily, which is equivalent to 2 cups (100 mg/240 mL) of ground coffee [4]. Caffeine action is thought to be mediated via several mechanisms: the antagonism of adenosine receptors, the inhibition of phosphodiesterase, the release of calcium from intracellular stores, and the antagonism of benzodiazepine receptors [5]. There are also reports that caffeine changes estrogen levels in women [6]. Since estrogen has a neuroprotective or neurotrophic effect and regulates the dopamine system of the black striatum [7], estrogen regulates the effect of caffeine on the dopamine system and suggests that a complex interaction between caffeine, estrogen, and dopamine exists in the basal ganglia system [8]. Furthermore, caffeine is a stimulant for the central nervous system that can penetrate biological membranes, including the blood–brain barrier and placental barrier, and it maintains arousal function in the brain as a nonspecific potent inhibitor of the A1 and A2A adenosine receptors that promote drowsiness [9]. Caffeine also has psychostimulant effects via modulation of the dopaminergic neuron [10], contributing to an attenuated risk for depression in coffee drinkers [7]. Many people consume caffeine to overcome headaches, owing to its vasoconstrictive properties restricting blood flow in the brain [11]. However, excessive caffeine consumption (1~1.5 g/day) can cause caffeine poisoning (caffeinism), which includes symptoms such as anxiety, agitation, insomnia, gastrointestinal disorders, tremors, and mental disorders [12]. Furthermore, depending on the sensitivity, in rare cases, it can also cause death [13]. Caffeine resistance and the rate of caffeine metabolism vary greatly from person to person, especially depending on the activity of the cytochrome P450 1A2 (CYP1A2) gene, encoding an enzyme that breaks down caffeine [6]. CYP1A2 is a major enzyme responsible for the metabolism of purine alkaloid (1,3,7-trimethylxanthine), a caffeine that occurs naturally in coffee beans, and plays an important role in the metabolism of estrogen and coffee [14]. Additionally, depending on endogenous and exogenous factors, the half-life of caffeine is 2 to 10 h (average 3.7 h), and is mainly excreted by urine after being metabolized in the liver [7]. Accumulating evidence has shown sex-specific differences in the activity and expression of many CYP isoforms [15–17]. Recent studies demonstrate that CYP1A2 and CYP2E1 activities are higher in men than in women, while the activity of CYP3A, one of the most clinically relevant CYP isoforms, is greater in women [15]. The activity of several other CYP (CYP2C16, CYP2C19, and CYP2D6) isozymes and the conjugation (glucuronidation) activity involved in drug metabolism are higher in men than in women [17]. According to the World Health Organization (WHO), about 6.8 million people worldwide die each year from various neurological and psychiatric disorders, including stroke, Alzheimer's disease (AD), Parkinson's disease (PD), and depression. Neurological and psychiatric disorders are not only expensive to treat, but patients have experienced serious stigma, social exclusion, and poor quality of life as a result of their affliction [18]. Over the years, caffeine has been investigated as a potential risk or protective factor for neurological and psychiatric disorders [19]. Some studies have shown that by drinking more than three cups of coffee a day, caffeine reduces the risk of developing AD and PD [20]. Meanwhile, the risk of developing anxiety and panic disorder has been reported to increase after consumption of more than six cups of coffee a day [21]. Interestingly, there are significant sex/gender differences in the prevalence or incidence of neurological and psychiatric disorders. Moreover, a recent study found that individuals with reduced CYP2D6 activity due to the mutated CYP2D6 * 4A (allelic variants of CYP2D6) genotype had a 2.5 times higher risk of PD than those with wild type, which was higher in men [22]. In addition, the presence of high-risk alleles in both CYP17 and CYP19 increased the risk of AD in menopausal women by almost four times [23,24]. From these studies, it has been suggested that the effects of caffeine on the prevalence/incidence of neurological and psychiatric disorders may vary depending on sex, but it is still not thoroughly understood. In the present review, we first review the sex differences in the prevalence and/or incidence of several neurological and psychiatric disorders. Further, this review summarizes the effect of caffeine intake as a risk or protection factor for these disorders in men and women.

2. Sex Differences in the Prevalence/Incidence of Neurological and Psychiatric Disorders

Millions of people worldwide are affected by neurological and psychiatric disorders. More than six million people die each year from stroke, and there are 7.7 million new cases of dementia each year [25]. The prevalence/incidence of several neurological and psychiatric disorders in men and women are discussed in the following sections and summarized in Table 1.

2.1. Stroke

Stroke is a disease in which the vessels that supply blood to the brain develop abnormalities and suddenly cause local brain dysfunction, accompanied by various neurological deficits such as consciousness disorders, unilateral paralysis, and/or speech disorders [26]. There are two main types of stroke: ischemic stroke, due to lack of blood flow (85%), and hemorrhagic stroke, due to bleeding (15%) [27–30]. It has been identified that the symptoms of stroke are different between men and women. Fatigue (women vs. men = 31.2% vs. 21.1%), disorientation (44.4% vs. 34.7%), and fever (12.1% vs. 5.3%) appear predominantly in women, while paresthesia (24.2% vs. 37.9%) and ataxia (61.4% vs. 74.7%) are more common in men [31]. In a systematic review by Appelros et. al, it was shown that there was high variance between age groups and countries, but on average, both the incidence and the prevalence of stroke were higher in men than in women [32]. On the other hand, mortality from stroke was greater in women (24.7%) than in men (19.7%). A prospective study from the USA conducted on 505 patients with first ischemic stroke (ischemic stroke genetics study) found that 270 patients (55%) were men and 229 (45%) were women [33]. In their study, no sex differences were found in stroke severity, stroke subtype, or infarct size and location, but a higher percentage of mortality was shown in women [27–30,33]. In 2009, a study conducted by the Beth Israel Deaconess Medical Center in the USA analyzed 1107 inpatients aged 21 and older who were diagnosed with neuro-ischemic stroke [28]. This study revealed no difference in the prevalence of stroke between men and women, but when comparing the age of patients, women were older than men and were more likely to have heart embolism [28]. Taken together, at most ages, women have a lower or similar risk of stroke than men. However, possibly due to the longer lifespan of women, the incidence of stroke in women gradually increases with age, and as a result, mortality rates in women are higher.

Table 1. Sex differences in the prevalence/incidence of selected neurological and psychiatric disorders.

Diseases	Note	Sex Difference in Incidence/Prevalence	Age	Case Number	Ref.
Stroke	No sex differences in the prevalence of stroke, but women are more likely to have heart attacks and embolism.	M = F	~73	1107	[25]
	No sex differences were found in stroke incidence, severity, or infarct size and location, but female mortality was higher.	M = F	19–94	505	[33]
	Stroke prevalence between ages of 65 and 85 is 41% higher in men than women, and the male/female prevalence ratio decreases with age.	M > F	65–85	30,414	[32]
	Although the incidence of stroke by age is higher in men than in women, the death rate from stroke each year is higher in women because women live longer and have the highest mortality rate at the oldest age (≥85 years).	M > F	56–	1136	[34]
Sleep disorder	Women over 65 have the highest risk of insomnia and have been reported to have increased risk of insomnia as life expectancy is longer in women than in men.	M < F	18–	4885	[35]
	Insomnia symptoms of two nights or more per week are reported in 30.5% in women and 24.5% in men, and for chronic insomnia, the incidence is higher in women (12.9%) than men (6.2%).	M < F	20–35	1395	[36]
	Women are more than twice as likely to be diagnosed with insomnia as men.	M < F	19–	817	[37]
	The diagnosis of insomnia was 9.0% for women and 5.9% for men.	M < F	20–100	1741	[38]
Dementia	A substantially larger number of women than men have AD worldwide.	M < F	65–	NA	[39]
	Rate of progression from MCI to AD was similar in men and women aged 70–79, but higher in women than men after age 80.	M < F	70–	4398	[40]
	In adults over 65, the risk of AD in women is twice as high as in men.	M < F	65–	2611	[41]
	Two-thirds of patients with AD are women.	M < F	65–	5976	[42]
Parkinson's disease	Incidence rates were consistently higher in men than in women at all ages for PD.	M > F	~90	NA	[43]
	Men had a risk of developing PD twice that of women.	M > F	65–84	4341	[44]
	Women showed higher cognitive abilities than men.	M > F	~80	1741	[45]
	PD is more common in men than women, with an approximate ratio of 2:1.	M > F	19–	902	[46]
Depression	The incidence of more severe depression is higher in women.	M < F	39–65	100	[47]
	In the HCV-infected female population, anxiety and depression were more common than in men.	M < F	41–62	38	[48]
	Greater risk for depression among women compared to men.	M < F	~60	2824	[49]
Anxiety	The incidence of the trait of anxiety is high in women.	M < F	20–23	108	[50]
	Stress-induced anxiety is higher in women than in men.	M < F	19–50	96	[51]
Neuromuscular disease	The incidence of MG was significantly higher in women under age 40, but higher in men over age 50.	M < F	~40	1976	[52]
		M > F	50–		
	Women with CMT1X have less severe consequences for almost all parameters of MNCS compared to men with CMT1X.	M < F	18–79	107	[53]
	The incidence and prevalence of ALS are greater in men than in women.	M > F	~30	NA	[54]

NA, not analyzed; Ref., reference; AD, Alzheimer's disease; MCI, mild cognitive impairment; PD, Parkinson's disease; HCV, hepatitis C virus; MG, myasthenia gravis; MNCS, motor nerve conduction studies; CMT1X, Charcot–Marie–Tooth type 1X; ALS, amyotrophic lateral sclerosis; F, female; M, male.

2.2. Sleep Disorder

Sleep mediates changes in various physiological functions, including brain activity, breathing, and heart rate, and sufficient sleep improves attention, creativity, memory, and learning [55]. Insufficient sleep or poor sleep quality can act as a risk factor for a variety of diseases, including dementia, psychosis, and diabetes [56,57]. Prevalence of sleep disorders is high, with about 25–30% of population worldwide having some form of inadequate sleep. Sleep disorders degrade the quality of life due to secondary psychological stress as well as promoting physical illness [58]. A recent study found that there was a difference in the prevalence of sleep disorders between sexes. Insomnia, the most common type of sleep disorder, is defined as a condition where it is difficult to initiate and maintain sleeping, resulting in difficulty in early rising [59]. Regarding sex differences in the prevalence of insomnia, many studies have reported that insomnia occurs more frequently in women [37]. In the USA, insomnia diagnosis is double in women compared with that in men, and insomnia symptoms for two nights or more per week have been reported to occur in 30.5% of women and 24.5% of men. In the case of chronic insomnia, the incidence rate was higher in women (12.9%) than in men (6.2%) [36]. In particular, women over 65 have the highest risk for insomnia and have been reported to have an increasing risk with age [35,38]. One of the reasons that women are more susceptible to insomnia than men is the changes in body hormones due to menstruation and menopause [60]. This is because estrogen, an important female hormone, decreases and body symptoms such as hot flashes and sweating are caused by an imbalance of hormones in the body.

2.3. Dementia

Dementia is a pathological neurodegenerative process characterized by a gradual decrease in cognitive, memory, and functional capacity that is severe enough to affect daily functioning [61]. Other symptoms include emotional problems, speech problems, and decreased motivation [62]. AD is the most common form of dementia and most studies do not distinguish AD from all-cause dementia [63]. Global estimates on the prevalence of dementia are up to 7% of the population aged 65 and over, and in developed countries with a longer lifespan, the prevalence is slightly higher still (8–10%) [64]. According to the World Alzheimer's Report 2015, there are currently 46.8 million people with dementia worldwide, with an estimated increase to 74.7 million by 2030 and 131.5 million by 2050 [65]. Age is a major risk factor for AD, and on average, women live longer than men. However, the difference in lifespan between men and women does not fully explain why two-thirds of Alzheimer's patients are women. Even after accounting for differences in longevity, some studies have found that women are still at a higher risk [66]. Recently, sex-related differences in neuroanatomy and function are being considered in patient diagnostics, and sex can be an important factor in stratified and personalized treatment in AD patients [39]. Consistent with this finding, analysis of longitudinal data from the Alzheimer's Disease Neuroimaging Initiative cohort showed that women had greater hippocampal atrophy and faster cognitive decline in the presence of AD biomarkers (Cerebrospinal fluid levels $A\beta1$-42 and total tau) compared to men [67]. Similarly, a study published in 2017 showed that in dementia patients who were classified as fast progressors, there was a faster rate of dementia in women than men, even when the diagnostic biomarker levels were similar [68]. Sex-related differences and treatment responses related to disease progression after AD diagnosis were also reported [40]. According to a Mayo Clinic study on aging, the progression from mild cognitive impairment (MCI) to AD was similar in men and women in the ages of 70–79, but higher in women than men after 80 years of age. This is likely due to the difference in brain anatomy between men and women, and it is reported that men are expected to withstand more pathologies because their heads are about 10% larger and have more brain volume compared to women, a hypothesis that was supported by autopsy. At the same level of pathology, the probability of clinical diagnosis of AD was found to be significantly higher in women than in men [69]. In the Framingham Study cohort, a study conducted in individuals aged between 65 and 100 years old, incidence of AD in women was twice as high as men [41], and another study reported that two-thirds of AD patients are women [42]. Overall, women showed higher incidence and prevalence of dementia than men, possibly due to various factors, such as longer life expectancy of women and different neuroanatomical function [42].

2.4. PD

PD is one of the neurodegenerative disorders with characteristic features, such as hand tremor, muscle stiffness, and postural instability [70]. PD is the second most frequent age-related neurodegenerative disorder, affecting about three percent of people over 65 and five percent over 85 years old [71]. The formation of the Lewy body (α-synuclein accumulation in neurons) in the stromal nigra pars compacta leads to basal ganglion circuit degeneration [46]. Patients under 40 years of age are rare, and prevalence increases with age, approaching three percent of the population over the age of 80 [72]. Increasing evidence has suggested that sex is an important factor in the development of PD. In PD, the onset age, severity, and type of symptoms vary by sex. According to several studies, the onset of PD in men occurs, on average, two years earlier than in women, and the incidence rate in men is twice as high as that in women [73]. It has also been reported that sex differences in PD are determined by the nigrostriatal dopamine system arising from genetic, environmental, and hormonal effects. Sex itself is a variable that can affect the manifestation of non-motor symptoms in PD patients [46]. Women have better cognitive performance than men in two measures: the Symbol Digit Modalities Test, a screening test for cognitive impairment, and Scales for Outcomes of Parkinson's disease-cognition, a measure of memory and learning, attention, executive function, and virtual space function [45]. Despite the higher incidence of PD in men at all ages, the difference in PD risk between men and women is reduced with age. In those aged 65 to 69, the incidence of PD was shown to be similar between men and women [44]. The reason is likely that women have a longer lifespan than men, and men are at greater risk of dying at a younger age [43]. In addition, motor improvement after deep brain stimulation is similar in men and women, but women are likely to show better improvement in daily living activities compared to men [74]. One of the reasons why the onset of PD is higher in men than in women may be due to the effect of estrogen on dopaminergic neurons and pathways in the brain [75].

2.5. Depression

Depression is a common and serious mental disorder that can have long-term consequences and affects all aspects of life. People with depression tend to feel sad, anxious, hopeless, irritable, and ashamed [76]. Severe cases of depression can lead to loss of appetite, sudden weight loss, sleeping problems, and frequent thoughts of death or suicide [77]. It is commonly comorbid with other chronic illnesses and/or mood disorders that make it a complicated disorder difficult to properly diagnose and treat [78]. Depression is more frequently experienced by women compared to men, with a peak in prevalence occurring in middle age. Gender differences in depression are known to be affected by several factors, such as biological, psychological, and environmental factors [79]. In 2018, in Canada, the THINC-integrated tool (THINC-it), a newly developed cognitive tool, was used to evaluate cognitive impairment in patients suffering from major depressive disorder (MDD). It was reported that women had a higher rate of severe depression than men [47]. Additionally, patients with chronic liver disease have a higher incidence of depression than the general population and depression is a common psychiatric comorbidity among individuals with hepatitis C virus (HCV) [80]. Studies have shown that 23% of women, but only 4.1% of men, with chronic HCV have depression. In conclusion, in those with chronic HCV infection, anxiety and depression were more common in women than in men [48]. The University of Michigan's survey center conducted a community-based study named "American Changing Lives (ACL)" that included two sets of data collected in 1986 and 1989. These data revealed that stressed women were more prone to depression than stressed men [49]. Recent evidence suggests that changes in ovarian hormone levels, especially biological factors such as decreased estrogen, may contribute to increased risk for depression in women [81].

2.6. Anxiety

Anxiety, which manifests as a sudden increase in alertness, excessive fear, and worry, is the most common mental health disorder and 1 in 9 individuals have experienced anxiety for a year. It is also known that women have a higher prevalence of anxiety than men [82,83]. Results of the State Trait Anxiety Inventory (STAT) score, a psychological inventory that determines individual anxiety and trait anxiety among healthy men and women volunteers at Utretch University Campus, confirmed that women have a high level of trait anxiety [50]. In 2017, a research team at Yale University in the USA conducted an experiment on stress-induced anxiety disorder in healthy adults between the ages of 19 and 50. Their results show that women are more susceptible to stress-induced anxiety [51]. That is, as a result of various anxiety measurement experiments, the incidence of anxiety was found likely to be higher in women than in men. Women have a higher incidence of anxiety disorders not only because they are more sensitive to the lower levels of hormones that make up the stress response, but also because women experience residual anxiety from sexual abuse/violence more often than men [84].

2.7. Neuromuscular Disease

Neuromuscular diseases are a broadly defined group of disorders that involve injury or dysfunction of the peripheral nerve or muscle and include wide variety of disorders, such as multiple sclerosis (MS), Charcot–Marie–Tooth (CMT) disease, amyotrophic lateral sclerosis (ALS), myasthenia gravis (MG), and neuropathic pain [85]. The most common of these diseases is MG, which is an autoimmune disease where the immune system produces antibodies that attach themselves to the neuromuscular junction and prevent transmission of the nerve impulse to the muscle [86]. The onset of MG occurs at any age, but significantly earlier in women than men. The incidence of MG has been reported to be significantly higher in women under age 40, but higher in men over age 50 [52]. CMT disease encompasses a group of disorders called hereditary sensory and motor neuropathies, which damage the peripheral nerves [87]. The highest prevalence of CMT disease occurs at ages 50–64, with men having a higher prevalence than women [53,88]. A study by Nivedita U. Jerath et al. reviewed the results of electrodiagnostic retrospectively in 45 women and 31 men. As a result, women with CMT1X have less severe outcomes for almost all parameters of motor nerve conduction studies (MNCS) (compound motor action potential amplitude, delay time on exercise, and conduction rate) compared to men with CMT1X [53]. ALS is a highly debilitating disease caused by progressive degeneration of motoneurons [89]. Both the incidence and the prevalence of ALS are greater in men than women. The reasons for the difference in the incidence of ALS between men and women is known as the differences in biological responses to exogenous toxins, various exposures to environmental toxins, and fundamental differences between male and female nervous systems and their ability to repair damage [54]. The prevalence/incidence of neuromuscular disease varies according to the age of men and women, but in most cases, it is higher in men than women. The difference in the incidence of ALS between men and women may be explained by differences in the biological response to exogenous toxins.

3. Effect of Caffeine Consumption on the Risk for Neurological and Psychiatric Disorders in Men and Women

According to a paper published in British Medical Journal (BMJ) in 2017, drinking 3–4 cups of coffee per day is associated with a reduced risk of various neurological disorders, including AD, PD, and depression [90]. However, few studies have been reported on sex differences in the effects of caffeine on neurological and psychiatric disorders. This review investigates the differential effects of caffeine on the incidence of symptoms of several neurological and psychiatric disorders in men and women (summarized in Table 2).

3.1. Stroke

According to the WHO, 15 million people worldwide suffer from stroke each year, five million of these people die, and another five million are permanently disabled [91]. The causative or protective effect of caffeine on stroke onset has been controversial, and moreover, sex differences have not been studied. In 2015, the National Health and Nutrition Examination Survey in the USA examined the association between coffee consumption and stroke in 19,994 participants (men 9374; women 10,620) over the age of 17. Multivariate analysis found that higher coffee consumption ($\geq$3 cups/day) reduced the incidence of stroke [92]. In 2017, data from the Health Examinees study, a large, prospective, community-based cohort study, were used to analyze the association between coffee consumption and stroke. A survey of about 15,000 men and women between 40 and 69 years of age did not show any significant association between coffee consumption and stroke risk among men. However, in the case of young women, the inverse relationship between coffee consumption and stroke risk was prominent. In other words, higher coffee consumption was found to be inversely proportional to the incidence rate of stroke in women [93]. Some studies show that coffee consumption temporarily increases the risk of ischemic stroke. Mostofsky's study showed that the incidence of stroke temporarily doubled in those who drank seven or more cups of coffee per week compared with non-drinkers, but there were no gender differences [94]. In summary, the effect of coffee intake on the risk for stroke showed controversial results, but more studies have shown that women have a lower risk of stroke incidence by caffeine intake, than men. As indirect evidence of the preventive effect of coffee consumption on stroke occurrence, there are papers reporting the preventive effect of coffee consumption on the onset of diabetes by maximizing insulin sensitivity, which is a risk factor for stroke, but no differences between sexes were revealed [95].

Table 2. Effect of caffeine consumption on the risk for selected neurological and psychiatric disorders in men and women.

Disease	Note	Risk for Neurological Disorder			Age	Case Number	Coffee Consumption	Ref.
		Men	Women	N.S.				
Stroke	The risk of temporary ischemic stroke increases for an hour after coffee consumption.			+	54–72	390	7 cups/week	[94]
	Higher daily coffee consumption and potential protection from strokes.	−			17–	19,994	≥3 cups/day	[92]
	Coffee consumption may modestly reduce risk of stroke.		−		55–	1800	≥4 cups/day	[96]
	Higher coffee consumption among middle-aged Korean women may have protective benefits with regard to stroke risk.		−		40–69	173,357	≥3 cups/day	[93]
Sleep disorder	Middle-aged sleep is more sensitive to increased caffeine dosage than young adults.			+	20–30 40–60	77	≥3 cups/day	[97]
	Caffeine decreased sleep efficiency, sleep time, slow-wave sleep, and REM sleep during the weekly recovery sleep.			+	20–30	24	165–205 mg/day	[98]
	Adolescent students who consumed high caffeine suffered higher sleep disturbances.			+	12–15	191	52.7 mg/day	[99]
	Short sleep is associated with more caffeine consumption, suggesting that adults with poor sleep quality consume more caffeine.	+	+		19–94	80	164.9 mg/day	[100]
	Habitual coffee intake decreases the efficiency and quality of sleep.	+	+		60–94	162	≥60 cups/year	[101]
Dementia	Moderate regular coffee consumption can have a neuroprotective effect on MCI.			−	65–84	1445	1–2 cup/day	[102]
	An inverse relationship exists between caffeine intake and the risk of dementia.			−	65–	587	200 mg/day	[103]
	Moderate coffee consumption in middle-aged individuals may reduce future risk of dementia/AD.				65–79	1409	3–5 cups/day	[104]
	Elderly women with high caffeine consumption are less likely to have dementia or cognitive impairment.		−		65–	6467	261 mg/day	[105]
	Caffeine appear to reduce cognitive decline in women, especially at higher ages.		−		65–	7017	>3 cups/day	[106]
	Lifetime coffee consumption was positively associated with cognitive performance in elderly women, but not in elderly men.		−		50–	1528	≥3 cups/day	[20]
Parkinson's disease	The PD risk decreased significantly before 3 cups/day, whereas it did not change materially after 3 cups/day of coffee consumption.	−			65–	5312	3 cups/day	[107]
	Coffee consumption is associated with reduced PD risk in men and women.	− −	−		69–	184,190	2 cups/day	[108]
	Coffee consumption reduces the risk of PD.	−			50–79	6710	>10 cups/week	[19]
	A U-shaped relationship exists between caffeine intake and PD in women.		+/−		40–75	135,916	1–3 cups/day	[110]
Depression	Men who consume moderate coffee have a significantly lower risk of PD than men who have never consumed coffee.	−			45–68	8004	28 oz/day	[111]
	The higher the caffeine intake, the lower the incidence of PD in men.	−			19–	9576	≥2 cups/day	[112]
	Korean adults who consume caffeine are less likely to become depressed.		−		30–55	50,739	>4 cups/day	[113]
	The risk of depression decreases as caffeine consumption increases.		−		18–	5563	309–425 mg/day	[114]
	Inverse association between caffeine intake and depressive symptoms.		−		11–17	2307	>1000 mg/week	[115]
Anxiety	In secondary school children's, the effect of caffeine on depression is higher in women than in men.	+	++		18–31	99	>150 mg/day	[116]
	Anxiety in men increased with increasing doses of caffeine.	+			11–17	2307	>1000 mg/week	[115]
Neuromuscular disease	In secondary school children, the effect of caffeine on anxiety is higher in males than in females.	++	+		18–69	1620	6 cups/day	[117]
	High caffeine intake is significantly associated with a decrease in developing MS.	−	−		25–42	258	0–5 cups/day	[118]
	Caffeine intake does not affect the risk of MS in white women.		−		26–94	1031	>1 cup/day	[119]
	People who drink more than one cup of coffee per day for at least 6 months have a lower risk of ALS compared to people who do not drink coffee at all.							

+: increase, ++: increase to a great extent, −: decrease, − −: decrease to a great extent. N.S.: not significant; Ref.: reference; REM, rapid eye movement; MCI, mild cognitive impairment; AD, Alzheimer's disease; PD, Parkinson's disease; MS, multiple sclerosis; ALS, amyotrophic lateral sclerosis.

3.2. Sleep Disorder

Caffeine overdose can delay sleep onset, reduce total sleep time, change normal sleep stages, and reduce sleep quality. Caffeine-induced sleep disorder is known as a psychiatric disorder caused by excessive caffeine consumption [120]. A double-blind cross-design study of 22 young participants (10 men, 12 women; 20–30 years old) and 25 middle-aged participants (12 men, 13 women; 40–60 years old) showed that in terms of sleep volume and efficiency, middle-aged participants in good health were more susceptible to increased caffeine doses compared to young adults [97]. In a study of 12 young and 12 middle-aged subjects who consumed one to three cups of coffee per day, caffeine intake was found to reduce sleep efficiency, sleep time, slow-wave sleep (SWS), and rapid eye movement (REM) sleep in both age groups. However, during the weekly recovery, middle-aged participants had significantly reduced sleep time and sleep efficiency compared to younger participants [98]. In addition, for 66 boys and 125 girls who consumed similar amounts of caffeine, the average sleep time decreased from 528.8 min (8.8 h) on Saturday nights, to 448.5 min on Sunday nights (7.5 h). Perhaps not surprisingly, teenagers who consumed large quantities of caffeine experienced interfered sleep [99]. Furthermore, a survey on the quality of sleep in 26 adult men and 54 women with an average daily caffeine intake of 164.9 mg, showed that 80% of respondents suffered from sleep disturbances once a week [100]. Finally, among 162 cognitively healthy Koreans aged 60–94 (85 men, 77 women), people who consumed more than 60 cups of coffee per year had a 20% lower volume of pineal parenchyma, a melatonin-producing region, than those who consumed less than 60 cups of coffee per year [101]. In summary, caffeine intake negatively affected the quality of sleep and the amount of sleep with age, with no differences seen between men and women.

3.3. Dementia

A number of studies report that caffeine consumption tends to decrease the incidence of dementia. Increased caffeine intake in white women aged 65–80 has been reported to lower the likelihood of dementia or cognitive impairment [105]. In addition, drinking a moderate amount of coffee (3~5 cups/day) lowers the incidence of dementia compared with not drinking coffee, and among coffee-drinkers, the incidence of dementia is lower in women than in men. Moreover, a later-life survey found that low consumers of coffee were more likely to develop depression (based on the Beck depression scale) compared to moderate coffee consumers [104]. According to a study by Vincenzo et al., individuals who habitually consumed moderate amounts of coffee (one to two cups of coffee a day) had a lower incidence of MCI than those who did not drink coffee [102]. A study of 587 people in a California retiree community found that those who consumed more than 200 mg of caffeine per day at the age of 90 and took extra vitamin C significantly reduced their risk for dementia [103]. Some studies have reported neuroprotective effects of caffeine by showing that women with high caffeine intake (more than three cups per day) have fewer speech retrieval and decreased spatiotemporal memory problems than women who consumed less than one cup of coffee per day [106]. The psycho-stimulating component of caffeine appears to reduce cognitive decline in women without dementia, especially in the elderly [106]. Retrospective observational studies have shown that lifetime coffee consumption tends to increase cognitive performance in aged women, but this is not the case in aged men [20]. Taken together, these studies show that caffeine intake did not help improve cognitive abilities in either men or women, although steady caffeine intake seems to reduce the risk of developing dementia for both men and women, with a greater effect in women.

3.4. PD

The possible relationship between caffeine intake and PD risk has attracted considerable attention since the early 1970s, and more and more observational studies have been conducted on this [107]. An inverse association between coffee consumption and PD risk has been found in several epidemiological studies [110,121–123]. Even though the evidence is increasing that caffeine intake can reduce the risk of PD, the number of cohort studies is still relatively small and is almost exclusively limited to the USA [109]. A meta-analysis of the Hui Qi research team found that consuming less than three cups of coffee per day significantly reduced the risk of PD, while consuming more than three cups of coffee per day did not significantly alter the risk for PD [107]. The link between caffeine consumption and the risk of developing PD was more pronounced in men than women. A study by Ascherio et al. reported that men who consumed a moderate amount of coffee had a significantly lower risk of PD than men who did not drink coffee at all [110]. For women, there is a U-shaped relationship between coffee consumption and Parkinson's disease risk, with women drinking 1–3 cups of coffee per day having the lowest risk. These results support the protective effect of moderate amounts of caffeine on Parkinson's disease risk. A cohort study conducted in the USA in 1992 found that in men, regular coffee consumption was associated with a reduced risk of PD [108]. In the case of women, the risk of PD was significantly reduced in the group with the highest caffeine intake (four or more cups per day) compared to the group with the lowest caffeine intake (less than one drink per day), but the decrease was lower than in men. According to a study published in 2000 by Ross et al., the incidence of PD observed among Japanese men participants aged 45 to 68 was two to three times higher in non-coffee drinkers than in coffee drinkers [111]. In summary, high caffeine intake is associated with a protective effect that suppresses PD incidence in men and women, significantly reduces the risk of PD in men, and only slightly reduces the risk in women. These results suggest that men and women respond differently to caffeine administration and that these gender differences may be mediated by changes in circulating steroid hormones [124].

3.5. Depression

Adequate caffeine intake has a positive effect on depression, but excessive caffeine intake can exacerbate depression by stimulating sympathetic nerves [125]. Moderate amounts of caffeine also help prevent an imbalance in brain neurotransmitters, such as serotonin and dopamine, that cause depression. The effect of caffeine intake on depression was investigated in students aged 11 to 17 years old (a total of 2307 students). As a result, consuming less than 1000 mg of caffeine per week increased the incidence of depression in girls compared to boys [115]. Unlike the above results, according to a survey conducted by the Centers for Disease Control and Prevention, the prevalence of depression decreased as caffeine intake increased. The incidence of depression among participants who drank more than two cups of coffee per day was reduced by 24% compared to those who didn't drink coffee [112]. In addition, as a result of analysis of data from the National Health and Nutrition Examination Survey conducted in 2019, it was found that the incidence of depression decreased as the amount of caffeine intake increased, but gender differences were not analyzed [114]. A 2011 cohort result from the US Nurses' Health Study found an inverse age-adjusted dose-response relationship between caffeine-containing coffee and depression risk in women. Compared with the group with the lowest caffeine consumption (<100 mg/d), the relative risk for depression was lower in the group with the highest caffeine consumption (≥550 mg/d). In other words, women who consumed more caffeine had a lower risk of depression than women who consumed less caffeine [113]. In summary, the risk of developing depression was decreased by caffeine intake to a greater extent in women than in men, and the effect of caffeine intake on depression incidence was different according to the age of women. In particular, in adolescence, caffeine decomposition ability is lower than that of adults, so the staying time in the body is relatively long and it can increase the risk of depression by inducing sleep disorders [126].

3.6. Anxiety

Generalized anxiety disorder is a serious mental illness that affects up to 6% of population in the world. Symptoms are complicated by the consequences of accompaniment with other mental disorders, such as MDD, panic disorder, and alcohol/substance abuse, resulting in worsening of symptoms and poor treatment responses [127]. Excessive caffeine can cause symptoms ranging from general anxiety to compulsive disorders [120]. However, few studies have been conducted on the incidence of anxiety in men and women, by caffeine. As a result from a cohort study of 3323 students aged 11–17 years (boys 48.5%, girl 51.5%), the effect of caffeine on anxiety was not significant in girls, but in boys, anxiety increased with caffeine intake [115]. Consistent with the above results, at the University of Valencia, Spain, a STAT test of 39 men and 60 women between 18 and 31 years of age showed that men had higher state anxiety than women [116]. As shown above, the effects of caffeine on anxiety were more pronounced in men than in women. However, very little research has been conducted to assess the association between caffeine intake and anxiety.

3.7. Neuromuscular Disease

There are only a few studies about the effect of caffeine on neuromuscular diseases, and little is known about its sex differences and mechanisms. A case-controlled study from the European ALS Consortium (EURALS Group) reported that people who drink more than one cup of coffee per day for at least six months have a lower risk of ALS than those who didn't drink coffee at all [119]. Similar findings of caffeine's impact on the risk of developing MS were found in two cohort studies conducted in the USA and Sweden in 2016 [117]. Compared to those who never had coffee, those with high coffee intakes in excess of six cups per day had a significantly reduced risk of MS in both men and women. However, a recent meta-analysis of five large cohort studies conducted in the USA showed no association between coffee consumption and ALS risk, in both males and female. Another large prospective study conducted by Massa et al. also reported no association between caffeine consumption and MS risk in white women [118].

4. Conclusions

This review has shown that the beneficial and/or risky effects of caffeine on several neurological and psychiatric disorders may vary depending on sex. In the case of stroke, caffeine intake has a greater protective effect in women than in men, and for sleep disorders, caffeine intake tends to increase the risk to a similar extent in both men and women. This review also shows that the risk for developing dementia is reduced to a greater extent in women than in men. In contrast, the protective effect of caffeine against PD was found to be greater in men than in women. Notably, in the case of anxiety and depression, the effect of caffeine on the risk for their incidence tends to be age dependent. In fact, the risk of depression has shown to decrease in adult women but not in men, while in adolescence, women have a much higher risk of depression than men. For anxiety, the risk seems to be increased primarily in adult men but not in women, while during adolescence, the risk increases in both men and women, but to a much greater extent in men. In other words, caffeine consumption not only has a positive effect of reducing the risk of stroke, dementia, and depression in women and reducing the risk of PD in men, but also has a negative effect of increasing sleep disorders and anxiety disorders in adolescence in both men and women. Moreover, there are not many research articles that analyzed individual sex/gender differences in the effect of caffeine on neurological disorders. Therefore, further studies focusing on sex/gender differences are needed to fully understand the positive and negative effects of coffee intake on neurological and psychiatric disorders in men and women, and to develop new strategies for sex-specific caffeine use.

Author Contributions: All authors participated in the literature review. S.G.L. and K.J.B. searched for the data. H.J.J. wrote the first draft. Y.-S.J. edited and revised the manuscript. All authors have read and agreed to the published version of the manuscript.

Funding: This research was supported by the Support Program for Women in Science, Engineering and Technology through the Center for Women In Science, Engineering and Technology (WISET) and funded by the Ministry of Science and ICT (No. WISET202003GI01); the Korea Health Technology R&D Project through the Korea Health Industry Development Institute (KHIDI), funded by the Ministry of Health and Welfare (HI18C0920); the Basic Science Research Program through the National Research Foundation of Korea (NRF), funded by the Ministry of Education (2018R1D1A1B07048729), Republic of Korea.

Conflicts of Interest: The authors declare no conflict of interest.

References

1. Heckman, M.A.; Weil, J.; De Mejia, E.G. Caffeine (1, 3, 7-trimethylxanthine) in Foods: A Comprehensive Review on Consumption, Functionality, Safety, and Regulatory Matters. *J. Food Sci.* **2010**, *75*, 77–87. [CrossRef] [PubMed]
2. Górecki, M.; Hallmann, E. The Antioxidant Content of Coffee and Its In Vitro Activity as an Effect of Its Production Method and Roasting and Brewing Time. *Antioxidants* **2020**, *9*, 308. [CrossRef] [PubMed]
3. DePaula, J.; Farah, A. Caffeine Consumption through Coffee: Content in the Beverage, Metabolism, Health Benefits and Risks. *Beverages* **2019**, *5*, 37. [CrossRef]
4. Lieberman, H.R.; Agarwal, S.; Fulgoni, V.L. Daily Patterns of Caffeine Intake and the Association of Intake with Multiple Sociodemographic and Lifestyle Factors in US Adults Based on the NHANES 2007-2012 Surveys. *J. Acad. Nutr. Diet.* **2018**, *119*, 106–114. [CrossRef] [PubMed]
5. Institute of Medicine. *Caffeine for the Sustainment of Mental Task Performance*; The National Academies Press: Washington, DC, USA, 2001.
6. Sisti, J.S.; Hankinson, S.E.; Caporaso, N.E.; Gu, F.; Tamimi, R.M.; Rosner, B.; Xu, X.; Ziegler, R.; Eliassen, A.H. Caffeine, coffee, and tea intake and urinary estrogens and estrogen metabolites in premenopausal women. *Cancer Epidemiol. Biomark. Prev.* **2015**, *24*, 1174–1183. [CrossRef]
7. Shulman, L.M. Is there a connection between estrogen and Parkinson's disease? *Park. Relat. Disord.* **2002**, *8*, 289–295. [CrossRef]
8. Cappelletti, S.; Daria, P.; Sani, G.; Aromatario, M. Caffeine: Cognitive and Physical Performance Enhancer or Psychoactive Drug? *Curr. Neuropharmacol.* **2015**, *13*, 71–88. [CrossRef]
9. Ribeiro, J.A.; Sebastião, A.M. Caffeine and Adenosine. *J. Alzheimer's Dis.* **2010**, *20*, 3–15. [CrossRef]
10. Ferré, S.; Ciruela, F.; Borycz, J.; Solinas, M.; Quarta, D.; Antoniou, K.; Quiroz, C.; Justinova, Z.; Lluis, C.; Franco, R.; et al. Adenosine A1-A2A receptor heteromers: New targets for caffeine in the brain. *Front. Biosci.* **2008**, *13*, 2391. [CrossRef]
11. Addicott, M.A.; Yang, L.L.; Peiffer, A.M.; Burnett, L.R.; Burdette, J.H.; Chen, M.Y.; Hayasaka, S.; Kraft, R.A.; Maldjian, J.A.; Laurienti, P.J. The effect of daily caffeine use on cerebral blood flow: How much caffeine can we tolerate? *Hum. Brain Mapp.* **2009**, *30*, 3102–3114. [CrossRef]
12. Willson, C. The clinical toxicology of caffeine: A review and case study. *Toxicol. Rep.* **2018**, *5*, 1140–1152. [CrossRef] [PubMed]
13. Cappelletti, S.; Piacentino, D.; Fineschi, V.; Frati, P.; Cipolloni, L.; Aromatario, M. Caffeine-Related Deaths: Manner of Deaths and Categories at Risk. *Nutrients* **2018**, *10*, 611. [CrossRef] [PubMed]
14. Guessous, I.; Dobrinas, M.; Kutalik, Z.; Pruijm, M.; Ehret, G.B.; Maillard, M.; Bergmann, S.; Beckmann, J.S.; Cusi, D.; Rizzi, F.; et al. Caffeine intake and CYP1A2 variants associated with high caffeine intake protect non-smokers from hypertension. *Hum. Mol. Genet.* **2012**, *21*, 3283–3292. [CrossRef] [PubMed]
15. Scandlyn, M.J.; Stuart, E.C.; Rosengren, R.J. Sex-specific differences in CYP450 isoforms in humans. *Expert Opin. Drug Metab. Toxicol.* **2008**, *4*, 413–424. [CrossRef]
16. Yang, L.; Li, Y.; Hong, H.; Chang, C.-W.; Guo, L.-W.; Lyn-Cook, B.; Shi, L.; Ning, B. Sex Differences in the Expression of Drug-Metabolizing and Transporter Genes in Human Liver. *J. Drug Metab. Toxicol.* **2012**, *3*, 1–9. [CrossRef]
17. Tanaka, E. Gender-related differences in pharmacokinetics and their clinical significance. *J. Clin. Pharm. Ther.* **1999**, *24*, 339–346. [CrossRef]
18. Calina, D.; Buga, A.M.; Mitroi, M.; Buha, A.; Caruntu, C.; Scheau, C.; Bouyahya, A.; El Omari, N.; El Menyiy, N.; Docea, A.O. The Treatment of Cognitive, Behavioural and Motor Impairments from Brain Injury and Neurodegenerative Diseases Through Cannabinoid System Modulation—Evidence from In Vivo Studies. *J. Clin. Med.* **2020**, *9*, 2395. [CrossRef]
19. Zwilling, M.; Theiss, C.; Matschke, V. Caffeine and NAD+ Improve Motor Neural Integrity of Dissociated Wobbler Cells In Vitro. *Antioxidants* **2020**, *9*, 460. [CrossRef]
20. Van Gelder, B.M.; Buijsse, B.; Tijhuis, M.; Kalmijn, S.; Giampaoli, S.; Nissinen, A.; Kromhout, D. Coffee consumption is inversely associated with cognitive decline in elderly European men: The FINE Study. *Eur. J. Clin. Nutr.* **2006**, *61*, 226–232. [CrossRef]

21. Kendler, K.S.; Myers, J.; Gardner, C.O. Caffeine intake, toxicity and dependence and lifetime risk for psychiatric and substance use disorders: An epidemiologic and co-twin control analysis. *Psychol. Med.* **2006**, *36*, 1717–1725. [CrossRef]
22. Anwarullah; Aslam, M.; Badshah, M.; Abbasi, R.; Sultan, A.; Khan, K.; Ahmad, N.; Von Engelhardt, J. Further evidence for the association of CYP2D6*4 gene polymorphism with Parkinson's disease: A case control study. *Genes Environ.* **2017**, *39*, 18. [CrossRef] [PubMed]
23. Chace, C.; Pang, D.; Weng, C.; Temkin, A.; Lax, S.; Silverman, W.; Zigman, W.B.; Ferin, M.; Lee, J.H.; Tycko, B.; et al. Variants in CYP17 and CYP19 Cytochrome P450 Genes are Associated with Onset of Alzheimer's Disease in Women with Down Syndrome. *J. Alzheimer's Dis.* **2012**, *28*, 601–612. [CrossRef] [PubMed]
24. Djelti, F.; Braudeau, J.; Hudry, E.; Dhenain, M.; Varin-Simon, J.; Bieche, I.; Marquer, C.; Chali, F.; Ayciriex, S.; Auzeil, N.; et al. CYP46A1 inhibition, brain cholesterol accumulation and neurodegeneration pave the way for Alzheimer's disease. *Brain* **2015**, *138*, 2383–2398. [CrossRef] [PubMed]
25. Duléry, R. Neurological Complications. In *The EBMT Handbook: Hematopoietic Stem Cell Transplantation and Cellular Therapies*; Carreras, E., Dufour, C., Mohty, M., Kröger, N., Eds.; Springer: Cham, Switzerland, 2019; pp. 403–407. [CrossRef]
26. Turnbull, D.; Rodricks, J.V.; Mariano, G.F.; Chowdhury, F. Caffeine and cardiovascular health. *Regul. Toxicol. Pharmacol.* **2017**, *89*, 165–185. [CrossRef] [PubMed]
27. Gall, S.; Donnan, G.; Dewey, H.M.; MacDonell, R.; Sturm, J.; Gilligan, A.; Srikanth, V.; Thrift, A.G. Sex differences in presentation, severity, and management of stroke in a population-based study. *Neurology* **2010**, *74*, 975–981. [CrossRef]
28. Stuart-Shor, E.M.; Wellenius, G.A.; DelloIacono, D.M.; Mittleman, M.A. Gender differences in presenting and prodromal stroke symptoms. *Stroke* **2009**, *40*, 1121–1126. [CrossRef]
29. Lisabeth, L.D.; Brown, D.L.; Hughes, R.; Majersik, J.J.; Morgenstern, L.B. Acute Stroke Symptoms. *Stroke* **2009**, *40*, 2031–2036. [CrossRef]
30. Jerath, N.U.; Reddy, C.; Freeman, W.D.; Jerath, A.U.; Brown, R.D. Gender Differences in Presenting Signs and Symptoms of Acute Ischemic Stroke: A Population-Based Study. *Gend. Med.* **2011**, *8*, 312–319. [CrossRef]
31. Appelros, P.; Stegmayr, B.; TereéntA. Sex Differences in Stroke Epidemiology. *Stroke* **2009**, *40*, 1082–1090. [CrossRef]
32. Barrett, K.M.; Brott, T.G.; Brown, R.D.; Frankel, M.R.; Worrall, B.B.; Silliman, S.L.; Case, L.D.; Rich, S.S.; Meschia, J.F.; Ischemic Stroke Genetics Study Group. Sex Differences in Stroke Severity, Symptoms, and Deficits After First-ever Ischemic Stroke. *J. Stroke Cerebrovasc. Dis.* **2007**, *16*, 34–39. [CrossRef]
33. Petrea, R.E.; Beiser, A.S.; Seshadri, S.; Kelly-Hayes, M.; Kase, C.S.; Wolf, P.A. Gender Differences in Stroke Incidence and Poststroke Disability in the Framingham Heart Study. *Stroke* **2009**, *40*, 1032–1037. [CrossRef] [PubMed]
34. Aurora, R.N.; Zak, R.S.; Maganti, R.K.; Auerbach, S.H.; Casey, K.R.; Chowdhuri, S.; Karippot, A.; Ramar, K.; Kristo, D.A.; Morgenthaler, T.I. Best Practice Guide for the Treatment of REM Sleep Behavior Disorder (RBD). *J. Clin. Sleep Med.* **2010**, *6*, 85–95. [CrossRef]
35. Singareddy, R.; Vgontzas, A.N.; Fernandez-Mendoza, J.; Liao, D.; Calhoun, S.; Shaffer, M.L.; Bixler, E.O. Risk factors for incident chronic insomnia: A general population prospective study. *Sleep Med.* **2012**, *13*, 346–353. [CrossRef]
36. Morphy, H.; Dunn, K.M.; Lewis, M.; Boardman, H.F.; Croft, P. Epidemiology of insomnia: A longitudinal study in a UK population. *Sleep* **2007**, *30*, 274–280. [CrossRef] [PubMed]
37. Jaussent, I.; Dauvilliers, Y.; Ancelin, M.-L.; Dartigues, J.-F.; Tavernier, B.; Touchon, J.; Ritchie, K.; Besset, A. Insomnia Symptoms in Older Adults: Associated Factors and Gender Differences. *Am. J. Geriatr. Psychiatry* **2011**, *19*, 88–97. [CrossRef] [PubMed]
38. Ferretti, M.T.; Iulita, M.F.; Cavedo, E.; Chiesa, P.A.; Schumacher, D.A.; Santuccione, C.A.; Baracchi, F.; Girouard, H.; Misoch, S.; Giacobini, E.; et al. Sex differences in Alzheimer disease—The gateway to precision medicine. *Nat. Rev. Neurol.* **2018**, *14*, 457–469. [CrossRef] [PubMed]
39. Mielke, M.M.; Vemuri, P.; Rocca, W.A. Clinical epidemiology of Alzheimer's disease: Assessing sex and gender differences. *Clin. Epidemiol.* **2014**, *6*, 37–48. [CrossRef]

40. Seshadri, S.; Wolf, P.A.; Beiser, A.S.; Au, R.; McNulty, K.; White, R.F.; D'Agostino, R.B. Lifetime risk of dementia and Alzheimer's disease: The impact of mortality on risk estimates in the Framingham Study. *Neurology* **1997**, *49*, 1498–1504. [CrossRef]
41. Nebel, R.A.; Aggarwal, N.T.; Barnes, L.L.; Gallagher, A.; Goldstein, J.M.; Kantarci, K.; Mallampalli, M.P.; Mormino, E.C.; Scott, L.; Yu, W.H.; et al. Understanding the impact of sex and gender in Alzheimer's disease: A call to action. *Alzheimer's Dement.* **2018**, *14*, 1171–1183. [CrossRef]
42. Elbaz, A.; Bower, J.H.; Maraganore, D.M.; McDonnell, S.K.; Peterson, B.J.; Ahlskog, J.E.; Schaid, D.; Rocca, W.A. Risk tables for parkinsonism and Parkinson's disease. *J. Clin. Epidemiol.* **2002**, *55*, 25–31. [CrossRef]
43. Baldereschi, M.; Di Carlo, A.; Rocca, W.A.; Vanni, P.; Maggi, S.; Perissinotto, E.; Grigoletto, F.; Amaducci, L.; Inzitari, D. Parkinson's disease and parkinsonism in a longitudinal study: Two-fold higher incidence in men. *Neurology* **2000**, *55*, 1358–1363. [CrossRef] [PubMed]
44. Augustine, E.F.; Pérez, A.; Dhall, R.; Umeh, C.C.; Videnovic, A.; Cambi, F.; Wills, A.-M.A.; Elm, J.J.; Zweig, R.M.; Shulman, L.M.; et al. Sex Differences in Clinical Features of Early, Treated Parkinson's Disease. *PLoS ONE* **2015**, *10*, 0133002. [CrossRef] [PubMed]
45. Jurado-Coronel, J.C.; Cabezas, R.; Avila-Rodriguez, M.F.; Echeverria, V.; Garcia-Segura, L.M.; Barreto, G.E. Sex differences in Parkinson's disease: Features on clinical symptoms, treatment outcome, sexual hormones and genetics. *Front. Neuroendocr.* **2018**, *50*, 18–30. [CrossRef] [PubMed]
46. Carmona, N.E.; Subramaniapillai, M.; Mansur, R.B.; Cha, D.S.; Lee, Y.; Fus, D.; McIntyre, R.S. Sex differences in the mediators of functional disability in Major Depressive Disorder. *J. Psychiatr. Res.* **2018**, *96*, 108–114. [CrossRef]
47. Rempel, J.D.; Krueger, C.; Uhanova, J.; Wong, S.; Minuk, G.Y. The Impact of Gender on Interferon-Associated Depression and Anxiety. *J. Interferon Cytokine Res.* **2019**, *39*, 416–420. [CrossRef]
48. Maciejewski, P.K.; Prigerson, H.G.; Mazure, C.M. Sex differences in event-related risk for major depression. *Psychol. Med.* **2001**, *31*, 593–604. [CrossRef]
49. De Visser, L.; Van Der Knaap, L.; Van De Loo, A.; Van Der Weerd, C.; Ohl, F.; Bos, R.V.D. Trait anxiety affects decision-making differently in healthy men and women: Towards gender-specific endophenotypes of anxiety. *Neuropsychologia* **2010**, *48*, 1598–1606. [CrossRef]
50. Seo, D.; Ahluwalia, A.; Potenza, M.N.; Sinha, R. Gender differences in neural correlates of stress-induced anxiety. *J. Neurosci. Res.* **2016**, *95*, 115–125. [CrossRef]
51. Grob, D.; Brunner, N.; Namba, T.; Pagala, M. Lifetime course of myasthenia gravis. *Muscle Nerve* **2007**, *37*, 141–149. [CrossRef]
52. Jerath, N.U.; Gutmann, L.; Reddy, C.G.; Shy, M.E. Charcot-marie-tooth disease type 1X in women: Electrodiagnostic findings. *Muscle Nerve* **2016**, *54*, 728–732. [CrossRef]
53. McCombe, P.A.; Henderson, R.D. Effects of gender in amyotrophic lateral sclerosis. *Gend. Med.* **2010**, *7*, 557–570. [CrossRef] [PubMed]
54. Krueger, J.M.; Frank, M.G.; Wisor, J.P.; Roy, S. Sleep function: Toward elucidating an enigma. *Sleep Med. Rev.* **2015**, *28*, 46–54. [CrossRef] [PubMed]
55. Jee, H.J.; Shin, W.; Jung, H.J.; Kim, B.; Lee, B.K.; Jung, Y.-S. Impact of Sleep Disorder as a Risk Factor for Dementia in Men and Women. *Biomol. Ther.* **2020**, *28*, 58–73. [CrossRef] [PubMed]
56. Autio, J.; Stenbäck, V.; Gagnon, D.D.; Leppäluoto, J.; Herzig, K.-H. (Neuro)Peptides, Physical Activity, and Cognition. *J. Clin. Med.* **2020**, *9*, 2592. [CrossRef]
57. Kiley, J.P.; Twery, M.J.; Gibbons, G.H. The National Center on Sleep Disorders Research—Progress and promise. *Sleep* **2019**, *42*. [CrossRef]
58. Hung, C.-M.; Li, Y.-C.; Chen, H.-J.; Lu, K.; Liang, C.-L.; LiLiang, P.-C.; Tsai, Y.-D.; Wang, K.-W. Risk of dementia in patients with primary insomnia: A nationwide population-based case-control study. *BMC Psychiatry* **2018**, *18*, 38. [CrossRef]
59. Nowakowski, S.; Meers, J.; Heimbach, E. Sleep and Women's Health. *Sleep Med. Res.* **2013**, *4*, 1–22. [CrossRef]
60. Kim, M.-Y.; Jung, M.; Noh, Y.; Shin, S.; Hong, C.H.; Lee, S.; Jung, Y.-S. Impact of Statin Use on Dementia Incidence in Elderly Men and Women with Ischemic Heart Disease. *Biomedicines* **2020**, *8*, 30. [CrossRef]
61. Kim, M.-Y.; Kim, K.; Hong, C.H.; Lee, S.Y.; Jung, Y.-S. Sex Differences in Cardiovascular Risk Factors for Dementia. *Biomol. Ther.* **2018**, *26*, 521–532. [CrossRef]

62. Podcasy, J.L.; Epperson, C.N. Considering sex and gender in Alzheimer disease and other dementias. *Dialogues Clin. Neurosci.* **2016**, *18*, 437–446.
63. Prince, M.; Bryce, R.; Albanese, E.; Wimo, A.; Ribeiro, W.; Ferri, C.P. The global prevalence of dementia: A systematic review and metaanalysis. *Alzheimer's Dement.* **2013**, *9*, 63–75. [CrossRef] [PubMed]
64. Wu, Y.-T.; Beiser, A.S.; Breteler, M.M.B.; Fratiglioni, L.; Helmer, C.; Hendrie, H.C.; Honda, H.; Ikram, M.A.; Langa, K.M.; Lobo, A.; et al. The changing prevalence and incidence of dementia over time—Current evidence. *Nat. Rev. Neurol.* **2017**, *13*, 327–339. [CrossRef] [PubMed]
65. Prince, M.; Ali, G.-C.; Guerchet, M.; Prina, A.M.; Albanese, E.; Wu, Y.-T. Recent global trends in the prevalence and incidence of dementia, and survival with dementia. *Alzheimer's Res. Ther.* **2016**, *8*, 23. [CrossRef] [PubMed]
66. Hebert, L.E.; Weuve, J.; Scherr, P.A.; Evans, D.A. Alzheimer disease in the United States (2010–2050) estimated using the 2010 census. *Neurology* **2013**, *80*, 1778–1783. [CrossRef]
67. Alzheimer's Association 2014 Alzheimer's disease facts and figures. *Alzheimer's Dement.* **2014**, *10*, 47–92. [CrossRef]
68. Roberts, R.O.; Knopman, D.S.; Mielke, M.M.; Cha, R.H.; Pankratz, V.S.; Christianson, T.J.; Geda, Y.E.; Boeve, B.F.; Ivnik, R.J.; Tangalos, E.G.; et al. Higher risk of progression to dementia in mild cognitive impairment cases who revert to normal. *Neurology* **2013**, *82*, 317–325. [CrossRef]
69. Noh, H.; Jang, J.; Kwon, S.; Cho, S.-Y.; Jung, W.S.; Moon, S.-K.; Park, J.-M.; Ko, C.-N.; Kim, H.; Park, S.-U. The Impact of Korean Medicine Treatment on the Incidence of Parkinson's Disease in Patients with Inflammatory Bowel Disease: A Nationwide Population-Based Cohort Study in South Korea. *J. Clin. Med.* **2020**, *9*, 2422. [CrossRef]
70. Mhyre, T.R.; Boyd, J.T.; Hamill, R.W.; Maguire-Zeiss, K.A. Parkinson's Disease. *Subcell. Biochem.* **2012**, *65*, 389–455. [CrossRef]
71. Dexter, D.T.; Jenner, P. Parkinson disease: From pathology to molecular disease mechanisms. *Free. Radic. Biol. Med.* **2013**, *62*, 132–144. [CrossRef]
72. Eeden, S.K.V.D.; Tanner, C.M.; Bernstein, A.L.; Fross, R.D.; Leimpeter, A.; Bloch, D.A.; Nelson, L.M. Incidence of Parkinson's Disease: Variation by Age, Gender, and Race/Ethnicity. *Am. J. Epidemiol.* **2003**, *157*, 1015–1022. [CrossRef]
73. Georgiev, D.; Hamberg, K.; Hariz, M.; Forsgren, L.; Hariz, G.-M. Gender differences in Parkinson's disease: A clinical perspective. *Acta Neurol. Scand.* **2017**, *136*, 570–584. [CrossRef] [PubMed]
74. Miller, I.N.; Cronin-Golomb, A. Gender differences in Parkinson's disease: Clinical characteristics and cognition. *Mov. Disord.* **2010**, *25*, 2695–2703. [CrossRef] [PubMed]
75. Colognesi, M.; Gabbia, D.; De Martin, S. Depression and Cognitive Impairment—Extrahepatic Manifestations of NAFLD and NASH. *Biomedicines* **2020**, *8*, 229. [CrossRef] [PubMed]
76. Huang, R.; Wang, K.; Hu, J. Effect of Probiotics on Depression: A Systematic Review and Meta-Analysis of Randomized Controlled Trials. *Nutrients* **2016**, *8*, 483. [CrossRef] [PubMed]
77. Ménard, C.; Hodes, G.; Russo, S.J. Pathogenesis of depression: Insights from human and rodent studies. *Neuroscience* **2015**, *321*, 138–162. [CrossRef]
78. Malhi, G.S.; Mann, J.J. Depression. *Lancet* **2018**, *392*, 2299–2312. [CrossRef]
79. Krueger, C.; Hawkins, K.; Wong, S.; Enns, M.W.; Minuk, G.; Rempel, J.D. Persistent pro-inflammatory cytokines following the initiation of pegylated IFN therapy in hepatitis C infection is associated with treatment-induced depression. *J. Viral Hepat.* **2010**, *18*, 284–291. [CrossRef]
80. Albert, P.R. Why is depression more prevalent in women? *J. Psychiatry Neurosci.* **2015**, *40*, 219–221. [CrossRef]
81. Craske, M.G.; Stein, M.B. Anxiety. *Lancet* **2016**, *388*, 3048–3059. [CrossRef]
82. Kandola, A.; Vancampfort, D.; Herring, M.; Rebar, A.; Hallgren, M.; Firth, J.; Stubbs, B. Moving to Beat Anxiety: Epidemiology and Therapeutic Issues with Physical Activity for Anxiety. *Curr. Psychiatry Rep.* **2018**, *20*, 63. [CrossRef]
83. Cerdá, M.; DiGangi, J.; Galea, S.; Koenen, K.C. Epidemiologic research on interpersonal violence and common psychiatric disorders: Where do we go from here? *Depress. Anxiety* **2012**, *29*, 359–385. [CrossRef] [PubMed]
84. Burgess, R.W.; Cox, G.A.; Seburn, K.L. Neuromuscular Disease Models and Analysis. *Adv. Struct. Saf. Stud.* **2016**, *1438*, 349–394.

85. Tanovska, N.; Novotni, G.; Sazdova-Burneska, S.; Kuzmanovski, I.; Boshkovski, B.; Kondov, G.; Jovanoski-Srceva, M.; Kokareva, A.; Isjanovska, R. Myasthenia Gravis and Associated Diseases. *Open Access Maced. J. Med Sci.* **2018**, *6*, 472–478. [CrossRef]
86. Szigeti, K.; Lupski, J.R. Charcot–Marie–Tooth disease. *Eur. J. Hum. Genet.* **2009**, *17*, 703–710. [CrossRef] [PubMed]
87. Theadom, A.; Roxburgh, R.; Macaulay, E.; O'Grady, G.; Burns, J.; Parmar, P.; Jones, K.; Rodrigues, M.; Impact CMT Research Group; Pal, M. Prevalence of Charcot-Marie-Tooth disease across the lifespan: A population-based epidemiological study. *BMJ Open* **2019**, *9*, 029240. [CrossRef] [PubMed]
88. Campanari, M.-L.; García-Ayllón, M.-S.; Ciura, S.; Sáez-Valero, J.; Kabashi, E. Neuromuscular Junction Impairment in Amyotrophic Lateral Sclerosis: Reassessing the Role of Acetylcholinesterase. *Front. Mol. Neurosci.* **2016**, *9*, 160. [CrossRef] [PubMed]
89. Poole, R.; Kennedy, O.J.; Roderick, P.; Fallowfield, J.; Hayes, P.C.; Parkes, J. Coffee consumption and health: Umbrella review of meta-analyses of multiple health outcomes. *BMJ* **2017**, *359*. [CrossRef] [PubMed]
90. Spychala, M.S.; Honarpisheh, P.; McCullough, L.D. Sex differences in neuroinflammation and neuroprotection in ischemic stroke. *J. Neurosci. Res.* **2016**, *95*, 462–471. [CrossRef]
91. Liebeskind, D.S.; Sanossian, N.; Fu, K.A.; Wang, H.-J.; Arab, L. The coffee paradox in stroke: Increased consumption linked with fewer strokes. *Nutr. Neurosci.* **2015**, *19*, 406–413. [CrossRef]
92. Lee, J.; Lee, J.-E.; Kim, Y. Relationship between coffee consumption and stroke risk in Korean population: The Health Examinees (HEXA) Study. *Nutr. J.* **2017**, *16*, 7. [CrossRef]
93. Mostofsky, E.; Schlaug, G.; Mukamal, K.J.; Rosamond, W.D.; Mittleman, M.A. Coffee and acute ischemic stroke onset: The Stroke Onset Study. *Neurology* **2010**, *75*, 1583–1588. [CrossRef] [PubMed]
94. Alperet, D.J.; Rebello, S.A.; Khoo, E.Y.-H.; Tay, Z.; Seah, S.S.-Y.; Tai, B.-C.; Tai, E.-S.; Emady-Azar, S.; Chou, C.J.; Darimont, C.; et al. The effect of coffee consumption on insulin sensitivity and other biological risk factors for type 2 diabetes: A randomized placebo-controlled trial. *Am. J. Clin. Nutr.* **2019**, *111*, 448–458. [CrossRef] [PubMed]
95. Lopez-Garcia, E.; Rodriguez-Artalejo, F.; Rexrode, K.; Logroscino, G.; Hu, F.B.; Van Dam, R.M. Coffee consumption and risk of stroke in women. *Circulation* **2009**, *119*, 1116–1123. [CrossRef] [PubMed]
96. Robillard, R.; Bouchard, M.; Cartier, A.; Nicolau, L.; Carrier, J. Sleep is more sensitive to high doses of caffeine in the middle years of life. *J. Psychopharmacol.* **2015**, *29*, 688–697. [CrossRef]
97. Carrier, J.; Paquet, J.; Fernandez-Bolanos, M.; Girouard, L.; Roy, J.; Selmaoui, B.; Filipini, D. Effects of caffeine on daytime recovery sleep: A double challenge to the sleep–wake cycle in aging. *Sleep Med.* **2009**, *10*, 1016–1024. [CrossRef]
98. Pollak, C.P.; Bright, D. Caffeine consumption and weekly sleep patterns in US seventh-, eighth-, and ninth-graders. *Pediatrics* **2003**, *111*, 42–46. [CrossRef]
99. Watson, E.J.; Coates, A.M.; Kohler, M.; Banks, S. Caffeine Consumption and Sleep Quality in Australian Adults. *Nutrients* **2016**, *8*, 479. [CrossRef]
100. Park, J.; Han, J.W.; Lee, J.R.; Byun, S.; Suh, S.W.; Kim, T.; Yoon, I.-Y.; Kim, K.W. Lifetime coffee consumption, pineal gland volume, and sleep quality in late life. *Sleep* **2018**, *41*, 41. [CrossRef]
101. Solfrizzi, V.; Panza, F.; Imbimbo, B.P.; D'Introno, A.; Galluzzo, L.; Gandin, C.; Misciagna, G.; Guerra, V.; Osella, A.; Baldereschi, M.; et al. Coffee Consumption Habits and the Risk of Mild Cognitive Impairment: The Italian Longitudinal Study on Aging. *J. Alzheimer's Dis.* **2015**, *47*, 889–899. [CrossRef]
102. Paganini-Hill, A.; Kawas, C.H.; Corrada, M.M. Lifestyle Factors and Dementia in the Oldest-old. *Alzheimer Dis. Assoc. Disord.* **2016**, *30*, 21–26. [CrossRef]
103. Eskelinen, M.H.; Ngandu, T.; Tuomilehto, J.; Soininen, H.; Kivipelto, M. Midlife Coffee and Tea Drinking and the Risk of Late-Life Dementia: A Population-Based CAIDE Study. *J. Alzheimer's Dis.* **2009**, *16*, 85–91. [CrossRef]
104. Driscoll, I.; Shumaker, S.A.; Snively, B.M.; Margolis, K.L.; Manson, J.E.; Vitolins, M.Z.; Rossom, R.C.; Espeland, M.A. Relationships Between Caffeine Intake and Risk for Probable Dementia or Global Cognitive Impairment: The Women's Health Initiative Memory Study. *J. Gerontol. Ser. A Biol. Sci. Med. Sci.* **2016**, *71*, 1596–1602. [CrossRef] [PubMed]

105. Ritchie, K.; Carriere, I.; De Mendonça, A.; Portet, F.; Dartigues, J.F.; Rouaud, O.; Barberger-Gateau, P.; Ancelin, M.-L. The neuroprotective effects of caffeine: A prospective population study (the Three City Study). *Neurology* **2007**, *69*, 536–545. [CrossRef] [PubMed]
106. Qi, H.; Li, S. Dose-response meta-analysis on coffee, tea and caffeine consumption with risk of Parkinson's disease. *Geriatr. Gerontol. Int.* **2013**, *14*, 430–439. [CrossRef] [PubMed]
107. Palacios, N.; Gao, X.; McCullough, M.L.; Schwarzschild, M.A.; Shah, R.; Gapstur, S.; Ascherio, A. Caffeine and risk of Parkinson's disease in a large cohort of men and women. *Mov. Disord.* **2012**, *27*, 1276–1282. [CrossRef]
108. Sääksjärvi, K.; Knekt, P.; Rissanen, H.; Laaksonen, M.A.; Reunanen, A.; Männistö, S. Prospective study of coffee consumption and risk of Parkinson's disease. *Eur. J. Clin. Nutr.* **2007**, *62*, 908–915. [CrossRef]
109. Ascherio, A.; Zhang, S.M.; Hernán, M.A.; Kawachi, I.; Colditz, G.A.; Speizer, F.E.; Willett, W.C. Prospective study of caffeine consumption and risk of Parkinson's disease in men and women. *Ann. Neurol.* **2001**, *50*, 56–63. [CrossRef]
110. Ross, G.W.; Abbott, R.D.; Petrovitch, H.; Morens, D.M.; Grandinetti, A.; Tung, K.-H.; Tanner, C.M.; Masaki, K.H.; Blanchette, P.L.; Curb, J.D.; et al. Association of coffee and caffeine intake with the risk of Parkinson disease. *JAMA* **2000**, *283*, 2674–2679. [CrossRef]
111. Kim, J.; Kim, J. Green Tea, Coffee, and Caffeine Consumption Are Inversely Associated with Self-Report Lifetime Depression in the Korean Population. *Nutrients* **2018**, *10*, 1201. [CrossRef]
112. Lucas, M.; Mirzaei, F.; Pan, A.; Okereke, O.I.; Willett, W.C.; O'Reilly, E.J.; Koenen, K.C.; Ascherio, A. Coffee, Caffeine, and Risk of Depression Among Women. *Arch. Intern. Med.* **2011**, *171*, 1571–1578. [CrossRef]
113. Iranpour, S.; Sabour, S. Inverse association between caffeine intake and depressive symptoms in US adults: Data from National Health and Nutrition Examination Survey (NHANES) 2005–2006. *Psychiatry Res.* **2019**, *271*, 732–739. [CrossRef] [PubMed]
114. Richards, G.; Smith, A. Caffeine consumption and self-assessed stress, anxiety, and depression in secondary school children. *J. Psychopharmacol.* **2015**, *29*, 1236–1247. [CrossRef] [PubMed]
115. Botella, P. Coffee increases state anxiety in males but not in females. *Hum. Psychopharmacol. Clin. Exp.* **2003**, *18*, 141–143. [CrossRef] [PubMed]
116. Hedström, A.K.; Mowry, E.M.; Gianfrancesco, M.A.; Shao, X.; Schaefer, C.A.; Shen, L.; Olsson, T.; Barcellos, L.F.; Alfredsson, L. High consumption of coffee is associated with decreased multiple sclerosis risk; results from two independent studies. *J. Neurol. Neurosurg. Psychiatry* **2016**, *87*, 454–460. [CrossRef] [PubMed]
117. Massa, J.; O'Reilly, E.; Munger, K.; Ascherio, A. Caffeine and alcohol intakes have no association with risk of multiple sclerosis. *Mult. Scler. J.* **2012**, *19*, 53–58. [CrossRef]
118. Beghi, E.; Pupillo, E.; Messina, P.; Giussani, G.; Chiò, A.; Zoccolella, S.; Moglia, C.; Corbo, M.; Logroscino, G. Coffee and Amyotrophic Lateral Sclerosis: A Possible Preventive Role. *Am. J. Epidemiol.* **2011**, *174*, 1002–1008. [CrossRef]
119. Winston, A.P.; Hardwick, E.; Jaberi, N. Neuropsychiatric effects of caffeine. *Adv. Psychiatr. Treat.* **2005**, *11*, 432–439. [CrossRef]
120. Benedetti, M.D.; Bower, J.H.; Maraganore, D.M.; McDonnell, S.K.; Peterson, B.J.; Ahlskog, J.E.; Schaid, D.J.; Rocca, W.A. Smoking, alcohol, and coffee consumption preceding Parkinson's disease: A case-control study. *Neurology* **2000**, *55*, 1350–1358. [CrossRef]
121. Paganini-Hill, A. Risk factors for parkinson's disease: The leisure world cohort study. *Neuroepidemiology* **2001**, *20*, 118–124. [CrossRef]
122. Ascherio, A.; Weisskopf, M.G.; O'Reilly, E.J.; McCullough, M.L.; Calle, E.E.; Rodriguez, C.; Thun, M.J. Coffee Consumption, Gender, and Parkinson's Disease Mortality in the Cancer Prevention Study II Cohort: The Modifying Effects of Estrogen. *Am. J. Epidemiol.* **2004**, *160*, 977–984. [CrossRef]
123. Mino, Y.; Yasuda, N.; Fujimura, T.; Ohara, H. Caffeine consumption and anxiety and depressive symptomatology among medical students. *Arukoru kenkyu yakubutsu izon Jpn. J. Alcohol Stud. Drug Depend.* **1990**, *25*, 486–496.
124. Park, S.; Lee, Y.; Lee, J.H. Association between energy drink intake, sleep, stress, and suicidality in Korean adolescents: Energy drink use in isolation or in combination with junk food consumption. *Nutr. J.* **2016**, *15*, 87. [CrossRef] [PubMed]
125. Maron, E.; Nutt, D. Biological Markers of Generalized Anxiety Disorder. *Focus* **2018**, *16*, 210–218. [CrossRef] [PubMed]

126. Petimar, J.; O'Reilly, E.; Adami, H.-O.; Brandt, P.A.V.D.; Buring, J.; English, D.; Freedman, D.M.; Giles, G.G.; Håkansson, N.; Kurth, T.; et al. Coffee, tea, and caffeine intake and amyotrophic lateral sclerosis mortality in a pooled analysis of eight prospective cohort studies. *Eur. J. Neurol.* **2018**, *26*, 468–475. [CrossRef] [PubMed]
127. Fondell, E.; O'Reilly, E.J.; Fitzgerald, K.C.; Falcone, G.J.; Kolonel, L.N.; Park, Y.; Gapstur, S.M.; Ascherio, A. Intakes of caffeine, coffee and tea and risk of amyotrophic lateral sclerosis: Results from five cohort studies. *Amyotroph. Lateral Scler. Front. Degener.* **2015**, *16*, 366–371. [CrossRef] [PubMed]

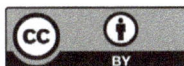

© 2020 by the authors. Licensee MDPI, Basel, Switzerland. This article is an open access article distributed under the terms and conditions of the Creative Commons Attribution (CC BY) license (http://creativecommons.org/licenses/by/4.0/).

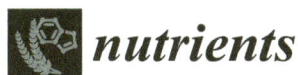 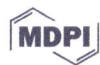

Review

The Ambiguous Role of Caffeine in Migraine Headache: From Trigger to Treatment

Magdalena Nowaczewska [1,*], Michał Wiciński [2] and Wojciech Kaźmierczak [3]

1. Department of Otolaryngology, Head and Neck Surgery, and Laryngological Oncology, Faculty of Medicine, Ludwik Rydygier Collegium Medicum in Bydgoszcz, Nicolaus Copernicus University, M. Curie 9, 85-090 Bydgoszcz, Poland
2. Department of Pharmacology and Therapeutics, Faculty of Medicine, Collegium Medicum in Bydgoszcz, Nicolaus Copernicus University, M. Curie 9, 85-090 Bydgoszcz, Poland; wicinski4@wp.pl
3. Department of Sensory Organs Examination, Faculty of Health Sciences, Collegium Medicum in Bydgoszcz, Nicolaus Copernicus University, M. Curie 9, 85-090 Bydgoszcz, Poland; wojciech.kazmierczak@umk.pl
* Correspondence: magy_mat@by.onet.pl; Tel.: +48-52-585-4716

Received: 7 July 2020; Accepted: 26 July 2020; Published: 28 July 2020

Abstract: Migraine is a chronic disorder, and caffeine has been linked with migraine for many years, on the one hand as a trigger, and on the other hand as a cure. As most of the population, including migraineurs, consume a considerable amount of caffeine daily, a question arises as to whether it influences their headaches. Indeed, drinking coffee before a migraine attack may not be a real headache trigger, but a consequence of premonitory symptoms, including yawning, diminished energy levels, and sleepiness that may herald a headache. Here, we aim to summarize the available evidence on the relationship between caffeine and migraines. Articles concerning this topic published up to June 2020 were retrieved by searching clinical databases, and all types of studies were included. We identified 21 studies investigating the prevalence of caffeine/caffeine withdrawal as a migraine trigger and 7 studies evaluating caffeine in acute migraine treatment. Among them, in 17 studies, caffeine/caffeine withdrawal was found to be a migraine trigger in a small percentage of participants (ranging from 2% to 30%), while all treatment studies found caffeine to be safe and effective in acute migraine treatment, mostly in combination with other analgesics. Overall, based on our review of the current literature, there is insufficient evidence to recommend caffeine cessation to all migraine patients, but it should be highlighted that caffeine overuse may lead to migraine chronification, and sudden caffeine withdrawal may trigger migraine attacks. Migraine sufferers should be aware of the amount of caffeine they consume and not exceed 200 mg daily. If they wish to continue drinking caffeinated beverages, they should keep their daily intake as consistent as possible to avoid withdrawal headache.

Keywords: migraine; headache; caffeine; coffee; trigger; withdrawal headache; adenosine; vasoconstriction; cerebral blood flow

---

1. Introduction

Migraine has emerged as a great public health concern, and the World Health Organization (WHO) has classified it as the third most common disease worldwide, with over a billion people estimated to suffer from it [1,2]. This type of primary headache usually presents with recurrent, typically unilateral and pulsating attacks of severe headaches, lasting from 4 to 72 h, with accompanying symptoms including photophobia, phonophobia, nausea, and vomiting [3]. Caffeine has been linked with migraine for many years, on the one hand as a trigger, and on the other as a cure [4–8]. As most of the population, including migraine sufferers, consume a considerable amount of coffee and other caffeinated drinks and foods daily, a question arises as to whether it influences their headaches. Besides, some migraine sufferers ask their doctors about dietary recommendations regarding their intake of caffeinated beverages. They demand specific information regarding whether they are allowed to drink coffee or should avoid it, and whether it will be beneficial for their migraine if they stop drinking it. The aim of this review is to examine the relationship between caffeine and migraine, and to check whether caffeine is a migraine trigger and avoiding it may be of benefit to certain patients, and to find out if caffeine may be helpful in migraine treatment.

1.1. Caffeine

Caffeine is the most popular and widely used active food ingredient, with up to 80% of the population consuming a caffeinated product every day [9]. One of the most popular caffeine drinks is coffee, and many people start their day with a cup of coffee. Caffeine also occurs in tea leaves, guarana, cocoa, chocolate, cola nuts, and wide variety of medications, dietary supplements, soft drinks, and energy drinks [10]. As the structure of caffeine is similar to adenosine, it works through nonselective antagonism of adenosine A1 and A2A receptors, causing their inhibition. It is important to note that adenosine is an inhibitor of neuronal activity in the nervous system; its receptors have been reported to be involved in antinociception, and enhancing them may lead to arousal, concentration, and vigilance [11]. However, caffeine has no influence on dopamine release, thus has no potential for abuse [12]. In humans, after oral intake, caffeine is rapidly and completely absorbed (max t 30–120 min) and freely crosses the blood–brain barrier [10]. Although a main component of coffee is caffeine, it should be pointed out that it is a complex drink including over 1000 compounds, most of them not yet identified. Haskell-Ramsay compared the effects of regular coffee, decaffeinated coffee, and placebo on mood and cognition, and discovered that decaffeinated coffee also increased alertness when compared to placebo. Thus, the behavioral activity of coffee seems to expand beyond its caffeine content, and the use of decaffeinated coffee as a placebo may be controversial [13]. It is reported that moderate daily caffeine intake (300–400 mg, around 4–5 cups of coffee) is safe and does not raise any health concerns (except in pregnant women and children) [14]. Nevertheless, higher doses may induce anxiety, nervousness, headache, drowsiness, nausea, insomnia, tremor, tachycardia, and increased blood pressure [10]. Interestingly, there is evidence that response to caffeine consumption may be genetically determined [12]. Besides, the amount of caffeine that produces adverse effects can vary and is influenced by the person's weight and sex, the presence of hypertension and hepatic disease, and metabolic induction and inhibition of cytochrome P-450 [15]. It is noteworthy that people who consume caffeine habitually have a lower risk of experiencing the adverse effects than those who do not frequently consume caffeine [10].

1.2. Caffeine's Influence on Health

Coffee consumption is associated with a number of health benefits in men and women. In an umbrella review, Grosso et al. demonstrated that caffeine was associated with a decreased risk of cancer, diabetes, cardiovascular disease and mortality, and Parkinson's disease but an increased risk of pregnancy loss [16]. On the other hand, coffee was linked with a rise in serum lipids and blood pressure. Overall, they concluded that coffee (moderate daily intake) can be part of a healthful diet [16]. A number of epidemiological studies confirmed a link between higher coffee consumption and better performance on cognitive tests in older adults, and an inverse relationship exists between coffee consumption and the risk of developing Parkinson's or Alzheimer's disease and a lower risk of stroke. Interestingly, regular coffee consumption does not affect patients with epilepsy [17]. It is reported thatcaffeine can enhance awareness, attention, and reaction time by stimulating wakefulness, increasing concentration, and decreasing the sensation of fatigue, but also may disturb sleep quality [14,17,18]. Moreover, caffeine in low doses (150–200 mg) can improve mood states and decreases the risk of depression and suicide [17].

1.3. Caffeine and Cerebral Blood Flow

The effect of caffeine on blood flow and arteries remains controversial. On the one hand, there is evidence that caffeine decreases the production of nitric oxide (NO, responsible for vasodilation) from the endothelial cells, and on the other hand, a number of studies showed increased NO production after caffeine administration [19,20]. Several studies investigated the direct effects of caffeine on endothelial function and concluded that caffeine augmented and improved endothelium-dependent but not endothelium-independent vasodilatation, suggesting that it has no effect on vascular smooth muscle function [21,22]. The reason for this ambiguous effect, called by Higashi the "coffee paradox," may be a different action of caffeine on endothelium and smooth muscles [21]. It is known that caffeine is an adenosine receptor antagonist. Interestingly, adenosine via the adenosine A2A receptor stimulates the production of NO with further vasodilatation, but contrary to this, via the adenosine A1 receptor, adenosine decreases NO release and produces vasoconstriction. Thus, depending on caffeine binding affinity and dose, it can cause either vasoconstriction or vasodilatation and sometimes even no change in vascular function [21]. It is important to note that methylxanthines such as caffeine usually induce vasodilatation except in the central nervous system, where they raise cerebrovascular resistance (CVR) and reduce cerebral blood flow (CBF) [23]. A number of studies demonstrated that by inducing vasoconstriction, caffeine reduces CBF in healthy people, but also in pathological conditions. Vidyasagar at al. discovered a global 20% reduction in gray matter CBF with caffeine and tea but not decaffeinated tea, which indicates that only caffeine change CBF. Moreover, the effect of caffeine was regionally specific. Interestingly, none of the interventions had an effect on CVR [24]. Haanes et al. investigated the effect of adenosine A2A receptor antagonists on the vasodilation of the middle meningeal artery. They found that antagonists did not influence neurogenic vasodilation, but blocked the vasodilation produced by A2A receptor agonists, suggesting that selective A2A receptor antagonists might be useful in migraine treatment by preventing meningeal arterial dilation [25]. Another study, using vascular information extracted from the blood-oxygen-level-dependent (BOLD) signal in functional MRI (fMRI) showed that shorter time delays and smaller standard deviations were detected in scans of caffeinated areas. This means that caffeine increased blood flow velocity by vasoconstriction [26]. The spatial distribution of adenosine receptors may be one reason for the region-dependent changes in brain activity induced by caffeine, thus, the average brain metabolic rate stays unchanged. Besides, caffeine's effects on arteries may be region-specific [27]. Blaha et al., in a transcranial Doppler (TCD) study, investigated the effects of caffeine on an already dilated cerebral circulation and found a significant decrease in CBF velocity after caffeine ingestion in a normal cerebrovascular bed as well as in peripheral vasodilatation. This means that caffeine may regulate CBF under various pathological conditions, with possible therapeutic effects in vasoparalysis [28]. Lunt et al., using two methods of cerebral blood flow measurement (transcranial Doppler and xenon clearance), demonstrated that 250 mg caffeine reduced CBF by an average of 22% in healthy volunteers as well as in patients recovering from stroke. Caffeine caused a smaller change in middle cerebral artery (MCA) blood flow velocity than in CBF, which indicates that caffeine reduces the MCA diameter [29]. Addicott et al. used perfusion magnetic resonance imaging to check the effect of caffeine on CBF in chronic users of low, moderate, and high amounts in an abstained state and the normal use (native) state. In each state, participants received either caffeine (250 mg) or placebo. It was found that in both states, caffeine reduced CBF by an average of 27%, but in the native placebo condition, users of high amounts of caffeine trended toward less CBF than those who consumed low and moderate amounts. These results suggest a limited ability of the cerebrovascular adenosine system to compensate for high amounts of daily caffeine [30]. Another TCD study examined whether controlled caffeine cessation would produce headache and changes in CBF velocity. After 24 h of caffeine abstinence, 10 individuals developed headache with an accompanying increase in CBF velocity. One hour after caffeine intake, the headache resolved and CBF velocity decreased. The study indicates a link between caffeine withdrawal, headache, and CBF [31]. Sigmon et al., in a double-blind study, demonstrated that acute caffeine abstinence increased mean, systolic, and diastolic velocity in the MCA and anterior cerebral artery (ACA) and decreased the pulsatility index in the MCA measured by TCD [32].

1.4. Caffeine's Effects on Pain and Non-Migraine Headache

There is evidence that caffeine may reduce pain sensation through its effects on adenosine receptors [12]. The antinociceptive effects of caffeine may be explained by an inhibition of cyclooxygenase activity as well as adenosine receptor antagonism. Caffeine acts not only by central blocking of adenosine receptors, which affects pain signaling, but also by blocking peripheral adenosine receptors on sensory afferents [12]. It was demonstrated that a 200 mg caffeine dose can inhibit the analgesic effects of transcutaneous electrical nerve stimulation [33]. Caffeine (≥100 mg) combined with a standard dose of analgesics led to an increased proportion of individuals with a satisfactory level of pain relief [34]. Laska et al. found that, in combination with paracetamol or aspirin, caffeine reduced the amount of analgesic needed to reach the same effect by approximately 40% [35]. Other clinical effects in these patients may be linked with the promotion of the absorption of analgesics by rapid lowering of gastric pH. Nevertheless, meta-analyses of caffeine combined with ibuprofen, paracetamol, or acetylic acid found only weak adjuvant effects in patients with postoperative pain [34].

It has been proved that caffeine and caffeine-containing analgesics are effective in the treatment of several types of primary and secondary headaches. For example, it is known to terminate hypnic headache, a sleep-related headache disorder that wakes people from sleep at a consistent time [36]. Based on observational studies, the most effective acute and prophylactic treatment of this rare disease is caffeine [37]. Another type of headache that may benefit from caffeine is post-dural puncture headache (PDPH), the most common complication of lumbar puncture and spinal anesthesia. A Cochrane review published in 2015 revealed that treatment with caffeine reduced PDPH in a number of participants and decreased the need for supplementary interventions compared to placebo [38]. This effect is probably due to increased production of cerebrospinal fluid (CSF), as one study demonstrated that long-term consumption of caffeine induced ventriculomegaly, and adenosine receptor signaling can regulate the production of CSF [39]. It has been reported that caffeine withdrawal can often produce headaches. According to the International Classification of Headache Disorders (ICHD-3), a withdrawal headache is a headache experienced by individuals who frequently consume caffeine (>200 mg/d for >2 weeks) and suddenly stop. They develop a headache within 24 h after their last caffeine intake, which is relieved within 1 h by ingesting caffeine (100 mg) or resolves within 7 days after caffeine withdrawal [3]. The higher the baseline level of caffeine ingestion, the greater the likelihood of withdrawal headache. The cause of this type of headache is probably increased CBF due to vasoconstriction [31]. It is important to note that caffeine withdrawal has been described as the cause of reversible cerebral vasoconstriction syndrome in several cases of this rare sudden thunderclap headache [40,41]. Ward et al., in a double-blind placebo-controlled trial, examined whether caffeine alone has independent analgesic effects on non-migraine headaches, and found equivalent effects to acetaminophen [8]. According to Mazzoni et al., overuse of caffeine was found in 36.6% of patients with chronic cluster headaches, compared to only 6.9% of patients with episodic headaches [42]. Interestingly, patients with chronic daily headaches were more likely to overuse caffeine before the onset of the headache, compared with controls with episodic headaches. Nevertheless, no association was found regarding present caffeine consumption [43]. Medication overuse headache (MOH) is a rebound headache that usually occurs with frequent use of analgesics to relieve headaches (more than 10–15 days a month). Kluonaitis et al. revealed that caffeine-containing combination analgesics were overused among 35.8% of patients with migraines [44]. Another study showed that combination analgesics were the most frequently overused medications by MOH patients, and caffeine was a component of 89.9% of these [45]. A randomized double-blind study conducted in patients with tension-type headache revealed that treatment with ibuprofen and caffeine provided significantly greater analgesic effect than ibuprofen alone, caffeine alone, or placebo. Notably, no analgesic effect of caffeine alone (200 mg) compared with placebo was found [46].

1.5. Caffeine and Migraine

1.5.1. Caffeine as Migraine Treatment: Potential Mechanism of Action 1

Although caffeine has been used for migraine headaches for many years, at the beginning its efficiency was linked with vascular properties. As caffeine produces cerebral vasoconstriction, it was thought that by this mechanism it may stop migraine attack. However, the role of vasodilatation in migraines is unclear, and recent findings challenge its necessity [47]. Nowadays, it is known that migraine is a neurological, not vascular, disorder, so the therapeutic effect of caffeine seems to be beyond its vascular effects. It is reported that adenosine is one of the neuromodulators that contribute to migraine pathophysiology. First of all, adenosine plasma levels increase during migraine attacks and exogenous adenosine may start migraine headaches [48]. Besides, an adenosine uptake inhibitor (dipyridamole) may increase the frequency of migraine attacks. Finally, as caffeine competitively antagonizes adenosine's effects by binding to some of the same receptors, it may be effective in migraine treatment [36]. On the other hand, it is important to note that regular use of caffeine-containing analgesics is associated with medication-overuse headaches. It was demonstrated that migraine sufferers have gastric stasis not only during, but also outside of acute migraine attacks [49]. This reduction in gastric motility slows the absorption of acute medications and diminishes their effectiveness [50]. As caffeine increases gastric motility, this may have important clinical implications for migraine patients, and may contribute to its effectiveness when combined with analgesics [34]. Caffeine, by inhibiting phosphodiesterases and blocking adenosine receptors, can potentially alter nitric oxide (NO) production. Bruce et al. demonstrated that caffeine diminished exhaled NO, probably by adenosine receptor antagonism or by altering levels of cGMP [19]. As NO levels increase in jugular venous plasma during a migraine attack and NO synthase inhibitors are effective in migraine treatment, it is possible that caffeine as a biologically active compound may decrease the frequency of migraine attacks by inhibiting NO synthase production [51]. Recently González at al. found that regular coffee consumption may be associated with changes in some intestinal microbiota groups [52]. As there is a relationship between migraine and the gut–brain axis and probiotics were found to be beneficial in migraine treatment, this can be another mechanism by which caffeine may influence migraines [53,54].

1.5.2. Caffeine as a Migraine Trigger: Potential Mechanism of Action

Trigger factors are events or exposures that increase the probability of an attack over a short period of time [55]. The 10 most frequent migraine triggers are stress; fatigue; fasting; auditory, visual, and olfactory triggers; hormonal triggers; sleep; weather; and alcohol [56]. Dietary triggers are less frequent, and include chocolate, coffee, red wine, nuts, cheeses, citrus fruits, processed meats, monosodium glutamate, and aspartame [57]. It is possible that an isolated trigger is insufficient to precipitate a migraine attack, thus, migraine sufferers usually recognize multiple dietary triggers [58]. Caffeine may act as a trigger in two possible ways: drinking coffee or other caffeinated beverages may start a migraine attack, and caffeine withdrawal is an even more frequent migraine trigger [59,60]. The prevalence of coffee as a migraine trigger in the reported literature ranges from 6.3% to 14.5% [36]. Moreover, caffeine overuse is one of the risk factors of migraine chronification, thus promoting the transformation of episodic migraine into its chronic form (when headaches persist for ≥15 days/month for >3 months) [61,62]. It is important to note that caffeine consumption was not significantly connected to medication overuse in chronic migraine patients [63]. A question arises: What is the exact mechanism by which caffeine can induce migraine headache? First, caffeine induces urinary loss of magnesium, probably by reducing its reabsorption [64]. As magnesium affects neuromuscular conduction and nerve transmission and plays a beneficial role in chronic pain conditions and migraines, caffeine, by decreasing the magnesium level, may induce headache [65]. Dehydration is one possible migraine trigger [66]. Caffeinated coffee in higher doses induces an acute diuretic effect, and subsequently may lead to dehydration [67]. Courturier et al. linked weekend migraine attacks to caffeine withdrawal. In their study, patients with high daily caffeine consumption on workdays and reduced or delayed intake on weekends (because of prolonged sleep) had an increased risk of weekend headache [68]. Thus, the observed higher frequency of migraines during weekends may be linked with caffeine withdrawal [68].

On the other hand, the methodological difficulties of investigating the influence of trigger factors on migraine are highlighted by many authors [58]. Premonitory features are defined as symptoms associated with an increased probability of aura or headache [55]. It is known that certain trigger factors can overlap with corresponding premonitory symptoms; for example, food craving in the premonitory phase may be responsible for eating chocolate or other foods, thus, they may be misinterpreted as migraine triggers [69]. It is possible that premonitory symptoms, including yawning, diminished energy levels, and sleepiness, may force migraineurs to drink coffee or caffeinated beverages, leading to the wrong conclusion that they triggered a migraine, while it was just a consequence of starting a migraine attack. On the other hand, premonitory sleepiness makes migraineurs prone to caffeine overuse, with further migraine chronification. Interestingly, according to Alstadhaug et al., the prodromal phase of migraine and caffeine withdrawal syndrome share the same or similar pathophysiological pathways [4].

A question arises as to whether caffeine may induce cortical spreading depression (CSD) in migraine aura sufferers. Yalcin at al. demonstrated that neither acute/chronic administration nor withdrawal of caffeine affected CSD susceptibility or related cortical blood flow changes in mice. Thus, they concluded that the influence of caffeine on headache is not linked with CSD pathophysiology, which may explain the non-migrainous presentation of caffeine-related headache [70].

Thus, should migraine patients strictly avoid all potential triggers, including caffeine? First of all, trigger avoidance create frustration, which may limit the beneficial effects or make the situation worse. Moreover, migraine is a disorder of the habituation of the CNS to sensory signals, thus, the brain should be trained to habituate to, not avoid triggers [71]. It is reported that short exposure to a headache trigger may increase sensitivity, while chronic exposure results in diminished sensitivity (leading to desensitization). According to Martin et al., patients with migraines should cope with triggers rather than avoid them [72].

If caffeine is a migraine trigger, does its cessation influence migraine attack frequency? Mikulec et al. demonstrated that only 14% of vestibular migraine patients reported an improvement in symptoms upon caffeine cessation [73]. Lee et al. evaluated the effect of caffeine cessation on the acute treatment of migraine. After controlling for covariates, caffeine cessation was independently connected with excellent efficacy of acute treatment. Indeed, 72.2% of those in the abstinence group reported excellent efficacy of triptans compared with only 40.3% in the non-abstinence group ($p = 0.002$). Besides, the abstinence group trended toward a greater reduction in headache impact test-6 (HIT-6) scores [74]. On the other hand, Mostofsky et al. revealed no association between one to two servings of caffeinated beverage intake and the odds of headaches on that day; only three or more servings were linked with higher odds of headache [75]. As caffeine dose per serving varies by type of drink and preparation method it may be difficult to assess the amount with increased risk. The average caffeine content of an 8 oz cup of coffee is around 100 mg [10]. It means that migraineurs may consume up to 200 mg caffeine without increased attacks risk.

All possible mechanisms regarding the influence of caffeine on migraine headache are summarized in Figure 1.

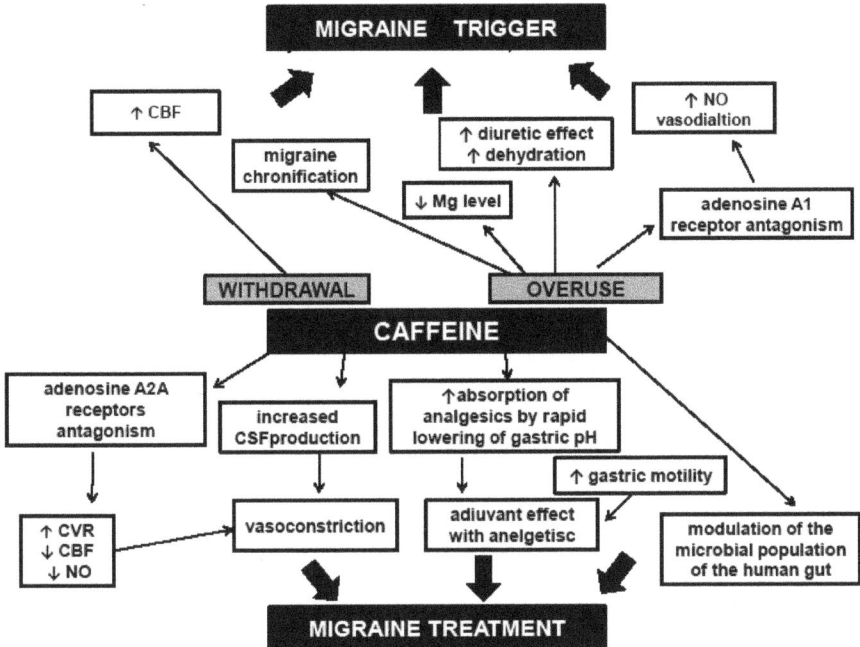

Figure 1. Possible mechanisms by which caffeine may trigger or stop migraine attacks (based on our literature review). Abbreviations: CBF—Cerebral blood flow, CVR—Cerebrovascular resistance, CSF—Cerebrospinal fluid, NO—Nitric oxide, Mg—Magnesium.

2. Materials and Methods

This review includes all articles concerning the association between migraines and caffeine/coffee published up to June 2020. The list was obtained by searching clinical databases, including the PubMed, MEDLINE, Google Scholar, and Cochrane Library databases. Papers regarding any connection between caffeine/coffee and migraine were identified through a literature search. The applied terminology and keywords included "caffeine", "coffee", "caffeine withdrawal", "adenosine", "migraine", "headache", "trigger factors", "treatment", and "pain". Each article was then cross-referenced to identify relevant studies. Only English language studies were eligible for inclusion. All types of articles, including clinical trials, observational, cross-sectional, and case-control studies, were involved and reviewed. Two independent investigators extracted data from each article.

3. Results and Discussion

3.1. Prevalence of Caffeine as a Migraine Trigger Factor

All studies investigating the prevalence of caffeine/coffee or caffeine withdrawal as a trigger factor in patients with migraines are summarized in Table 1.

Table 1. Overview of studies investigating the prevalence of caffeine/coffee as a trigger factor in migraineurs. TTH, tension-type headache; MWA, migraine without aura; MA, migraine with aura; EM, episodic migraine; CM, chronic migraine; TF, trigger factor.

Author (Year)	Study Design	Study Design (Method of Identifying Trigger Factors)	Study Group: Type of Headache (Number of Participants)	Study Population Age (Years)	Coffee/Caffeine Reported as a Trigger Factor (%)	Additional Information
Beh 2019 [76]	Retrospective cross-sectional	Retrospective chart review	Vestibular migraine (n = 131)	No data	11.5	
Tai 2018 [77]	Prospective cross-sectional	Comprehensive dietary checklist	Migraine (n = 319) TTH (n = 365) MWA (n = 188) MA (n = 128) CM (n = 91)	Migraine 37.1 ± 14.3 TTH 46.5 ± 18.1	Migraine 25.4 TTH 15.1	Caffeine significantly associated with migraines compared to TTH
Taheri 2017 [78]	Prospective observational case series	Food diary	Migraine (n = 65) TTH (n = 50)	Range 10-15 Mean 10.5	28	87% of patients achieved complete resolution of headaches by exclusion of 1-3 triggers
Park 2016 [79]	Prospective cross-sectional	Smartphone headache diary application	Episodic migraine (n = 62) MWA (n = 60) MA (n = 2)	Mean 37.7 ± 8.6	2.4	
Peris 2016 [80]	Prospective cross-sectional	Detailed 90-day paper diary database from PAMINA migraine study	Migraine (n = 326)	No data	7.7	
Rist 2014 [81]	Cross-sectional study among participants in the Women's Health Study	Semi-quantitative food frequency questionnaire	Non-migraine headache (n = 5573) Migraine (n = 7042) MWA (n = 2972) MA (n = 1974)	Mean 53.6	Not applicable	Patients with non-migraine headache more likely to have low intake of coffee; women who experienced migraine were less likely to have low intake of coffee compared to those with non-migraine headache
Mollaoglu 2013 [57]	Prospective cross-sectional	Interview TF checklist	Migraine (n = 146) MWA (n = 73) MA (n = 53)	Mean 36.32	6.3	
Fraga 2013 [82]	Prospective cross-sectional	Predetermined list of trigger factors	Migraine (n = 100) EM (n = 50) CM (n = 50)	Range 10-20	Total 14 EM female 17.85 EM male 0 CM female 19.51 CM male 12.5	
Camboim Rockett 2012 [60]	Cross-sectional	Predetermined list of 22 dietary factors	Migraine (n = 123) MWA (n = 84) MA (n = 39)	Mean 43.2 ± 13.9	Migraine after caffeine consumption Occasional 10-15 Consistent <10 Caffeine withdrawal Occasional 10-15 Consistent 20-30	

Table 1. Cont.

Author (Year)	Study Design	Study Design (Method of Identifying Trigger Factors)	Study Group: Type of Headache (Number of Participants)	Study Population Age (Years)	Coffee/Caffeine Reported as a Trigger Factor (%)	Additional Information
Neut 2012 [83]	Retrospective	Predetermined list of TFs	Migraine (n = 102) MWA (n = 71) MA (n = 22)	Mean 12 Range 7–16	Cola drinks 8.8	
Schürks 2011 [84]	Cross-sectional	Mailed migraine-specific questionnaire	Women's Health Study (n = 1675)	No data	Coffee 8.1 Cola drinks 5	
Yadav 2010 [85]	Prospective cross-sectional	Questionnaire	Migraine without aura (n = 182)	Mean 30.7 Range 14–58	None	No subjects reported coffee or caffeine withdrawal as a trigger
Hauge 2010 [86]	Cross-sectional	Questionnaire listing 16 trigger factors	Migraine with aura (n = 347)	Mean 51	Caffeine withdrawal 20–30	
Andress-Rothrock 2010 [87]	Prospective cross-sectional	Headache trigger checklist	Migraine (n = 200) EM (n = 56) CM (n = 144)	Mean 41.1 Range 16–75	8	
Chakravarty 2009 [88]	Prospective and retrospective cross-sectional	Migraine trigger checklist	Migraine (n = 200) MWA (n = 197) MA (n = 3)	Range 7–15	Caffeinated drinks Retrospective study 0 Prospective study 0	
Fukui 2008 [89]	Prospective cross-sectional	Predetermined list of TGGs	Migraine (n = 200)	Mean 37.7	14.5 (12.96% females, 21.05% males)	
Wöber 2006 [90]	Cross-sectional	Two predetermined TF checklists (patients' personal experience and theoretical knowledge)	Migraine (n = 71) TTH (n = 49)	Range 18–65 Migraine 36.8 ± 11.4 TTH 39.5 ± 12.7	Theoretical knowledge 25 Personal experience 10	Difference between theoretical knowledge and personal experience of coffee was statistically significant
Takeschima 2004 [91]	Door-to-door survey	Structured questionnaires	Headache (n = 1628) migraine (n = 342) MWA (n = 301) MA (n = 41)	No data	None	Odds ratio of coffee and tea consumption significantly higher in migraineurs compared to TTH sufferers
Bank 2000 [92]	Population-based epidemiological survey	Self-administered headache questionnaire	Migraine (n = 62)	Mean Women 41 Men 43	None	
Van Den Bergh 1987 [93]	Retrospective	Unstructured recall/free self-report	Migraine (n = 217)	Mean 40	6.4	

123

Twenty-one studies evaluated the prevalence of caffeine as a migraine trigger. Among them, four studies failed to find any participant who reported caffeine as a trigger. In other studies, caffeine was reported to be a migraine trigger in a small percentage of participants (ranging from 2.4% to 30%). Only two studies examined caffeine withdrawal as a trigger factor, both with a relatively high percentage of patients (ranging from 10% to 30%) [60,86]. However, it is worth noting that in most of the studies, patients were asked retrospectively to recall their usual headache triggers using a predetermined list, thus they mostly assessed beliefs about triggers rather than facts. Only one study used an electronic diary (supposedly one of the best trigger factor study designs) and found coffee as a trigger in a very small percentage of migraineurs. Unfortunately, we found no provocative studies evaluating whether caffeine can provoke migraine attacks. It is reported that a high level of caffeinated beverage intake may induce a migraine attack on that day. Mostofsky et al., in a prospective cohort study, found that although consuming one or two caffeinated beverages was not associated with the odds of having a migraine on that day, ≥3 beverages was connected to higher odds of having a headache, even after accounting for potential confounding by other triggers. Moreover, a nonlinear association between caffeine intake and the odds of migraine occurrence on that day was found [75]. Taheri et al. examined the effects of dietary exclusion on the course of primary headache including migraine in a group of children. Interestingly, caffeine was reported as the most common trigger in this group (28%). After excluding one to three of the identified food triggers, 87% of patients achieved complete resolution of their headaches, meaning that the cumulative effect of food rather than a single ingestion influences headaches [78]. In the Head-HUNT study, chronic headaches were more prevalent among individuals with low caffeine intake compared to those with moderate or high intake. Besides, a significant association was found between high caffeine consumption and the prevalence of infrequent headache (OR = 1.16, 95% CI 1.09–1.23). The authors concluded that high caffeine intake may change chronic headache into episodic headache due to the analgesic properties of caffeine. Another explanation is that chronic headache sufferers tend to avoid caffeine so as to not aggravate their headaches [94]. Couturier et al. revealed that weekend headaches are linked to caffeine withdrawal. They examined 151 patients with migraine or tension-type headache (TTH) and found that 21.9% of them had weekend headaches. Weekend headache sufferers consumed significantly more caffeine daily (mean 734 mg/day) and slept longer on weekends compared with those without weekend headaches. Prolonged weekend sleep delayed the usual cup of coffee, thus produced headache [68]. Camboim Rockett et al., in a very interesting study, found that coffee withdrawal was more frequently reported as a migraine trigger than coffee intake. Besides, participants reported that coffee intake produced migraine attack occasionally, but coffee withdrawal did so frequently. Moreover, coffee withdrawal was a more prevalent trigger in migraines with aura, and coffee intake was a common trigger in migraines without aura [60].

3.2. Caffeine as Acute Migraine Treatment

Only one prospective study evaluated separate doses of caffeine in the treatment of acute migraine attack. Baratloo et al. compared the effectiveness of either 60 mg intravenous caffeine or 2 g intravenous magnesium sulfate in migraine attacks. Although both treatment options diminished pain scores significantly, after one hour magnesium was more effective than caffeine [95]. A number of studies examined the usefulness of caffeine in combination with other analgesics. In a double-blind randomized placebo-controlled study, a combination of acetaminophen, acetylsalicylic acid, and caffeine (130 mg) was compared with ibuprofen and placebo for treatment of acute migraine in patients with severe baseline migraine pain. The combination of drugs relieved the pain and associated symptoms of severe migraine significantly better and faster than ibuprofen ($p \leq 0.05$) [96]. Another randomized double-blind study compared the efficacy and tolerability of the combination of paracetamol and caffeine (130 mg) with sumatriptan (50 mg) for migraine attacks. Surprisingly, both treatments were equally effective and safe with respect to the baseline, with no differences between the two [97]. In a different double-blind randomized trial, patients treated two migraine attacks, one with almotriptan

12.5 mg and one with ergotamine plus caffeine (200 mg). Almotriptan was associated with significantly greater efficacy in treating migraine compared to the combined drug, and moreover was well tolerated and associated with greater treatment satisfaction [98]. The effectiveness of a combination analgesic containing acetaminophen, aspirin, and caffeine (65 mg) was compared with ibuprofen and placebo for migraine attacks. Although both active treatments were significantly better than placebo in relieving the pain and associated symptoms of migraine, the combination product provided superior efficacy and speed of onset compared with ibuprofen [99]. Another study compared the combination of acetaminophen, aspirin, and caffeine (130 mg) with sumatriptan (50 mg) for treatment of migraine attacks. The combination product was significantly more effective ($p > 0.05$) than sumatriptan in the early treatment of migraine [100]. A randomized double-blind study evaluated the efficacy of 100 mg diclofenac sodium softgel with or without 100 mg caffeine versus placebo during migraine attacks. Headache relief at 60 min was reported by 14% of the placebo group versus 27% of the diclofenac group and 41% of the diclofenac plus caffeine group. Diclofenac softgel plus caffeine produced statistically significant benefits when compared to placebo at 60 min, while diclofenac softgel alone did not differ significantly from placebo. Nonsignificant trends support the analgesic adjuvant benefit of caffeine when added to diclofenac softgels [101].

3.3. Recommendations for Migraine Patients Regarding Caffeine Use

1. Individuals with migraines must be aware of the amount of caffeine they consume daily. They should carefully identify all caffeine products consumed daily, including coffee, tea, soft drinks, energy drinks, and medications.
2. Migraine sufferers who are regular caffeine consumers and wish to continue drinking caffeinated beverages, should keep their daily caffeine intake as consistent as possible. They should also choose coffee as a preferable caffeine source because of the additional health benefit. Those who wish to cease caffeine consumption should gradually taper their intake over several weeks.
3. Daily intake of caffeine should be limited to less than 200 mg/day (about two servings of caffeinated beverage).
4. Patients should continue to consume caffeine regularly every day, preferably at a consistent time, and should not discontinue it during the weekend. They should avoid sleeping longer on weekends to prevent caffeine withdrawal headache.
5. Caffeine-containing analgesics are safe and effective in treating migraine attacks, but their consumption should be limited to two days during the week to avoid medication overuse headache.

4. Conclusions

Although caffeine has been connected to migraine for many years, its effect on headache is ambiguous. Caffeine or coffee consumption as well as caffeine withdrawal were found to be migraine trigger factors in a small proportion of migraine patients. However, it may be challenging to distinguish between migraine triggers and premonitory symptoms, as drinking coffee or an energy drink before an attack may be due to yawning, diminished energy levels, and sleepiness that may herald a headache. Besides, no provocative studies have been conducted to confirm that caffeine can trigger migraines. On the other hand, caffeine alone or as a drug compound was found to be safe and effective in treating acute migraines. Caffeine may influence migraines through many possible mechanisms, mostly by adenosine receptor antagonism with further vasoconstriction and reduced CBF. Although there is a link between caffeine and migraines, a larger prospective study based on electronic diaries should be performed to assess the connection. Based on our review of the current literature, there is insufficient evidence to show that a single dose of caffeine is a migraine trigger; however, it should be emphasized that chronic caffeine overuse may lead to migraine chronification and sudden caffeine cessation may trigger migraine attacks. Migraine sufferers should be aware of the amount of caffeine they consume so that they do not exceed 200 mg daily. If they wish to continue drinking caffeinated beverages, they should keep their daily intake as consistent as possible to avoid withdrawal headache.

Author Contributions: M.N. contributed to data analysis, interpretation of the findings, and drafting of the article. M.N. and M.W. participated in data collection. M.W. and W.K. participated in the critical revision and final approval. All authors have read and agreed to the published version of the manuscript.

Funding: This research received no external funding.

Conflicts of Interest: The authors declare no conflict of interest.

References

1. Steiner, T.J.; Stovner, L.J.; Birbeck, G.L. Migraine: The seventh disabler. *Headache* **2013**, *53*, 227–229. [CrossRef] [PubMed]
2. Collaborators, G.H. Global, regional, and national burden of migraine and tension-type headache, 1990–2016: A systematic analysis for the Global Burden of Disease Study 2016. *Lancet Neurol.* **2018**, *17*, 954–976.
3. Headache Classification Committee of the International Headache Society (IHS). The International Classification of Headache Disorders 3rd edition. *Cephalalgia* **2018**, *38*, 1–211. [CrossRef] [PubMed]
4. Alstadhaug, K.B.; Andreou, A.P. Caffeine and Primary (Migraine) Headaches-Friend or Foe? *Front. Neurol.* **2019**, *10*, 1275. [CrossRef] [PubMed]
5. Hindiyeh, N.A.; Zhang, N.; Farrar, M.; Banerjee, P.; Lombard, L.; Aurora, S.K. The Role of Diet and Nutrition in Migraine Triggers and Treatment: A Systematic Literature Review. *Headache* **2020**. [CrossRef]
6. Lipton, R.B.; Diener, H.C.; Robbins, M.S.; Garas, S.Y.; Patel, K. Caffeine in the management of patients with headache. *J. Headache Pain* **2017**, *18*, 107. [CrossRef]
7. Spencer, B. Caffeine withdrawal: A model for migraine? *Headache* **2002**, *42*, 561–562. [CrossRef]
8. Ward, N.; Whitney, C.; Avery, D.; Dunner, D. The analgesic effects of caffeine in headache. *Pain* **1991**, *44*, 151–155. [CrossRef]
9. Ogawa, N.; Ueki, H. Clinical importance of caffeine dependence and abuse. *Psychiatry Clin. Neurosci.* **2007**, *61*, 263–268. [CrossRef]
10. Heckman, M.A.; Weil, J.; Gonzalez de Mejia, E. Caffeine (1, 3, 7-trimethylxanthine) in foods: A comprehensive review on consumption, functionality, safety, and regulatory matters. *J. Food Sci.* **2010**, *75*, R77–R87. [CrossRef]
11. Fried, N.T.; Elliott, M.B.; Oshinsky, M.L. The Role of Adenosine Signaling in Headache: A Review. *Brain Sci.* **2017**, *7*, 30. [CrossRef]
12. Baratloo, A.; Rouhipour, A.; Forouzanfar, M.M.; Safari, S.; Amiri, M.; Negida, A. The Role of Caffeine in Pain Management: A Brief Literature Review. *Anesth Pain Med.* **2016**, *6*, e33193. [CrossRef] [PubMed]
13. Haskell-Ramsay, C.F.; Jackson, P.A.; Forster, J.S.; Dodd, F.L.; Bowerbank, S.L.; Kennedy, D.O. The Acute Effects of Caffeinated Black Coffee on Cognition and Mood in Healthy Young and Older Adults. *Nutrients* **2018**, *10*, 1386. [CrossRef]
14. Nawrot, P.; Jordan, S.; Eastwood, J.; Rotstein, J.; Hugenholtz, A.; Feeley, M. Effects of caffeine on human health. *Food Addit. Contam.* **2003**, *20*, 1–30. [CrossRef]
15. Miners, J.O.; Birkett, D.J. The use of caffeine as a metabolic probe for human drug metabolizing enzymes. *Gen. Pharmacol.* **1996**, *27*, 245–249. [CrossRef]
16. Grosso, G.; Godos, J.; Galvano, F.; Giovannucci, E.L. Coffee, Caffeine, and Health Outcomes: An Umbrella Review. *Annu. Rev. Nutr.* **2017**, *37*, 131–156. [CrossRef] [PubMed]
17. Nehlig, A. Effects of coffee/caffeine on brain health and disease: What should I tell my patients? *Pract. Neurol.* **2016**, *16*, 89–95. [CrossRef] [PubMed]
18. Cornelis, M.C. The Impact of Caffeine and Coffee on Human Health. *Nutrients* **2019**, *11*, 416. [CrossRef]
19. Bruce, C.; Yates, D.H.; Thomas, P.S. Caffeine decreases exhaled nitric oxide. *Thorax* **2002**, *57*, 361–363. [CrossRef]
20. Umemura, T.; Ueda, K.; Nishioka, K.; Hidaka, T.; Takemoto, H.; Nakamura, S.; Jitsuiki, D.; Soga, J.; Goto, C.; Chayama, K.; et al. Effects of acute administration of caffeine on vascular function. *Am. J. Cardiol.* **2006**, *98*, 1538–1541. [CrossRef]
21. Higashi, Y. Coffee and Endothelial Function: A Coffee Paradox? *Nutrients* **2019**, *11*, 2104. [CrossRef] [PubMed]
22. Joris, P.J.; Mensink, R.P.; Adam, T.C.; Liu, T.T. Cerebral Blood Flow Measurements in Adults: A Review on the Effects of Dietary Factors and Exercise. *Nutrients* **2018**, *10*, 530. [CrossRef] [PubMed]

23. Gererd, D. *Coffee and Health*; John Libbey Eurotext: Esher, UK, 1994.
24. Vidyasagar, R.; Greyling, A.; Draijer, R.; Corfield, D.R.; Parkes, L.M. The effect of black tea and caffeine on regional cerebral blood flow measured with arterial spin labeling. *J. Cereb. Blood Flow Metab.* **2013**, *33*, 963–968. [CrossRef] [PubMed]
25. Haanes, K.A.; Labastida-Ramírez, A.; Chan, K.Y.; de Vries, R.; Shook, B.; Jackson, P.; Zhang, J.; Flores, C.M.; Danser, A.H.J.; Villalón, C.M.; et al. Characterization of the trigeminovascular actions of several adenosine A. *J. Headache Pain* **2018**, *19*, 41. [CrossRef]
26. Yang, H.S.; Liang, Z.; Yao, J.F.; Shen, X.; Frederick, B.D.; Tong, Y. Vascular effects of caffeine found in BOLD fMRI. *J. Neurosci. Res.* **2019**, *97*, 456–466. [CrossRef] [PubMed]
27. Xu, F.; Liu, P.; Pekar, J.J.; Lu, H. Does acute caffeine ingestion alter brain metabolism in young adults? *Neuroimage* **2015**, *110*, 39–47. [CrossRef]
28. Blaha, M.; Benes, V.; Douville, C.M.; Newell, D.W. The effect of caffeine on dilated cerebral circulation and on diagnostic CO2 reactivity testing. *J. Clin. Neurosci.* **2007**, *14*, 464–467. [CrossRef]
29. Lunt, M.J.; Ragab, S.; Birch, A.A.; Schley, D.; Jenkinson, D.F. Comparison of caffeine-induced changes in cerebral blood flow and middle cerebral artery blood velocity shows that caffeine reduces middle cerebral artery diameter. *Physiol. Meas.* **2004**, *25*, 467–474. [CrossRef]
30. Addicott, M.A.; Yang, L.L.; Peiffer, A.M.; Burnett, L.R.; Burdette, J.H.; Chen, M.Y.; Hayasaka, S.; Kraft, R.A.; Maldjian, J.A.; Laurienti, P.J. The effect of daily caffeine use on cerebral blood flow: How much caffeine can we tolerate? *Hum. Brain Mapp.* **2009**, *30*, 3102–3114. [CrossRef]
31. Couturier, E.G.; Laman, D.M.; van Duijn, M.A.; van Duijn, H. Influence of caffeine and caffeine withdrawal on headache and cerebral blood flow velocities. *Cephalalgia* **1997**, *17*, 188–190. [CrossRef]
32. Sigmon, S.C.; Herning, R.I.; Better, W.; Cadet, J.L.; Griffiths, R.R. Caffeine withdrawal, acute effects, tolerance, and absence of net beneficial effects of chronic administration: Cerebral blood flow velocity, quantitative EEG, and subjective effects. *Psychopharmacology (Berl.)* **2009**, *204*, 573–585. [CrossRef] [PubMed]
33. Marchand, S.; Li, J.; Charest, J. Effects of caffeine on analgesia from transcutaneous electrical nerve stimulation. *N. Engl. J. Med.* **1995**, *333*, 325–326. [CrossRef] [PubMed]
34. Derry, C.J.; Derry, S.; Moore, R.A. Caffeine as an analgesic adjuvant for acute pain in adults. *Cochrane Database Syst. Rev.* **2014**. [CrossRef]
35. Laska, E.M.; Sunshine, A.; Mueller, F.; Elvers, W.B.; Siegel, C.; Rubin, A. Caffeine as an analgesic adjuvant. *JAMA* **1984**, *251*, 1711–1718. [CrossRef]
36. Zaeem, Z.; Zhou, L.; Dilli, E. Headaches: A Review of the Role of Dietary Factors. *Curr. Neurol. Neurosci. Rep.* **2016**, *16*, 101. [CrossRef] [PubMed]
37. Liang, J.F.; Wang, S.J. Hypnic headache: A review of clinical features, therapeutic options and outcomes. *Cephalalgia* **2014**, *34*, 795–805. [CrossRef]
38. Basurto Ona, X.; Osorio, D.; Bonfill Cosp, X. Drug therapy for treating post-dural puncture headache. *Cochrane Database Syst. Rev.* **2015**. [CrossRef] [PubMed]
39. Han, M.E.; Kim, H.J.; Lee, Y.S.; Kim, D.H.; Choi, J.T.; Pan, C.S.; Yoon, S.; Baek, S.Y.; Kim, B.S.; Kim, J.B.; et al. Regulation of cerebrospinal fluid production by caffeine consumption. *BMC Neurosci.* **2009**, *10*, 110. [CrossRef]
40. Kalladka, D.; Siddiqui, A.; Tyagi, A.; Newman, E. Reversible cerebral vasoconstriction syndrome secondary to caffeine withdrawal. *Scott. Med. J.* **2018**, *63*, 22–24. [CrossRef] [PubMed]
41. Chattha, N.; Webb, T.; Hargroves, D.; Balogun, I.; Bertoni, M. Reversible cerebral vasoconstriction syndrome after sudden caffeine withdrawal. *Br. J. Hosp. Med. (Lond.)* **2019**, *80*, 730–731. [CrossRef]
42. Manzoni, G.C. Cluster headache and lifestyle: Remarks on a population of 374 male patients. *Cephalalgia* **1999**, *19*, 88–94. [CrossRef] [PubMed]
43. Scher, A.I.; Stewart, W.F.; Lipton, R.B. Caffeine as a risk factor for chronic daily headache: A population-based study. *Neurology* **2004**, *63*, 2022–2027. [CrossRef]
44. Kluonaitis, K.; Petrauskiene, E.; Ryliskiene, K. Clinical characteristics and overuse patterns of medication overuse headache: Retrospective case-series study. *Clin. Neurol. Neurosurg.* **2017**, *163*, 124–127. [CrossRef] [PubMed]
45. Dong, Z.; Chen, X.; Steiner, T.J.; Hou, L.; Di, H.; He, M.; Dai, W.; Pan, M.; Zhang, M.; Liu, R.; et al. Medication-overuse headache in China: Clinical profile, and an evaluation of the ICHD-3 beta diagnostic criteria. *Cephalalgia* **2015**, *35*, 644–651. [CrossRef] [PubMed]

46. Diamond, S.; Balm, T.K.; Freitag, F.G. Ibuprofen plus caffeine in the treatment of tension-type headache. *Clin. Pharmacol. Ther.* **2000**, *68*, 312–319. [CrossRef]
47. Jacobs, B.; Dussor, G. Neurovascular contributions to migraine: Moving beyond vasodilation. *Neuroscience* **2016**, *338*, 130–144. [CrossRef]
48. Guieu, R.; Devaux, C.; Henry, H.; Bechis, G.; Pouget, J.; Mallet, D.; Sampieri, F.; Juin, M.; Gola, R.; Rochat, H. Adenosine and migraine. *Can. J. Neurol. Sci.* **1998**, *25*, 55–58. [CrossRef]
49. Aurora, S.K.; Kori, S.H.; Barrodale, P.; McDonald, S.A.; Haseley, D. Gastric stasis in migraine: More than just a paroxysmal abnormality during a migraine attack. *Headache* **2006**, *46*, 57–63. [CrossRef]
50. Silberstein, S. Gastrointestinal manifestations of migraine: Meeting the treatment challenges. *Headache* **2013**, *53*, 1–3. [CrossRef]
51. Messlinger, K.; Lennerz, J.K.; Eberhardt, M.; Fischer, M.J. CGRP and NO in the trigeminal system: Mechanisms and role in headache generation. *Headache* **2012**, *52*, 1411–1427. [CrossRef]
52. González, S.; Salazar, N.; Ruiz-Saavedra, S.; Gómez-Martín, M.; de Los Reyes-Gavilán, C.G.; Gueimonde, M. Long-Term Coffee Consumption is Associated with Fecal Microbial Composition in Humans. *Nutrients* **2020**, *12*, 1287. [CrossRef]
53. Arzani, M.; Jahromi, S.R.; Ghorbani, Z.; Vahabizad, F.; Martelletti, P.; Ghaemi, A.; Sacco, S.; Togha, M.; On behalf of the School of Advanced Studies of the European Headache Federation (EHF-SAS). Gut-brain Axis and migraine headache: A comprehensive review. *J. Headache Pain* **2020**, *21*, 15. [CrossRef] [PubMed]
54. Martami, F.; Togha, M.; Seifishahpar, M.; Ghorbani, Z.; Ansari, H.; Karimi, T.; Jahromi, S.R. The effects of a multispecies probiotic supplement on inflammatory markers and episodic and chronic migraine characteristics: A randomized double-blind controlled trial. *Cephalalgia* **2019**, *39*, 841–853. [CrossRef]
55. Lipton, R.B.; Pavlovic, J.M.; Haut, S.R.; Grosberg, B.M.; Buse, D.C. Methodological issues in studying trigger factors and premonitory features of migraine. *Headache* **2014**, *54*, 1661–1669. [CrossRef] [PubMed]
56. Peroutka, S.J. What turns on a migraine? A systematic review of migraine precipitating factors. *Curr. Pain Headache Rep.* **2014**, *18*, 454. [CrossRef] [PubMed]
57. Mollaoğlu, M. Trigger factors in migraine patients. *J. Health Psychol.* **2013**, *18*, 984–994. [CrossRef] [PubMed]
58. Hoffmann, J.; Recober, A. Migraine and triggers: Post hoc ergo propter hoc? *Curr. Pain Headache Rep.* **2013**, *17*, 370. [CrossRef]
59. Wöber, C.; Wöber-Bingöl, C. Triggers of migraine and tension-type headache. *Handb. Clin. Neurol.* **2010**, *97*, 161–172.
60. Rockett, F.C.; Castro, K.; de Oliveira, V.R.; da Silveira, P.A.; Chaves, M.L.F.; Perry, I.D.S. Perceived migraine triggers: Do dietary factors play a role? *Nutr. Hosp.* **2012**, *27*, 483–489.
61. Aguggia, M.; Saracco, M.G. Pathophysiology of migraine chronification. *Neurol. Sci.* **2010**, *31*, S15–S17. [CrossRef]
62. Bigal, M.E.; Lipton, R.B. Modifiable risk factors for migraine progression. *Headache* **2006**, *46*, 1334–1343. [CrossRef]
63. Guendler, V.Z.; Mercante, J.P.; Ribeiro, R.T.; Zukerman, E.; Peres, M.F. Factors associated with acute medication overuse in chronic migraine patients. *Einstein (Sao Paulo)* **2012**, *10*, 312–317. [CrossRef]
64. Bergman, E.A.; Massey, L.K.; Wise, K.J.; Sherrard, D.J. Effects of dietary caffeine on renal handling of minerals in adult women. *Life Sci.* **1990**, *47*, 557–564. [CrossRef]
65. Kirkland, A.E.; Sarlo, G.L.; Holton, K.F. The Role of Magnesium in Neurological Disorders. *Nutrients* **2018**, *10*, 730. [CrossRef] [PubMed]
66. Wöber, C.; Brannath, W.; Schmidt, K.; Kapitan, M.; Rudel, E.; Wessely, P.; Wöber-Bingöl, C.; Group, P.S. Prospective analysis of factors related to migraine attacks: The PAMINA study. *Cephalalgia* **2007**, *27*, 304–314. [CrossRef] [PubMed]
67. Seal, A.D.; Bardis, C.N.; Gavrieli, A.; Grigorakis, P.; Adams, J.D.; Arnaoutis, G.; Yannakoulia, M.; Kavouras, S.A. Coffee with High but Not Low Caffeine Content Augments Fluid and Electrolyte Excretion at Rest. *Front. Nutr.* **2017**, *4*, 40. [CrossRef]
68. Couturier, E.G.; Hering, R.; Steiner, T.J. Weekend attacks in migraine patients: Caused by caffeine withdrawal? *Cephalalgia* **1992**, *12*, 99–100. [CrossRef]
69. Schulte, L.H.; Jürgens, T.P.; May, A. Photo-, osmo- and phonophobia in the premonitory phase of migraine: Mistaking symptoms for triggers? *J. Headache Pain* **2015**, *16*, 14. [CrossRef]

70. Yalcin, N.; Chen, S.P.; Yu, E.S.; Liu, T.T.; Yen, J.C.; Atalay, Y.B.; Qin, T.; Celik, F.; van den Maagdenberg, A.M.; Moskowitz, M.A.; et al. Caffeine does not affect susceptibility to cortical spreading depolarization in mice. *J. Cereb. Blood Flow Metab.* **2019**, *39*, 740–750. [CrossRef]
71. Goadsby, P.J.; Silberstein, S.D. Migraine triggers: Harnessing the messages of clinical practice. *Neurology* **2013**, *80*, 424–425. [CrossRef]
72. Martin, P.R. Managing headache triggers: Think 'coping' not 'avoidance'. *Cephalalgia* **2010**, *30*, 634–637. [CrossRef] [PubMed]
73. Mikulec, A.A.; Faraji, F.; Kinsella, L.J. Evaluation of the efficacy of caffeine cessation, nortriptyline, and topiramate therapy in vestibular migraine and complex dizziness of unknown etiology. *Am. J. Otolaryngol.* **2012**, *33*, 121–127. [CrossRef] [PubMed]
74. Lee, M.J.; Choi, H.A.; Choi, H.; Chung, C.S. Caffeine discontinuation improves acute migraine treatment: A prospective clinic-based study. *J. Headache Pain* **2016**, *17*, 71. [CrossRef] [PubMed]
75. Mostofsky, E.; Mittleman, M.A.; Buettner, C.; Li, W.; Bertisch, S.M. Prospective Cohort Study of Caffeinated Beverage Intake as a Potential Trigger of Headaches among Migraineurs. *Am. J. Med.* **2019**, *132*, 984–991. [CrossRef] [PubMed]
76. Beh, S.C.; Masrour, S.; Smith, S.V.; Friedman, D.I. The Spectrum of Vestibular Migraine: Clinical Features, Triggers, and Examination Findings. *Headache* **2019**, *59*, 727–740. [CrossRef] [PubMed]
77. Tai, M.S.; Yap, J.F.; Goh, C.B. Dietary trigger factors of migraine and tension-type headache in a South East Asian country. *J. Pain Res.* **2018**, *11*, 1255–1261. [CrossRef]
78. Taheri, S. Effect of exclusion of frequently consumed dietary triggers in a cohort of children with chronic primary headache. *Nutr. Health* **2017**, *23*, 47–50. [CrossRef]
79. Park, J.W.; Chu, M.K.; Kim, J.M.; Park, S.G.; Cho, S.J. Analysis of Trigger Factors in Episodic Migraineurs Using a Smartphone Headache Diary Applications. *PLoS ONE* **2016**, *11*, e0149577. [CrossRef]
80. Peris, F.; Donoghue, S.; Torres, F.; Mian, A.; Wöber, C. Towards improved migraine management: Determining potential trigger factors in individual patients. *Cephalalgia* **2017**, *37*, 452–463. [CrossRef]
81. Rist, P.M.; Buring, J.E.; Kurth, T. Dietary patterns according to headache and migraine status: A cross-sectional study. *Cephalalgia* **2015**, *35*, 767–775. [CrossRef]
82. Fraga, M.D.; Pinho, R.S.; Andreoni, S.; Vitalle, M.S.; Fisberg, M.; Peres, M.F.; Vilanova, L.C.; Masruha, M.R. Trigger factors mainly from the environmental type are reported by adolescents with migraine. *Arq. Neuropsiquiatr.* **2013**, *71*, 290–293. [CrossRef] [PubMed]
83. Neut, D.; Fily, A.; Cuvellier, J.C.; Vallée, L. The prevalence of triggers in paediatric migraine: A questionnaire study in 102 children and adolescents. *J. Headache Pain* **2012**, *13*, 61–65. [CrossRef] [PubMed]
84. Schürks, M.; Buring, J.E.; Kurth, T. Migraine features, associated symptoms and triggers: A principal component analysis in the Women's Health Study. *Cephalalgia* **2011**, *31*, 861–869. [CrossRef]
85. Yadav, R.K.; Kalita, J.; Misra, U.K. A study of triggers of migraine in India. *Pain Med.* **2010**, *11*, 44–47. [CrossRef] [PubMed]
86. Hauge, A.W.; Kirchmann, M.; Olesen, J. Trigger factors in migraine with aura. *Cephalalgia* **2010**, *30*, 346–353. [CrossRef]
87. Andress-Rothrock, D.; King, W.; Rothrock, J. An analysis of migraine triggers in a clinic-based population. *Headache* **2010**, *50*, 1366–1370. [CrossRef]
88. Chakravarty, A.; Mukherjee, A.; Roy, D. Trigger factors in childhood migraine: A clinic-based study from eastern India. *J. Headache Pain* **2009**, *10*, 375–380. [CrossRef]
89. Fukui, P.T.; Gonçalves, T.R.; Strabelli, C.G.; Lucchino, N.M.; Matos, F.C.; Santos, J.P.; Zukerman, E.; Zukerman-Guendler, V.; Mercante, J.P.; Masruha, M.R.; et al. Trigger factors in migraine patients. *Arq. Neuropsiquiatr.* **2008**, *66*, 494–499. [CrossRef]
90. Wöber, C.; Holzhammer, J.; Zeitlhofer, J.; Wessely, P.; Wöber-Bingöl, C. Trigger factors of migraine and tension-type headache: Experience and knowledge of the patients. *J. Headache Pain* **2006**, *7*, 188–195. [CrossRef]
91. Takeshima, T.; Ishizaki, K.; Fukuhara, Y.; Ijiri, T.; Kusumi, M.; Wakutani, Y.; Mori, M.; Kawashima, M.; Kowa, H.; Adachi, Y.; et al. Population-based door-to-door survey of migraine in Japan: The Daisen study. *Headache* **2004**, *44*, 8–19. [CrossRef]
92. Bánk, J.; Márton, S. Hungarian migraine epidemiology. *Headache* **2000**, *40*, 164–169. [CrossRef] [PubMed]

93. Van den Bergh, V.; Amery, W.K.; Waelkens, J. Trigger factors in migraine: A study conducted by the Belgian Migraine Society. *Headache* **1987**, *27*, 191–196. [CrossRef] [PubMed]
94. Hagen, K.; Thoresen, K.; Stovner, L.J.; Zwart, J.A. High dietary caffeine consumption is associated with a modest increase in headache prevalence: Results from the Head-HUNT Study. *J. Headache Pain* **2009**, *10*, 153–159. [CrossRef] [PubMed]
95. Baratloo, A.; Mirbaha, S.; Delavar Kasmaei, H.; Payandemehr, P.; Elmaraezy, A.; Negida, A. Intravenous caffeine citrate vs. magnesium sulfate for reducing pain in patients with acute migraine headache; a prospective quasi-experimental study. *Korean J. Pain* **2017**, *30*, 176–182. [CrossRef] [PubMed]
96. Goldstein, J.; Hagen, M.; Gold, M. Results of a multicenter, double-blind, randomized, parallel-group, placebo-controlled, single-dose study comparing the fixed combination of acetaminophen, acetylsalicylic acid, and caffeine with ibuprofen for acute treatment of patients with severe migraine. *Cephalalgia* **2014**, *34*, 1070–1078.
97. Pini, L.A.; Guerzoni, S.; Cainazzo, M.; Ciccarese, M.; Prudenzano, M.P.; Livrea, P. Comparison of tolerability and efficacy of a combination of paracetamol + caffeine and sumatriptan in the treatment of migraine attack: A randomized, double-blind, double-dummy, cross-over study. *J. Headache Pain* **2012**, *13*, 669–675. [CrossRef]
98. Láinez, M.J.; Galván, J.; Heras, J.; Vila, C. Crossover, double-blind clinical trial comparing almotriptan and ergotamine plus caffeine for acute migraine therapy. *Eur. J. Neurol.* **2007**, *14*, 269–275. [CrossRef]
99. Goldstein, J.; Silberstein, S.D.; Saper, J.R.; Ryan, R.E.; Lipton, R.B. Acetaminophen, aspirin, and caffeine in combination versus ibuprofen for acute migraine: Results from a multicenter, double-blind, randomized, parallel-group, single-dose, placebo-controlled study. *Headache* **2006**, *46*, 444–453. [CrossRef]
100. Goldstein, J.; Silberstein, S.D.; Saper, J.R.; Elkind, A.H.; Smith, T.R.; Gallagher, R.M.; Battikha, J.P.; Hoffman, H.; Baggish, J. Acetaminophen, aspirin, and caffeine versus sumatriptan succinate in the early treatment of migraine: Results from the ASSET trial. *Headache* **2005**, *45*, 973–982. [CrossRef]
101. Peroutka, S.J.; Lyon, J.A.; Swarbrick, J.; Lipton, R.B.; Kolodner, K.; Goldstein, J. Efficacy of diclofenac sodium softgel 100 mg with or without caffeine 100 mg in migraine without aura: A randomized, double-blind, crossover study. *Headache* **2004**, *44*, 136–141. [CrossRef] [PubMed]

© 2020 by the authors. Licensee MDPI, Basel, Switzerland. This article is an open access article distributed under the terms and conditions of the Creative Commons Attribution (CC BY) license (http://creativecommons.org/licenses/by/4.0/).

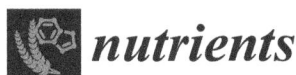

Article

Interactions of Habitual Coffee Consumption by Genetic Polymorphisms with the Risk of Prediabetes and Type 2 Diabetes Combined

Taiyue Jin [1], Jiyoung Youn [1], An Na Kim [1], Moonil Kang [2], Kyunga Kim [3,4], Joohon Sung [5] and Jung Eun Lee [1,6,*]

1. Department of Food and Nutrition, College of Human Ecology, Seoul National University, Seoul 08826, Korea; taewol@snu.ac.kr (T.J.); ji0youn@snu.ac.kr (J.Y.); ank1101@snu.ac.kr (A.N.K.)
2. Institute of Health and Environment, Graduate School of Public Health, Seoul National University, Seoul 08826, Korea; kmihoho1@snu.ac.kr
3. Statistics and Data Center, Research Institute for Future Medicine, Samsung Medical Center, Seoul 03181, Korea; kyunga.j.kim@samsung.com
4. Department of Digital Health, Samsung Advanced Institute for Health Sciences & Technology, Sungkyunkwan University, Seoul 06351, Korea
5. Department of Epidemiology, Graduate School of Public Health, Seoul National University, Seoul 08826, Korea; jsung@snu.ac.kr
6. The Research Institute of Human Ecology, Seoul National University, Seoul 08826, Korea
* Correspondence: jungelee@snu.ac.kr; Tel.: +82-2-880-6834

Received: 2 July 2020; Accepted: 23 July 2020; Published: 26 July 2020

Abstract: Habitual coffee consumption and its association with health outcomes may be modified by genetic variation. Adults aged 40 to 69 years who participated in the Korea Association Resource (KARE) study were included in this study. We conducted a genome-wide association study (GWAS) on coffee consumption in 7868 Korean adults, and examined whether the association between coffee consumption and the risk of prediabetes and type 2 diabetes combined was modified by the genetic variations in 4054 adults. In the GWAS for coffee consumption, a total of five single nucleotide polymorphisms (SNPs) located in 12q24.11-13 (rs2074356, rs11066015, rs12229654, rs11065828, and rs79105258) were selected and used to calculate weighted genetic risk scores. Individuals who had a larger number of minor alleles for these five SNPs had higher genetic risk scores. Multivariate logistic regression models were used to estimate the odds ratios (ORs) and 95% confidence intervals (95% CIs) to examine the association. During the 12 years of follow-up, a total of 2468 (60.9%) and 480 (11.8%) participants were diagnosed as prediabetes or type 2 diabetes, respectively. Compared with non-black-coffee consumers, the OR (95% CI) for ≥2 cups/day by black-coffee consumers was 0.61 (0.38–0.95; p for trend = 0.023). Similarly, sugared coffee showed an inverse association. We found a potential interaction by the genetic variations related to black-coffee consumption, suggesting a stronger association among individuals with higher genetic risk scores compared to those with lower scores; the ORs (95% CIs) were 0.36 (0.15–0.88) for individuals with 5 to 10 points and 0.87 (0.46–1.66) for those with 0 points. Our study suggests that habitual coffee consumption was related to genetic polymorphisms and modified the risk of prediabetes and type 2 diabetes combined in a sample of the Korean population. The mechanisms between coffee-related genetic variation and the risk of prediabetes and type 2 diabetes combined warrant further investigation.

Keywords: coffee consumption; type 2 diabetes; prediabetes; genome-wide association analysis (GWAS); single nucleotide polymorphism (SNP)

1. Introduction

The incidence rate and prevalence of type 2 diabetes have steadily increased in Asian populations. The International Diabetes Federation (IDF) estimated that 163 million people (35.2% of global diabetic population) in the Western Pacific region had prevalent type 2 diabetes in 2019 [1], contributing the most to type 2 diabetes in the world. In Korea, the prevalence of type 2 diabetes has increased from 6.9% in 1998 to 10.8% in 2017 [2,3]. Additionally, type 2 diabetes contributed to 17.1% of the total deaths in Korea in 2018 [4].

Coffee consumption has been suggested to lower several chronic diseases, including type 2 diabetes [5], metabolic syndrome [6], coronary heart disease [7], liver disorders [8], and several types of cancers [9]. The bioactive compounds in coffee, such as caffeine and chlorogenic acids, have been investigated as potential compounds that lower the risk of type 2 diabetes. Caffeine has been shown to stimulate the metabolic rate [10,11], and its thermogenic effect has been hypothesized to decrease the risk of metabolic disease development. Antioxidants, including chlorogenic acids, commonly found in coffee, have also been highlighted as a preventing factor for type 2 diabetes by inhibiting the generation of free radicals and removing hyperglycemia-induced oxidative stress [12–14].

A heritability study on caffeine [15] and genome-wide association studies (GWASs) have suggested that coffee consumption behavior may be linked to genetic polymorphisms. The first genome-wide meta-analysis of coffee consumption was conducted in a European population and identified two independent loci, rs4410790 nears *AHR* and rs2470893 between *CYP1A1* and *CYP1A2*, which are caffeine metabolism-related genes [16]. Additional European/Caucasian GWASs also discovered single nucleotide polymorphisms (SNPs) located in *AHR*, *CYP1A1* and *CYP1A2* as well as *ABCG2*, *POR*, *BDNF*, *SLC6A4*, *GCKR* and *MLXIPL* [17], near *NRCAM* or *ULK3* [18]. A Japanese GWAS, the first GWAS of coffee consumption in Asia, identified 24 SNPs on chromosome 12, showing rs2074356 in *HECTD4* as the strongest significant SNP [19]. Another Japanese GWAS found two loci located in *CUX2* (rs7910258) and *AHR* (rs10251701) [20]. The few GWASs in Asia warrant further investigation of the coffee-related genetic polymorphisms in Asian populations because there has been an increase in coffee consumption and type 2 diabetes in Asia. Because coffee consumption has the potential to prevent type 2 diabetes [21], it is important to investigate whether coffee consumption is linked to a lower risk of type 2 diabetes and whether this association is modified by genetic variations common in Asian populations.

The objective of this study was to identify genetic polymorphisms associated with habitual coffee consumption and examine whether the association between coffee consumption and the risk of prediabetes and type 2 diabetes combined was modified by these genetic variants in Korean population.

2. Materials and Methods

2.1. Study Population

Participants were recruited from the Korea Association Resource (KARE) study, which is part of the Korean Genome and Epidemiology Study (KoGES), a community-based cohort study. A total of 5012 and 5018 participants aged 40–69 years were enrolled from Ansan and Ansung, respectively, between 2001 and 2002. Socio-demographic status, anthropometric indices, dietary lifestyle, physical activity, and disease history were examined at baseline and follow-up phase every 2 years. In this study, we included data from baseline to the 6th follow-up (2001–2014). The details of the KoGES project have been described elsewhere [22].

Among the 10,030 participants of this study, DNA samples from a total of 8840 participants were genotyped at baseline. We excluded participants who did not have genetic information ($n = 1190$); those who were diagnosed with a type 2 diabetes by physicians or had been treated with oral hypoglycemic medication or insulin therapy at baseline ($n = 619$); those who had a history of cardiovascular disease including myocardial infarction and stroke ($n = 150$) or cancer ($n = 20$) at baseline; and those who did not provide daily coffee consumption frequency ($n = 129$) or amount (*n* = 54). In summary, 7868 participants (3685 men and 4183 women) were included in the GWAS (Table S1).

When we examined the association between habitual coffee consumption and the incident risk of prediabetes and type 2 diabetes combined, we further excluded participants who had prevalent type 2 diabetes (*n* = 666) or prediabetes (*n* = 2099) determined by the fasting plasma glucose (FPG) test, a 2-h oral glucose tolerance test (OGTT) and a hemoglobin A1c (HbA1c) test at baseline. We also excluded those who attended neither fifth nor sixth follow-up examination (*n* = 1049). As a result, a total of 4054 participants (1904 men and 2150 women) were included in the association analysis. This study was approved by the Institutional Review Board of Seoul National University (IRB No. E1911/003-011).

2.2. Dietary Assessment

A 103-item semi-quantitative food frequency questionnaire (FFQ) for the KoGES was used to assess the habitual coffee consumption at baseline. The validity of the FFQ was evaluated by 3-day diet records [23,24]. Participants were asked to answer the frequency of coffee consumption over the last year (almost none, 1 time/month, 2–3 times/month, 1–2 times/week, 3–4 times/week, 5–6 times/week, 1 time/day, 2 times/day or 3 times/day) as well as the amount of coffee (0.5, 1 or 2 cups per time). The amount of sugar added in coffee was also investigated (1, 2 or 3 teaspoons per time). We multiplied the frequency and the amount of the daily consumption of coffee to obtain the number of cups consumed per day. Coffee consumption was categorized into non-coffee consumers, <1 cup/day, 1 to <2 cups/day and ≥2 cups/day. Among coffee consumers, participants who consumed coffee without sugar were defined as black-coffee consumers and those who consumed coffee with sugar as sugared-coffee consumers.

We calculated the amount of caffeine consumption of each participant by using the caffeine database published by the Korea Ministry of Food and Drug Safety (MFDS) [25] or the United States Department of Agriculture (USDA) [26] or by contacting the product companies. The foods considered to contain caffeine were as follows: beverages (coffee, tea and soft drinks) and foods made with cocoa (chocolate, chocolate candies, chocolate ice cream, chocolate milk, chocolate pies, and chocolate cakes).

2.3. Ascertainment of Cases

Participants underwent a 2-h 75 g OGTT and HbA1c test at baseline and each follow-up. The concentrations of FPG and 2-h plasma glucose were measured by the hexokinase method (ADVIA 1650; Bayer, Berkley, MI, USA). Incident cases of prediabetes and type 2 diabetes were defined according to the American Diabetes Association (ADA) criteria [27]. Incident type 2 diabetes was ascertained if a participant had one of the following during the follow-up examination: had been diagnosed with a type 2 diabetes by physicians or had been treated with oral hypoglycemic medication or insulin therapy; had an FPG ≥ 126 mg/dL (≥7.0 mmol/L); had a 2-h plasma glucose ≥ 200 mg/dL (≥11.1 mmol/L); or had a HbA1c ≥ 6.5%. Prediabetes incidence was defined as an FPG ≥ 100 mg/dL (≥5.6 mmol/L) or 2-h plasma glucose ≥ 140 mg/dL (≥7.8 mmol/L) or HbA1c ≥ 6.0%.

2.4. Genotyping and Quality Control

DNA samples were genotyped using the Affymetrix Genome-Wide Human SNP Array 5.0 (Affymetrix, Santa Clara, CA, USA). The Bayesian Robust Linear Modeling using Mahalanobis Distance (BRLMM) Genotyping Algorithm was used for the genotype calling of 500,568 SNPs [28]. After quality control filtering, a total of 352,228 SNPs remained for analysis. Details about quality control criteria have been described elsewhere [29].

2.5. GWAS on Coffee Consumption

We identified SNPs related to habitual coffee consumption in the GWAS. Participants were grouped into non-coffee consumers and coffee consumers, and this group information was used as a binary outcome variable in a logistic regression model for each SNP. We adjusted for age (years, continuous), sex, and alcohol consumption (g/day, continuous) in the GWAS. We also adjusted for baseline BMI in the secondary GWAS. In addition, we replicated a GWAS using a continuous variable of coffee consumption. A GWAS on continuous caffeine intake was also conducted. A box-cox transformed coffee or caffeine intake and a linear regression model were used for continuous analysis. A Manhattan plot and quantile-quantile (Q-Q) plot were generated, and the inflation factor (λ) was calculated. The GWAS was performed using PLINK version 1.07, and SNPs with a p-value $< 1 \times 10^{-5}$ were considered suggestive significant. A regional association plot of the significant SNPs was generated using the LocusZoom program (http://locuszoom.org). The linkage disequilibrium (LD) between the significant SNPs was examined using the HaploView program [30].

2.6. Statistical Analysis

To calculate the genetic risk scores, each coffee-related SNP identified from the GWAS was assigned 0, 1, or 2 according to the number of minor alleles and then weighted by its relative effective size (β coefficient obtained from the GWAS). The genetic risk scores were calculated as following the equation: $5 \times (\beta_1 \times SNP_1 + \beta_2 \times SNP_2 + \beta_3 \times SNP_3 + \beta_4 \times SNP_4 + \beta_5 \times SNP_5)/(\beta_1 + \beta_2 + \beta_3 + \beta_4 + \beta_5)$ [31]. The genetic risk scores ranged from 0 to 10 points, and the median value was 5 points among those with at least one minor allele. Participants were categorized into 3 groups: 0 point, 0.1 to <5 points, and 5 to 10 points. We examined the association between coffee consumption and the risk of prediabetes and type 2 diabetes combined in black coffee and sugared coffee. Non-coffee consumers and sugared-coffee consumers combined were regarded as reference group for black-coffee consumers. For sugared-coffee consumers, non-coffee consumers and black-coffee consumers combined were regarded as a reference group. Odds ratios (ORs) and 95% confidence intervals (CIs) for the association between coffee consumption and the risk of prediabetes and type 2 diabetes combined were calculated using multivariate logistic regression models among men and women combined or separately. The median cups of coffee consumed per day were assigned to each coffee group and used to test the linear trends. We also examined whether the association varied by genetic risk scores. The interaction analysis was performed by comparing the models with or without interaction term using a likelihood ratio test. All of the analyses were adjusted for age (years, continuous), sex (for men and women combined), body mass index (BMI, <23, 23 to <25, 25 to <30 and ≥30 kg/m^2), smoking status (never smokers, ≤10 and >10 pack-years for black-coffee consumers; never smokers, ≤10, 10.1 to ≤20, 20.1 to ≤30 and >30 pack-years for sugared-coffee consumers), alcohol consumption (non-drinkers, ≤5, 5.1 to ≤10 and >10 g/day for black-coffee consumers; non-drinkers, ≤5, 5.1 to ≤10, 10.1 to ≤20 and >20 g/day for sugared-coffee consumers), family history of type 2 diabetes (yes or no), and total energy intake (kcal/day, continuous). Additionally, we also adjusted for the amount of sugar added in coffee when analyzing the association between black coffee consumption and the risk of prediabetes and type 2 diabetes combined (0, ≤5, 5.1 to ≤10, 10.1 to ≤15 and >15 g/day). SAS version 9.4 (SAS Institute, Cary, NC, USA) was used for all analyses, and p-value < 0.05 in two-sided tests was defined as a significant difference.

3. Results

3.1. Baseline Characteristics

Of the 4054 participants in the association analysis, a total of 480 (11.8%) and 2468 (60.9%) participants developed type 2 diabetes and prediabetes during the 12-year follow-up period, respectively. Table 1 shows the baseline characteristics of the study population according to habitual coffee consumption. Compared with non-coffee consumers, participants who consumed either black coffee or sugared coffee were more likely to be younger, smoke, drink alcohol, and have a higher BMI.

Table 1. Baseline characteristics of study population according to habitual coffee consumption.

	Non-Coffee Consumers ($n = 864$)	Black-Coffee Consumers		
		<1 Cup/Day ($n = 100$)	1 to <2 Cups/Day ($n = 70$)	≥2 Cups/Day ($n = 105$)
Age, mean ± SD (years)	53.3 ± 8.7	49.7 ± 7.5	47.4 ± 6.9	46.9 ± 5.7
Sex, n (%)				
Men	299 (34.6)	32 (32.0)	21 (30.0)	47 (44.8)
Women	565 (65.4)	68 (68.0)	49 (70.0)	58 (55.2)
BMI, mean ± SD (kg/m^2)	23.8 ± 3.0	24.3 ± 2.8	24.6 ± 3.1	24.7 ± 3.1
Smoking status, n (%)				
Never smokers	638 (73.8)	76 (76.0)	49 (70.0)	57 (54.3)
Past smokers	103 (11.9)	9 (9.0)	11 (15.7)	14 (13.3)
Current smokers	123 (14.2)	15 (15.0)	10 (14.3)	34 (32.4)
Alcohol consumption, n (%)				
Never drinkers	588 (68.1)	55 (55.0)	44 (62.9)	46 (43.8)
≤5 g/day	104 (12.0)	15 (15.0)	12 (17.1)	23 (21.9)
5 to ≤10 g/day	36 (4.2)	8 (8.0)	4 (5.7)	8 (7.6)
10 to ≤20 g/day	46 (5.3)	10 (10.0)	6 (8.6)	11 (10.5)
>20 g/day	90 (10.4)	12 (12.0)	4 (5.7)	17 (16.2)
Family history of type 2 diabetes, n (%)				
Yes	65 (7.5)	11 (11.0)	5 (7.1)	14 (13.3)
No	799 (92.5)	89 (89.0)	65 (92.9)	91 (86.7)
Sugar added in coffee, mean ± SD (g/day)	0.1 ± 0.9	0 ± 0	0 ± 0	0 ± 0
Total energy intake, mean ± SD (kcal/day)	1882.1 ± 762.5	1981.1 ± 747.6	1863.9 ± 718.0	2143.7 ± 1121.4
	Non-Coffee Consumers ($n = 864$)	Sugared-coffee Consumers		
		<1 Cup/Day ($n = 892$)	1 to <2 Cups/Day ($n = 986$)	≥2 Cups/Day ($n = 1037$)
Age, mean ± SD (years)	53.3 ± 8.7	51.4 ± 8.5	50.0 ± 8.4	49.2 ± 8.0
Sex, n (%)				
Men	299 (34.6)	442 (49.6)	425 (43.1)	638 (61.5)
Women	565 (65.4)	450 (50.5)	561 (56.9)	399 (38.5)
BMI, mean ± SD (kg/m^2)	23.8 ± 3.0	24.4 ± 2.9	24.3 ± 2.9	24.3 ± 3.0
Smoking status, n (%)				
Never smokers	638 (73.8)	555 (62.2)	626 (63.5)	458 (44.2)
Past smokers	103 (11.9)	147 (16.5)	129 (13.1)	188 (18.1)
Current smokers	123 (14.2)	190 (21.3)	231 (23.4)	391 (37.7)
Alcohol consumption, n (%)				
Never drinkers	588 (68.1)	435 (48.8)	488 (49.5)	459 (44.3)
≤5 g/day	104 (12.0)	166 (18.6)	196 (19.9)	204 (19.7)
5 to ≤10 g/day	36 (4.2)	77 (8.6)	59 (6.0)	85 (8.2)
10 to ≤20 g/day	46 (5.3)	90 (10.1)	88 (8.9)	91 (8.8)
>20 g/day	90 (10.4)	124 (13.9)	155 (15.7)	198 (19.1)
Family history of type 2 diabetes, n (%)				
Yes	65 (7.5)	104 (11.7)	91 (9.2)	96 (9.3)
No	799 (92.5)	788 (88.3)	895 (90.8)	941 (90.7)
Sugar added in coffee, mean ± SD (g/day)	0.1 ± 0.9	1.6 ± 1.5	4.9 ± 1.2	11.9 ± 4.4
Total energy intake, mean ± SD (kcal/day)	1882.1 ± 762.5	1881.2 ± 638.6	1969.5 ± 596.2	2115.8 ± 749.4

Abbreviations: SD, standard deviation; BMI, body mass index.

3.2. Genetic Polymorphisms Associated with Coffee Consumption

In the GWAS of habitual coffee consumption, a total of 18 SNPs located in 12q24 achieved a suggestive significance ($p < 1 \times 10^{-5}$) (Table S2). When we additionally adjusted for baseline BMI, the same 18 significant SNPs were identified as well (Table S3). SNPs identified based on habitual coffee consumption were the same when we additionally conducted a GWAS for continuous caffeine intake.

Figures 1 and 2 show the Manhattan plot and regional association plot, respectively. Figure 3 shows the Q-Q plot, and the genomic inflation factor (λ) of the GWAS was 1.0103, suggesting that the study population structure was well-adjusted [32]. Among the SNPs achieved suggestive significance at $p < 1 \times 10^{-5}$, we selected SNPs as follows, which were used later for calculating the genetic risk scores. First, pairwise correlations were examined and high correlation was declared when $r^2 > 0.8$ (Figure 4). Then, we excluded all imputed SNPs having a high correlation with any genotyped SNP, and selected the SNPs among highly-correlated genotyped SNPs. As a result, three genotyped SNPs (rs2074356, rs11066015, and rs12229654) and two imputed SNPs (rs11065828 and rs79105258) were considered as coffee-related SNPs and used for calculating the genetic risk scores. Table 2 presents the information on these five SNPs related to coffee consumption. The SNPs were located in genes HECTD4, ACAD10, MYL2, and CUX2, and the minor allele frequency ranged from 0.143 to 0.172 in our population.

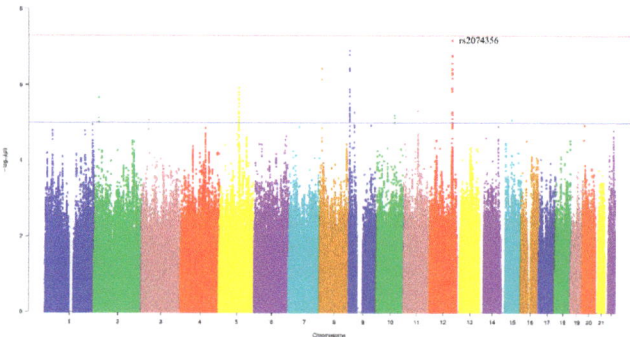

Figure 1. Manhattan plot of the genome-wide association study (GWAS) on coffee consumption. Each color represents a different chromosome. The strongest significant SNP was rs2074356 in chromosome 12 (p-value = 6.62×10^{-8}).

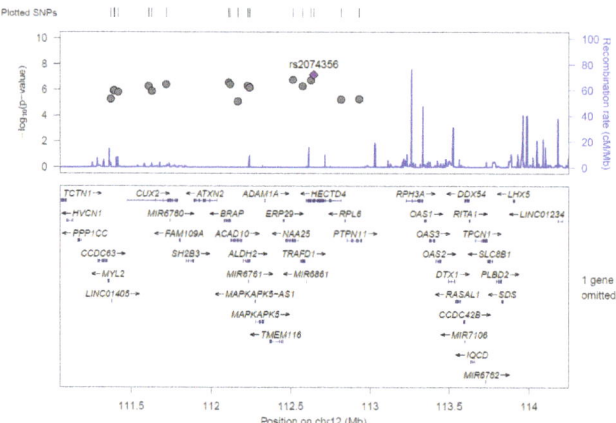

Figure 2. Regional association plot of the 18 significant single nucleotide polymorphisms (SNPs) discovered from the GWAS on coffee consumption. The strongest significant SNP, rs2074356, was shown in purple, and the gray dots represent chromosomal positions of other SNPs near the rs2074356.

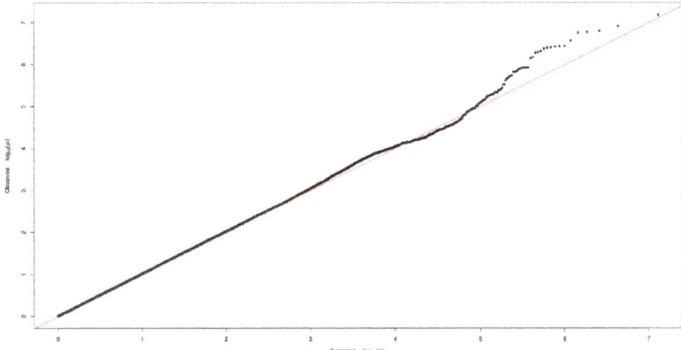

Figure 3. Quantile-quantile (Q-Q) plot of the GWAS on coffee consumption.

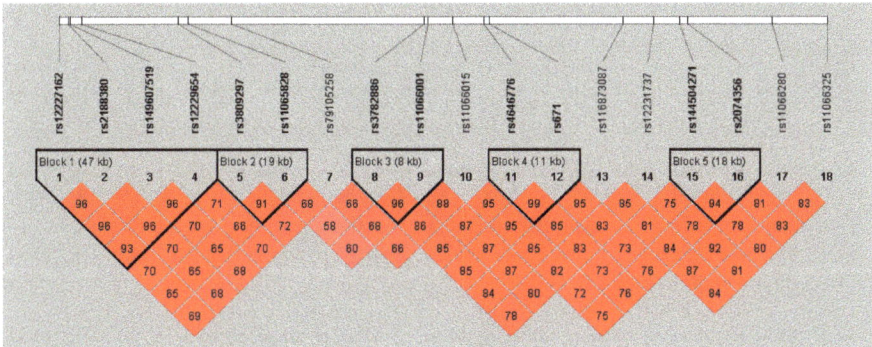

Figure 4. Linkage disequilibrium (LD) plot of the 18 significant SNPs discovered from the GWAS on coffee consumption. Values shown in the red boxes represent the LD (r^2) between the SNPs.

Table 2. SNPs related to coffee consumption (p-value $< 1 \times 10^{-5}$).

Chr	SNP	Position	Gene	Alleles [1]	MAF [2]	MAF [3]	Beta [4]	p-Value [5]
12	rs2074356	112,645,401	HECTD4	A/G	0.149	0.129	0.3185	6.62×10^{-8}
12	rs11066015	112,168,009	ACAD10	A/G	0.172	0.176	0.2469	7.79×10^{-6}
12	rs12229654	111,414,461	MYL2	G/T	0.143	0.159	0.2867	1.49×10^{-6}
12	rs11065828	111,629,389	CUX2	A/C	0.172	0.214	0.2654	1.26×10^{-6}
12	rs79105258	111,718,231	CUX2	A/C	0.156	0.216	0.2912	3.89×10^{-7}

Abbreviations: Chr, chromosome; SNP, single nucleotide polymorphism; MAF, minor allele frequency. [1] Alleles are presented as minor allele/major allele; [2] minor allele frequency in this study population; [3] minor allele frequency in the 1000Genomes, East Asian; [4] the beta (β) coefficient was obtained from the GWAS; [5] the p-value was calculated using a Wald test from logistic regression model adjusted for age (years; continuous), sex, and alcohol consumption (g/day; continuous).

3.3. Coffee Consumption and the Risk of Prediabetes and Type 2 Diabetes Combined

We examined the association between black coffee consumption and the risk of prediabetes and type 2 diabetes combined (Table 3). Compared with non-black-coffee consumers, participants who consumed ≥2 cups/day of black coffee had a 39% lower risk of prediabetes and type 2 diabetes combined among men and women combined (95% CI = 0.38–0.95; p for trend = 0.023). When we separated men and women, compared with non-black-coffee consumers, participants who consumed ≥2 cups/day of black coffee had a 54% lower risk of prediabetes and type 2 diabetes combined among men (95% CI = 0.23–0.94; p for trend = 0.026). Although the association was not statistically significant among women, an inverse trend was observed (OR = 0.74; 95% CI = 0.41–1.34).

Table 3. Multivariate-adjusted ORs and 95% CIs for the risk of prediabetes and type 2 diabetes combined according to black coffee consumption.

	Non-Black-Coffee Consumers [1]	Black-Coffee Consumers			p for Trend
		<1 Cup/Day	1 to <2 Cups/Day	≥2 Cups/Day	
Men and women combined					0.023
Case/total	2759/3779	73/100	47/70	69/105	
ORs (95% CIs) [2]	Reference	0.96 (0.59, 1.55)	0.75 (0.44, 1.28)	0.61 (0.38, 0.95)	
Men					0.026
Case/total	1394/1804	26/32	15/21	32/47	
ORs (95% CIs) [2]	Reference	1.18 (0.45, 3.15)	0.69 (0.25, 1.93)	0.46 (0.23, 0.94)	
Women					0.271
Case/total	1365/1975	47/68	32/49	37/58	
ORs (95% CIs) [2]	Reference	0.91 (0.52, 1.59)	0.78 (0.41, 1.47)	0.74 (0.41, 1.34)	

Abbreviations: OR, odds ratio; 95% CI, 95% confidence interval. [1] For black-coffee consumers, non-coffee consumers and sugared-coffee consumers combined were regarded as reference group; [2] the ORs (95% CIs) were adjusted for age (years, continuous), sex (for men and women combined), body mass index (BMI, <23, 23 to <25, 25 to <30 and ≥30 kg/m^2), smoking status (never smokers, ≤10 and >10 pack-years), alcohol consumption (non-drinkers, ≤5, 5.1 to ≤10 and >10 g/day), family history of type 2 diabetes (yes or no), total energy intake (kcal/day, continuous), and the amount of sugar added in coffee (0, ≤5, 5.1 to ≤10, 10.1 to ≤15 and >15 g/day).

Table 4 presents the association between sugared coffee consumption and the risk of prediabetes and type 2 diabetes combined. The ORs (95% CIs) of prediabetes and type 2 diabetes combined comparing sugared-coffee consumers with non-sugared-coffee consumers were 0.73 (0.60–0.89; p for trend = 0.005) for men and women combined, 0.71 (0.52–0.97; p for trend = 0.015) for men, and 0.75 (0.57–0.99; p for trend = 0.080) for women.

Table 4. Multivariate-adjusted ORs and 95% CIs for the risk of prediabetes and type 2 diabetes combined according to sugared coffee consumption.

	Non-Sugared-Coffee Consumers [1]	Sugared-Coffee Consumers			p for Trend
		<1 Cup/Day	1 to <2 Cups/Day	≥2 Cups/Day	
Men and women combined					0.005
Case/total	834/1139	644/892	749/986	721/1037	
ORs (95% CIs) [2]	Reference	0.84 (0.68, 1.03)	1.11 (0.90, 1.35)	0.73 (0.60, 0.89)	
Men					0.015
Case/total	310/399	335/442	357/425	465/638	
ORs (95% CIs) [2]	Reference	0.83 (0.59, 1.15)	1.45 (1.01, 2.08)	0.71 (0.52, 0.97)	
Women					0.080
Case/total	524/740	309/450	392/561	256/399	
ORs (95% CIs) [2]	Reference	0.84 (0.64, 1.09)	0.96 (0.75, 1.23)	0.75 (0.57, 0.99)	

Abbreviations: OR, odds ratio; 95% CI, 95% confidence interval. [1] For sugared-coffee consumers, non-coffee consumers and black-coffee consumers combined were regarded as reference group; [2] the ORs (95% CIs) were adjusted for age (years, continuous), sex (for men and women combined), body mass index (BMI, <23, 23 to <25, 25 to <30 and ≥30 kg/m^2), smoking status (never smokers, ≤10, 10.1 to ≤20, 20.1 to ≤30 and >30 pack-years), alcohol consumption (non-drinkers, ≤5, 5.1 to ≤10, 10.1 to ≤20 and >20 g/day), family history of type 2 diabetes (yes or no), and total energy intake (kcal/day, continuous).

3.4. Associations Modified by Genetic Risk Scores

We analyzed whether the association between habitual coffee consumption and the risk of prediabetes and type 2 diabetes combined varied by genetic polymorphisms. For black-coffee consumers, we found that an inverse association was more pronounced among individuals with high genetic risk scores, but the interaction was not statistically significant (p for interaction = 0.261) (Table 5). The ORs

(95% CIs) for ≥2 cups/day of black coffee vs. non-black-coffee consumers were 0.87 (0.46–1.66) for participants with 0 points, 0.49 (0.17–1.44) for those with 0.1 to <5 points, and 0.36 (0.15–0.88) for those with 5 to 10 points for their genetic risk scores. For sugared coffee consumption, the associations with the risk of prediabetes and type 2 diabetes combined were similar across genetic risk scores (p for interaction = 0.608) (Table 6). When we conducted an interaction analysis for each coffee-related SNP for black coffee consumption, the association between black coffee consumption and the risk of prediabetes and type 2 diabetes combined was inverse for the minor allele of each SNP (Table 7).

Table 5. Multivariate-adjusted ORs and 95% CIs for the risk of prediabetes and type 2 diabetes combined by genetic risk scores according to black coffee consumption.

Genetic Risk Scores [1]	Non-Black-Coffee Consumers [2]	Black-Coffee Consumers			p for Interaction
		<1 Cup/Day	1 to <2 Cups/Day	≥2 Cups/Day	
0 point					
Case/total	1639/2204	47/61	25/39	46/61	
ORs (95% CIs) [3]	Reference	1.03 (0.54, 1.97)	0.67 (0.33, 1.35)	0.87 (0.46, 1.66)	
0.1 to <5 points					0.261
Case/total	524/721	12/18	8/11	9/17	
ORs (95% CIs) [3]	Reference	1.00 (0.33, 3.06)	0.90 (0.21, 3.94)	0.49 (0.17, 1.44)	
5 to 10 points					
Case/total	596/854	14/21	14/20	14/27	
ORs (95% CIs) [3]	Reference	0.78 (0.28, 2.15)	0.89 (0.31, 2.58)	0.36 (0.15, 0.88)	

Abbreviations: OR, odds ratio; 95% CI, 95% confidence interval. [1] Genetic risk scores were calculated by 5 SNPs related to coffee consumption weighted by relative effect size (β coefficient); [2] for black-coffee consumers, non-coffee consumers and sugared-coffee consumers combined were regarded as reference group; [3] the ORs (95% CIs) were adjusted for age (years, continuous), sex (for men and women combined), body mass index (BMI, <23, 23 to <25, 25 to <30 and ≥30 kg/m^2), smoking status (never smokers, ≤10 and >10 pack-years), alcohol consumption (non-drinkers, ≤5, 5.1 to ≤10 and >10 g/day), family history of type 2 diabetes (yes or no), total energy intake (kcal/day, continuous), and the amount of sugar added in coffee (0, ≤5, 5.1 to ≤10, 10.1 to ≤15 and >15 g/day).

Table 6. Multivariate-adjusted ORs and 95% CIs for the risk of prediabetes and type 2 diabetes combined by genetic risk scores according to sugared coffee consumption.

Genetic Risk Scores [1]	Non-Sugared-Coffee Consumers [2]	Sugared-Coffee Consumers			p for Interaction
		<1 Cup/Day	1 to <2 Cups/Day	≥2 Cups/Day	
0 point					
Case/total	521/698	397/544	442/571	397/552	
ORs (95% CIs) [3]	Reference	0.79 (0.61, 1.04)	1.11 (0.85, 1.46)	0.74 (0.56, 0.97)	
0.1 to <5 points					0.608
Case/total	139/196	121/162	151/196	142/213	
ORs (95% CIs) [3]	Reference	1.02 (0.62, 1.67)	1.28 (0.79, 2.07)	0.71 (0.45, 1.12)	
5 to 10 points					
Case/total	174/245	126/186	156/219	182/272	
ORs (95% CIs) [3]	Reference	0.79 (0.51, 1.22)	1.03 (0.68, 1.57)	0.74 (0.49, 1.12)	

Abbreviations: OR, odds ratio; 95% CI, 95% confidence interval. [1] Genetic risk scores were calculated by 5 SNPs related to coffee consumption weighted by relative effect size (β coefficient); [2] for sugared-coffee consumers, non-coffee consumers and black-coffee consumers combined were regarded as reference group; [3] the ORs (95% CIs) were adjusted for age (years, continuous), sex (for men and women combined), body mass index (BMI, <23, 23 to <25, 25 to <30 and ≥30 kg/m^2), smoking status (never smokers, ≤10, 10.1 to ≤20, 20.1 to ≤30 and >30 pack-years), alcohol consumption (non-drinkers, ≤5, 5.1 to ≤10, 10.1 to ≤20 and >20 g/day), family history of type 2 diabetes (yes or no), and total energy intake (kcal/day, continuous).

Table 7. Multivariate-adjusted ORs and 95% CIs for the risk of prediabetes and type 2 diabetes combined by 5 coffee-related SNPs according to black coffee consumption.

	Non-Black-Coffee Consumers [1]	Black-Coffee Consumers			p for Interaction
		<1 Cup/Day	1 to <2 Cups/Day	≥2 Cups/Day	
rs2074356					0.171
GG					
Case/total	1989/2694	54/71	33/48	52/73	
ORs (95% CIs) [2]	Reference	1.07 (0.59, 1.94)	0.83 (0.43, 1.61)	0.77 (0.44, 1.35)	
GA+AA					
Case/total	770/1085	19/29	14/22	17/32	
ORs (95% CIs) [2]	Reference	0.72 (0.31, 1.71)	0.65 (0.25, 1.70)	0.37 (0.16, 0.84)	
rs11066015					0.143
GG					
Case/total	1894/2557	54/69	29/43	51/70	
ORs (95% CIs) [2]	Reference	1.24 (0.67, 2.30)	0.81 (0.41, 1.62)	0.84 (0.47, 1.51)	
GA+AA					
Case/total	865/1222	19/31	18/27	18/35	
ORs (95% CIs) [2]	Reference	0.56 (0.25, 1.27)	0.68 (0.28, 1.65)	0.35 (0.16, 0.75)	
rs12229654					0.366
TT					
Case/total	2049/2765	55/73	31/47	52/72	
ORs (95% CIs) [2]	Reference	1.02 (0.57, 1.83)	0.69 (0.36, 1.32)	0.75 (0.42, 1.33)	
TG+GG					
Case/total	710/1014	18/27	16/23	17/33	
ORs (95% CIs) [2]	Reference	0.82 (0.33, 2.01)	0.94 (0.35, 2.52)	0.42 (0.19, 0.93)	
rs11065828					0.460
CC					
Case/total	1909/2575	51/70	26/42	52/71	
ORs (95% CIs) [2]	Reference	0.88 (0.49, 1.56)	0.60 (0.31, 1.18)	0.81 (0.45, 1.45)	
CA+AA					
Case/total	850/1204	22/30	21/28	17/34	
ORs (95% CIs) [2]	Reference	1.17 (0.48, 2.87)	1.19 (0.46, 3.06)	0.36 (0.17, 0.80)	
rs79105258					0.395
CC					
Case/total	1986/2672	52/70	31/48	51/70	
ORs (95% CIs) [2]	Reference	0.98 (0.55, 1.77)	0.66 (0.35, 1.25)	0.79 (0.44, 1.42)	
CA+AA					
Case/total	773/1107	21/30	16/22	18/35	
ORs (95% CIs) [2]	Reference	0.91 (0.38, 2.17)	1.04 (0.37, 2.92)	0.40 (0.18, 0.87)	

Abbreviations: OR, odds ratio; 95% CI, 95% confidence interval. [1] For black-coffee consumers, non-coffee consumers and sugared-coffee consumers combined were regarded as reference group; [2] the ORs (95% CIs) were adjusted for age (years, continuous), sex (for men and women combined), body mass index (BMI, <23, 23 to <25, 25 to <30 and ≥30 kg/m^2), smoking status (never smokers, ≤10 and >10 pack-years), alcohol consumption (non-drinkers, ≤5, 5.1 to ≤10 and >10 g/day), family history of type 2 diabetes (yes or no), total energy intake (kcal/day, continuous), and the amount of sugar added in coffee (0, ≤5, 5.1 to ≤10, 10.1 to ≤15 and >15 g/day).

4. Discussion

Our first GWAS of coffee consumption in the Korean population identified five SNPs (rs2074356 in *HECTD4*, rs11066015 in *ACAD10*, rs12229654 in *MYL2*, rs11065828 and rs79105258 in *CUX2*) related to habitual coffee consumption. Compared with non-coffee consumers, the risk of prediabetes and type 2 diabetes being combined was inversely associated with habitual coffee consumption, either black coffee or sugared coffee. Individuals with black coffee consumption had a lower risk of prediabetes and type 2 diabetes combined compared with non-black-coffee consumers among those with multiple minor alleles for these five SNPs.

The significant SNPs discovered to be related to habitual coffee consumption in our GWAS were all introns. Although the introns were noncoding regions of genes, they may affect the transcription rate and translation efficiency, further regulating gene expression [33]. Recent GWASs have identified several loci on the *AHR*, *CYP1A1*, and *CYP1A2* genes associated with coffee consumption [16,17]. However, most of the GWASs on coffee consumption were conducted in European populations, only two GWASs, to our knowledge, reported SNPs related to coffee consumption in Asian populations. A GWAS in the Japan Multi-Institutional Collaborative Cohort (J-MICC) study, the first GWAS on coffee consumption in Asia, found that rs2074356 located in 12q24 was most strongly associated with habitual coffee consumption ($p = 2.2 \times 10^{-6}$) [19]. Similarly, in our GWAS, a total of 18 SNPs were associated with coffee consumption at $p < 1 \times 10^{-5}$, all of which were found to be related to habitual coffee consumption in the J-MICC study, and the strongest significant variant was rs2074356 as well. Another Japanese coffee GWAS identified two independent loci (rs79105258 in 12q24 and rs10252701 in 7p21) that were associated with coffee consumption [20]. rs79105258 was also selected as a coffee-related variant in our study. In addition to the association with habitual coffee consumption, these SNPs were associated with type 2 diabetes [34], blood glucose levels [35], blood pressure levels [36], and obesity [37]. rs2074356 in *HECTD4* was associated with prevalent type 2 diabetes and blood glucose level in a Korean population [34,35]. Three SNPs (rs12229654, rs11066015 and rs2074356) were also identified to be linked with both systolic and diastolic blood pressure in a Japanese GWAS [36].

Previous epidemiologic studies have shown that coffee consumption was inversely associated with the risk of type 2 diabetes. A meta-analysis of 28 cohort and nested case-control studies reported that participants who consumed 5 cups/day of coffee had a 30% lower risk of type 2 diabetes compared with almost non-consumers, and the associations were similar between men and women [5]. Although we found a stronger inverse association among men than among women, further investigation is needed to explore a larger amount of coffee consumption, e.g., 3 or more cups/day, and whether the inverse association holds for women.

The lower risk of type 2 diabetes linked to coffee consumption could be linked to several biological mechanisms. As a main polyphenolic compound in coffee, chlorogenic acids have been shown as inhibitors of hepatic glucose-6-phosphatase, the rate-limiting enzyme of glucose hydrolysis [38]. Reduced hepatic glucose-6-phosphatase may affect the glucose output and thus decrease the blood glucose concentration. In addition, chlorogenic acids act as antioxidants to lower oxidative stress shown in both in vitro and in vivo studies [39]. Additionally, caffeine and magnesium, both of which are commonly found in coffee, have been suggested to have roles in type 2 diabetes prevention by improving insulin resistance. Previous studies suggested that caffeine could improve insulin resistance by stimulating insulin secretion from pancreatic β cells [40]. In addition to insulin secretion, caffeine increases thermogenesis, lipolysis, and β-oxidation [41]. Magnesium supplementation has reduced the development of type 2 diabetes and improved glucose disposal in experimental studies [42,43], and cohort studies have reported a significant inverse association between magnesium intake and type 2 diabetes risk [44].

In this study, we observed that both black coffee and sugared coffee decreased the risk of prediabetes and type 2 diabetes combined for individuals who consumed more than 2 cups of coffee per day. But participants who consumed 1 to <2 cups/day of sugared coffee had a 45% higher risk of prediabetes and type 2 diabetes combined among men alone, but not among women. Although sugar-sweetened beverage intake including carbonated beverages has been positively associated with the risk of type 2 diabetes [45,46], the results of coffee with sugar remained equivocal. In a French cohort study, compared to non-coffee consumers, the incident type 2 diabetes decreased by 40% and 31% among participants consuming more than 1.1 cups of coffee per lunch with or without sugar, respectively [47]. In a small clinical trial, where eight lean, young and healthy adults drank six types of beverages or water 1 h before a potato-based meal, postprandial hyperglycemia, an early abnormality of type 2 diabetes [48], was significantly reduced when they drank sweetened coffee before their meals [49]. Further studies are needed to examine whether the benefit of coffee remains even after adding a small amount of sugar.

To our knowledge, this study is the first GWAS of habitual coffee consumption in a Korean population. The strengths of this study include good ascertainment of prediabetes and type 2 diabetes, adjustment for potential confounding factors, and a 12-year follow-up. The incidence of prediabetes and type 2 diabetes were identified based on the circulating levels of FPG, 2-h plasma glucose, and HbA1c, which could minimize the misclassification. Adjustment for potential confounding factors, including smoking status and alcohol consumption, may enable us to remove the effect of the confounding factors. However, we cannot rule out the possibility that residual confounding factors remained. There are several limitations to our study. First, the rate of revisits to the clinic for the blood draw decreased to 60% in the last sixth follow-up. Therefore, our study may not be representative of the full cohort of KARE study. However, the internal validity may not be impaired as we obtained relatively accurate information on the incidence of prediabetes and type 2 diabetes during the 12-year follow-up. Second, we could not distinguish caffeinated and decaffeinated coffee or boiled and filtered coffee. However, previous studies have shown that the associations between coffee and type 2 diabetes were similar by the amount of caffeine [5] or preparation methods [50]. Third, we were not able to examine high coffee consumption (e.g., 3 or more cups/day) because only a few participants consumed more than 3 cups/day. Fourth, we did not consider medicinal caffeine intake when we performed a GWAS. However, beverages may mainly contribute to daily caffeine intake in Korea.

5. Conclusions

In our study, we conducted a GWAS and discovered five SNPs (rs2074356 in *HECTD4*, rs11066015 in *ACAD10*, rs12229654 in *MYL2*, rs11065828 and rs79105258 in *CUX2*) associated with habitual coffee consumption in a Korean population. We observed that moderate black coffee and sugared coffee consumption reduced the risk of prediabetes and type 2 diabetes combined. We found that an inverse association was stronger among black-coffee consumers with minor alleles of five SNPs related to coffee consumption compared to those with major alleles. Further Asian GWASs and epidemiological studies are needed to elucidate the effects of coffee-related genetic variation and high coffee consumption on chronic disease risk.

Supplementary Materials: The following are available online at http://www.mdpi.com/2072-6643/12/8/2228/s1. Table S1: Baseline characteristics of the participants included in the GWAS on coffee consumption; Table S2: The significant SNPs discovered from the GWAS on coffee consumption; Table S3: The significant SNPs discovered from the GWAS on coffee consumption after additionally adjusted for BMI.

Author Contributions: Conceptualization, T.J. and J.E.L.; data curation, T.J., J.Y., K.K., J.S. and J.E.L.; formal analysis, T.J., J.Y. and J.E.L.; investigation, T.J., J.Y., A.N.K., M.K., K.K., J.S. and J.E.L.; methodology, T.J., J.Y., M.K., K.K., J.S. and J.E.L.; project administration, J.S. and J.E.L.; supervision, J.E.L.; writing—original draft, T.J. and J.E.L.; writing—review & editing, T.J., J.Y., A.N.K., M.K., K.K., J.S. and J.E.L. All authors have read and agreed to the published version of the manuscript.

Funding: This research received no external funding.

Acknowledgments: This study was conducted with bioresources from National Biobank of Korea, the Center for Disease Control and Prevention, Republic of Korea (KBN-2018-044).

Conflicts of Interest: The authors declare no conflict of interest.

References

1. Saeedi, P.; Petersohn, I.; Salpea, P.; Malanda, B.; Karuranga, S.; Unwin, N.; Colagiuri, S.; Guariguata, L.; Motala, A.A.; Ogurtsova, K.; et al. Global and regional diabetes prevalence estimates for 2019 and projections for 2030 and 2045: Results from the International Diabetes Federation Diabetes Atlas, 9th edition. *Diabetes Res. Clin. Pract.* **2019**, *157*, 107843. [CrossRef] [PubMed]
2. Ko, B.; Lim, J.; Kim, Y.Z.; Park, H.S. Trends in type 2 diabetes prevalence according to income levels in Korea (1998–2012). *Diabetes Res. Clin. Pract.* **2016**, *115*, 137–139. [CrossRef] [PubMed]
3. Shin, J.-Y. Trends in the prevalence and management of diabetes in Korea: 2007–2017. *Epidemiol. Health* **2019**, *41*, e2019029. [CrossRef] [PubMed]
4. Statistics Korea. *Causes of Death Statistics in 2018*; Statistics Korea: Daejeon, Korea, 2019.

5. Ding, M.; Bhupathiraju, S.N.; Chen, M.; van Dam, R.M.; Hu, F.B. Caffeinated and decaffeinated coffee consumption and risk of type 2 diabetes: A systematic review and a dose-response meta-analysis. *Diabetes Care* **2014**, *37*, 569–586. [CrossRef] [PubMed]
6. Shang, F.; Li, X.; Jiang, X. Coffee consumption and risk of the metabolic syndrome: A meta-analysis. *Diabetes Metab.* **2016**, *42*, 80–87. [CrossRef]
7. Wu, J.-N.; Ho, S.C.; Zhou, C.; Ling, W.-H.; Chen, W.-Q.; Wang, C.-L.; Chen, Y.-M. Coffee consumption and risk of coronary heart diseases: A meta-analysis of 21 prospective cohort studies. *Int. J. Cardiol.* **2009**, *137*, 216–225. [CrossRef]
8. Saab, S.; Mallam, D.; Cox Ii, G.A.; Tong, M.J. Impact of coffee on liver diseases: A systematic review. *Liver Int.* **2014**, *34*, 495–504. [CrossRef]
9. Arab, L. Epidemiologic Evidence on Coffee and Cancer. *Nutr. Cancer* **2010**, *62*, 271–283. [CrossRef]
10. Acheson, K.J.; Zahorska-Markiewicz, B.; Pittet, P.; Anantharaman, K.; Jéquier, E. Caffeine and coffee: Their influence on metabolic rate and substrate utilization in normal weight and obese individuals. *Am. J. Clin. Nutr.* **1980**, *33*, 989–997. [CrossRef]
11. Astrup, A.; Toubro, S.; Cannon, S.; Hein, P.; Breum, L.; Madsen, J. Caffeine: A double-blind, placebo-controlled study of its thermogenic, metabolic, and cardiovascular effects in healthy volunteers. *Am. J. Clin. Nutr.* **1990**, *51*, 759–767. [CrossRef]
12. Liang, N.; Kitts, D.D. Role of Chlorogenic Acids in Controlling Oxidative and Inflammatory Stress Conditions. *Nutrients* **2015**, *8*, 16. [CrossRef] [PubMed]
13. Ludwig, I.A.; Clifford, M.N.; Lean, M.E.J.; Ashihara, H.; Crozier, A. Coffee: Biochemistry and potential impact on health. *Food Funct.* **2014**, *5*, 1695–1717. [CrossRef] [PubMed]
14. Ceriello, A.; Testa, R.; Genovese, S. Clinical implications of oxidative stress and potential role of natural antioxidants in diabetic vascular complications. *Nutr. Metab. Cardiovasc. Dis.* **2016**, *26*, 285–292. [CrossRef] [PubMed]
15. Yang, A.; Palmer, A.A.; de Wit, H. Genetics of caffeine consumption and responses to caffeine. *Psychopharmacology* **2010**, *211*, 245–257. [CrossRef] [PubMed]
16. Cornelis, M.C.; Monda, K.L.; Yu, K.; Paynter, N.; Azzato, E.M.; Bennett, S.N.; Berndt, S.I.; Boerwinkle, E.; Chanock, S.; Chatterjee, N.; et al. Genome-wide meta-analysis identifies regions on 7p21 (AHR) and 15q24 (CYP1A2) as determinants of habitual caffeine consumption. *PLoS Genet.* **2011**, *7*, e1002033. [CrossRef] [PubMed]
17. Cornelis, M.C.; Byrne, E.M.; Esko, T.; Nalls, M.A.; Ganna, A.; Paynter, N.; Monda, K.L.; Amin, N.; Fischer, K.; Renstrom, F.; et al. Genome-wide meta-analysis identifies six novel loci associated with habitual coffee consumption. *Mol. Psychiatry* **2015**, *20*, 647–656. [CrossRef] [PubMed]
18. Amin, N.; Byrne, E.; Johnson, J.; Chenevix-Trench, G.; Walter, S.; Nolte, I.M.; kConFab, I.; Vink, J.M.; Rawal, R.; Mangino, M.; et al. Genome-wide association analysis of coffee drinking suggests association with CYP1A1/CYP1A2 and NRCAM. *Mol. Psychiatry* **2012**, *17*, 1116–1129. [CrossRef]
19. Nakagawa-Senda, H.; Hachiya, T.; Shimizu, A.; Hosono, S.; Oze, I.; Watanabe, M.; Matsuo, K.; Ito, H.; Hara, M.; Nishida, Y.; et al. A genome-wide association study in the Japanese population identifies the 12q24 locus for habitual coffee consumption: The J-MICC Study. *Sci. Rep.* **2018**, *8*, 1493. [CrossRef]
20. Jia, H.; Nogawa, S.; Kawafune, K.; Hachiya, T.; Takahashi, S.; Igarashi, M.; Saito, K.; Kato, H. GWAS of habitual coffee consumption reveals a sex difference in the genetic effect of the 12q24 locus in the Japanese population. *BMC Genet.* **2019**, *20*, 61. [CrossRef]
21. Carlström, M.; Larsson, S.C. Coffee consumption and reduced risk of developing type 2 diabetes: A systematic review with meta-analysis. *Nutr. Rev.* **2018**, *76*, 395–417. [CrossRef]
22. Kim, Y.; Han, B.-G.; KoGES Group. Cohort Profile: The Korean Genome and Epidemiology Study (KoGES) Consortium. *Int. J. Epidemiol.* **2017**, *46*, e20. [CrossRef] [PubMed]
23. Ahn, Y.; Kwon, E.; Shim, J.E.; Park, M.K.; Joo, Y.; Kimm, K.; Park, C.; Kim, D.H. Validation and reproducibility of food frequency questionnaire for Korean genome epidemiologic study. *Eur. J. Clin. Nutr.* **2007**, *61*, 1435. [CrossRef] [PubMed]
24. Kim, J.; Kim, Y.; Ahn, Y.O.; Paik, H.Y.; Ahn, Y.; Tokudome, Y.; Hamajima, N.; Inoue, M.; Tajima, K. Development of a food frequency questionnaire in Koreans. *Asia Pac. J. Clin. Nutr.* **2003**, *12*, 243–250. [PubMed]

25. Ministry of Food and Drug Safety (KR). Food Composition Database. Available online: http://www.foodsafetykorea.go.kr/fcdb/ (accessed on 5 March 2020).
26. United States Department of Agriculture (USDA), A.R.S. Abridged List Ordered by Nutrient Content in Household Measure, Nutrients: Caffeine(mg). Available online: https://www.nal.usda.gov/sites/www.nal.usda.gov/files/caffeine.pdf (accessed on 17 February 2020).
27. American Diabetes Association. Diagnosis and Classification of Diabetes Mellitus. *Diabetes Care* **2014**, *37*, S81. [CrossRef] [PubMed]
28. Rabbee, N.; Speed, T.P. A genotype calling algorithm for affymetrix SNP arrays. *Bioinformatics* **2005**, *22*, 7–12. [CrossRef] [PubMed]
29. Cho, Y.S.; Go, M.J.; Kim, Y.J.; Heo, J.Y.; Oh, J.H.; Ban, H.J.; Yoon, D.; Lee, M.H.; Kim, D.J.; Park, M.; et al. A large-scale genome-wide association study of Asian populations uncovers genetic factors influencing eight quantitative traits. *Nat. Genet.* **2009**, *41*, 527–534. [CrossRef] [PubMed]
30. Barrett, J.C.; Fry, B.; Maller, J.; Daly, M.J. Haploview: Analysis and visualization of LD and haplotype maps. *Bioinformatics* **2005**, *21*, 263–265. [CrossRef]
31. Wang, T.; Huang, T.; Heianza, Y.; Sun, D.; Zheng, Y.; Ma, W.; Jensen, M.K.; Kang, J.H.; Wiggs, J.L.; Pasquale, L.R.; et al. Genetic Susceptibility, Change in Physical Activity, and Long-term Weight Gain. *Diabetes* **2017**, *66*, 2704–2712. [CrossRef]
32. Zeng, P.; Zhao, Y.; Qian, C.; Zhang, L.; Zhang, R.; Gou, J.; Liu, J.; Liu, L.; Chen, F. Statistical analysis for genome-wide association study. *J. Biomed. Res.* **2015**, *29*, 285–297. [CrossRef]
33. Shaul, O. How introns enhance gene expression. *Int. J. Biochem. Cell Biol.* **2017**, *91*, 145–155. [CrossRef]
34. Go, M.J.; Hwang, J.Y.; Kim, Y.J.; Hee Oh, J.; Kim, Y.J.; Heon Kwak, S.; Soo Park, K.; Lee, J.; Kim, B.J.; Han, B.G.; et al. New susceptibility loci in MYL2, C12orf51 and OAS1 associated with 1-h plasma glucose as predisposing risk factors for type 2 diabetes in the Korean population. *J. Hum. Genet.* **2013**, *58*, 362–365. [CrossRef] [PubMed]
35. Go, M.J.; Hwang, J.Y.; Park, T.J.; Kim, Y.J.; Oh, J.H.; Kim, Y.J.; Han, B.G.; Kim, B.J. Genome-wide association study identifies two novel Loci with sex-specific effects for type 2 diabetes mellitus and glycemic traits in a korean population. *Diabetes Metab. J.* **2014**, *38*, 375–387. [CrossRef] [PubMed]
36. Yamada, Y.; Sakuma, J.; Takeuchi, I.; Yasukochi, Y.; Kato, K.; Oguri, M.; Fujimaki, T.; Horibe, H.; Muramatsu, M.; Sawabe, M.; et al. Identification of polymorphisms in 12q24.1, ACAD10, and BRAP as novel genetic determinants of blood pressure in Japanese by exome-wide association studies. *Oncotarget* **2017**, *8*, 43068–43079. [CrossRef] [PubMed]
37. Wen, W.; Zheng, W.; Okada, Y.; Takeuchi, F.; Tabara, Y.; Hwang, J.Y.; Dorajoo, R.; Li, H.; Tsai, F.J.; Yang, X.; et al. Meta-analysis of genome-wide association studies in East Asian-ancestry populations identifies four new loci for body mass index. *Hum. Mol. Genet.* **2014**, *23*, 5492–5504. [CrossRef]
38. Arion, W.J.; Canfield, W.K.; Ramos, F.C.; Schindler, P.W.; Burger, H.J.; Hemmerle, H.; Schubert, G.; Below, P.; Herling, A.W. Chlorogenic acid and hydroxynitrobenzaldehyde: New inhibitors of hepatic glucose 6-phosphatase. *Arch. Biochem. Biophys.* **1997**, *339*, 315–322. [CrossRef]
39. Sato, Y.; Itagaki, S.; Kurokawa, T.; Ogura, J.; Kobayashi, M.; Hirano, T.; Sugawara, M.; Iseki, K. In vitro and in vivo antioxidant properties of chlorogenic acid and caffeic acid. *Int. J. Pharm.* **2011**, *403*, 136–138. [CrossRef]
40. Keijzers, G.B.; De Galan, B.E.; Tack, C.J.; Smits, P. Caffeine Can Decrease Insulin Sensitivity in Humans. *Diabetes Care* **2002**, *25*, 364. [CrossRef]
41. Greenberg, J.A.; Boozer, C.N.; Geliebter, A. Coffee, diabetes, and weight control. *Am. J. Clin. Nutr.* **2006**, *84*, 682–693. [CrossRef]
42. Schulze, M.B.; Schulz, M.; Heidemann, C.; Schienkiewitz, A.; Hoffmann, K.; Boeing, H. Fiber and Magnesium Intake and Incidence of Type 2 Diabetes: A Prospective Study and Meta-analysis. *Arch. Intern. Med.* **2007**, *167*, 956–965. [CrossRef]
43. Balon, T.W.; Gu, J.L.; Tokuyama, Y.; Jasman, A.P.; Nadler, J.L. Magnesium supplementation reduces development of diabetes in a rat model of spontaneous NIDDM. *Am. J. Physiol.-Endocrinol. Metab.* **1995**, *269*, E745–E752. [CrossRef]
44. Larsson, S.C.; Wolk, A. Magnesium intake and risk of type 2 diabetes: A meta-analysis. *J. Intern. Med.* **2007**, *262*, 208–214. [CrossRef] [PubMed]

45. Drouin-Chartier, J.P.; Zheng, Y.; Li, Y.; Malik, V.; Pan, A.; Bhupathiraju, S.N.; Tobias, D.K.; Manson, J.E.; Willett, W.C.; Hu, F.B. Changes in Consumption of Sugary Beverages and Artificially Sweetened Beverages and Subsequent Risk of Type 2 Diabetes: Results from Three Large Prospective U.S. Cohorts of Women and Men. *Diabetes Care* **2019**, *42*, 2181–2189. [CrossRef] [PubMed]
46. Schulze, M.B.; Manson, J.E.; Ludwig, D.S.; Colditz, G.A.; Stampfer, M.J.; Willett, W.C.; Hu, F.B. Sugar-Sweetened Beverages, Weight Gain, and Incidence of Type 2 Diabetes in Young and Middle-Aged Women. *JAMA* **2004**, *292*, 927–934. [CrossRef] [PubMed]
47. Sartorelli, D.S.; Fagherazzi, G.; Balkau, B.; Touillaud, M.S.; Boutron-Ruault, M.-C.; de Lauzon-Guillain, B.; Clavel-Chapelon, F. Differential effects of coffee on the risk of type 2 diabetes according to meal consumption in a French cohort of women: The E3N/EPIC cohort study. *Am. J. Clin. Nutr.* **2010**, *91*, 1002–1012. [CrossRef]
48. American Diabetes Association. Postprandial Blood Glucose. *Diabetes Care* **2001**, *24*, 775. [CrossRef]
49. Louie, J.C.; Atkinson, F.; Petocz, P.; Brand-Miller, J.C. Delayed effects of coffee, tea and sucrose on postprandial glycemia in lean, young, healthy adults. *Asia Pac. J. Clin. Nutr.* **2008**, *17*, 657–662.
50. Tuomilehto, J.; Hu, G.; Bidel, S.; Lindström, J.; Jousilahti, P. Coffee Consumption and Risk of Type 2 Diabetes Mellitus Among Middle-aged Finnish Men and Women. *JAMA* **2004**, *291*, 1213–1219. [CrossRef]

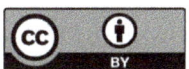

© 2020 by the authors. Licensee MDPI, Basel, Switzerland. This article is an open access article distributed under the terms and conditions of the Creative Commons Attribution (CC BY) license (http://creativecommons.org/licenses/by/4.0/).

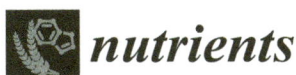 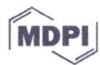

Article

Effects of Coffee Intake on Dyslipidemia Risk According to Genetic Variants in the *ADORA* Gene Family among Korean Adults

Jihee Han [1], Jinyoung Shon [1], Ji-Yun Hwang [2] and Yoon Jung Park [1,*]

1. Department of Nutritional Science and Food Management, Ewha Womans University, Seoul 03760, Korea; jiheehan61@gmail.com (J.H.); shon.jinyoung.layla@gmail.com (J.S.)
2. Department of Foodservice Management and Nutrition, Sangmyung University, Seoul 03016, Korea; jiyunhk@smu.ac.kr
* Correspondence: park.yoonjung@ewha.ac.kr; Tel.: +82-2-3277-6533

Received: 18 December 2019; Accepted: 11 February 2020; Published: 14 February 2020

Abstract: Current evidence on the effects of coffee intake on cardiovascular diseases is not consistent, in part contributed by the genetic variability of the study subjects. While adenosine receptors (ADORAs) are involved in caffeine signaling, it remains unknown how genetic variations at the *ADORA* loci correlate the coffee intake with cardiovascular diseases. The present study examined the associations of coffee intake with dyslipidemia risk depending on genetic variants in the *ADORA* gene family. The study involved a population-based cohort of 4898 Korean subjects. Consumption of more than or equal to a cup of coffee per day was associated with lower dyslipidemia risk in females carrying the *ADORA2B* minor allele rs2779212 (OR: 0.645, 95% CI: 0.506–0.823), but not in those with the major allele. At the *ADORA2A* locus, male subjects with the minor allele of rs5760423 showed instead an increased risk of dyslipidemia when consuming more than or equal to a cup of coffee per day (OR: 1.352, 95% CI: 1.014–1.802). The effect of coffee intake on dyslipidemia risk differs depending on genetic variants at the *ADORA* loci in a sex-specific manner. Our study suggests that a dietary guideline for coffee intake in the prevention and management of dyslipidemia ought to consider ADORA-related biomarkers carefully.

Keywords: Adenosine receptors; genetic variants; coffee; dyslipidemia; Korean Genome and Epidemiology Study (KoGES)

1. Introduction

While coffee consumption has increased globally, the research on biological function and effects of coffee intake remain controversial [1]. A meta-analysis of randomized controlled trials stated that coffee intake changed blood lipid profiles, including increase of cholesterol and triglyceride (TG) [2], which are clinical indicators for cardiovascular disease risk. On the contrary, other meta-analysis on observational and interventional studies suggested that high coffee consumption was associated with reduced risks of cardiovascular disease and mortality [3–5].

Genetic variation has been suggested as one of the main reasons why individuals respond differently to coffee intake [6]. Focused studies have been conducted on the ADORA locus and its genetic variants because their expression is antagonized by caffeine and, in turn, play a role in transmitting the effects of coffee intake throughout the body [7].

Studies investigating the association between coffee intake and the ADORA gene family have focused on neuronal effects such as habitual coffee intake [8], arousal [9], sleep disorders [10], and anxiety [11], or on blood pressure [6]. The *ADORA* gene family, composed of *ADORA1*, *ADORA2A*, *ADORA2B*, and *ADORA3*, are differently expressed in a tissue-specific manner and show unique properties in regulating multiple physiological statuses [7]. A recent review highlighted that the *ADORA* gene members are modulators of lipid availability [12]. The physiological role of the ADORAs has been reported to be associated with lipid-related diseases, including cardiovascular disease [13], coronary blood flow [14], chronic heart failure [15], atherosclerosis, and dyslipidemia [16].

While the association of the *ADORA* gene family between coffee intake and multiple lipid-related diseases have been investigated in several studies, we hypothesized that the discrepancies in the findings of coffee intake with regard to dyslipidemia might be explained by genetic variants, which henceforth motivated this study.

2. Materials and Methods

2.1. Study Population

This study was conducted with a local community-based cohort emanating from the Korean population-based cohorts of the Korean Genome and Epidemiology Study [17]. The local community-based cohort included residents living in rural Ansung and urban Ansan since 2001. All subjects provided informed consent at baseline. The cohort was examined by follow-up surveys every two years, and the eighth follow-up survey was performed in 2018. This study used data from the second follow-up survey conducted from 2005 to 2006.

From a total of 7515 subjects, aged 43–74 years, we excluded 2617 subjects with missing data, those with daily energy consumption <500 kcal or >4500 kcal, those with previous history and presence of diabetes, renal disease, thyroid disease, cardiovascular disease, cancer, hysterectomy, and ovariectomy, and those who received medications for those diseases. Finally, 2527 male and 2371 female subjects were included in this study (Figure 1).

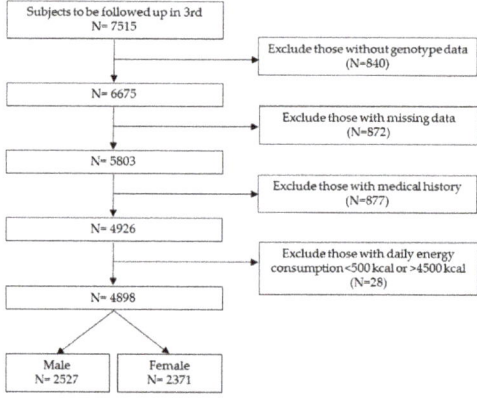

Figure 1. A flow chart of subject selection.

Dyslipidemia was defined as dyslipidemia diagnosis, related drug use, and abnormal lipid profile (low-density lipoprotein-cholesterol ≥ 160 mg/dL, TG ≥ 200 mg/dL, total cholesterol (TC) ≥ 240 mg/dL, and high-density lipoprotein-cholesterol <40 mg/dL). Blood pressure was the average of three measurements with five minutes interval, taken in the morning after 10 min of rest in sitting position. Coffee intake was assessed using the food-frequency questionnaire. Depending on the amounts of coffee intake per week, the subjects were divided into those who consumed less than one cup of coffee per day (low coffee intake group) and those who consumed more than or equal to one cup of coffee per day (high coffee intake group). A cup was estimated as much as 150 mL. This study was approved by the Institutional Review Board of Ewha Womans University, Seoul, Korea (IRB No. 129-17).

2.2. Genotyping and Analysis of Single Nucleotide Polymorphisms

Genomic DNA was collected from peripheral blood samples of the subjects and genotyped on Affymetrix Genome-Wide Human SNP Array 5.0, as previously described [18]. Among SNPs in four loci encoding ADORAs, 79 SNPs were included in the platform. The missing call rate (>5%), deviation from Hardy–Weinberg equilibrium (HWE) ($p < 1 \times 10^6$), or minor allele frequency ($p < 0.05$) was used to eliminate 38 inadequate SNPs in the sample population. Among the remaining 38 SNPs, 30 SNPs were removed due to high levels of pairwise linkage disequilibrium (LD) (Figure 2). Finally, eight of the 79 SNPs were used for further analysis (Table 1).

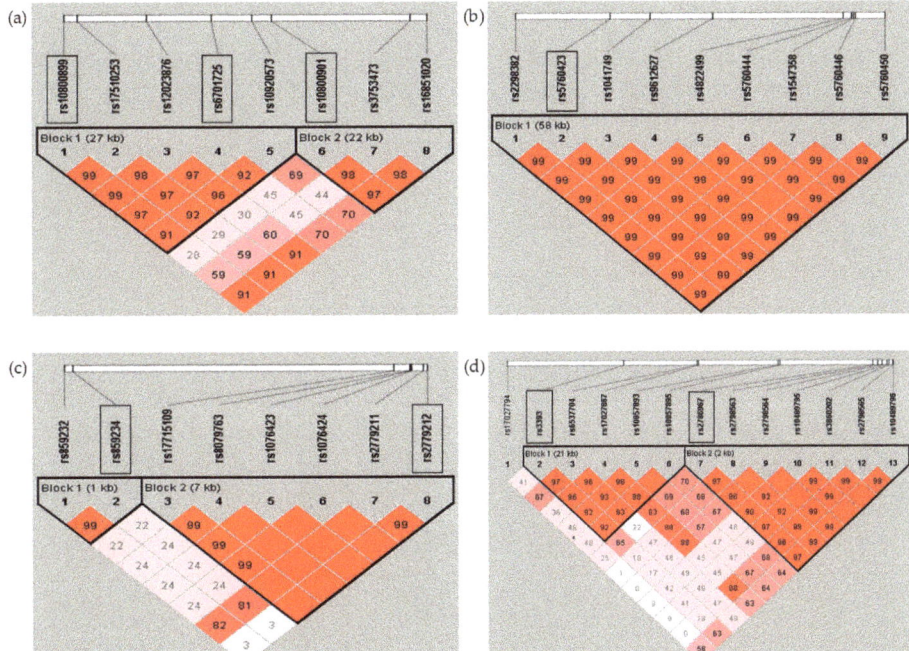

Figure 2. Linkage Disequilibrium (LD) block of genetic variants in the *Adenosine Receptor* (*ADORA*) gene family. The LD blocks are for variants in (**a**) *ADORA1*, (**b**) *ADORA2A*, (**c**) *ADORA2B*, and (**d**) *ADORA3* loci, respectively. Square boxes indicate SNPs used for further analysis.

Table 1. The list of selected SNPs in the *Adenosine Receptor* (*ADORA*) gene family.

Gene	SNP ID	Chr	Physical Position	Location	Regulatory Element	Alleles [1]	MAF	HWE
ADORA1	rs10800899	1	203081125	intron		A/G	0.1607	0.2697
	rs6701725		203102728	intron		A/G	0.1735	0.1381
	rs10800901		203111304	intron		G/A	0.4486	0.7471
ADORA2A	rs5760423	22	24840118	intron		T/G	0.4439	0.2536
ADORA2B	rs17715109	17	15869557	intron	H3K4me1, Dnase1	T/G	0.0517	0.5145
	rs2779212		15876655	intron	H3K4me1, eQTL	C/T	0.2287	0.4510
ADORA3	rs3393	1	112042149	UTR-3	Dnase1	T/C	0.4457	0.7306
	rs2786967		112075948	intron		G/A	0.8891	0.8767

[1] Alleles are presented as minor/major alleles. SNP, single nucleotide polymorphism; Chr, chromosome; MAF, minor allele frequency; HWE, Hardy–Weinberg equilibrium.

2.3. Statistical Analysis

Statistical analyses were performed using the SAS program (SAS 9.4, 2016, SAS Institute, Cary, NC, USA). Data are presented as mean with standard deviation (SD). The numbers in brackets are percentages in the column. To compare differences between groups, we used Student's *t*-test for numeric variables after log transformation and the chi-square test for categorical variables. Odds ratio (OR) and 95% confidence interval (CI) were calculated to evaluate te associations among variables by using logistic regression analysis. OR and 95% CI were adjusted with the following confounders: age, marital status, income, education, smoking behavior, energy intake, systolic blood pressure, and body mass index (BMI) in male subjects and age, income, education, drinking behavior, smoking behavior, energy intake, BMI, menopause, female hormone treatment, and hypertension in female subjects. The *p*-value for the interaction between genetics and coffee intake was calculated. Findings were considered significant at $p < 0.05$. Calculation of allele frequencies and HWE and variant pruning based on LD were conducted using the software package PLINK v1.09 [19]. Pairwise LD blocks of genetic variants in the ADORA gene family were produced by Haploview 4.2 [20]. After testing different genetic models, including dominant, recessive, and additive models, the recessive model was selected for this study.

3. Results

3.1. Basic Characteristics Depending on Coffee Consumption

Table 2 shows the basic characteristics of the subjects according to sex and the amount of coffee intake. In both male and female subjects, those in the high coffee intake group were younger, had a higher income, had a longer duration of education, and were more frequently current smokers when compared with the findings in the low coffee intake group. Energy consumption was higher in the high coffee intake group than in the low coffee intake group. Additionally, the high coffee intake group showed a significantly lower consumption of sugar and the proportion of carbohydrates in energy distribution when compared with the findings in the low coffee intake group.

Table 2. Basic Characteristics depending on the amount of coffee intake in male and female [1].

	Male			Female		
Coffee	<1 cup/d	≥1 cup/d	p^2	<1 cup/d	≥1 cup/d	p^2
	(n = 837)	(n = 1690)		(n = 1112)	(n = 1259)	
Age (year)	56.62 ± 8.90	53.95 ± 8.13	<0.0001	57.28 ± 8.75	54.55 ± 8.73	<0.0001
Marriage [3]						
Married	798 (95.34)	1639 (96.98)	0.0361	939 (84.44)	1071 (85.07)	0.6725
Monthly income (×10⁴ KRW)						
Low (<100)	251 (29.99)	351 (20.77)	<0.0001	524 (47.12)	468 (37.17)	<0.0001
Medium (100–199)	199 (23.78)	356 (21.07)		268 (24.10)	254 (20.17)	
High (≥200)	387 (46.24)	983 (58.17)		320 (28.78)	537 (42.65)	
Education (year)						
Low (0–6)	217 (25.93)	313 (18.52)	<0.0001	619 (55.67)	508 (40.35)	<0.0001
Medium ((7–9)	171 (20.43)	348 (20.59)		222 (19.96)	264 (20.97)	
High (≥10)	449 (53.64)	1029 (60.89)		271 (24.37)	487 (36.68)	
Alcohol drinking behavior						
Never	154 (18.40)	335 (19.82)	0.6875	869 (78.15)	817 (64.89)	<0.0001
Former	70 (8.36)	136 (8.05)		22 (1.98)	19 (1.51)	
Current	613 (73.24)	1219 (72.13)		221 (19.87)	423 (33.60)	

Table 2. Cont.

Coffee	Male			Female		
	<1 cup/d	≥1 cup/d	p^2	<1 cup/d	≥1 cup/d	p^2
	(n = 837)	(n = 1690)		(n = 1112)	(n = 1259)	
Alcohol intake (g/day) [4]	25.77 ± 36.07	25.00 ± 31.27	0.5934	3.99 ± 8.89	4.88 ± 11.01	<0.0001
Smoking behavior						
Never	287 (34.29)	346 (20.47)	<0.0001	1094 (98.38)	1219 (96.82)	0.0489
Former	304 (36.32)	642 (37.99)		5 (0.45)	12 (0.95)	
Current	246 (29.39)	702 (41.54)		13 (1.17)	28 (2.22)	
Tobacco consumption (pack/years) [5]	16.61 ± 14.57	20.25 ± 18.42	<0.0001	7.38 ± 6.04	7.42 ± 8.31	0.0289
Nutrient intakes						
Energy (Kcal)	1,772.21 ± 510.35	1984.88 ± 527.16	<0.0001	1594.52 ± 497.34	1753.07 ± 532.77	<0.0001
Sugar (g/per 1000 Kcal)	180.35 ± 16.89	177.75 ± 14.54	<0.0001	186.28 ± 16.97	182.06 ± 15.48	<0.0001
Fat (g/per 1000 Kcal)	14.72 ± 5.89	16.44 ± 5.13	<0.0001	12.68 ± 5.89	14.85 ± 5.44	<0.0001
Protein (g/per 1000 Kcal)	32.52 ± 5.93	32.48 ± 5.13	0.8755	31.88 ± 5.30	32.44 ± 5.97	0.0269
Energy distribution (%)						
Carbohydrate	73.35 ± 7.20	71.93 ± 6.13	<0.0001	75.56 ± 7.32	73.47 ± 6.63	<0.0001
Fat	13.44 ± 5.31	14.94 ± 4.61	<0.0001	11.53 ± 5.29	13.45 ± 4.85	<0.0001
Protein	13.21 ± 2.35	13.13 ± 2.03	0.4204	12.91 ± 2.45	13.07 ± 2.33	0.0946
SBP (mmHg)	117.73 ± 15.80	116.12 ± 14.87	0.0147	116.00 ± 17.26	113.95 ± 16.84	0.0030
DBP (mmHg)	79.74 ± 10.11	79.18 ± 10.10	0.1838	76.61 ± 10.37	75.58 ± 10.53	0.0131
Waist circumference (cm)	84.22 ± 7.76	84.77 ± 7.46	0.0692	83.98 ± 9.68	82.76 ± 9.45	0.0022
Hip circumference (cm)	90.90 ± 5.23	92.32 ± 5.21	<0.0001	91.13 ± 5.35	92.18 ± 5.25	<0.0001
Height (cm)	166.32 ± 5.95	167.15 ± 5.83	0.0008	153.23 ± 5.84	153.94 ± 5.63	0.0026
Weight (kg)	65.71 ± 9.27	68.04 ± 9.57	<0.0001	57.55 ± 8.45	58.76 ± 8.03	0.0004
BMI (kg/m^2) [6]						
Underweight (<18.5)	26 (3.11)	29 (1.72)	0.0003	18 (1.62)	15 (1.19)	0.0739
Normal (18.5–22.9)	290 (34.65)	502 (29.70)		364 (32.73)	356 (28.28)	
Overweight (23–24.9)	253 (30.23)	485 (28.70)		284 (25.54)	356 (28.28)	
Obese (≥25)	268 (32.02)	674 (39.88)		446 (40.11)	532 (42.26)	
HbA1C (%)	5.41 ± 0.41	5.41 ± 0.39	0.9575	5.47 ± 0.40	5.44 ± 0.40	0.0628
Total cholesterol (mg/dL)	183.12 ± 34.42	191.06 ± 32.64	<0.0001	193.01 ± 34.56	196.65 ± 33.53	0.0060
HDL-Cholesterol (mg/dL)	43.90 ± 10.86	43.04 ± 10.24	0.0614	44.83 ± 9.77	46.75 ± 10.16	<0.0001
Triglyceride (mg/dL)	144.81 ± 107.99	150.9 ± 117.12	0.0385	124.89 ± 69.71	116.24 ± 66.91	0.0001
Menopause				789 (70.95)	712 (56.55)	<0.0001
Female hormone treatment				25 (2.25)	34 (2.70)	0.4804
Hypertension [7]	259 (30.94)	482 (28.52)	0.2079	367 (33.00)	333 (26.45)	0.0005

[1] Data are presented as the means ± SDs or n (%). [2] Statistical significance was calculated with Student's t-tests for continuous variables after log transformation and chi-square tests for categorical variables. [3] Married included married and cohabitation. [4] Data were collected from current alcohol consumers without missing responders; n = 610, 1216 in male and 220, 421 in female, respectively. [5] Data were collected from former and current smokers without missing responders; n = 189, 372 in male and 13, 24 in female, respectively. [6] Degree of obesity was categorized into four stages according to the criterion of World Health Organization (WHO) Asia-Pacific Area [21]. [7] Subjects with diagnosis in medical history.

In contrast, the mean intake of fat was higher in the high coffee intake group than in the low coffee intake group, and the finding was in accordance with an increased ratio of energy distribution. Systolic blood pressure was lower in the high coffee intake group than in the low coffee intake group. However, hip circumference, height, and weight were higher in the high coffee intake group than in the low coffee intake group. Among both male and female subjects, the TC level was higher in the high coffee intake group than in the low coffee intake group. However, the TG level was higher among male subjects and lower among female subjects in the high coffee intake group than in the low coffee intake group. Among female subjects, the prevalence of hypertension and menopause were lower in the high coffee intake group than in the low coffee intake group.

3.2. Association of Coffee Intake with the Risk of Dyslipidemia

We next examined the effect of coffee intake on dyslipidemia risk. There was an inverse correlation between coffee intake and the prevalence of dyslipidemia in female subjects (OR: 0.768, 95% CI: 0.645–0.914, p = 0.0030) but not in male subjects (p = 0.2635) after adjusting for confounders (Table 3).

Table 3. Associations between coffee intake and the risk of dyslipidemia.

Coffee	Male				Female			
	Healthy (n = 1215)	DLP (n = 1312)	Adjusted Model [1]		Healthy (n = 1330)	DLP (n = 1041)	Adjusted Model [2]	
			OR (95% CI)	p [3]			OR (95% CI)	p [3]
<1 cup/d	427 (35.14)	410 (31.25)	1		571 (42.93)	541 (51.97)	1	
≥1 cup/d	788 (64.86)	902 (68.75)	1.107 (0.926–1.323)	0.2635	759 (57.07)	500 (48.03)	0.768 (0.645–0.914)	0.0030

[1] Adjusted for age, marital status, income, education, smoking behavior, energy intake, systolic blood pressure, and BMI. [2] Adjusted for age, income, education, drinking and smoking behavior, energy intake, BMI, menopause, treatment of female hormone, and hypertension. [3] Odds ratio (OR), 95% confidence interval (95% CI), and statistical significance were calculated with logistic regression analysis. DLP, dyslipidemia.

3.3. Effects of Coffee Intake on the Risk of Dyslipidemia Depending on ADORA Gene Family

Finally, we performed a logistic regression analysis to confirm the genetic effect of the *ADORA* gene family on the association between coffee intake and dyslipidemia risk (Tables 4 and 5). Interestingly, among female subjects, a favorable effect of consuming more coffee on dyslipidemia risk showed only those with the minor alleles of *ADORA1* rs10800901 (OR: 0.727, 95% CI: 0.560–0.944, p = 0.0168), and *ADORA2B* rs2779212 (OR: 0.645, 95% CI: 0.506–0.823, p = 0.0004) and the major alleles of *ADORA3* rs2786967 (OR: 0.818, 95% CI: 0.676–0.989, p = 0.0384), but not in those with alternative alleles. Among male subjects, there was instead an increased dyslipidemia risk on consuming more coffee carrying the minor alleles of *ADORA2A* rs57604223 (OR: 1.352, 95% CI: 1.014–1.802, p = 0.0402). Male subjects with the minor allele of *ADORA3A* rs3393 also showed lower risk on dyslipidemia (Table S1), and the favorable effects did not occur when they consumed more coffee. Overall, these results indicate that the effect of coffee intake on dyslipidemia risk depends on genetic variants in the *ADORA* gene family in a sex-specific manner.

Table 4. Risk of dyslipidemia depending on the coffee intake and genotype in ADORA gene family in male.

Genes SNPs	Alleles	Coffee Intake	Healthy (n = 1215)	Dyslipidemia (n = 1312)	Adjusted Model [1]		
					Odds Ratios (95% CI)	p	p [2]
ADORA1							
rs10800899	GG	<1 cup/d	299 (24.61)	274 (20.88)	1		0.8839
		≥1 cup/d	541 (44.53)	641 (48.86)	1.176 (0.952–1.453)	0.1327	
	AG/AA	<1 cup/d	128 (10.53)	136 (10.37)	1.103 (0.816–1.493)	0.5231	
		≥1 cup/d	247 (20.33)	261 (19.89)	1.064 (0.828–1.368)	0.6267	
rs6701725	GG	<1 cup/d	294 (24.20)	277 (21.11)	1		0.3714
		≥1 cup/d	534 (43.95)	625 (47.64)	1.127 (0.911–1.394)	0.2723	
	AG/AA	<1 cup/d	133 (10.95)	133 (10.14)	0.991 (0.733–1.341)	0.9542	
		≥1 cup/d	254 (20.91)	277 (21.11)	1.056 (0.823–1.355)	0.6691	
rs10800901	AA	<1 cup/d	131 (10.78)	118 (8.99)	1		0.6906
		≥1 cup/d	246 (20.25)	265 (20.20)	1.115 (0.812–1.532)	0.5003	
	GA/GG	<1 cup/d	296 (24.36)	292 (22.26)	1.132 (0.833–1.540)	0.4277	
		≥1 cup/d	542 (44.61)	637 (48.55)	1.250 (0.938–1.665)	0.1276	

Table 4. Cont.

Genes SNPs	Alleles	Coffee Intake	Healthy (n = 1215)	Dyslipidemia (n = 1312)	Adjusted Model [1] Odds Ratios (95% CI)	p	p [2]
ADORA2A							
rs5760423	GG	<1 cup/d	138 (11.36)	111 (8.46)	1		0.8317
		≥1 cup/d	264 (21.73)	283 (21.57)	1.246 (0.910–1.706)	0.1699	
	TG/TT	<1 cup/d	289 (23.79)	299 (22.79)	1.282 (0.942–1.744)	0.1139	
		≥1 cup/d	524 (43.13)	619 (47.18)	1.352 (1.014–1.802)	0.0402	
ADORA2B							
rs17715109	GG	<1 cup/d	381 (31.36)	360 (27.44)	1		0.8732
		≥1 cup/d	712 (58.60)	817 (62.27)	1.130 (0.936–1.365)	0.2020	
	TG/TT	<1 cup/d	46 (3.79)	50 (3.81)	1.149 (0.738–1.786)	0.5389	
		≥1 cup/d	76 (6.26)	85 (6.48)	1.076 (0.753–1.536)	0.6878	
rs2779212	TT	<1 cup/d	252 (20.74)	226 (17.23)	1		0.0336
		≥1 cup/d	494 (40.66)	555 (42.30)	1.187 (0.943–1.494)	0.1433	
	CT/CC	<1 cup/d	175 (14.40)	184 (14.02)	1.155 (0.870–1.534)	0.3182	
		≥1 cup/d	294 (24.20)	347 (26.45)	1.165 (0.906–1.497)	0.2345	
ADORA3							
rs3393	CC	<1 cup/d	122 (10.04)	147 (11.20)	1		0.5917
		≥1 cup/d	228 (18.77)	284 (21.65)	0.990 (0.725–1.350)	0.9477	
	TC/TT	<1 cup/d	305 (25.10)	263 (20.05)	0.731 (0.541–0.989)	0.0423	
		≥1 cup/d	560 (46.09)	618 (47.10)	0.856 (0.647–1.133)	0.2767	
rs2786967	AA	<1 cup/d	361 (29.71)	357 (27.21)	1		0.2144
		≥1 cup/d	676 (55.64)	752 (57.32)	1.036 (0.856–1.255)	0.7152	
	GA/GG	<1 cup/d	66 (5.43)	53 (4.04)	0.771 (0.514–1.155)	0.2066	
		≥1 cup/d	112 (9.22)	150 (11.43)	1.257 (0.933–1.694)	0.1324	

[1] Adjusted for age, marital status, income, education, smoking behavior, energy intake, systolic blood pressure, and BMI. [2] p for interaction.

Table 5. Risk of dyslipidemia depending on the coffee intake and genotype in ADORA gene family in female.

Genes SNPs	Alleles	Coffee Intake	Healthy (n = 1215)	Dyslipidemia (n = 1312)	Adjusted Model [1] Odds ratios (95% CI)	p	p [2]
ADORA1							
rs10800899	GG	<1 cup/d	392 (29.47)	374 (35.93)	1		0.2012
		≥1 cup/d	537 (40.38)	366 (35.16)	0.789 (0.643–0.968)	0.0233	
	AG/AA	<1 cup/d	179 (13.46)	167 (16.04)	0.989 (0.761–1.286)	0.9356	
		≥1 cup/d	222 (16.69)	134 (12.87)	0.705 (0.537–0.924)	0.0115	
rs6701725	GG	<1 cup/d	393 (29.55)	367 (35.25)	1		0.3393
		≥1 cup/d	520 (37.10)	346 (33.24)	0.784 (0.636–0.966)	0.0225	
	AG/AA	<1 cup/d	178 (13.38)	174 (16.71)	1.031 (0.794–1.339)	0.8196	
		≥1 cup/d	239 (17.97)	154 (14.79)	0.758 (0.585–0.982)	0.0356	
rs10800901	AA	<1 cup/d	180 (13.53)	172 (16.52)	1		0.3401
		≥1 cup/d	210 (15.79)	160 (15.37)	0.891 (0.656–1.210)	0.4956	
	GA/GG	<1 cup/d	391 (29.40)	369 (35.45)	1.008 (0.777–1.309)	0.9504	
		≥1 cup/d	549 (41.28)	340 (32.66)	0.727 (0.560–0.944)	0.0168	
ADORA2A							
rs5760423	GG	<1 cup/d	194 (14.59)	173 (16.62)	1		0.3188
		≥1 cup/d	224 (16.84)	149 (14.31)	0.836 (0.617–1.134)	0.2497	
	TG/TT	<1 cup/d	377 (28.35)	368 (35.35)	1.124 (0.869–1.456)	0.3736	
		≥1 cup/d	535 (40.23)	351 (33.72)	0.829 (0.641–1.073)	0.1539	

Table 5. Cont.

Genes SNPs	Alleles	Coffee Intake	Healthy (n = 1215)	Dyslipidemia (n = 1312)	Adjusted Model [1] Odds ratios (95% CI)	p	p [2]
ADORA2B							
rs17715109	GG	<1 cup/d	508 (38.20)	486 (46.69)	1		0.7766
		≥1 cup/d	671 (50.45)	461 (44.28)	0.795 (0.662–0.956)	0.0146	
	TG/TT	<1 cup/d	63 (4.74)	55 (5.28)	0.903 (0.608–1.339)	0.6107	
		≥1 cup/d	88 (6.62)	39 (3.75)	0.500 (0.332–0.754)	0.0009	
rs2779212	TT	<1 cup/d	343 (25.79)	335 (32.18)	1		0.8210
		≥1 cup/d	421 (31.65)	301 (28.91)	0.839 (0.671–1.049)	0.1226	
	CT/CC	<1 cup/d	228 (17.14)	206 (19.79)	0.943 (0.735–1.210)	0.6469	
		≥1 cup/d	338 (25.41)	199 (19.12)	0.645 (0.506–0.823)	0.0004	
ADORA3							
rs3393	CC	<1 cup/d	179 (13.46)	163 (15.66)	1		0.9277
		≥1 cup/d	247 (18.57)	157 (15.08)	0.776 (0.572–1.053)	0.1035	
	TC/TT	<1 cup/d	392 (29.47)	378 (36.31)	1.053 (0.809–1.370)	0.7011	
		≥1 cup/d	512 (38.50)	343 (32.95)	0.806 (0.618–1.051)	0.1109	
rs2786967	AA	<1 cup/d	486 (36.54)	444 (42.65)	1		0.0308
		≥1 cup/d	617 (46.39)	411 (39.48)	0.818 (0.676–0.989)	0.0384	
	GA/GG	<1 cup/d	85 (6.39)	97 (9.32)	1.306 (0.939–1.816)	0.1125	
		≥1 cup/d	142 (10.68)	89 (8.55)	0.737 (0.542–1.002)	0.0515	

[1] Adjusted for age, income, education, drinking and smoking behavior, energy intake, BMI, menopause, treatment of female hormone, Hypertension. [2] p for interaction.

4. Discussion

The present study aimed to investigate whether genetic variants in the ADORA gene family influence the effect of coffee intake on dyslipidemia risk. Coffee intake was associated with decreased dyslipidemia risk in female subjects but not in male subjects. Furthermore, with regard to the genetic effect on the association, the favorable effect of coffee intake among female subjects depends on a subset of genetic variants in ADORA gene family. The risk of dyslipidemia was also increased among male subjects in the high coffee intake group based on genetic variation of the ADORA gene family, indicating that a subset of genetic variants in the ADORA gene family modulates the effect of coffee intake on dyslipidemia risk in a sex-specific manner.

The ADORA gene family has been reported to play a role in regulating the lipid profile [12]. For instance, ADORA1 deficiency in ApoE KO mice was associated with increased plasma lipid levels [22], and ADORA2B knockout mice showed increased TG and TC levels compared to the wildtype [23]. Disturbed lipid levels via modulation of ADORA2B also influenced the development of dyslipidemia and atherosclerosis, known risk factors of cardiovascular mortality [16]. ADORA2B also showed a close relationship with cholesterol regulation by formation of foam cells and inflammation, which are mediator of cardiovascular disease [13,16]. In addition to the functional relevance of the ADORAs in blood lipid profiles and lipid-related chronic diseases, a genetic variant of ADORA2A showed association with the severity of chronic heart failure in Asians [15]. The evidence proposed that variations in the ADORA gene family might influence lipid regulation and cardiovascular disease. We also observed a subset of genetic variants in the ADORA gene family associated with the risk of dyslipidemia (Table S1).

Despite the interesting finding of an association between the ADORA gene family and dyslipidemia itself, the novelty here is that the ADORAs modulates the effect of coffee intake on dyslipidemia. A meta-analysis showed coffee intake increase blood lipid level [2], but not all of the included studies satisfied the result [3–5]. We identified different effects of coffee intake in the risk of dyslipidemia linked to their genetic variants in the ADORA gene family. Even though there was no association between coffee intake and dyslipidemia in male, we confirmed the increased risk of dyslipidemia when subjects with the minor allele of rs5760423 in *ADORA2A* consumed more than one cup of coffee. While we did not experimentally examine the association, instead only focusing on the association of genetic variants in *ADORA* gene family with coffee intake in dyslipidemia, we identified a subset of genetic variants in the *ADORA* gene family located at regulatory elements which could play a role as eQTLs influencing gene expression in various tissues [24] (Table 1). Indeed, a recent study suggested that genetic variation could contribute to altered gene expression by changing epigenetic enhancer activity, which, in turn, is linked to five different vascular diseases [25]. Given the previous reports, genetic variants in ADORA gene family might modify gene expression through epigenetic regulation, possibly modulating the lipid profile and the effect of coffee intake in dyslipidemia pathogenesis. Further studies are needed to elucidate their possible functional mechanisms.

We also observed a favorable association between coffee intake and the prevalence of dyslipidemia in female subjects but not in male subjects. Inconsistent results of coffee intake between male and female individuals [26,27], including a Korean population [28], obscure the view. Female individuals responded favorably to coffee concerning cardiovascular health. It has been proposed that the female sex hormone estrogen plays a role in the sensitivity of female individuals to the effects of coffee intake [29]. Estrogen is synthesized from cholesterol in the ovary, and it influences lipid metabolism by increasing lipoprotein lipase activity and is directly interacting with specific estrogen receptors in the adipose tissue. Thus, susceptibility to cardiovascular diseases is lower in premenopausal women than in men of the same age and postmenopausal women [30]. A previous finding that coffee intake increases the concentration of estrogen in Asian female individuals could explain the sex-specific differences in the effect of coffee intake on dyslipidemia [29].

The most interesting of our findings is that increased coffee intake had beneficial effects in female subjects but harmful effects in male subjects significantly associated with a subset of genetic variants in the *ADORA* gene family. This could suggest that the response to environmental factors of the ADORAs differs according to sex. Several previous studies showed different influences of environmental factors related to the *ADORA* genotypes depending on sex. Treatment with the ADORA antagonist ATL444 was shown to have a preventive effect on cocaine addiction in male individuals but not in female individuals [31]. Additionally, locomotor activity in response to administration of caffeine was higher in male WT mice than in male *ADORA2A* knockout mice, however, this difference was not noted in female mice. Although the reason why the *ADORA* genotype causes a difference in the environmental response depending on sex is not known, a possible explanation may be that dopamine receptor 2 (D2) and the ADORA2A system are more sensitive in female than in male individuals [32,33]. Dopamine signaling has been suggested as a therapeutic target of dyslipidemia, showing cardioprotective effects [32]. Caffeine treatment has been shown to increase the expression of D2 protein in female but not in male individuals [33]. Based on our data, we suggest that not only do D2 but also the ADORAs modulate the environmental response of the sex-specific physiological mechanism.

We found a novel gene-environment interaction of the *ADORA* genetic variants and coffee intake on dyslipidemia in a Korean population. However, further, larger studies are warranted to replicate the findings. In addition, while our study did not consider how subjects consumed coffee and how much caffeine was present owing to the limited information in the original cohort, we appreciate the importance of further studies including those parameters. Although it has been reported that the addition of milk, the type of coffee bean, and the type of roasting method do not alter antioxidant activity [34], it may be important to consider these factors to perform an in-depth analysis. Lastly, our analysis did not consider physical activity as a confounding factor, although it has been shown to influence blood lipid profiles [35,36]. Additional confounding factors, such as physical activity, may need to be considered for further analysis.

5. Conclusions

This study demonstrated that a subset of genetic variants in the *ADORA* gene family influences the association between coffee intake and dyslipidemia risk in a sex-specific manner. As a first study to elucidate the effect of coffee intake on dyslipidemia risk in terms of genetic variability in the *ADORA* gene family, important avenues of detailed research are available. This includes deep understanding of the functional mechanisms on the genetic variants in the *ADORA* gene family in response to coffee intake, potentially aiding prevention and management of dyslipidemia among individuals vulnerable to the disease.

Supplementary Materials: The following are available online at http://www.mdpi.com/2072-6643/12/2/493/s1, Table S1. Association between genetic variants in ADORA gene family and the risk of dyslipidemia.

Author Contributions: Conceptualization and investigation: J.H. and Y.J.P.; data curation and formal analysis: J.H., J.S. and J.-Y.H.; writing—original draft preparation: J.H.; writing—review and editing: J.S., Y.J.P., and J.-Y.H.; funding acquisition: Y.J.P. All authors have read and agreed to the published version of the manuscript.

Funding: This study was supported by Basic Science Research Programs through the National Research Foundation (NRF) funded by the Korea government (2018R1D1A1B07051274) to Y.J.P., J.H. and J.S. were supported by Brain Korea 21 plus project (22A20130012143).

Acknowledgments: Data in this study were from the Korean Genome and Epidemiology Study (KoGES; 4851-302). National Research Institute of Health, Centers for Disease Control and Prevention, Ministry for Health and Welfare, Republic of Korea.

Conflicts of Interest: The authors declare no conflict of interest.

References

1. Cano-Marquina, A.; Tarin, J.J.; Cano, A. The impact of coffee on health. *Maturitas* **2013**, *75*, 7–21. [CrossRef] [PubMed]
2. Cai, L.; Ma, D.; Zhang, Y.; Liu, Z.; Wang, P. The effect of coffee consumption on serum lipids: A meta-analysis of randomized controlled trials. *Eur. J. Clin. Nutr.* **2012**, *66*, 872–877. [CrossRef] [PubMed]
3. Poole, R.; Kennedy, O.J.; Roderick, P.; Fallowfield, J.A.; Hayes, P.C.; Parkes, J. Coffee consumption and health: Umbrella review of meta-analyses of multiple health outcomes. *BMJ* **2017**, *359*, j5024. [CrossRef] [PubMed]
4. Ding, M.; Bhupathiraju, S.N.; Satija, A.; Van Dam, R.M.; Hu, F.B. Long-term coffee consumption and risk of cardiovascular disease: A systematic review and a dose–response meta-analysis of prospective cohort studies. *Circulation* **2014**, *129*, 643–659. [CrossRef] [PubMed]
5. Wu, J.N.; Ho, S.C.; Zhou, C.; Ling, W.H.; Chen, W.Q.; Wang, C.L.; Chen, Y.M. Coffee consumption and risk of coronary heart diseases: A meta-analysis of 21 prospective cohort studies. *Int. J. Cardiol.* **2009**, *137*, 216–225. [CrossRef] [PubMed]
6. Renda, G.; Zimarino, M.; Antonucci, I.; Tatasciore, A.; Ruggieri, B.; Bucciarelli, T.; Prontera, T.; Stuppia, L.; De Caterina, R. Genetic determinants of blood pressure responses to caffeine drinking. *Am. J. Clin. Nutr.* **2012**, *95*, 241–248. [CrossRef] [PubMed]
7. Fredholm, B.B.; AP, I.J.; Jacobson, K.A.; Linden, J.; Muller, C.E. International Union of Basic and Clinical Pharmacology. LXXXI. Nomenclature and classification of adenosine receptors—An update. *Pharmacol. Rev.* **2011**, *63*, 1–34. [CrossRef]
8. Cornelis, M.C.; El-Sohemy, A.; Campos, H. Genetic polymorphism of the adenosine A2A receptor is associated with habitual caffeine consumption. *Am. J. Clin. Nutr.* **2007**, *86*, 240–244. [CrossRef]
9. Huang, Z.L.; Qu, W.M.; Eguchi, N.; Chen, J.F.; Schwarzschild, M.A.; Fredholm, B.B.; Urade, Y.; Hayaishi, O. Adenosine A2A, but not A1, receptors mediate the arousal effect of caffeine. *Nat. Neurosci.* **2005**, *8*, 858–859. [CrossRef]
10. Retey, J.V.; Adam, M.; Khatami, R.; Luhmann, U.F.; Jung, H.H.; Berger, W.; Landolt, H.P. A genetic variation in the adenosine A2A receptor gene (ADORA2A) contributes to individual sensitivity to caffeine effects on sleep. *Clin. Pharmacol. Ther.* **2007**, *81*, 692–698. [CrossRef]
11. Alsene, K.; Deckert, J.; Sand, P.; de Wit, H. Association between A2a receptor gene polymorphisms and caffeine-induced anxiety. *Neuropsychopharmacology* **2003**, *28*, 1694–1702. [CrossRef] [PubMed]
12. Leiva, A.; Guzman-Gutierrez, E.; Contreras-Duarte, S.; Fuenzalida, B.; Cantin, C.; Carvajal, L.; Salsoso, R.; Gutierrez, J.; Pardo, F.; Sobrevia, L. Adenosine receptors: Modulators of lipid availability that are controlled by lipid levels. *Mol. Asp. Med.* **2017**, *55*, 26–44. [CrossRef]
13. Eisenstein, A.; Patterson, S.; Ravid, K. The Many Faces of the A2b Adenosine Receptor in Cardiovascular and Metabolic Diseases. *J. Cell. Physiol.* **2015**, *230*, 2891–2897. [CrossRef] [PubMed]

14. Long, X.; Mokelke, E.A.; Neeb, Z.P.; Alloosh, M.; Edwards, J.M.; Sturek, M. Adenosine receptor regulation of coronary blood flow in Ossabaw miniature swine. *J. Pharmacol. Exp. Ther.* **2010**, *335*, 781–787. [CrossRef] [PubMed]
15. Zhai, Y.J.; Liu, P.; He, H.R.; Zheng, X.W.; Wang, Y.; Yang, Q.T.; Dong, Y.L.; Lu, J. The association of ADORA2A and ADORA2B polymorphisms with the risk and severity of chronic heart failure: A case-control study of a northern Chinese population. *Int. J. Mol. Sci.* **2015**, *16*, 2732–2746. [CrossRef]
16. Koupenova, M.; Johnston-Cox, H.; Vezeridis, A.; Gavras, H.; Yang, D.; Zannis, V.; Ravid, K. A2b adenosine receptor regulates hyperlipidemia and atherosclerosis. *Circulation* **2012**, *125*, 354–363. [CrossRef] [PubMed]
17. Kim, Y.; Han, B.G.; KoGES Group. Cohort Profile: The Korean Genome and Epidemiology Study (KoGES) Consortium. *Int. J. Epidemiol.* **2017**, *46*, e20. [CrossRef] [PubMed]
18. Cho, Y.S.; Go, M.J.; Kim, Y.J.; Heo, J.Y.; Oh, J.H.; Ban, H.J.; Yoon, D.; Lee, M.H.; Kim, D.J.; Park, M.; et al. A large-scale genome-wide association study of Asian populations uncovers genetic factors influencing eight quantitative traits. *Nat. Genet.* **2009**, *41*, 527–534. [CrossRef]
19. Purcell, S.; Neale, B.; Todd-Brown, K.; Thomas, L.; Ferreira, M.A.; Bender, D.; Maller, J.; Sklar, P.; de Bakker, P.I.; Daly, M.J.; et al. PLINK: A tool set for whole-genome association and population-based linkage analyses. *Am. J. Hum. Genet.* **2007**, *81*, 559–575. [CrossRef]
20. Barrett, J.C.; Fry, B.; Maller, J.; Daly, M.J. Haploview: Analysis and visualization of LD and haplotype maps. *Bioinformatics* **2005**, *21*, 263–265. [CrossRef]
21. World Health Organization. *The Asia-Pacific Perspective: Redefining Obesity and Its Treatment*; Health Communications Australia: Sydney, Australia, 2000.
22. Teng, B.; Smith, J.D.; Rosenfeld, M.E.; Robinet, P.; Davis, M.E.; Morrison, R.R.; Mustafa, S.J. A(1) adenosine receptor deficiency or inhibition reduces atherosclerotic lesions in apolipoprotein E deficient mice. *Cardiovasc. Res.* **2014**, *102*, 157–165. [CrossRef] [PubMed]
23. Csoka, B.; Koscso, B.; Toro, G.; Kokai, E.; Virag, L.; Nemeth, Z.H.; Pacher, P.; Bai, P.; Hasko, G. A2B adenosine receptors prevent insulin resistance by inhibiting adipose tissue inflammation via maintaining alternative macrophage activation. *Diabetes* **2014**, *63*, 850–866. [CrossRef] [PubMed]
24. Consortium, G. The Genotype-Tissue Expression (GTEx) project. *Nat. Genet.* **2013**, *45*, 580–585. [CrossRef]
25. Gupta, R.M.; Hadaya, J.; Trehan, A.; Zekavat, S.M.; Roselli, C.; Klarin, D.; Emdin, C.A.; Hilvering, C.R.E.; Bianchi, V.; Mueller, C.; et al. A Genetic Variant Associated with Five Vascular Diseases Is a Distal Regulator of Endothelin-1 Gene Expression. *Cell* **2017**, *170*, 522–533. [CrossRef]
26. Bidel, S.; Hu, G.; Qiao, Q.; Jousilahti, P.; Antikainen, R.; Tuomilehto, J. Coffee consumption and risk of total and cardiovascular mortality among patients with type 2 diabetes. *Diabetologia* **2006**, *49*, 2618–2626. [CrossRef]
27. Grosso, G.; Micek, A.; Godos, J.; Sciacca, S.; Pajak, A.; Martinez-Gonzalez, M.A.; Giovannucci, E.L.; Galvano, F. Coffee consumption and risk of all-cause, cardiovascular, and cancer mortality in smokers and non-smokers: A dose-response meta-analysis. *Eur. J. Epidemiol.* **2016**, *31*, 1191–1205. [CrossRef]
28. Shin, S.; Lim, J.; Lee, H.W.; Kim, C.E.; Kim, S.A.; Lee, J.K.; Kang, D. Association between the prevalence of metabolic syndrome and coffee consumption among Korean adults: Results from the Health Examinees study. *Appl. Physiol. Nutr. Metab.* **2019**, *44*, 1371–1378. [CrossRef]
29. Schliep, K.C.; Schisterman, E.F.; Mumford, S.L.; Pollack, A.Z.; Zhang, C.; Ye, A.; Stanford, J.B.; Hammoud, A.O.; Porucznik, C.A.; Wactawski-Wende, J. Caffeinated beverage intake and reproductive hormones among premenopausal women in the BioCycle Study. *Am. J. Clin. Nutr.* **2012**, *95*, 488–497. [CrossRef]
30. Kolovou, G.D.; Kolovou, V.; Kostakou, P.M.; Mavrogeni, S. Body mass index, lipid metabolism and estrogens: Their impact on coronary heart disease. *Curr. Med. Chem.* **2014**, *21*, 3455–3465. [CrossRef]
31. Doyle, S.E.; Breslin, F.J.; Rieger, J.M.; Beauglehole, A.; Lynch, W.J. Time and sex-dependent effects of an adenosine A2A/A1 receptor antagonist on motivation to self-administer cocaine in rats. *Pharmacol. Biochem. Behav.* **2012**, *102*, 257–263. [CrossRef]
32. Gupta, V.; Goyal, R.; Sharma, P.L. Preconditioning offers cardioprotection in hyperlipidemic rat hearts: Possible role of Dopamine (D2) signaling. *BMC Cardiovasc. Disord.* **2015**, *15*, 77. [CrossRef] [PubMed]
33. Stonehouse, A.H.; Adachi, M.; Walcott, E.C.; Jones, F.S. Caffeine regulates neuronal expression of the dopamine 2 receptor gene. *Mol. Pharmacol.* **2003**, *64*, 1463–1473. [CrossRef] [PubMed]

34. Richelle, M.; Tavazzi, I.; Offord, E. Comparison of the antioxidant activity of commonly consumed polyphenolic beverages (coffee, cocoa, and tea) prepared per cup serving. *J. Agric. Food Chem.* **2001**, *49*, 3438–3442. [CrossRef] [PubMed]
35. Ohta, T.; Nagashima, J.; Sasai, H.; Ishii, N. Relationship of Cardiorespiratory Fitness and Body Mass Index with the Incidence of Dyslipidemia among Japanese Women: A Cohort Study. *Int. J. Environ. Res. Public Health* **2019**, *16*, 4647. [CrossRef]
36. Watanabe, N.; Sawada, S.S.; Shimada, K.; Lee, I.M.; Gando, Y.; Momma, H.; Kawakami, R.; Miyachi, M.; Hagi, Y.; Kinugawa, C.; et al. Relationship between Cardiorespiratory Fitness and Non-High-Density Lipoprotein Cholesterol: A Cohort Study. *J. Atheroscler. Thromb.* **2018**, *25*, 1196–1205. [CrossRef]

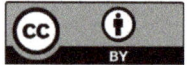

© 2020 by the authors. Licensee MDPI, Basel, Switzerland. This article is an open access article distributed under the terms and conditions of the Creative Commons Attribution (CC BY) license (http://creativecommons.org/licenses/by/4.0/).

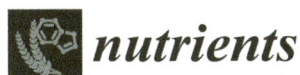
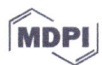

Article

Interaction between Coffee Drinking and TRIB1 rs17321515 Single Nucleotide Polymorphism on Coronary Heart Disease in a Taiwanese Population

Yin-Tso Liu [1,2], Disline Manli Tantoh [3,4], Lee Wang [4], Oswald Ndi Nfor [4], Shu-Yi Hsu [4], Chien-Chang Ho [5,6], Chia-Chi Lung [4], Horng-Rong Chang [7,8,*] and Yung-Po Liaw [3,4,*]

1. Institute of Medicine, Chung Shan Medical University, Taichung City 40201, Taiwan; cvsliu0325@gmail.com
2. Department of Cardiovascular Surgery, Asia University Hospital, Taichung 41354, Taiwan
3. Department of Medical Imaging, Chung Shan Medical University Hospital, Taichung City 40201, Taiwan; tantohdisline@gmail.com
4. Department of Public Health and Institute of Public Health, Chung Shan Medical University, Taichung 40201, Taiwan; wl@csmu.edu.tw (L.W.); nforoswald22@gmail.com (O.N.N.); sui0209@gmail.com (S.-Y.H.); dinoljc@csmu.edu.tw (C.-C.L.)
5. Department of Physical Education, Fu Jen Catholic University, New Taipei 24205, Taiwan; ccho1980@gmail.com
6. Research and Development Center for Physical Education, Health, and Information Technology, Fu Jen Catholic University, New Taipei 24205, Taiwan
7. Division of Nephrology, Department of Internal Medicine, Chung Shan Medical University Hospital, Taichung 40201, Taiwan
8. School of Medicine, Chung Shan Medical University, Taichung 40201, Taiwan
* Correspondence: chrcsmu@gmail.com (H.-R.C.); Liawyp@csmu.edu.tw (Y.-P.L.); Tel.: +886-424730022 (ext. 11838) (Y.-P.L.); Fax: +886-423248179 (Y.-P.L.)

Received: 5 March 2020; Accepted: 27 April 2020; Published: 2 May 2020

Abstract: A complex interplay of several genetic and lifestyle factors influence coronary heart disease (CHD). We determined the interaction between coffee consumption and the *tribbles pseudokinase 1* (*TRIB1*) rs17321515 variant on coronary heart disease (CHD). Data on CHD were obtained from the National Health Insurance Research Database (NHIRD) while genotype data were collected from the Taiwan Biobank (TWB) Database. From the linked electronic health record data, 1116 individuals were identified with CHD while 7853 were control individuals. Coffee consumption was associated with a lower risk of CHD. The multivariate-adjusted odds ratio (OR) and 95% confidence interval (CI) was 0.84 (0.72–0.99). Association of CHD with the *TRIB1* rs17321515 variant was not significant. The OR (95% CI) was 1.01 (0.72–0.99). There was an interaction between *TRIB1* rs17321515 and coffee consumption on CHD risk (p for interaction = 0.0330). After stratification by rs17321515 genotypes, coffee drinking remained significantly associated with a lower risk of CHD only among participants with GG genotype (OR, 0.62; 95% CI, 0.45–0.85). In conclusion, consumption of coffee was significantly associated with a decreased risk of CHD among Taiwanese adults with the *TRIB1* GG genotype.

Keywords: coffee drinking; TRIB1; rs17321515; CHD; Taiwan Biobank

1. Introduction

Coronary heart disease, also known as ischemic heart disease (IHD) or coronary artery disease (CAD) is the top cause of global mortality [1,2]. It remains the second leading cause of death in Taiwan [3]. The global coronary heart disease (CHD) mortality is projected to grow from 7.594 million in 2016 to about 9.245 million in 2030 [4].

A complex interplay of numerous genetic and lifestyle factors influence the onset of CHD [5–7]. Genotypes are nonmodifiable factors, so they cannot be confounded by other factors. As such, they are capable of playing direct causal roles in disease development [8,9]. Identification of genetic variants associated with diseases and the underlying pathophysiological mechanisms is an important step in the development of potential drug targets [8].

Genetic predisposition accounts for about 30%–60% of CHD [10,11]. Despite this, most underlying genes and molecular pathways are yet to be fully explored and therefore a significant portion of CHD heritability is not clearly understood [2]. For instance, SNPs account for just a minute fraction (approximately 10–15%) of CHD heritability [1,2,5,12,13]. The *TRIB1* is among the top genes having genome-wide significant single nucleotide polymorphisms (SNPs) for CHD [14]. It is located on chromosome 8q24 and is greatly involved in cholesterol metabolism and atherosclerosis process [15]. One of its variants, rs17321515, has been associated with variations in plasma lipid levels and CHD [14,16–18].

Coffee is a popular beverage that is widely consumed in the world [19]. In Taiwan, coffee consumption has grown rapidly in recent years. So far, the local coffee industry has expanded significantly [20]. Several studies have investigated the effects of coffee consumption on CHD. However, results have been controversial. For instance, in one of the studies, excessive consumption was significantly associated with a moderate increase in the risk of CHD [21]. However, in another study, CHD risk was higher among moderate than for excessive coffee consumers [22]. Cardioprotective effects of coffee may stem from its richness in bioactive compounds like polyphenols that possess hypocholesterolemic, antihypertensive, anti-inflammatory, and antioxidant properties [23,24]. The antioxidant content in coffee was found to be higher than that in tea, vegetables, and fruits [25].

It is well known that interactions between genes and the environment influence disease outcomes [26]. So far, there is substantial information on genetic variation and dietary patterns (including but not limited to coffee consumption) and the risk of CHD. Results from a previous study indicated that a variant in the *cytochrome P450 1A2 gene (CYP1A2)* modifies the association between caffeinated coffee consumption and the risk of myocardial infection [27]. Nevertheless, pinpointing a specific polymorphic variant is challenging considering that individual differences may exist in response to coffee or caffeine. To our knowledge, no prior study has discussed specific genotypes that can modify the association between coffee intake and the risk of CHD in Taiwan. In light of this, we determined the interaction between coffee consumption and the *TRIB1* rs17321515 variant on CHD.

2. Materials and Methods

2.1. Data Source and Participants

We used electronic data of Taiwan Biobank (TWB) participants recruited between 2008 and 2015. Participants provided blood samples for DNA extraction and completed questionnaires covering a wide range of medical, social, and lifestyle information. All participants provided informed consent. Genotyping was done using the Axiom™ Genome-Wide TWB 2.0 Array plate (Santa Clara, CA, USA). Data on CHD between 1998 and 2015 were obtained from the National Health Insurance Research Database (NHIRD). The TWB database was linked to the NHIRD using encrypted personal identification numbers. This study was approved by the Institutional Review Board of Chung Shan Medical University (CS2-16114).

In total, 9001 biobank participants were recruited. After excluding persons with incomplete questionnaires ($n = 13$) and genotype information ($n = 19$), 1116 coronary heart disease patients and 7853 controls were included in the study.

2.2. Assessment of Variables

Coronary heart disease was identified based on either two outpatient visits or one admission with reported International Classification of Diseases, Ninth Revision, Clinical Modification (ICD-9-CM) code 410–414. Participants were classified as regular coffee drinkers if they drank coffee at least three days per week in the last 6 months. Details of the covariates and physical measures used in the text have been described in our recent publication [28].

2.3. Selection of the Polymorphic Variant

The rs17321515 variant in the *TRIB1* gene was selected based on the literature search. This variant was selected because of its previous associations with CHD and dyslipidemia, especially in Han Chinese populations [16,17]. We also searched Google Scholar and selected rs762551 variant in the CYP1A2 gene which has been associated with caffeine metabolism and increased risk of myocardial infarction. We followed a standard quality control procedure and excluded SNPs with (1) a low call rate (<95%), (2) p-value of $<1.0 \times 10^{-3}$ for the Hardy–Weinberg equilibrium test, and (3) minor allele frequency of <0.05. Moreover, we removed one individual from the pair of related samples based on pairwise identity-by-descent (IBD).

2.4. Statistical Analysis

We used the statistical analysis system (SAS) software (version 9.4, SAS Institute, Cary, NC, USA) and PLINK (v1.09, http://pngu.mgh.harvard.edu/purcell/plink/) to perform analyses. Differences between groups were compared using the chi-square test. Associations of coffee and the rs17321515 variant with CHD were determined using logistic regression analysis. Adjusted variables included sex, age, educational level, smoking, alcohol intake, tea consumption, vegetarian diet, body mass index (BMI), diabetes, hypertension, hyperlipidemia, atrial fibrillation, and *CYP1A2* rs762551 variant. Odds ratios with their 95% confidence intervals were estimated.

3. Results

The descriptive data of 1116 participants with CHD and 7863 control individuals are shown in Table 1. Significant differences existed between patients and controls for coffee drinking, sex, age, educational level, cigarette smoking, exercise, body mass index (BMI), diabetes, hypertension, hyperlipidemia, atrial fibrillation, and vegetarian diet ($p < 0.05$). However, there were no significant differences between patients and controls for the *TRIB1* rs17321515 and *CYP1A2* rs762551 genotypes, alcohol, and tea consumption. Differences in coffee consumption habits between men and women as well as between those in different age groups are shown in Table 2.

Table 1. Descriptive data of the study participants.

Variable	Controls (n = 7853) n (%)	CHD Patients (n = 1116) n (%)	p-Value
Coffee drinking			<0.0001
No	5269 (67.10)	824 (73.84)	
Yes	2584 (32.90)	292 (26.16)	
TRIB1 rs17321515			0.9920
GG	2362 (30.08)	335 (30.02)	
GA+AA	5491 (69.92)	781 (69.98)	
CYP1A2 rs762551			0.1490
AA	3326 (42.35)	500 (44.80)	
AC+CC	4527 (57.65)	616 (55.20)	
Sex			<0.0001
Women	4275 (54.44)	520 (46.59)	
Men	3578 (45.56)	596 (53.41)	
Age (years)			<0.0001
30–39	2042 (26.00)	46 (4.12)	
40–49	2337 (29.76)	111 (9.95)	
50–59	2217 (28.23)	415 (37.19)	
60–70	1257 (16.01)	544 (48.75)	

Table 1. Cont.

Variable	Controls (n = 7853) n (%)	CHD Patients (n = 1116) n (%)	p-Value
Educational level			<0.0001
Elementary school	493 (6.28)	170 (15.23)	
Junior and senior high school	3258 (41.49)	498 (44.62)	
University and above	4102 (52.23)	448 (40.14)	
Cigarette smoking			0.0060
No	6117 (77.89)	828 (74.19)	
Yes	1736 (22.11)	288 (25.81)	
Alcohol drinking			0.3540
No	7031 (89.53)	989 (88.62)	
Yes	822 (10.47)	127 (11.38)	
Exercise			<0.0001
No	4702 (59.88)	474 (42.47)	
Yes	3151 (40.12)	642 (57.53)	
BMI (kg/m^2)			<0.0001
BMI < 18.5 (Underweight)	215 (2.74)	11 (0.99)	
18.5 ≤ BMI < 24 (Normal weight)	3870 (49.28)	396 (35.48)	
24 ≤ BMI < 27 (Overweight)	2283 (29.07)	415 (37.19)	
BMI ≥ 27 (Obesity)	1485 (18.91)	294 (26.34)	
Diabetes			<0.0001
No	6943 (88.41)	738 (66.13)	
Yes	910 (11.59)	378 (33.87)	
Hypertension			<0.0001
No	6424 (81.80)	391 (35.04)	
Yes	1429 (18.20)	725 (64.96)	
Hyperlipidemia			<0.0001
No	5828 (74.21)	372 (33.33)	
Yes	2025 (25.79)	744 (66.67)	
Atrial fibrillation			<0.0001
No	7833 (99.75)	1089 (97.58)	
Yes	20 (0.25)	27 (2.42)	
Tea consumption			0.1110
No	4894 (62.30)	723 (64.78)	
Yes	2959 (37.68)	393 (35.22)	
Vegetarian diet			0.0090
No	7011 (89.28)	1025 (91.85)	
Yes	842 (10.72)	91 (8.15)	

CHD: Coronary heart disease, BMI: Body mass index, TRIB1: tribbles pseudokinase 1; CYP1A2: cytochrome P450 1A2. GG, GA, and AA represent genotypes in the TRIB1 rs17321515 variant while AA, AC, and CC represent genotypes in the CYP1A2 rs762551 variant.

Table 2. Characteristics of study participants based on coffee consumption.

	No Coffee Drinking				Coffee Drinking				p-Value
	Controls		CHD Patients		Controls		CHD Patients		
	n	%	n	%	n	%	n	%	
TRIB1 rs17321515									0.4130
GG	1574	29.87	261	31.67	788	30.50	74	25.34	
GA	2564	48.66	396	48.06	1272	49.23	148	50.68	
AA	1131	21.47	167	20.27	524	20.28	70	23.97	
CYP1A2 rs762551									0.5160
AA	2229	42.30	361	43.81	1097	42.45	139	47.60	
AC	2411	45.76	375	45.51	1176	45.51	126	43.15	
CC	629	11.94	88	10.68	311	12.04	27	9.25	
Sex									<0.0001
Women	2785	52.86	391	47.45	1490	57.66	129	44.18	
Men	2484	47.14	433	52.55	1094	42.34	163	55.82	
Age									<0.0001
30–39	1340	25.43	31	3.76	702	27.17	15	5.14	
40–49	1485	28.18	77	9.34	852	32.97	34	11.64	
50–59	1521	28.87	310	37.62	696	26.93	105	35.96	
60–70	923	17.52	406	49.27	334	12.93	138	47.26	
Education									<0.0001
Elementary school	379	7.19	143	17.35	114	4.41	27	9.25	
Junior and Senior high school	2259	42.87	375	45.51	999	38.66	123	42.12	
University and above	2631	49.93	306	37.14	1471	56.93	142	48.63	
Cigarette smoking									<0.0001
No	4174	79.22	628	76.21	1943	75.19	200	68.49	
Yes	1095	20.78	196	23.79	641	24.81	92	31.51	
Alcohol drinking									0.1890
No	4734	89.85	737	89.44	2297	88.89	252	86.30	
Yes	535	10.15	87	10.56	287	11.11	40	13.70	
Physical activity									<0.0001
No	3142	59.63	353	42.84	1560	60.37	121	41.44	
Yes	2127	40.37	471	57.16	1024	39.63	171	58.56	
BMI (kg/m^2)									<0.0001
BMI < 18.5	156	2.96	9	1.09	59	2.28	2	0.68	
18.5 ≤ BMI < 24	2629	49.90	308	37.38	1241	48.03	88	30.14	
24 ≤ BMI < 27	1491	28.30	294	35.68	792	30.65	121	41.44	
BMI ≥ 27	993	18.85	213	25.85	492	19.04	81	27.74	
Diabetes									<0.0001
No	4631	87.89	538	65.29	2312	89.47	200	68.49	
Yes	638	12.11	286	34.71	272	10.53	92	31.51	
Hypertension									<0.0001
No	4237	80.41	280	33.98	2187	84.64	111	38.01	
Yes	1032	19.59	544	66.02	397	15.36	181	61.99	
Hyperlipidemia									<0.0001
No	3873	73.51	285	34.59	1955	75.66	87	29.79	
Yes	1396	26.49	539	65.41	629	24.34	205	70.21	
Atrial fibrillation									<0.0001
No	5255	99.73	804	97.57	2578	99.77	285	97.60	
Yes	14	0.27	20	2.43	6	0.23	7	2.40	
Tea consumption									<0.0001
No	3518	66.77	571	69.3	1376	53.25	152	52.05	
Yes	1751	33.23	253	30.7	1208	46.75	140	47.95	
Vegetarian diet									<0.0001
No	4646	88.18	761	92.35	2365	91.52	264	90.41	
Yes	623	11.82	63	7.65	219	8.48	28	9.59	

CHD: Coronary heart disease, BMI: Body mass index, TRIB1: tribbles pseudokinase 1, CYP1A2: cytochrome P450 1A2.

Coffee drinking was associated with a lower risk of CHD (OR, 0.84; 95% CI, 0.72–0.99), as shown in Table 3. Association with the TRIB1 rs17321515 variant was not significant; the OR was 1.01, 95% CI = 0.87–1.18. However, for the CYP1A2 rs762551 variant, the OR was 0.86 with a 95% CI of 0.74–0.99 for AC+CC, compared to the AA genotype. Corresponding ORs (95% CI) for CHD were 1.53 (1.07–2.19) for ages 40–49 years, 3.92 (2.82–5.46) for ages 50–59 years, 6.46 (4.59–9.09) for ages 60–70 years, 1.23 (1.04–1.46) for overweight, 1.35 (1.11–1.63) for obesity, 1.19 (1.01–1.41) for diabetes, 3.40 (2.91–3.98) for hypertension, 2.25 (1.91–2.63) for hyperlipidemia, and 4.09 (2.14–7.82) for atrial fibrillation.

Table 3. Association of CHD with associated variables.

Variable	OR	95% CI
Coffee drinking (ref: No)		
Yes	0.84	0.72–0.99
TRIB1 rs17321515 (ref: GG)		
GA+AA	1.01	0.87–1.18
CYP1A2 rs762551 (ref: AA)		
AC+CC	0.86	0.74–0.99
Sex (ref: Women)		
Men	1.17	0.98–1.39
Age (ref: 30–39)		
40–49	1.53	1.07–2.19
50–59	3.92	2.82–5.46
60–70	6.46	4.59–9.09
Educational level (ref: Elementary school)		
Junior and senior high school	0.97	0.77–1.21
University and above	1.01	0.80–1.28
Cigarette smoking (ref: No)		
Yes	1.07	0.88–1.30
Alcohol drinking (ref: No)		
Yes	0.79	0.62–1.01
Exercise (ref: No)		
Yes	1.07	0.92–1.24
BMI (ref: $18.5 \leq BMI < 24$)		
BMI < 18.5	0.78	0.40–1.51
$24 \leq BMI < 27$	1.23	1.04–1.46
$BMI \geq 27$	1.35	1.11–1.63
Diabetes (ref: No)		
Yes	1.19	1.01–1.41
Hypertension (ref: No)		
Yes	3.40	2.91–3.98
Hyperlipidemia (ref: No)		
Yes	2.25	1.91–2.63
Atrial fibrillation (ref: No)		
Yes	4.09	2.14–7.82
Tea consumption (ref: No)		
Yes	0.97	0.83–1.13
Vegetarian diet (ref: No)		
Yes	0.96	0.75–1.24

Ref: reference, CHD: Coronary heart disease, BMI: Body mass index, OR: odds ratio, CI: confidence interval, *TRIB1*: tribbles pseudokinase 1, *CYP1A2*: cytochrome P450 1A2.

There was a significant interaction ($p = 0.0330$) between *TRIB1* rs17321515 and coffee drinking on CHD risk (Table 4). After stratification by rs17321515 genotypes, coffee drinking remained significantly associated with a lower risk of CHD only among those with the GG genotype (OR, 0.62; 95% CI, 0.45–0.85). There was no interaction between the *CYP1A2* rs762551 variant and coffee consumption.

Table 4. Association of CHD with coffee drinking stratified by rs17321515 genotypes.

Variable	TRIB1 rs17321515 (GG)		TRIB1 rs17321515 (GA+AA)	
	OR	95% CI	OR	95% CI
Coffee drinking (ref: No)				
Yes	0.62	0.45–0.85	0.95	0.79–1.15
CYP1A2 rs762551 (ref: AA)				
AC+CC	0.83	0.64–1.08	0.86	0.72–1.02
Sex (ref: Women)				
Men	1.26	0.91–1.74	1.13	0.92–1.38
Age (ref: 30–39)				
40–49	0.79	0.41–1.54	2.01	1.30–3.10
50–59	3.46	1.96–6.12	4.21	2.79–6.35
60–70	5.52	3.05–10.00	7.10	4.66–10.84
Educational level (ref: Elementary school)				
Junior and senior high school	1.16	0.76–1.77	0.91	0.69–1.18
University and above	1.22	0.78–1.89	0.94	0.71–1.25
Cigarette smoking (ref: No)				
Yes	0.90	0.63–1.30	1.15	0.91–1.45
Alcohol drinking (ref: No)				
Yes	0.74	0.47–1.17	0.81	0.61–1.08
Exercise (ref: No)				
Yes	1.04	0.79–1.36	1.08	0.90–1.29
BMI (ref: 18.5 ≤ BMI < 24)				
BMI < 18.5	1.91	0.68–5.40	0.51	0.21–1.21
24 ≤ BMI < 27	1.49	1.09–2.05	1.15	0.94–1.40
BMI ≥ 27	2.03	1.43–2.88	1.14	0.90–1.43
Diabetes (ref: No)				
Yes	1.12	0.82–1.53	1.22	1.00–1.49
Hypertension (ref: No)				
Yes	3.84	2.87–5.12	3.28	2.72–3.96
Hyperlipidemia (ref: No)				
Yes	1.94	1.44–2.60	2.40	1.99–2.90
Atrial fibrillation (ref: No)				
Yes	8.13	2.44–27.09	3.10	1.42–6.77
Tea consumption (ref: No)				
Yes	1.14	0.86–1.52	0.91	0.75–1.09
Vegetarian diet (ref: No)				
Yes	0.88	0.54–1.42	0.99	0.74–1.33
rs17321515*coffee	$p = 0.0330$			

Ref: reference, CHD: Coronary heart disease, BMI: Body mass index, OR: odds ratio, CI: confidence interval, TRIB1: tribbles pseudokinase 1, CYP1A2: cytochrome P450 1A2.

4. Discussion

In the current study, we determined whether an interactive association exists between coffee intake and the TRIB1 rs17321515 variant with the risk of CHD. Our findings offered unique evidence that coffee intake might have a protective effect on CHD. We also found that contrary to previous findings [17,29], rs17321515 was not associated with CHD. Importantly, we found evidence of an interaction between rs17321515 and coffee intake. After stratification by rs17321515 genotypes, we found that CHD risk was significantly lower among those with GG genotype who consumed coffee relative to their non-coffee-drinking counterparts. However, there was no association among those with the GA+AA genotype, indicating that the genotype may not have any effect on CHD. TRIB1 rs17321515 has been associated with a decreased risk of CAD among Europeans, Malays, and Asian Indians [15,30,31]. However, their analyses were not performed based on coffee intake.

So far, several studies have investigated the independent effects of coffee intake and TRIB1 rs17321515 on cardiovascular disease risk. Of the studies, those investigating coffee consumption and cardiovascular disease risk have shown conflicting results. Contrary to findings from case–control studies which suggested that coffee intake was detrimental to coronary arteries [32], umbrella reviews of observational and intervention studies have found it to be beneficial even in little amounts [33,34]. An increased risk of CHD previously reported among heavy coffee drinkers was attributed to smoking [35]. In light of this, we included smoking in our analysis.

Regarding the rs17321515 polymorphism, its AA+GA genotypes were previously associated with an increased risk of CHD among Han Chinese [36]. In a Singapore Malay Eye study of 3280 adults aged 40–79 years old, the odds ratio for CHD among carriers of this variant was 1.23 for each copy of the A allele [31]. Even though the rs17321515 variant has been assessed in Asian populations as noted above, attempts have not been made to replicate it in Taiwan. This was the motivation behind the selection of this variant for the current study.

As stated earlier, lifestyle changes and genetic factors play a substantial role in the development of cardiovascular diseases. Of note, the interactive associations of both factors with CHD have not been widely reported. When coffee intake and the *TRIB1* rs17321515 variant were included in our model with adjustments for smoking and other lifestyle variables, we found that the GG genotype was significantly protective against CHD disease in individuals who consumed coffee compared to those who did not. The underlying mechanisms of interaction between coffee drinking and *TRIB1* rs17321515 SNP on CHD are not completely understood. However, metabolites in coffee are believed to influence protective endogenous pathways by modulation of gene expression [37].

One of the main variables included in our model was the rs762551 variant in the *CYP1A2* gene. We chose this variant based on its previous association with caffeine metabolism and its role in modifying the association between caffeinated coffee and the risk of heart disease [27]. Contrary to expectation, we found that AC+CC, compared to the AA genotype was protective against CHD in both the adjusted (OR, 0.86; 95% CI (0.74–0.99) and the separate model (Supplementary Table S1). By performing stratified analyses, we found that associations of *CYP1A2* rs762551 genotypes with CHD were not significant (Supplementary Table S2). Besides, there was no interaction between the variant and coffee consumption. Given that our findings are based on a limited number of coffee consumers, further investigations would be needed to clarify these associations.

In this study, we also observed that coffee consumption habits between cases and controls differed significantly based on gender and different age groups. However, differences in consumption based on gender and age are yet to be adequately determined, particularly in Taiwan.

We believe that these results will help to enhance the knowledge on the role of coffee in the association between rs17321515 variant and CHD among Taiwanese adults. However, the current study is just a first step to examine this association, which remains a fundamental issue for future research.

This study was limited in several ways. First, about 70% of the population studied did not consume any coffee. Such a limited number of coffee drinkers may preclude the possibility of observing meaningful associations between coffee and CHD. Next, our questionnaire did not have information on the type of coffee, caffeine content (that is, caffeinated or decaffeinated), methods of preparation, and the daily amount of consumption. We understand that these attributes may have different effects on CHD. Therefore, we recommend further research in this area. Second, well-established risk factors such as smoking, exercise, education, male sex, diabetes, tea-drinking, and vegetarian diet were not associated with the risk of CHD in the current population. This is an indication that our study population might not be representative of typical CHD study populations. Third, there is a possibility of nondifferential misclassification bias as information on coffee intake was based on self-report Lastly, even though the TWB is representative of the general population, only individuals who are 30–70 years old were recruited in the project. Therefore, we could not analyze data of adults under 30 or over 70 years of age.

5. Conclusions

In conclusion, our findings highlight the interactive association of coffee drinking and *TRIB1* rs17321515 polymorphism on coronary heart disease in Taiwanese adults. Taken together, we found that the risk of CHD was significantly lower among those with GG genotype who consumed coffee compared to their non-coffee-drinking counterparts. These results have provided considerable knowledge on gene–nutrient interaction in relation to cardiovascular disease.

Supplementary Materials: The following are available online at http://www.mdpi.com/2072-6643/12/5/1301/s1. Table S1: Association of CHD with rs762551 variant and associated factors, Table S2: Association of CHD with coffee drinking stratified by rs762551 genotypes.

Author Contributions: Conceptualization, Y.-T.L., D.M.T., L.W., O.N.N., S.-Y.H., C.-C.H., C.-C.L., H.-R.C., and Y.-P.L.; formal analysis, S.-Y.H., C.-C.L., and Y.-P.L.; methodology, Y.-T.L., D.M.T., L.W., O.N.N., S.-Y.H., C.-C.H., C.-C.L., H.-R.C., and Y.-P.L.; supervision, H.-R.C., and Y.-P.L.; writing–original draft, Y.-T.L., D.M.T., L.W., and O.N.N., writing–review and editing Y.-T.L., D.M.T., L.W., O.N.N., S.-Y.H., C.-C.H., C.-C.L., H.-R.C., and Y.-P.L. All authors have read and agreed to the published version of the manuscript.

Funding: The Ministry of Science and Technology (MOST), Taiwan partly funded this work (MOST 107-2627-M-040-002, 108-2621-M-040-00, and 107-EPA-F-017-002).

Acknowledgments: Authors would like to thank the Ministry of Science and Technology for the financial support.

Conflicts of Interest: The authors declare no conflict of interest.

Abbreviations

SNP: single nucleotide polymorphism, CHD: coronary heart disease, TWB: Taiwan Biobank, NHIRD: National Health Insurance Research Database, OR: odds ratio, CI: confidence interval, BMI: body mass index, *ICD-9-CM:* International Classification of Diseases, Ninth Revision, Clinical Modification.

References

1. Deloukas, P.; Kanoni, S.; Willenborg, C.; Farrall, M.; Assimes, T.L.; Thompson, J.R.; Ingelsson, E.; Saleheen, D.; Erdmann, J.; the CARDIoGRAMplusC4D Consortium; et al. Large-Scale association analysis identifies new risk loci for coronary artery disease. *Nat. Genet.* **2012**, *45*, 25–33. [CrossRef] [PubMed]
2. Mäkinen, V.-P.; Civelek, M.; Meng, Q.; Zhang, B.; Zhu, J.; Levian, C.; Huan, T.; Segrè, A.V.; Ghosh, S.; Vivar, J.; et al. Integrative genomics reveals novel molecular pathways and gene networks for coronary artery disease. *PLoS Genet.* **2014**, *10*, e1004502. [CrossRef]
3. Li, Y.-H.; Chen, J.-W.; Lin, T.-H.; Wang, Y.-C.; Wu, C.-C.; Yeh, H.-I.; Huang, C.-C.; Chang, K.-C.; Wu, C.-K.; Chen, P.-W.; et al. A performance guide for major risk factors control in patients with atherosclerotic cardiovascular disease in Taiwan. *J. Formos. Med. Assoc.* **2020**, *119*, 674–684. [CrossRef] [PubMed]
4. WHO. Projections of Mortality and Causes of Death, 2016 to 2060. Available online: https://www.who.int/healthinfo/global_burden_disease/projections/en/ (accessed on 5 February 2019).
5. Said, M.A.; Van De Vegte, Y.; Zafar, M.; Van Der Ende, Y.; Raja, G.K.; Verweij, N.; Van Der Harst, P. Contributions of interactions between lifestyle and genetics on coronary artery disease risk. *Curr. Cardiol. Rep.* **2019**, *21*, 89. [CrossRef]
6. Said, M.A.; Verweij, N.; Van Der Harst, P. Associations of combined genetic and lifestyle risks with incident cardiovascular disease and diabetes in the UK Biobank study. *JAMA Cardiol.* **2018**, *3*, 693. [CrossRef]
7. Khera, A.V.; Emdin, C.A.; Drake, I.; Natarajan, P.; Bick, A.; Cook, N.R.; Chasman, D.I.; Baber, U.; Mehran, R.; Rader, D.J.; et al. Genetic risk, adherence to a healthy lifestyle, and coronary disease. *N. Engl. J. Med.* **2016**, *375*, 2349–2358. [CrossRef]
8. Kingsmore, S.F.; Lindquist, I.E.; Mudge, J.; Gessler, D.D.; Beavis, W.D. Genome-wide association studies: Progress and potential for drug discovery and development. *Nat. Rev. Drug Discov.* **2008**, *7*, 221–230. [CrossRef]
9. Stein, E.A.; Mellis, S.; Yancopoulos, G.D.; Stahl, N.; Logan, D.; Smith, W.B.; Lisbon, E.; Gutierrez, M.; Webb, C.; Wu, R.; et al. Effect of a monoclonal antibody to PCSK9 on LDL cholesterol. *N. Engl. J. Med.* **2012**, *366*, 1108–1118. [CrossRef]
10. Peden, J.F.; Farrall, M. Thirty-five common variants for coronary artery disease: The fruits of much collaborative labour. *Hum. Mol. Genet.* **2011**, *20*, R198–R205. [CrossRef]
11. Marenberg, M.E.; Risch, N.; Berkman, L.F.; Floderus, B.; De Faire, U. Genetic susceptibility to death from coronary heart disease in a study of twins. *N. Engl. J. Med.* **1994**, *330*, 1041–1046. [CrossRef]

12. Schunkert, H.; König, I.R.; Kathiresan, S.; Reilly, M.; Assimes, T.L.; Holm, H.; Preuss, M.; Stewart, A.F.; Barbalić, M.; Gieger, C.; et al. Large-scale association analysis identifies 13 new susceptibility loci for coronary artery disease. *Nat. Genet.* **2011**, *43*, 333–338. [CrossRef] [PubMed]
13. Clarke, R.; Peden, J.F.; Hopewell, J.C.; Kyriakou, T.; Goel, A.; Heath, S.; Parish, S.; Barlera, S.; Franzosi, M.G.; Rust, S.; et al. Genetic variants associated with Lp(a) Lipoprotein level and coronary disease. *N. Engl. J. Med.* **2009**, *361*, 2518–2528. [CrossRef]
14. The IBC 50K CAD consortium correction: Large-scale gene-centric analysis identifies novel variants for coronary artery disease. *PLoS Genet.* **2012**, *8*, 7. [CrossRef]
15. Aung, L.H.H.; Yin, R.-X.; Wu, D.-F.; Li, Q.; Yan, T.-T.; Wang, Y.-M.; Li, H.; Wei, D.-X.; Shi, Y.-L.; Dezhai, Y. Association of the TRIB1 tribbles homolog 1 gene rs17321515 A>G polymorphism and serum lipid levels in the Mulao and Han populations. *Lipids Heal. Dis.* **2011**, *10*, 230. [CrossRef] [PubMed]
16. Liu, Q.; Xue, F.; Meng, J.; Liu, S.-S.; Chen, L.-Z.; Gao, H.; Geng, N.; Jin, W.-W.; Xin, Y.-N.; Xuan, S.-Y. TRIB1 rs17321515 and rs2954029 gene polymorphisms increase the risk of non-alcoholic fatty liver disease in Chinese Han population. *Lipids Heal. Dis.* **2019**, *18*, 61. [CrossRef] [PubMed]
17. Wang, L.; Jing, J.; Fu, Q.; Tang, X.; Su, L.; Wu, S.; Li, G.; Zhou, L. Association study of genetic variants at newly identified lipid gene TRIB1 with coronary heart disease in Chinese Han population. *Lipids Heal. Dis.* **2015**, *14*, 46. [CrossRef] [PubMed]
18. Wang, J.; Ban, M.R.; Zou, G.Y.; Cao, H.; Lin, T.; Kennedy, B.A.; Anand, S.; Yusuf, S.; Huff, M.W.; Pollex, R.L.; et al. Polygenic determinants of severe hypertriglyceridemia. *Hum. Mol. Genet.* **2008**, *17*, 2894–2899. [CrossRef]
19. Loftfield, E.; Cornelis, M.C.; Caporaso, N.; Yu, K.; Sinha, R.; Freedman, N. Association of Coffee Drinking with Mortality by Genetic Variation in Caffeine Metabolism: Findings From the UK Biobank. *JAMA Intern. Med.* **2018**, *178*, 1086–1097. [CrossRef]
20. Wann, J.-W.; Kao, C.-Y.; Yang, Y.-C. Consumer Preferences of Locally Grown Specialty Crop: The Case of Taiwan Coffee. *Sustainability* **2018**, *10*, 2396. [CrossRef]
21. Zhou, A.; Hyppönen, E. Long-term coffee consumption, caffeine metabolism genetics, and risk of cardiovascular disease: A prospective analysis of up to 347,077 individuals and 8368 cases. *Am. J. Clin. Nutr.* **2019**, *109*, 509–516. [CrossRef]
22. Ding, M.; Bhupathiraju, S.; Satija, A. Long-term coffee consumption and risk of cardiovascular disease: A systematic review and a dose-response meta-analysis of prospective cohort studies. *J. Vasc. Surg.* **2014**, *59*, 1471. [CrossRef]
23. Larsson, S.C. Coffee, tea, and cocoa and risk of stroke. *Stroke* **2014**, *45*, 309–314. [CrossRef] [PubMed]
24. Butt, M.S.; Sultan, M.T. Coffee and its consumption: Benefits and risks. *Crit. Rev. Food Sci. Nutr.* **2011**, *51*, 363–373. [CrossRef] [PubMed]
25. Svilaas, A.; Sakhi, A.K.; Andersen, L.F.; Svilaas, T.; Ström, E.C.; Jacobs, D.R.; Ose, L.; Blomhoff, R. Intakes of antioxidants in coffee, wine, and vegetables are correlated with plasma carotenoids in humans. *J. Nutr.* **2004**, *134*, 562–567. [CrossRef] [PubMed]
26. Rappaport, S. Genetic factors are not the major causes of chronic diseases. *PLoS ONE* **2016**, *11*, e0154387. [CrossRef]
27. Cornelis, M.C.; El-Sohemy, A.; Kabagambe, E.; Campos, H. Coffee, CYP1A2 genotype, and risk of myocardial infarction. *JAMA* **2006**, *295*, 1135. [CrossRef]
28. Liu, Y.-T.; Nfor, O.N.; Wang, L.; Hsu, S.-Y.; Lung, C.-C.; Tantoh, D.M.; Wu, M.-C.; Chang, H.-R.; Liaw, Y.-P. Interaction between sex and LDLR rs688 polymorphism on hyperlipidemia among Taiwan Biobank adult participants. *Biomolecules* **2020**, *10*, 244. [CrossRef]
29. Willer, C.J.; Sanna, S.; Jackson, A.U.; Scuteri, A.; Bonnycastle, L.L.; Clarke, R.; Heath, S.; Timpson, N.J.; Najjar, S.S.; Stringham, H.M.; et al. Newly identified loci that influence lipid concentrations and risk of coronary artery disease. *Nat. Genet.* **2008**, *40*, 161–169. [CrossRef]
30. Teslovich, T.M.; Musunuru, K.; Smith, A.V.; Edmondson, A.C.; Stylianou, I.M.; Koseki, M.; Pirruccello, J.P.; Ripatti, S.; Chasman, D.I.; Willer, C.J.; et al. Biological, clinical and population relevance of 95 loci for blood lipids. *Nature* **2010**, *466*, 707–713. [CrossRef]
31. Tai, E.S.; Sim, X.L.; Ong, T.H.; Wong, T.Y.; Saw, S.M.; Aung, T.; Kathiresan, S.; Orho-Melander, M.; Ordovas, J.M.; Tan, J.T.; et al. Polymorphisms at newly identified lipid-associated loci are associated with

blood lipids and cardiovascular disease in an Asian Malay population. *J. Lipid Res.* **2008**, *50*, 514–520. [CrossRef]
32. Sofi, F.; Conti, A.A.; Gori, A.M.; Luisi, M.L.E.; Casini, A.; Abbate, R.; Gensini, G.F. Coffee consumption and risk of coronary heart disease: A meta-analysis. *Nutr. Metab. Cardiovasc. Dis.* **2007**, *17*, 209–223. [CrossRef] [PubMed]
33. Grosso, G.; Godos, J.; Galvano, F.; Giovannucci, E.L. Coffee, Caffeine, and Health Outcomes: An Umbrella Review. *Annu. Rev. Nutr.* **2017**, *37*, 131–156. [CrossRef] [PubMed]
34. Poole, R.; Kennedy, O.J.; Roderick, P.; Fallowfield, J.; Hayes, P.C.; Parkes, J. Coffee consumption and health: Umbrella review of meta-analyses of multiple health outcomes. *BMJ* **2017**, *359*, 5024–5042. [CrossRef] [PubMed]
35. Kleemola, P.; Jousilahti, P.; Pietinen, P. Coffee consumption and the risk of coronary heart disease and death. *ACC Curr. J. Rev.* **2001**, *10*, 25. [CrossRef]
36. Liu, Q.; Liu, S.-S.; Zhao, Z.-Z.; Zhao, B.-T.; Du, S.-X.; Jin, W.-W.; Xin, Y.-N. TRIB1 rs17321515 gene polymorphism increases the risk of coronary heart disease in general population and non-alcoholic fatty liver disease patients in Chinese Han population. *Lipids Heal. Dis.* **2019**, *18*, 165–169. [CrossRef]
37. Bøhn, S.K.; Ward, N.C.; Hodgson, J.M.; Croft, K.D. Effects of tea and coffee on cardiovascular disease risk. *Food Funct.* **2012**, *3*, 575. [CrossRef]

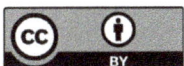

© 2020 by the authors. Licensee MDPI, Basel, Switzerland. This article is an open access article distributed under the terms and conditions of the Creative Commons Attribution (CC BY) license (http://creativecommons.org/licenses/by/4.0/).

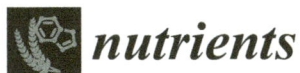 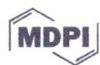

Review

Coffee Consumption and C-Reactive Protein Levels: A Systematic Review and Meta-Analysis

Elizabeth D. Moua [1], Chenxiao Hu [2], Nicole Day [3], Norman G. Hord [4] and Yumie Takata [4,*]

1. College of Pharmacy, Oregon State University/Oregon Health & Science University, Corvallis, OR 97331, USA; mouae@oregonstate.edu
2. Department of Statistics, College of Science, Oregon State University, Corvallis, OR 97331, USA; huche@oregonstate.edu
3. College of Engineering, School of Chemical, Biological, and Environmental Engineering, Oregon State University, Corvallis, OR 97331, USA; Nicole.B.Day@colorado.edu
4. College of Public Health and Human Sciences, School of Biological and Population Health Sciences, Oregon State University, Corvallis, OR 97331, USA; norman.hord@oregonstate.edu
* Correspondence: yumie.takata@oregonstate.edu; Tel.: +1-541-737-1606

Received: 23 March 2020; Accepted: 6 May 2020; Published: 8 May 2020

Abstract: Coffee contains bioactive compounds with anti-inflammatory properties, and its consumption may reduce c-reactive protein (CRP) levels, a biomarker of chronic inflammation. A previous meta-analysis reported no overall association between blood CRP level and coffee consumption by modeling the coffee consumption in categories, with substantial heterogeneity. However, the coffee cup volume was not considered. We conducted a systematic review and dose–response meta-analysis investigating the association between coffee consumption and CRP levels reported in previous observational studies. A dose–response meta-analysis was conducted by mixed-effects meta-regression models using the volume of coffee consumed as metric. Eleven studies from three continents were identified using the PubMed database, totaling 61,047 participants. Three studies with the largest sample sizes observed a statistically significant association between coffee and CRP levels, which was inverse among European and United States (US) women and Japanese men (1.3–5.5% decrease in CRP per 100 mL of coffee consumed) and positive among European men (2.2% increase). Other studies showed no statistically significant associations. When all studies were combined in the dose–response meta-analysis, no statistically significant associations were observed among all participants or when stratified by gender or geographic location, reflecting the conflicting associations reported in the included studies. Further studies are warranted to explore these inconsistent associations.

Keywords: coffee consumption; c-reactive protein; cross-sectional studies; systematic review and meta-analysis

---

1. Introduction

Coffee is a well-known beverage around the world and the most popular caffeinated drink choice [1,2]. A recent meta-analysis of 31 cohort studies reported that coffee consumption is associated with decreased risk of total mortality and cause-specific mortality from cardiovascular disease (CVD) and cancer [3]. C-reactive protein (CRP) is considered a biomarker of chronic inflammation [4] and of disease risk and progression [5], including for CVD. The association between coffee and mortality reported in the meta-analysis may be mediated through CRP.

Coffee contains many bioactive components such as chlorogenic acids, polyphenols, diterpenes, micronutrients and caffeine [2,6–8], which may exert beneficial health effects through antioxidant and anti-inflammatory properties [6–8]. There are also bioactive compounds that may negatively affect health; for instance, the high amount of lipids in unfiltered coffee may increase blood cholesterol [9,10].

In this analysis, we investigated the associations between coffee consumption and CRP levels among adults in observational studies by conducting a systematic literature review and a dose-response meta-analysis. A previous meta-analysis of 24,863 participants from nine studies modeled coffee consumption by categories and reported no overall statistically significant association with CRP level, but there was evidence of substantial heterogeneity [11]. The cup volume varied by geographic location, which affects the amount of bioactive compounds consumed and, consequently, their biological effects [7,8,12–14]. Hence, we modeled the volume of coffee consumed and hypothesized that higher coffee consumption is associated with lower levels of CRP.

2. Materials and Methods

2.1. Registration

This study was reported according to the Preferred Reporting Items for Systematic Reviews and Meta-Analyses (PRISMA) [15] and is registered with the PROSPERO International Prospective Register of Systematic Reviews (CRD42018108351).

2.2. Literature Search

A systematic literature review was conducted using the electronic database PubMed to collect data from published studies. The following search terms were used: ("coffee" [MeSH Terms] OR "coffee"[All Fields]) AND ("c-reactive protein"[MeSH Terms] OR ("c-reactive"[All Fields] AND "protein"[All Fields]) OR "c-reactive protein"[All Fields] OR "c reactive protein"[All Fields]). The last search was conducted in March 2020, and a total of 61 abstracts were identified and reviewed independently by two authors (E.D.M. and Y.T.). A full-text article was not obtained if the title and/or abstract met one or more of the following exclusion criteria: (1) animal study; (2) study among children; (3) no mention of coffee or other beverages, or of associations between food or beverage intake other than coffee and CRP or other inflammatory biomarkers; (4) no mention of CRP or other inflammatory markers/biomarkers, or of associations between beverage consumption and outcome variables other than CRP; (5) non-original study such as review or commentary. After removing abstracts that met those exclusions, the full-text articles of the remaining abstracts were obtained, reviewed, and excluded if they met one of the following additional exclusion criteria: (1) not reporting the association between coffee consumption and CRP level; (2) overlapping study populations; (3) not reporting enough data, such as coffee consumption categories (at least three) and levels of CRP within those categories; (4) meeting any of the previous exclusion criteria that could not be determined from the abstract alone, but was determined based on the full-text article. A total of 10 articles that did not meet any of the exclusion criteria were included in the systematic literature review. We found three meta-analysis/systematic review articles in our PubMed search [4,11,16] and compared the list of original research studies included in the article, finding no additional studies to the 10 articles we identified that met our inclusion criteria. Data were extracted independently by two authors (E.D.M. and Y.T.) and inconsistencies were discussed and brought to consensus.

The following information was extracted, compiled and summarized for each study: first author; year of publication; study name; country; study design; calendar years when the study was conducted and questionnaire information and blood samples were collected; number of participants; age; gender; coffee consumption assessment (questionnaire validated or not) and methods of questionnaire administration (interview or self-administered); cup volume conversion and/or frequency of consumption; study results such as CRP levels (mean and standard deviations/error or 95% confidence intervals (CI)) by coffee consumption categories.

Not all of the information described above could be extracted from each of the 10 articles. In such cases, articles that might provide missing information were examined by examining references cited by the studies, searching for articles about the study or questionnaire through PubMed, or contacting the corresponding author of the articles. For instance, information on cup volume conversion was available for nine studies [17–24], but not for the Kyushu University cohort and the Dose-Response to Exercise in Women (DREW) trial [25,26]. When we contacted the corresponding authors of these two studies, we either received confirmation of the lack of information [26] or no response [25]; hence, we estimated the cup conversion based on the other studies conducted in similar location and calendar years, such as the Aichi Workers' study [20] and Nurses' Health Study (NHS) [18], respectively. Data on high-sensitivity CRP levels were obtained from all studies, but two studies needed to be converted to milligram per liter [20,22]. For all 11 studies, high-sensitivity CRP was measured using blood samples collected throughout each study.

The risk of bias for each study was assessed by both authors (E.D.M. and Y.T.) independently using the modified Newcastle–Ottawa Scale for cross-sectional studies [27]; any discrepancies were discussed and a consensus reached.

2.3. Meta-Analysis

A meta-analysis of associations between coffee consumption volume and CRP level was conducted through the Metafor package from R. Based on the cup conversion information we collected and the range of cups of coffee consumed in each category reported in each article, we estimated the mid-point volume (in mL) of coffee consumption in each category; we then re-calculated the *p*-trend to test a linear association between coffee consumption and CRP level by treating coffee volume as continuous in a model.

The estimated weighted mean changes in CRP level (per 100 mL of coffee) and 95% CI were calculated through a mixed-effects meta-regression model. We used log-transformed CRP levels in our meta-analysis. Due to incomparability of the reported values, the ATTICA study was excluded from the meta-analysis. The heterogeneity across studies was assessed by I^2 statistics [28]. To explore the source of heterogeneity, we pre-specified and stratified analyses by gender and geographic location.

3. Results

Our study identified 61 abstracts published in March 2020 or earlier with search terms identified previously. After reviewing articles based on the title and abstract (Figure 1), 47 were selected to obtain full-text articles. Among them, 37 of the published studies were excluded: 26 for not reporting the association between coffee consumption and CRP level, four for using the same study population [29–32], five for not providing enough data [33–37], and two for being a non-original article [38,39]. In total, 10 published articles reporting associations between coffee consumption and CRP levels in 11 study populations (one article reported results from two cohorts [18]) were selected and included in the current systematic review and meta-analysis.

The 11 studies were conducted between 1976 and 2007 in various locations: three in the United States (US) [18,26], three in Asia [19,20,25], and the rest in Europe [17,21–24] (Table 1). These 11 studies involved a total of 61,047 participants. Most studies had over 500 participants each [17–20,22,23,25], with the exception of two studies which had 344 and 61 participants, respectively [21,26]. Among the 11 studies, six included both men and women [17,19,20,22,23,25]. Of the other five studies, two included only women [18,26] and three included only men [18,21,24].

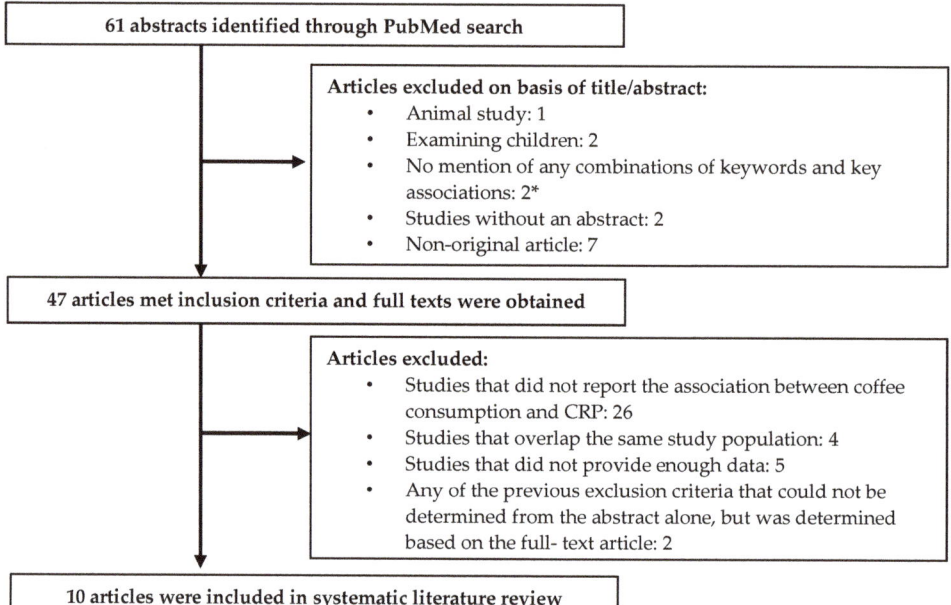

Figure 1. Flow chart of systematic literature review. * no mention of coffee or other beverages, or of associations between food or beverage intake other than coffee and c-reactive protein (CRP) or other inflammatory biomarkers; no mention of CRP or other inflammatory markers/biomarkers, or of associations between beverage consumption and outcome variables other than CRP.

The age of study participants varied from 18 to 87 years old. The mean body mass index (BMI) of each study was between 22.8 kg/m^2 and 36.1 kg/m^2, with the exception of one that did not report BMI values, but reported instead that 17.7% of participants were obese [17]. Six studies reported that the mean alcohol consumption ranged from 1.7–27.3 g/day [18,20–24,26], while four studies reported that 18.6–72.7% of participants drank alcohol [19,25]. One study did not provide information on alcohol consumption [17]. As for smoking, one study of women and one study of men consisted of only non-smokers [21,26]. Hence, the percentage of current smokers ranged from 0% (due to recruitment criterion) in the DREW trial and United Kingdom (UK) study [21,26] to 53.3% in the ATTICA study [17]. Of the three studies that included postmenopausal women and reported hormone therapy use [18,22,26], the proportion of users ranged from 25.9% in the European Prospective Investigation into Cancer and Nutrition (EPIC) study [22] to 46.5% in the DREW trial [26].

All studies used questionnaires to assess coffee consumption, through self-administration, interview, or both. Each study had 3–5 coffee consumption categories including "no", "low", "medium", "high", and "very high" coffee consumption. The consumption amount considered "low" or "high" varied across studies, ranging from 1 cup/month to <6 cups/week for low consumption and 2 to ≥6 cups/day for high consumption. Two studies included the fifth ("very high") consumption category as high as ≥7 cups/day [22,25]. As the studies were conducted in various locations, the volume of a cup for each region ranged from 150 mL in the Aichi Workers' cohort in Japan [20] and the Finnish Diabetic Nephropathy (FinnDiane) study in Finland [23] to 237 mL in NHS and Health Professional Follow-Up Study (HPFS) studies in the US [18] and EPIC and UK studies in Europe [21,22].

Table 1. Participant characteristics by study *.

Study Name	Study Years	Gender	Number of Participants	Age (Years Old)	BMI	Current Smokers (%)	Alcohol	Hormone Therapy Use (%)	Coffee Consumption	Cup Conversion
DREW trial [26]	2001–2005	Women	344	57.1 ± 6.4 45–75	36.1 ± 3.9 kg/m²	0%	1.7 ± 2.4 g/day	46.5%	55.2% consumed < 1 cup/day	No data (used 237 mL)
NHS [18]	1976	Women	15,551	57.3	25.5 kg/m²	13.4%	6 g/day	41.3%	28.9% consumed ≤ 1 cup/day	1 cup = 237 mL
HPFS [18]	1986	Men	7397	62.4	25.7 kg/m²	6.2%	11.8 g/day	-	36.1% consumed ≤ 1 cup/day	1 cup = 237 mL
EPIC Study [22]	1992–2000	Women Men	10,520 4280	51.7 (45.3–58.4) 53.3 (46.6–59.6)	24.2 kg/m² 26.3 kg/m²	17% 30%	4.2 g/day 14.5 g/day	25.9% -	300 mL/day 380 mL/day	1 cup = 237 mL
Kyushu University Cohort Study [25]	2004–2007	Women Men	5918 4407	62 49–76	22.5 kg/m² 23.5 kg/m²	6% 32.4%	27.1% 72.7%	No data	Median: 2 cups/day	No data (used 150 mL)
ATTICA study [17]	2001–2002	Women Men	1528 1514	45.5 ± 13 18–87	15.6% 19.7%	45.5% 62.4%	No data	No data	24% consumed < 1 cup/day 9% consumed < 1 cup/day	1 cup = 150 mL
Singapore Prospective Study [19]	2003–2007	Both	4139	48.8 ± 11.3	23.2 kg/m²	11.7%	18.6%	No data	40% consumed < 1 cup/day	1 cup = 215 mL
Aichi Workers' Cohort Study [20]	2002	Both	3317	47.6 ± 7.1 35–69	22.8 ± 2.7 kg/m²	29.6%	14.2 g/day	No data	Median: 1 cup/day	1 cup = 150 mL
United Kingdom Study [21]	2003–2004	Men	61	32.7	25.3 kg/m²	0%	14.7 g/day	No data	Mean: 1.1 cup/day	1 cup = 237 mL
FinnDiane Study [23]	1997	Both	1040	46.7 ± 0.4	25.6 kg/m²	13.3%	2.7 g/day	No data	12.9% consumed < 1 cup/day Mean: 3.8 ± 2.8 cups/day	1 cup = 150 mL
BELSTRESS [24]	1994–1998	Men	1031	49.0	27.0 kg/m²	34.9%	27.3 g/day	-	16% consumed < 1 cup/day	1 cup = 150 mL

* Mean or mean ± standard deviation; range; and/or median (25th–75th percentiles) are provided for age; mean, median, or percentage of obesity is provided for BMI; mean or percentage of alcohol consumers is provided for alcohol consumption; percentage of hormone therapy users among postmenopausal women is provided for hormone therapy use; mean, median, and/or percentage of those who consumed specific numbers of cups per day are provided for coffee consumption. Study years/calendar year(s) when the study was conducted were obtained as follows when not mentioned in the article: (1) extracting the years when participants enrolled in the study or provided information through questionnaires and other data collection procedures for cross-sectional study (ATTICA study [17]) or analysis of intervention trials or prospective studies (DREW [26], EPIC [22], Kyushu University cohort study [25], Singapore Prospective study [19], and Aichi Workers' study [20]); (2) extracting from another article of the same study (UK study [40] and the FinnDiane study [41,42] and BELSTRESS study [43]); or (3) extracting years when blood draw and coffee intake assessments through a food frequency questionnaire (FFQ) (NHS and HPFS [18]). Lifestyle factors and median (25th–75th percentiles) age by gender for EPIC were taken from other EPIC study publications [44,45], and lifestyle factors for BELSTRESS study were taken from another BELSTRESS study publication [46].

When the linear association was assessed taking the volume of coffee consumed into account, three of the 11 studies observed statistically significant inverse or positive associations between coffee consumption and CRP levels, although the rest reported no significant association (Table 2). These three studies examined associations separately by gender, and different associations were observed by gender and study [18,22,25]. Among women, the EPIC and NHS included 10,520 and 15,551 women, respectively, and they had a statistically significant inverse association (EPIC: p-trend = 0.002, 2.7% decrease in CRP per 100 mL of coffee consumption; NHS: p-trend = 0.02, 5.5% decrease in CRP) [18,22]. Among men, the Kyushu University cohort included 4407 men and also showed a statistically significant inverse association (p-trend = 0.03, 1.3% decrease in CRP) [25]. In contrast, the EPIC study had 4280 men and showed a statistically significant positive association between coffee consumption and CRP levels (p-trend = 0.01, 2.2% increase in CRP) [22].

When the 10 studies that reported compatible CRP levels were combined through the dose–response meta-analysis, no statistically significant association was observed among all participants (mean change in CRP level: −2.4%; 95% CI: −8.7% to 4.4%; p = 0.49) with no evidence of heterogeneity (I^2 < 0.01%). Similarly, no significant associations (mean change in CRP level; 95% CI; p-value) were observed when we stratified by gender (men: 0.9%; −9.7% to 8.8%; p = 0.85; women: −6.3%; −16.4% to 5.0%; p = 0.26), or geographic location (US: −6.7%; −6.5% to 8.3%; p = 0.54; Europe: 0.6%; −6.5% to 8.3%; p = 0.83; Asia: −1.6%; −12.1% to 10.2%; p = 0.78) with no evidence of heterogeneity (I^2 < 0.01%). Given that BELSTRESS study [24] was based on crude estimates, we repeated the analyses without the BELSTRESS study, which did not materially change the results (data not shown).

Regarding risk of bias, assessed through the modified Newcastle–Ottawa Scale for cross-sectional studies [27], all studies had scores of six or higher (Supplementary Table S1). Five studies [20–23,25] scored seven, which is considered good quality. Two studies [24,26] scored six (satisfactory quality), three [18,19] scored eight (good quality), and another [17] scored 10 (very good quality).

Table 2. C-reactive protein levels by coffee consumption by study.

Study Name	Gender	Categories in the Original Study: Median or Mid-Point Volume (mL)					P-Trend *
		None	Low	Medium	High	Very High	
		Number of Participants					
		Geometric Mean c-Reactive Protein (95% Confidence Intervals) (mg/L)					
DREW trial [26]	Women	None: 0 mL	1 cup/month to 6 cups/week: 104 mL	1 cup/day to 13 cups/week: 339 mL	≥2 cups/day: 533 mL	—	0.05
		104	86	89	65	—	
		4.1 (3.4, 4.9)	4.1 (3.3, 5.0)	3.1 (2.6, 3.8)	3 (2.4, 3.8)	—	
NHS [18]	Women	None: 0 mL	<1 cup/day: 119 mL	2–3 cups/day: 356 mL	≥4 cups/day: 1037 mL	—	0.02
		3433	4178	5653	2287	—	
		4.18 (3.55, 4.92)	4.04 (3.60, 4.52)	3.25 (3.03, 3.48)	2.37 (2.16, 2.59)	—	
HPFS [18]	Men	1723	2341	2354	979	—	0.37
		1.09 (0.92, 1.29)	1.07 (0.95, 1.21)	0.97 (0.88, 1.06)	1.00 (0.88, 1.12)	—	
EPIC study [22]	Men	None: 0 mL	Low: 103 mL	Medium-low: 297 mL	Medium-high: 451 mL	High: 745 mL	0.01
		212	1078	977	1078	935	
		1.15 (1.13, 1.16)	1.16 (1.15, 1.18)	1.18 (1.17, 1.20)	1.21 (1.19, 1.22)	1.34 (1.33, 1.36)	
	Women	832	2730	2171	2730	2057	0.002
		1.42 (1.40, 1.45)	1.39 (1.36, 1.41)	1.28 (1.26, 1.30)	1.26 (1.24, 1.30)	1.16 (1.14, 1.17)	
Kyushu University Cohort Study [25]		None: 0 mL	<1 cup/day: 75 mL	1–3 cups/day: 300 mL	4–6 cups/day: 750 mL	≥7 cups/day: 1305 mL	
	Men	721	1145	1986	469	86	0.03
		0.55 (0.51, 0.59)	0.53 (0.50, 0.56)	0.51 (0.49, 0.53)	0.5 (0.46, 0.55)	0.44 (0.35, 0.55)	
	Women	892	1578	2944	444	60	0.50
		0.40 (0.38, 0.43)	0.40 (0.38, 0.42)	0.39 (0.38, 0.41)	0.41 (0.37, 0.45)	0.31 (0.24, 0.39)	
ATTICA study [17]		None: 0 mL	<200 mL/day: 100 mL	200–400 mL/day: 300 mL	>400 mL/day: 650 mL	—	
	Men	133	758	521	27	—	0.11
		2.3 (0.76, 3.84)	2.2 (0.76, 3.64)	2.9 (−0.56, 6.36)	3.1 (1.85, 4.35)	—	
	Women	366	922	211	19	—	0.21
		2.1 (0.66, 3.54)	2.0 (0.56, 3.44)	2.7 (−0.76, 6.16)	2.9 (1.36, 4.44)	—	

Table 2. Cont.

Study Name	Gender	Categories in the Original Study: Median or Mid-Point Volume (mL)					P-Trend *
		None	Low	Medium	High	Very High	
		Number of Participants					
		Geometric Mean c-Reactive Protein (95% Confidence Intervals) (mg/L)					
Singapore Prospective Study [19]	Both	Never/rarely: 0 mL 1202 1.31 (1.16, 1.49)	<1 cup/day: 123 mL 475 1.43 (1.25, 1.65)	1–2 cups/day: 323 mL 2118 1.28 (1.14, 1.44)	≥3 cups/day: 860 mL 344 1.23 (1.05, 1.44)	—	0.37
Aichi Workers' Cohort Study [20]	Both	<1 cup: 75 mL 949 0.43 (0.41, 0.47)	1 cup: 150 mL 803 0.4 (0.37, 0.43)	2–3 cups: 375 mL 1336 0.37 (0.35, 0.40)	≥4 cups/day: 750 mL 229 0.42 (0.36, 0.48)	—	0.51
United Kingdom study [21]	Men	— —	<1 cup/day: 45 mL 16 0.97 (0.77, 1.17)	1–2 cups/day: 195 mL 20 0.83 (0.64, 1.02)	>2 cups/day: 435 mL 41 0.94 (0.82, 1.06)	—	0.94
FinnDiane Study [23]	Both	<1 cup/day: 75 mL 134 1.93 (1.56, 2.30)	≥1 cup/day < 3: 300 mL 230 1.88 (1.61, 2.16)	≥3 cups/day < 5: 600 mL 371 1.62 (1.41, 1.82)	≥5 cups/day: 1013 mL 305 1.68 (1.44, 1.91)	—	0.27
BELSTRESS [24]	Men	None 168 0.89 (0.75, 1.04)	1–3 cups/day: 300 mL 415 0.95 (0.81, 1.11)	>3cups/day: 750 mL 448 0.97 (0.82, 1.14)	—	—	0.30

* P-trend was re-calculated based on the estimated mid-point volume (in mL) of coffee consumption in each category and obtained by treating coffee volume as continuous in a model testing a linear association between coffee consumption and CRP level.

4. Discussion

To our knowledge, this is the first dose–response meta-analysis of the association between coffee consumption and CRP level in cross-sectional analyses that considered the volume of coffee consumed instead of categorical data, as employed in a previous meta-analysis [11]. Hence, our analysis is more robust in assessing the effects of volume of coffee consumed, which reflects the amount of bioactive compounds in coffee better than considering categories alone [12–14]. This is important as cup volume varied across studies (150 to 237 mL). When studies were combined through the dose–response meta-analysis, no statistically significant associations were observed between coffee consumption and CRP levels among all studies or after stratifying by gender or geographic location. To further elucidate this finding, we examined associations of CRP level with coffee consumption by modeling the volume of coffee and re-calculating the p-value for linear associations for each study. We found that the three studies with the largest sample sizes, NHS, EPIC study, and Kyushu University cohort, had statistically significant inverse or positive associations between coffee consumption and CRP levels, while others reported no statistically significant association. These inconsistent associations across studies may be explained by differences in study populations as discussed below.

The characteristics related to coffee preference and preparation methods common in each study population may have affected the associations between coffee consumption and CRP level due to variation in the amount of bioactive compounds [12,13,47,48]. Around the time when coffee consumption was assessed in the included countries, instant coffees were popular in all countries. Unfiltered coffee was more commonly consumed in European countries than in the United States, Japan, and Singapore, where filtered coffee was more common [49]. Among the 11 included studies, three investigated associations separately by coffee preparation methods or types—filtered and unfiltered coffees in the ATTICA study [17] and decaffeinated and caffeinated coffees in the NHS and HPFS [18]. However, all studies found similar associations for either method [17,18]. Moreover, previous coffee intervention trials reported no difference in CRP levels by different types or preparation methods of coffee [34,50,51]. Nevertheless, a previous animal study provided evidence of anti-inflammatory effects of caffeine, given that a three-week caffeine administration (7.5 to 15 mg/kg of body weight) resulted in decreased CRP level in rats [7]. Therefore, previous human studies [34,50,51] may not have had a sufficiently large variation in coffee consumption (due to small sample sizes or homogeneous coffee consumption within a single study population) to observe differences in CRP levels comparable to the animal study [7]. Our meta-analysis had a limited ability to further explore associations by coffee preparation methods or types given that only three of the included studies conducted separate analyses [17,18]. In addition to caffeine, chlorogenic acid was reported to decrease inflammation in vitro, and its content varies by roasting levels [52]. To provide greater insight, future human studies may need to assess type, preparation methods and roasting types, along with the volume of coffee consumed.

In addition, discrepant results between studies could be due to participants' characteristics common in groups defined by gender and geographic location. These characteristics might have contributed to their interactions with coffee consumption or have confounded the observed associations. Firstly, BMI may have affected the inconsistent results between European men and women and Japanese men. Given the pro-inflammatory nature of CRP, a positive association of CRP levels with BMI and body fat composition was reported previously [53]. The EPIC study, with a positive association, had a higher average BMI (26.3 kg/m^2) [44] than the Kyushu University cohort (23.5 kg/m^2) [25], which reported an inverse association. Similarly, within the same EPIC study population, opposing associations (a positive association for men and an inverse association for women) were reported, which suggests that BMI (26.3 kg/m^2 for men and 24.2 kg/m^2 for women on average) [44] might have played a role rather than other factors such as coffee type. Hence, it is possible that BMI or body fat mass may have contributed to conflicting associations of coffee consumption with CRP levels in the EPIC and Kyushu University cohort studies. To further elucidate potential involvement of body fat mass, future studies need to use other anthropometric measures that are more reflective of body fat mass than BMI and stratify results by these anthropometric factors.

Secondly, smoking might have contributed to discrepant results. CRP levels were higher among smokers than non-smokers [54], and smoking tends to be more common among men than women, especially in Japan [25,55] and Singapore [56]. In addition, confounding effects of smoking in the association between coffee and CRP level are possible as previously reported for coronary artery disease or CVD mortality [3,57], which were closely linked to CRP levels. For the studies with statistically significant associations, the proportion of current smokers was 32% for men in the Kyushu University cohort [25], 30% for men and 17% for women in the EPIC study [45], and 13% in the NHS [18]. Hence, the relatively low proportion of current smokers might partially explain the inverse association for European and US women. However, other factors may play a role in conflicting associations between European and Japanese men, which warrants further investigations.

Alcohol intake may have also been an influential variable in gender differences with regard to the association between coffee consumption and CRP level. Among women, studies with a significant inverse association tended to have a higher alcohol consumption (6.0 g/day in NHS [18] and 4.2 g/day in EPIC women [22]) than studies with a non-significant association (1.7 g/day in DREW trial [26] and 27.1% as alcohol consumers in women in Kyushu University Cohort [25]). Among men, however, this trend was not clearly observed; EPIC men with a significant positive association reported consumption of 14.5 g/day [22]; Kyushu University Cohort men with a significant inverse association reported 72.7% of current alcohol consumers [25]; other studies with non-significant associations reported consumption in the range of 11.8 g/day in HPFS [18] and 27.3 g/day in BELSTRESS [24]. Among men in the Kyushu University Cohort, the inverse association between coffee and CRP was strongest among high current alcohol consumers [25], which might have driven the overall inverse association when all men in this study were combined. In the EPIC study, the association between coffee and CRP was not reported by alcohol consumption level. Biological effects may be influenced by consumption differences between genders, suggesting that the inverse association may be stronger for drinkers than non-drinkers. The positive association observed in EPIC men [22] may be partially explained by a previously reported U-shaped association between alcohol consumption and CRP [58], which warrants further investigation. The stronger inverse association between coffee and CRP in high alcohol consumers among Japanese men [25] is not consistent with the reported U-shaped association; however, relatively lower BMI in Japanese men than European men might have contributed to this difference. Additionally, the proportion of smokers was similar between Japanese and European men, which may not explain the opposing associations reported. Taken together, other potential factors (e.g., types of alcoholic beverages) that may explain the discrepant associations between European and Japanese men need to be explored in future studies.

Strengths of this current analysis include the large number of participants (a total of 61,047), with a majority of the included studies comprising over 500 participants. This analysis included a diverse population of apparently healthy men and women, overweight and postmenopausal women, and men and women with known diabetes or metabolic syndrome. Additionally, this analysis obtained results from over 15 different countries in Europe, North America, and Asia. This diversity in study populations allowed us to cover a wide range of coffee consumption levels (the estimated median volume of coffee consumed ranged from 150 mL in Aichi Workers' cohort [20] to 570 mL in the FinnDiane study [23]) that could not be achieved within a single study, and it allowed us to conduct a thorough examination of the association between coffee consumption and CRP levels. We also estimated the volume of coffee consumed in our analysis, instead of the pre-defined category or number of cups consumed, which better reflects the amount of hypothesized bioactive compounds in coffee. In addition, the comparability of CRP values across studies is a strength as all studies measured high-sensitivity CRP. The duration of blood sample storage varied by study; however, CRP values were reported to be highly stable over time (spanning several years) when blood samples were stored under the well-kept conditions [59] that all included studies followed. There may be slight variations in blood collection and handling procedures (such as temperature or time between blood collection and storage), which were also reported not to affect CRP values [60].

A limitation of this analysis is that the sample size ranged from 61 to 15,551, although a majority of the studies had over 500 participants. This may have affected the number of coffee consumption categories and statistical power within a single study. Hence, we conducted a dose–response meta-analysis including all eligible studies. Secondly, regarding CRP levels, two studies of women in the United States (i.e., DREW trial and NHS) had relatively higher levels than the rest of the studies. Previously, obesity and hormone therapy use were reported as determinants of high CRP level [38,53,61]. Both studies [18,26] had the two highest proportions of hormone therapy users (46.5% and 41.3% for the DREW trial and NHS, respectively), and the DREW trial included only overweight and obese women, while the NHS had a higher average BMI than other studies; these two characteristics may explain their high CRP levels. Thirdly, except for sex, we had limited ability to explore effects of potential confounding factors such as smoking and BMI. This is due to the fact that we did not have participant-level data and we relied on the reported associations adjusted for a set of confounding variables chosen by study investigators. Moreover, our study was limited in exploring the confounding effect of age because age ranges of study participants overlapped among the included studies and no study conducted analyses stratified by age group. Fourthly, all studies were based on cross-sectional analyses, which cannot infer temporal association, and future prospective analyses are warranted. Fifthly, our analysis only included one biomarker of chronic inflammation, CRP. Thus, other biomarkers such as interleukin-6 and tumor necrosis factor-alpha need to be explored in future studies. These biomarkers were linked to coffee extracts in previous in vitro [52] and human studies [17,18]. Furthermore, there is recent development in isoforms of CRP, such as pentameric and monomeric isoforms, linked to cardiovascular diseases and inflammatory conditions [62], which need to be considered in future studies. Sixthly, all the included studies used a food frequency questionnaire (FFQ) to assess coffee consumption. Although most were previously validated and reported correlation coefficients of coffee intake between FFQ and other dietary assessment instruments as high as 0.78 [31], the use of FFQs may have impacted the coffee consumption data due to inherent self-reporting errors [63]. Nonetheless, it is an efficient way to assess dietary intake in a large sample size. Future studies could use biomarkers of coffee consumption (e.g., urinary furoylglycine [64,65], N-methylpyridinium, and trigonelline [66]) to overcome limitations in self-reporting methods. Additionally, these biomarker studies would address the potential difference in the amount of bioactive compounds resulting from differences in coffee preparation, brew strength, roasting and beans, which cannot be construed solely by the volume of coffee consumed. Future studies measuring biomarkers of coffee consumption or collecting detailed information on coffee type and preparation method are warranted.

5. Conclusions

Our results from the dose–response meta-analysis suggest no statistically significant association between coffee consumption and CRP level among all studies combined or after stratification by gender and geographic location. The three individual studies with the largest sample sizes among the 11 included studies support an inverse or positive association between coffee consumption and CRP levels among European men and women, US women, and Japanese men. Given these conflicting associations, factors such as smoking and BMI may be attributable to these variations, and the potential interaction with gender needs to be explored further.

Supplementary Materials: The following are available online at http://www.mdpi.com/2072-6643/12/5/1349/s1, Table S1: Risk of Bias Assessment.

Author Contributions: Conceptualization, E.D.M. and Y.T.; methodology, Y.T. and C.H.; formal analysis C.H.; writing—Original draft preparation, E.D.M. and Y.T.; writing—Review and editing, C.H., N.D., and N.G.H.; supervision, Y.T.; project administration, Y.T. All authors have read and agreed to the published version of the manuscript.

Funding: This study received no funding.

Acknowledgments: E.D.M. completed this work as part of her Honors' thesis in the College of Public Health and Human Sciences at Oregon State University.

Conflicts of Interest: None declared by all authors (E.D.M., C.H., N.D., N.G.H., and Y.T.).

Abbreviations

BMI	body mass index
CI	confidence intervals
CRP	c-reactive protein
CVD	cardiovascular disease
DREW	Dose-Response to Exercise in Women
EPIC	European Prospective Investigation into Cancer and Nutrition
FFQ	food frequency questionnaire
FinnDiane	Finnish Diabetic Nephropathy
HPFS	Health Professional Follow-Up Study
NHS	Nurses' Health Study
UK	United Kingdom
US	United States

References

1. Frost-Meyer, N.J.; Logomarsino, J.V. Impact of coffee components on inflammatory markers: A review. *J. Funct. Foods* **2012**, *4*, 819–830. [CrossRef]
2. Nieber, K. The Impact of Coffee on Health. *Planta Med.* **2017**. [CrossRef]
3. Grosso, G.; Micek, A.; Godos, J.; Sciacca, S.; Pajak, A.; Martinez-Gonzalez, M.A.; Giovannucci, E.L.; Galvano, F. Coffee consumption and risk of all-cause, cardiovascular, and cancer mortality in smokers and non-smokers: A dose-response meta-analysis. *Eur. J. Epidemiol.* **2016**, *31*, 1191–1205. [CrossRef]
4. Rodrigues, I.M.; Klein, L.C. Boiled or filtered coffee? Effects of coffee and caffeine on cholesterol, fibrinogen and C-reactive protein. *Toxicol. Rev.* **2006**, *25*, 55–69. [CrossRef]
5. Ansar, W.; Ghosh, S. C-reactive protein and the biology of disease. *Immunol. Res.* **2013**, *56*, 131–142. [CrossRef]
6. Santana-Galvez, J.; Cisneros-Zevallos, L.; Jacobo-Velazquez, D.A. Chlorogenic Acid: Recent Advances on Its Dual Role as a Food Additive and a Nutraceutical against Metabolic Syndrome. *Molecules* **2017**, *22*, 358. [CrossRef]
7. Owoyele, B.V.; Oyewole, A.L.; Biliaminu, S.A.; Alashi, Y. Effect of taurine and caffeine on plasma c-reactive protein and calcium in Wistar rats. *Afr. J. Med. Med. Sci.* **2015**, *44*, 229–236. [PubMed]
8. Kim, H.G.; Kim, J.Y.; Hwang, Y.P.; Lee, K.J.; Lee, K.Y.; Kim, D.H.; Kim, D.H.; Jeong, H.G. The coffee diterpene kahweol inhibits tumor necrosis factor-alpha-induced expression of cell adhesion molecules in human endothelial cells. *Toxicol. Appl. Pharmacol.* **2006**, *217*, 332–341. [CrossRef]
9. Bak, A.A.; Grobbee, D.E. The effect on serum cholesterol levels of coffee brewed by filtering or boiling. *N. Engl. J. Med.* **1989**, *321*, 1432–1437. [CrossRef]
10. Zock, P.L.; Katan, M.B.; Merkus, M.P.; van Dusseldorp, M.; Harryvan, J.L. Effect of a lipid-rich fraction from boiled coffee on serum cholesterol. *Lancet* **1990**, *335*, 1235–1237. [CrossRef]
11. Zhang, Y.; Zhang, D.Z. Is coffee consumption associated with a lower level of serum C-reactive protein? A meta-analysis of observational studies. *Int. J. Food Sci. Nutr.* **2018**. [CrossRef]
12. Arisseto, A.P.; Vicente, E.; Ueno, M.S.; Tfouni, S.A.; Toledo, M.C. Furan levels in coffee as influenced by species, roast degree, and brewing procedures. *J. Agric. Food Chem.* **2011**, *59*, 3118–3124. [CrossRef]
13. Moon, J.K.; Shibamoto, T. Role of roasting conditions in the profile of volatile flavor chemicals formed from coffee beans. *J. Agric. Food Chem.* **2009**, *57*, 5823–5831. [CrossRef]
14. Yanagimoto, K.; Ochi, H.; Lee, K.G.; Shibamoto, T. Antioxidative activities of fractions obtained from brewed coffee. *J. Agric. Food Chem.* **2004**, *52*, 592–596. [CrossRef]
15. Moher, D.; Liberati, A.; Tetzlaff, J.; Altman, D.G.; Group, P. Preferred reporting items for systematic reviews and meta-analyses: The PRISMA statement. *PLoS. Med.* **2009**, *6*, e1000097. [CrossRef]

16. Paiva, C.; Beserra, B.; Reis, C.; Dorea, J.G.; Da Costa, T.; Amato, A.A. Consumption of coffee or caffeine and serum concentration of inflammatory markers: A systematic review. *Crit. Rev. Food Sci. Nutr.* **2019**, *59*, 652–663. [CrossRef]
17. Zampelas, A.; Panagiotakos, D.B.; Pitsavos, C.; Chrysohoou, C.; Stefanadis, C. Associations between coffee consumption and inflammatory markers in healthy persons: The ATTICA study. *Am. J. Clin. Nutr.* **2004**, *80*, 862–867. [CrossRef]
18. Hang, D.; Kvaerner, A.S.; Ma, W.; Hu, Y.; Tabung, F.K.; Nan, H.; Hu, Z.; Shen, H.; Mucci, L.A.; Chan, A.T.; et al. Coffee consumption and plasma biomarkers of metabolic and inflammatory pathways in US health professionals. *Am. J. Clin. Nutr.* **2019**, *109*, 635–647. [CrossRef]
19. Rebello, S.A.; Chen, C.H.; Naidoo, N.; Xu, W.; Lee, J.; Chia, K.S.; Tai, E.S.; van Dam, R.M. Coffee and tea consumption in relation to inflammation and basal glucose metabolism in a multi-ethnic Asian population: A cross-sectional study. *Nutr. J.* **2011**, *10*, 61. [CrossRef]
20. Yamashita, K.; Yatsuya, H.; Muramatsu, T.; Toyoshima, H.; Murohara, T.; Tamakoshi, K. Association of coffee consumption with serum adiponectin, leptin, inflammation and metabolic markers in Japanese workers: A cross-sectional study. *Nutr. Diabetes* **2012**, *2*, e33. [CrossRef]
21. Hamer, M.; Williams, E.D.; Vuononvirta, R.; Gibson, E.L.; Steptoe, A. Association between coffee consumption and markers of inflammation and cardiovascular function during mental stress. *J. Hypertens.* **2006**, *24*, 2191–2197. [CrossRef]
22. Gunter, M.J.; Murphy, N.; Cross, A.J.; Dossus, L.; Dartois, L.; Fagherazzi, G.; Kaaks, R.; Kuhn, T.; Boeing, H.; Aleksandrova, K.; et al. Coffee Drinking and Mortality in 10 European Countries: A Multinational Cohort Study. *Ann. Intern. Med.* **2017**, *167*, 236–247. [CrossRef]
23. Stutz, B.; Ahola, A.J.; Harjutsalo, V.; Forsblom, C.; Groop, P.H.; FinnDiane Study, G. Association between habitual coffee consumption and metabolic syndrome in type 1 diabetes. *Nutr. Metab. Cardiovasc. Dis.* **2018**, *28*, 470–476. [CrossRef]
24. De Bacquer, D.; Clays, E.; Delanghe, J.; De Backer, G. Epidemiological evidence for an association between habitual tea consumption and markers of chronic inflammation. *Atherosclerosis* **2006**, *189*, 428–435. [CrossRef]
25. Maki, T.; Pham, N.M.; Yoshida, D.; Yin, G.; Ohnaka, K.; Takayanagi, R.; Kono, S. The relationship of coffee and green tea consumption with high-sensitivity C-reactive protein in Japanese men and women. *Clin. Chem. Lab. Med.* **2010**, *48*, 849–854. [CrossRef]
26. Arsenault, B.J.; Earnest, C.P.; Despres, J.P.; Blair, S.N.; Church, T.S. Obesity, coffee consumption and CRP levels in postmenopausal overweight/obese women: Importance of hormone replacement therapy use. *Eur. J. Clin. Nutr.* **2009**, *63*, 1419–1424. [CrossRef]
27. Herzog, R.; Alvarez-Pasquin, M.J.; Diaz, C.; Del Barrio, J.L.; Estrada, J.M.; Gil, A. Are healthcare workers' intentions to vaccinate related to their knowledge, beliefs and attitudes? A systematic review. *BMC Public Health* **2013**, *13*, 154. [CrossRef]
28. Higgins, J.P.; Thompson, S.G. Quantifying heterogeneity in a meta-analysis. *Stat. Med.* **2002**, *21*, 1539–1558. [CrossRef]
29. Pham, N.M.; Wang, Z.; Morita, M.; Ohnaka, K.; Adachi, M.; Kawate, H.; Takayanagi, R.; Kono, S. Combined effects of coffee consumption and serum gamma-glutamyltransferase on serum C-reactive protein in middle-aged and elderly Japanese men and women. *Clin. Chem. Lab. Med.* **2011**, *49*, 1661–1667. [CrossRef]
30. Jacobs, S.; Kroger, J.; Floegel, A.; Boeing, H.; Drogan, D.; Pischon, T.; Fritsche, A.; Prehn, C.; Adamski, J.; Isermann, B.; et al. Evaluation of various biomarkers as potential mediators of the association between coffee consumption and incident type 2 diabetes in the EPIC-Potsdam Study. *Am. J. Clin. Nutr.* **2014**, *100*, 891–900. [CrossRef]
31. Lopez-Garcia, E.; van Dam, R.M.; Qi, L.; Hu, F.B. Coffee consumption and markers of inflammation and endothelial dysfunction in healthy and diabetic women. *Am. J. Clin. Nutr.* **2006**, *84*, 888–893. [CrossRef]
32. Williams, C.J.; Fargnoli, J.L.; Hwang, J.J.; van Dam, R.M.; Blackburn, G.L.; Hu, F.B.; Mantzoros, C.S. Coffee consumption is associated with higher plasma adiponectin concentrations in women with or without type 2 diabetes: A prospective cohort study. *Diabetes Care* **2008**, *31*, 504–507. [CrossRef]
33. Martinez-Lopez, S.; Sarria, B.; Mateos, R.; Bravo-Clemente, L. Moderate consumption of a soluble green/roasted coffee rich in caffeoylquinic acids reduces cardiovascular risk markers: Results from a randomized, cross-over, controlled trial in healthy and hypercholesterolemic subjects. *Eur J. Nutr.* **2018**. [CrossRef]

34. Kempf, K.; Kolb, H.; Gartner, B.; Bytof, G.; Stiebitz, H.; Lantz, I.; Lang, R.; Hofmann, T.; Martin, S. Cardiometabolic effects of two coffee blends differing in content for major constituents in overweight adults: A randomized controlled trial. *Eur. J. Nutr.* **2015**, *54*, 845–854. [CrossRef]
35. Hu, G.; Jousilahti, P.; Tuomilehto, J.; Antikainen, R.; Sundvall, J.; Salomaa, V. Association of serum C-reactive protein level with sex-specific type 2 diabetes risk: A prospective finnish study. *J. Clin. Endocrinol. Metab.* **2009**, *94*, 2099–2105. [CrossRef]
36. Raaska, K.; Raitasuo, V.; Laitila, J.; Neuvonen, P.J. Effect of caffeine-containing versus decaffeinated coffee on serum clozapine concentrations in hospitalised patients. *Basic Clin. Pharmacol. Toxicol.* **2004**, *94*, 13–18. [CrossRef]
37. Kotani, K.; Sakane, N.; Yamada, T.; Taniguchi, N. Association between coffee consumption and the estimated glomerular filtration rate in the general Japanese population: Preliminary data regarding C-reactive protein concentrations. *Clin. Chem. Lab. Med.* **2010**, *48*, 1773–1776. [CrossRef]
38. de Maat, M.P.; Kluft, C. Determinants of C-reactive protein concentration in blood. *Ital. Heart J.* **2001**, *2*, 189–195. [CrossRef]
39. Coffee linked to increased levels of heart risk markers. *Health News* **2005**, *11*, 15.
40. Hamer, M.; Williams, E.; Vuonovirta, R.; Giacobazzi, P.; Gibson, E.L.; Steptoe, A. The effects of effort-reward imbalance on inflammatory and cardiovascular responses to mental stress. *Psychosom Med.* **2006**, *68*, 408–413. [CrossRef]
41. Ahola, A.J.; Lassenius, M.I.; Forsblom, C.; Harjutsalo, V.; Lehto, M.; Groop, P.H. Dietary patterns reflecting healthy food choices are associated with lower serum LPS activity. *Sci. Rep.* **2017**, *7*, 6511. [CrossRef]
42. Ahola, A.J.; Mikkila, V.; Makimattila, S.; Forsblom, C.; Freese, R.; Groop, P.H.; FinnDiane Study, G. Energy and nutrient intakes and adherence to dietary guidelines among Finnish adults with type 1 diabetes. *Ann. Med.* **2012**, *44*, 73–81. [CrossRef]
43. Moreau, M.; Valente, F.; Mak, R.; Pelfrene, E.; de Smet, P.; De Backer, G.; Kornitzer, M. Obesity, body fat distribution and incidence of sick leave in the Belgian workforce: The Belstress study. *Int. J. Obes. Relat. Metab. Disord.* **2004**, *28*, 574–582. [CrossRef]
44. McKenzie, F.; Biessy, C.; Ferrari, P.; Freisling, H.; Rinaldi, S.; Chajes, V.; Dahm, C.C.; Overvad, K.; Dossus, L.; Lagiou, P.; et al. Healthy Lifestyle and Risk of Cancer in the European Prospective Investigation Into Cancer and Nutrition Cohort Study. *Medicine (Baltimore)* **2016**, *95*, e2850. [CrossRef]
45. Ferrari, P.; Licaj, I.; Muller, D.C.; Kragh Andersen, P.; Johansson, M.; Boeing, H.; Weiderpass, E.; Dossus, L.; Dartois, L.; Fagherazzi, G.; et al. Lifetime alcohol use and overall and cause-specific mortality in the European Prospective Investigation into Cancer and nutrition (EPIC) study. *BMJ Open* **2014**, *4*, e005245. [CrossRef]
46. Verdaet, D.; Dendale, P.; De Bacquer, D.; Delanghe, J.; Block, P.; De Backer, G. Association between leisure time physical activity and markers of chronic inflammation related to coronary heart disease. *Atherosclerosis* **2004**, *176*, 303–310. [CrossRef]
47. Ratnayake, W.M.; Hollywood, R.; O'Grady, E.; Stavric, B. Lipid content and composition of coffee brews prepared by different methods. *Food Chem. Toxicol.* **1993**, *31*, 263–269. [CrossRef]
48. Smrke, S.; Opitz, S.E.; Vovk, I.; Yeretzian, C. How does roasting affect the antioxidants of a coffee brew? Exploring the antioxidant capacity of coffee via on-line antioxidant assays coupled with size exclusion chromatography. *Food Funct.* **2013**, *4*, 1082–1092. [CrossRef]
49. IARC Working Group. *Monogr.: Eval. of Carcinogenic Risks to Humans: Coffee, Tea, Mate, Methylxanthines and Methylglyoxal*; International Agency for Research on Cancer: Lyon, France, 1991.
50. Ohnaka, K.; Ikeda, M.; Maki, T.; Okada, T.; Shimazoe, T.; Adachi, M.; Nomura, M.; Takayanagi, R.; Kono, S. Effects of 16-week consumption of caffeinated and decaffeinated instant coffee on glucose metabolism in a randomized controlled trial. *J. Nutr. Metab.* **2012**, *2012*, 207426. [CrossRef]
51. Wedick, N.M.; Brennan, A.M.; Sun, Q.; Hu, F.B.; Mantzoros, C.S.; van Dam, R.M. Effects of caffeinated and decaffeinated coffee on biological risk factors for type 2 diabetes: A randomized controlled trial. *Nutr. J.* **2011**, *10*, 93. [CrossRef]
52. Jung, S.; Kim, M.H.; Park, J.H.; Jeong, Y.; Ko, K.S. Cellular Antioxidant and Anti-Inflammatory Effects of Coffee Extracts with Different Roasting Levels. *J. Med. Food* **2017**, *20*, 626–635. [CrossRef] [PubMed]
53. Kao, T.W.; Lu, I.S.; Liao, K.C.; Lai, H.Y.; Loh, C.H.; Kuo, H.K. Associations between body mass index and serum levels of C-reactive protein. *SAMJ S. Afr. Med. J.* **2009**, *99*, 326–330. [PubMed]

54. Ahonen, T.M.; Kautiainen, H.J.; Keinanen-Kiukaanniemi, S.M.; Kumpusalo, E.A.; Vanhala, M.J. Gender Difference Among Smoking, Adiponectin, and High-Sensitivity C-Reactive Protein. *Am. J. Prev. Med.* **2008**, *35*, 598–601. [CrossRef] [PubMed]
55. Yamada, H.; Kawado, M.; Aoyama, N.; Hashimoto, S.; Suzuki, K.; Wakai, K.; Suzuki, S.; Watanabe, Y.; Tamakoshi, A.; Group, J.S. Coffee consumption and risk of colorectal cancer: The Japan Collaborative Cohort Study. *J. Epidemiol.* **2014**, *24*, 370–378. [CrossRef]
56. Ainslie-Waldman, C.E.; Koh, W.P.; Jin, A.; Yeoh, K.G.; Zhu, F.; Wang, R.; Yuan, J.M.; Butler, L.M. Coffee intake and gastric cancer risk: The Singapore Chinese health study. *Cancer Epidemiol. Biomark. Prev.* **2014**, *23*, 638–647. [CrossRef] [PubMed]
57. Klatsky, A.L.; Koplik, S.; Kipp, H.; Friedman, G.D. The confounded relation of coffee drinking to coronary artery disease. *Am. J. Cardiol.* **2008**, *101*, 825–827. [CrossRef]
58. Bell, S.; Mehta, G.; Moore, K.; Britton, A. Ten-year alcohol consumption typologies and trajectories of C-reactive protein, interleukin-6 and interleukin-1 receptor antagonist over the following 12 years: A prospective cohort study. *J. Intern. Med.* **2017**, *281*, 75–85. [CrossRef]
59. Doumatey, A.P.; Zhou, J.; Adeyemo, A.; Rotimi, C. High sensitivity C-reactive protein (Hs-CRP) remains highly stable in long-term archived human serum. *Clin. Biochem.* **2014**, *47*, 315–318. [CrossRef]
60. Sugden, K.; Danese, A.; Shalev, I.; Williams, B.S.; Caspi, A. Blood Substrate Collection and Handling Procedures under Pseudo-Field Conditions: Evaluation of Suitability for Inflammatory Biomarker Measurement. *Biodemography Soc. Biol.* **2015**, *61*, 273–284. [CrossRef]
61. Sas, A.A.; Vaez, A.; Jamshidi, Y.; Nolte, I.M.; Kamali, Z.; T, D.S.; Riese, H.; Snieder, H. Genetic and environmental influences on stability and change in baseline levels of C-reactive protein: A longitudinal twin study. *Atherosclerosis* **2017**, *265*, 172–178. [CrossRef]
62. Boncler, M.; Wu, Y.; Watala, C. The Multiple Faces of C-Reactive Protein-Physiological and Pathophysiological Implications in Cardiovascular Disease. *Molecules* **2019**, *24*, 2062. [CrossRef] [PubMed]
63. Subar, A.F.; Freedman, L.S.; Tooze, J.A.; Kirkpatrick, S.I.; Boushey, C.; Neuhouser, M.L.; Thompson, F.E.; Potischman, N.; Guenther, P.M.; Tarasuk, V.; et al. Addressing Current Criticism Regarding the Value of Self-Report Dietary Data. *J. Nutr.* **2015**, *145*, 2639–2645. [CrossRef]
64. Heinzmann, S.S.; Holmes, E.; Kochhar, S.; Nicholson, J.K.; Schmitt-Kopplin, P. 2-Furoylglycine as a Candidate Biomarker of Coffee Consumption. *J. Agric. Food Chem.* **2015**, *63*, 8615–8621. [CrossRef] [PubMed]
65. Stalmach, A.; Mullen, W.; Barron, D.; Uchida, K.; Yokota, T.; Cavin, C.; Steiling, H.; Williamson, G.; Crozier, A. Metabolite profiling of hydroxycinnamate derivatives in plasma and urine after the ingestion of coffee by humans: Identification of biomarkers of coffee consumption. *Drug Metab. Dispos.* **2009**, *37*, 1749–1758. [CrossRef] [PubMed]
66. Lang, R.; Wahl, A.; Stark, T.; Hofmann, T. Urinary N-methylpyridinium and trigonelline as candidate dietary biomarkers of coffee consumption. *Mol. Nutr. Food Res.* **2011**, *55*, 1613–1623. [CrossRef]

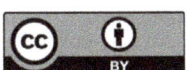 © 2020 by the authors. Licensee MDPI, Basel, Switzerland. This article is an open access article distributed under the terms and conditions of the Creative Commons Attribution (CC BY) license (http://creativecommons.org/licenses/by/4.0/).

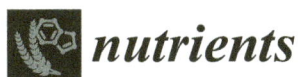 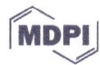

Article

Exploring the Association between Urine Caffeine Metabolites and Urine Flow Rate: A Cross-Sectional Study

Shou En Wu [1,2] and Wei-Liang Chen [1,2,3,]*

1. Division of Family Medicine, Department of Family and Community Medicine, Tri-Service General Hospital and School of Medicine, National Defense Medical Center, Taipei 114, Taiwan; grace830115@gmail.com
2. Division of Geriatric Medicine, Department of Family and Community Medicine, Tri-Service General Hospital, and School of Medicine, National Defense Medical Center, Taipei 114, Taiwan
3. Department of Biochemistry, National Defense Medical Center, Taipei 114, Taiwan
* Correspondence: weiliang0508@gmail.com; Tel.: +886-2-8792-3311 (ext. 16567); Fax: +886-2-8792-7057

Received: 6 August 2020; Accepted: 9 September 2020; Published: 13 September 2020

Abstract: Examination of urine excretion of caffeine metabolites has been a simple but common way to determine the metabolism and effect of caffeine, but the relationship between urinary metabolites and urine flow rate is less discussed. To explore the association between urinary caffeine metabolite levels and urine flow rate, 1571 participants from the National Health and Nutrition Examination Survey (NHANES) 2011–2012 were enrolled in this study. We examined the association between urinary caffeine metabolites and urine flow rate with linear regression models. Separate models were constructed for males and females and for participants aged <60 and ≥60 years old. A positive association was found between concentrations of several urinary caffeine metabolites and urine flow rate. Three main metabolites, namely, paraxanthine, theobromine, and caffeine, showed significance across all subgroups. The number of caffeine metabolites that revealed flow-dependency was greater in males than in females and was also greater in the young than in the elderly. Nevertheless, the general weakness of NHANES data, a cross-sectional study, is that the collection is made at one single time point rather than a long-term study. In summary, urinary concentrations of several caffeine metabolites showed a positive relationship with the urine flow rate. The trend is more noticeable in males and in young subgroups.

Keywords: urine caffeine metabolites; urine flow rate

1. Introduction

Caffeine is a common psychoactive stimulant that can be found in daily beverages such as coffee, tea, and cocoa. Its impact on various aspects has aroused the interest of researchers from different fields. In the field of physiology, the impact of caffeine on the central nervous system and peripheral organs has been widely discussed [1]. The most noticeable one is the antagonism of adenosine receptors A1 and A2 [2], which play a famous role in arousal, vigilance, and anxiety [3]. In regard to neurotransmitters, caffeine seems to affect norepinephrine, dopamine, and serotonin, which contribute to alertness [4]. In the cardiovascular system, caffeine increases heart rate and affects blood pressure, cardiac rhythm, and various cardiac diseases [5,6]. In kidneys, caffeine induces diuresis and natriuresis [7]. In the field of psychology, sleep disturbance, learning and memory, addiction, and withdrawal are popular topics related to caffeine [8–10].

In the field of pharmacology, enzyme assays, including CYP1A2, N-acetyltransferase, and xanthine oxidase, utilize caffeine and its urinary metabolites as the means of evaluation [11,12]. There are various ways of evaluating caffeine metabolism. Urine levels, serum levels, and metabolite ratios of caffeine act as biomarkers for diseases [13], targets for drugs [14], and probes for enzyme activity [15]. Factors that may confound the results of examinations should be taken into account when interpreting related data. Urine flow rate is undoubtedly a crucial factor when interpreting data regarding urinary caffeine metabolism, and thus the association between urinary caffeine metabolite concentrations and urine flow rate deserves attention. Previous literature discussing flow-dependency put more focus on theophylline, one of the caffeine metabolites that is well known for its therapeutic effects on asthma and chronic obstructive pulmonary disease (COPD) [16–18]. However, comprehensive studies about other caffeine metabolites are lacking. Therefore, the purpose of our study is to investigate the relationship between 14 main urinary caffeine metabolites and the urine flow rate.

2. Materials and Methods

2.1. Design and Participants

The NHANES study, a nationally representative study of population in the United States, is a cross-sectional survey based on a national sample of randomly-selected residents in the USA. It is administered by the National Center for Health Statistics (NCHS) of the Centers for Disease Control and Prevention (CDC). The survey combines three main parts. Initial screening questions determine qualified participants. Afterward, an extensive interview is held at home, which includes information such as age, gender, race, medical history, and health status. Further physical examination or clinical evaluations are performed at specially designed mobile examination centers (MECs). All interviewers received training programs and met the required standards. NHANES started in 1999 and remains a continuous annual survey, with data released every 2 years. Detailed questionnaire instruments, procedure manuals, brochures, and consent documents for the 2011–2012 NHANES are described on the NHANES website. This study gained Institutional Review Board (IRB; project identification code protocol #2011-17) approval by the National Center for Health Statistics (NCHS) in line with the revised Helsinki Declaration. Informed consents were collected from all research participants before the data-gathering procedure and examinations were carried out.

There were 9756 participants in the NHANES dataset from 2011–2012. Data from 2009–2010 also performed urinary caffeine analysis but was abandoned due to the instrument used not being suitable for analyzing both positive and negative ions simultaneously, so each urine specimen was analyzed twice. Data from 2011–2012 was from an improved instrument so that the measurement of each specimen was done in a single analysis. After excluding those under 18 years old and those with missing data such as urine flow rate, urinary caffeine analysis, and those taking medication of benign prostatic hyperplasia and diuretics, 1410 eligible participants were involved in our analysis. Figure 1 shows a scheme of the flow chart of participant recruitment. We performed our analyses in three stages: categorizing participants as a whole population, by gender (male and female), and by age (cutoff value set at 60 years old to refer to the elderly population [19,20]).

2.2. Measurement of Caffeine Metabolites in Urine

Spot urine samples were collected by experienced operators at the MECs. Recorded documents included the date and time of sampling and the volume of urine collection. Samples were stored at ≤ -70 °C based on the Laboratory Procedures Manual before transportation to the National Center for Environmental Health (Centers for Disease Control and Prevention, Atlanta, GA, USA) for testing. Urinary metabolite quantification was determined by ultra-high performance liquid chromatography–electrospray ionization–tandem quadrupole mass spectrometry (UHPLC–ESI–MS/MS) (Agilent Technologies, Palo Alta, CA, USA) with stable isotope-labeled internal standards. More detailed methods are reported on the NHANES website.

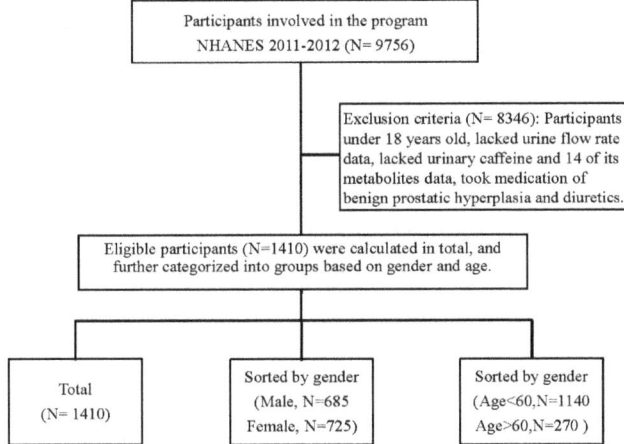

Figure 1. Flow chart of participant recruitment.

Caffeine and 14 of its urinary metabolites, 15 in total, were examined, including 1-methyluric acid, 3-methyluric acid, 7-methyluric acid, 1,3-dimethyluric acid, 1,7-dimethyluric acid, 3,7-dimethyluric acid, 1,3,7-trimethyluric acid, 1-methylxanthine, 3-methylxanthine, 7-methylxanthine, 1,3-dimethylxanthine (theophylline), 1,7-dimethylxanthine (paraxanthine), 3,7-dimethylxanthine (theobromine), 1,3,7-trimethylxanthine (caffeine), and 5-acetylamino-6-amino-3-methyluracil (AAMU). AAMU is the decomposition product of the relatively unstable caffeine metabolite 5-acetylamino-6-formylamino-3-methyluracil (AFMU). Samples were allowed to incubate for at least 30 min at room temperature so that conversion of all AFMU to the more stable AAMU was ensured.

The lower limit of detection (LLOD in umol/L) for caffeine and caffeine metabolites can be obtained from the NHANES website. For analytes with results below the lower limit of detection, the value is the lower limit of detection divided by the square root of 2 (LLOD/sqrt [2]). All presented data satisfied quality control (QC) procedures, which were performed by a multirule quality control system. Samples examined were collected from 3 QC pools (low-, medium-, and high-quality control pools). Urine analyte concentrations were adjusted to urinary creatinine (uCr) by dividing urine concentration of metabolites by uCr values.

2.3. Measurement of Urine Flow Rate

Urinary flow rate was not a regular examined item in every cycle of NHANES. We collected our data from NHANES 2011–2012. Upon visiting MECs, participants reported the time of the last urinary void at home. At the center, the urinary volume was measured, and the time of sample collection was recorded. Up to three voids could be collected if the initial two voiding volumes were insufficient for the clinical and laboratory analyses. Conceptually, the calculation of urine flow rate is by dividing the volume of the present urine sample by the time duration between the former urination and the present urine collection, i.e., (total urine volume)/(total time duration).

2.4. Covariates

The self-reported demographic details of all subjects comprise gender, age, race/ethnicity, smoking history, and medical history. Race was sorted into groups including Mexican American, other Hispanic, non-Hispanic whites and blacks, and other races. Both former and current smokers were defined as having a habit of smoking. The formula of body mass index (BMI) is weight in kilograms divided by height in meters squared (kg/m^2). Heart disease was defined as ever been diagnosed with congestive heart failure, coronary heart disease, angina, or heart attack. Biochemical data are measured as follows:

aspartate aminotransferase (AST) were detected by the Beckman Coulter UniCel DxC 800 Synchron Clinical System; fasting plasma glucose (FPG) levels and urine creatinine (Cr) were measured by Roche/Hitachi Modular P Chemistry Analyzer. Further details about collection procedures are available on the NHANES website.

2.5. Statistical Analysis

We conducted a statistical analysis using SPSS (IBM SPSS Statistics for Windows, version 22.0, released 2013; IBM Corp., Armonk, NY). Qualitative data and quantitative variables were reported in percentages and medians and interquartile ranges (IQRs), respectively. A p-value of ≤ 0.05 was considered statistically significant. The urine flow rates deviated from normality, and, thus, log-transformation was performed to achieve normalization. Subsequently, we applied linear regression models to investigate the relationship between urine levels of caffeine metabolite levels and the log-transformed urine flow rate.

Four models were provided in each analytic group to adjust for relevant covariates. The unadjusted model was numbered Model 1; Model 2 was adjusted for age, gender, and race; Model 3 was further adjusted for BMI, serum fasting glucose, AST, and urine creatinine; Model 4 was further adjusted for experiences of heart disease, smoking status, water intake, and caffeine intake.

3. Results

3.1. Characteristics of the Study Population

The demographic information of the eligible subjects in the study is shown in Table 1. The mean age of the participants was 47.7 ± 17.79 years old, and 49.8% of participants were male and 43.5% were ever-smokers. Median of baseline variables is as follows: BMI 28.89 kg/m^2, AST 25.54 U/L, uCr 0.89 mg/dL, and FPG 102.92 mg/dL.

3.2. Urinary Caffeine Metabolite Concentrations and Urine Flow Rate

Associations between urinary caffeine metabolite concentrations and urine flow rate are demonstrated in Table 2. Positive correlations were discovered by linear regression analysis in caffeine and several of its metabolites: 1-methyluric acid (β coefficient = 0.068, $p < 0.001$), 1,7-dimethyluric acid (β coefficient = 0.091, $p = 0.047$), 1,3,7-trimethyluric acid (β coefficient = 1.806, $p = 0.007$), 1-methylxanthine (β coefficient = 0.152, $p < 0.001$), 7-methylxanthine (β coefficient = 0.07, $p = 0.005$), 1,3-dimethylxanthine (theophylline, β coefficient = 1.177, $p < 0.001$), 1,7-dimethylxanthine (paraxanthine, β coefficient = 0.587, $p < 0.001$), 3,7-dimethylxanthine (theobromine, β coefficient = 0.316, $p < 0.001$), 1,3,7-trimethylxanthine (caffeine, β coefficient = 1.102, $p < 0.001$), and 5-acetylamino-6-amino-3-methyluracil (β coefficient = 0.053, $p = 0.004$). Notably, additional adjustments for all covariates did not affect the statistical significance in the aforementioned metabolites. We further categorized our participants into subgroups by gender in Table 3 and by age in Table 4. Paraxanthine ($p < 0.001$ in total population, male, female, under and over 60 years old), theobromine ($p < 0.001$ in total population, male, female, under 60 years old; $p = 0.011$ over 60 years old), and caffeine ($p < 0.001$ in total population, male, female, under and over 60 years old) were the three showing significant positive correlations in all subgroups.

Table 1. Characteristics of participants.

Variables	Median (IQR) or Percent (%)
Continuous variables	
Age (years)	47.70 ± 17.79
BMI (kg/m^2)	28.89 ± 6.85
Aspartate aminotransferase (AST)(U/L)	25.54 ± 14.01
urine creatinine (mg/dL)	0.89 ± 0.29
serum fasting glucose (mg/dL)	102.92 ± 41.51
1-methyluric acid (umol/L)	0.91 ± 1.19
3-methyluric acid (umol/L)	0.01 ± 0.02
7-methyluric acid (umol/L)	0.22 ± 0.34
1,3-dimethyluric acid (umol/L)	0.11 ± 0.26
1,7-dimethyluric acid (umol/L)	0.42 ± 0.49
3,7-dimethyluric acid (umol/L)	0.01 ± 0.02
1,3,7-trimethyluric acid (umol/L)	0.03 ± 0.03
1-methylxanthine (umol/L)	0.48 ± 0.68
3-methylxanthine (umol/L)	0.42 ± 0.61
7-methylxanthine (umol/L)	0.67 ± 0.92
1,3-dimethylxanthine (theophylline) (umol/L)	0.03 ± 0.07
1,7-dimethylxanthine (paraxanthine) (umol/L)	0.29 ± 0.40
3,7-dimethylxanthine (theobromine) (umol/L)	0.28 ± 0.44
1,3,7-trimethylxanthine (caffeine) (umol/L)	0.09 ± 0.18
5-acetylamino-6-amino-3-methyluracil (uM/L)	0.96 ± 1.25
Caffeine intake on the exam day (mg)	142.74 ± 192.73
Total plain water drank the day before exam (mg)	1130.95 ± 1213.59
Categorical variables	
Gender	
Male	49.8
Female	50.2
Race	
Mexican American	9.5
Other Hispanic	10.5
Non-Hispanic White	36.9
Non-Hispanic Black	26.8
Other Race—including Multi-Racial	16.4
Heart disease—ever had a diagnosis	
Congestive heart failure	3.5
Coronary heart disease	4
Angina	2.6
Heart attack	3.8
Smoking	43.5

interquartile range (IQR).

Table 2. Association between urinary caffeine metabolites and urine flow rate.

Variables	Model 1 β(95% CI)	p Value	Model 2 β(95% CI)	p Value	Model 3 β(95% CI)	p Value	Model 4 β(95% CI)	p Value
1-methyluric acid	0.072 (0.035, 0.110)	<0.001	0.074 (0.037, 0.112)	<0.001	0.083 (0.045, 0.121)	<0.001	0.055 (0.011, 0.099)	0.015
3-methyluric acid	1.472 (−1.373, 4.318)	0.310	2.048 (−0.833, 4.930)	0.163	2.651 (−0.244, 5.546)	0.073	1.281 (−1.698, 4.260)	0.399
7-methyluric acid	0.083 (−0.061, 0.228)	0.260	0.114 (−0.032, 0.260)	0.126	0.125 (−0.021, 0.271)	0.092	0.042 (−0.108, 0.192)	0.582
1,3-dimethyluric acid	0.048 (−0.116, 0.213)	0.565	0.046 (−0.118, 0.210)	0.585	0.055 (−0.109, 0.219)	0.510	−0.012 (−0.177, 0.153)	0.885
1,7-dimethyluric acid	0.108 (0.017, 0.200)	0.020	0.135 (0.041, 0.228)	0.005	0.147 (0.053, 0.240)	0.002	0.054 (−0.053, 0.161)	0.322
3,7-dimethyluric acid	2.291 (−0.022, 4.604)	0.052	2.825 (0.527, 5.123)	0.016	2.720 (0.427, 5.013)	0.02	1.802 (−0.507, 4.110)	0.126
1,3,7-trimethyluric acid	1.936 (0.598, 3.274)	0.005	2.400 (1.049, 3.751)	0.001	2.637 (1.287, 3.988)	<0.001	1.508 (0.029, 2.987)	0.046
1-methylxanthine	0.164 (0.100, 0.229)	<0.001	0.170 (0.105, 0.234)	<0.001	0.170 (0.105, 0.235)	<0.001	0.130 (0.056, 0.204)	0.001
3-methylxanthine	0.098 (0.013, 0.183)	0.024	0.125 (0.040, 0.211)	0.004	0.120 (0.035, 0.206)	0.006	0.078 (−0.010, 0.165)	0.081
7-methylxanthine	0.080 (0.029, 0.131)	0.002	0.091 (0.040, 0.141)	<0.001	0.087 (0.035, 0.138)	0.001	0.063 (0.010, 0.115)	0.019
1,3-dimethylxanthine (theophylline)	1.146 (0.549, 1.743)	<0.001	1.187 (0.594, 1.780)	<0.001	1.173 (0.579, 1.766)	<0.001	0.941 (0.343, 1.540)	0.002
1,7-dimethylxanthine (paraxanthine)	0.590 (0.483, 0.697)	<0.001	0.607 (0.500, 0.713)	<0.001	0.609 (0.502, 0.717)	<0.001	0.607 (0.488, 0.725)	<0.001
3,7-dimethylxanthine (theobromine)	0.368 (0.256, 0.479)	<0.001	0.398 (0.287, 0.509)	<0.001	0.386 (0.275, 0.498)	<0.001	0.347 (0.235, 0.459)	<0.001
1,3,7-trimethylxanthine (caffeine)	1.091 (0.855, 1.327)	<0.001	1.177 (0.942, 1.413)	<0.001	1.186 (0.950, 1.422)	<0.001	1.097 (0.845, 1.348)	<0.001
5-acetylamino-6-amino-3-methyluracil	0.061 (0.025, 0.097)	0.001	0.064 (0.028, 0.100)	0.001	0.065 (0.029, 0.102)	<0.001	0.029 (−0.014, 0.073)	0.188

Model 1 = unadjusted. Model 2 = Model 1 + age, gender, and race/ethnicity. Model 3 = Model 2 + BMI, serum fasting glucose, aspartate aminotransferase (AST), and urine creatinine. Model 4 = Model 3 + congestive heart failure, coronary heart disease, angina, heart attack, smoking, caffeine intake, and water intake. CI, confidence interval.

Table 3. Association between urinary caffeine metabolites and urine flow rate as categorized by gender.

Variables		Male				Female			
		Model 1	Model 2	Model 3	Model 4	Model 1	Model 2	Model 3	Model 4
1-methyluric acid	β (95% CI)	0.094 (0.046, 0.142)	0.099 (0.050, 0.148)	0.110 (0.061, 0.159)	0.089 (0.028, 0.149)	0.051 (−0.006, 0.108)	0.050 (−0.007, 0.108)	0.053 (−0.006, 0.111)	0.026 (−0.039, 0.091)
	p value	<0.001	<0.001	<0.001	0.004	0.078	0.087	0.078	0.436
3-methyluric acid	β (95% CI)	2.721 (−0.861, 6.303)	2.878 (−0.771, 6.526)	3.305 (−0.353, 6.962)	2.007 (−1.785, 5.798)	1.262 (−3.159, 5.683)	1.089 (−3.441, 5.620)	1.492 (−3.083, 6.067)	−0.043 (−4.770, 4.685)
	p value	0.136	0.122	0.077	0.299	0.575	0.637	0.522	0.986
7-methyluric acid	β (95% CI)	0.203 (−0.005, 0.412)	0.214 (0.002, 0.426)	0.231 (0.020, 0.443)	0.130 (−0.094, 0.354)	0.052 (−0.147, 0.252)	0.045 (−0.158, 0.249)	0.043 (−0.160, 0.246)	−0.024 (−0.236, 0.187)
	p value	0.056	0.048	0.032	0.256	0.607	0.661	0.677	0.823
1,3-dimethyluric acid	β (95% CI)	0.012 (−0.145, 0.170)	0.013 (−0.145, 0.171)	0.021 (−0.136, 0.179)	0.015 (−0.173, 0.142)	0.433 (−0.175, 1.042)	0.428 (−0.195, 1.052)	0.468 (−0.160, 1.096)	0.039 (−0.679, 0.758)
	p value	0.876	0.869	0.789	0.847	0.163	0.178	0.144	0.915
1,7-dimethyluric acid	β (95% CI)	0.254 (0.129, 0.378)	0.271 (0.143, 0.400)	0.281 (0.153, 0.409)	0.205 (0.051, 0.359)	0.032 (−0.100, 0.163)	0.027 (−0.108, 0.162)	0.032 (−0.103, 0.167)	−0.061 (−0.212, 0.091)
	p value	<0.001	<0.001	<0.001	0.009	0.637	0.695	0.644	0.433
3,7-dimethyluric acid	β (95% CI)	3.537 (0.185, 6.889)	3.551 (0.192, 6.910)	3.487 (0.139, 6.836)	2.580 (−0.812, 5.973)	2.357 (−0.829, 5.542)	2.377 (−0.814, 5.568)	2.123 (−1.061, 5.308)	1.214 (−2.026, 4.453)
	p value	0.039	0.038	0.041	0.136	0.147	0.144	0.191	0.462
1,3,7-trimethyluric acid	β (95% CI)	3.807 (1.895, 5.720)	4.005 (2.046, 5.965)	4.325 (2.365, 6.284)	3.194 (0.958, 5.431)	1.367 (−0.496, 3.229)	1.340 (−0.542, 3.222)	1.439 (−0.445, 3.323)	0.431 (−1.559, 2.482)
	p value	<0.001	<0.001	<0.001	0.005	0.150	0.162	0.134	0.654
1-methylxanthine	β (95% CI)	0.218 (0.133, 0.303)	0.221 (0.135, 0.306)	0.223 (0.137, 0.309)	0.190 (0.088, 0.292)	0.125 (0.030, 0.221)	0.125 (0.029, 0.221)	0.119 (0.022, 0.217)	0.088 (−0.018, 0.194)
	p value	<0.001	<0.001	<0.001	<0.001	0.010	0.011	0.017	0.103
3-methylxanthine	β (95% CI)	0.169 (0.048, 0.290)	0.173 (0.051, 0.295)	0.170 (0.051, 0.295)	0.123 (−0.002, 0.249)	0.093 (−0.026, 0.213)	0.092 (−0.029, 0.212)	0.081 (−0.040, 0.202)	0.042 (−0.082, 0.167)
	p value	0.006	0.006	0.007	0.054	0.126	0.135	0.191	0.503

Table 3. Cont.

Variables		Male				Female			
		Model 1	Model 2	Model 3	Model 4	Model 1	Model 2	Model 3	Model 4
7-methylxanthine	β (95% CI)	0.129 (0.052,0.205)	0.129 (0.052,0.206)	0.129 (0.052,0.207)	0.101 (0.021,0.182)	0.068 (0.000,0.137)	0.069 (0.000,0.137)	0.060 (−0.009,0.130)	0.043 (−0.029,0.115)
	p value	0.001	0.001	0.001	0.013	0.050	0.050	0.088	0.238
1,3-dimethylxanthine (theophylline)	β (95% CI)	0.515 (−0.072,1.101)	0.519 (−0.070,1.109)	0.530 (−0.057,1.118)	0.403 (−0.182,0.988)	5.657 (3.490,7.373)	5.696 (3.967,7.425)	5.681 (3.922,7.440)	5.309 (3.376,7.242)
	p value	0.085	0.084	0.077	0.177	<0.001	<0.001	<0.001	<0.001
1,7-dimethylxanthine (paraxanthine)	β (95% CI)	0.596 (0.460,0.732)	0.607 (0.470,0.744)	0.602 (0.465,0.740)	0.607 (0.453, 0.760)	0.609 (0.446,0.773)	0.609 (0.445,0.774)	0.610 (0.442,0.777)	0.605 (0.421,0.789)
	p value	<0.001	<0.001	<0.001	<0.001	<0.001	<0.001	<0.001	<0.001
3,7-dimethylxanthine (theobromine)	β (95% CI)	0.436 (0.279,0.593)	0.439 (0.282,0.597)	0.425 (0.267,0.583)	0.409 (0.249,0.568)	0.370 (0.213,0.527)	0.371 (0.214,0.529)	0.356 (0.198,0.514)	0.308 (0.147,0.468)
	p value	<0.001	<0.001	<0.001	<0.001	<0.001	<0.001	<0.001	<0.001
1,3,7-trimethylxanthine (caffeine)	β (95% CI)	1.496 (1.136,1.856)	1.526 (1.163,1.890)	1.514 (1.152,1.876)	1.429 (1.033,1.826)	0.983 (0.670,1.297)	0.989 (0.672,1.306)	0.988 (0.670,1.307)	0.890 (0.552,1.227)
	p value	<0.001	<0.001	<0.001	<0.001	<0.001	<0.001	<0.001	<0.001
5-acetylamino-6-amino-3-methyluracil	β (95% CI)	0.094 (0.051,0.138)	0.098 (0.054,0.143)	0.097 (0.052,0.141)	0.074 (0.019,0.129)	0.023 (−0.034,0.080)	0.022 (−0.037,0.080)	0.023 (−0.037,0.082)	−0.025 (−0.095,0.044)
	p value	<0.001	<0.001	<0.001	0.008	0.429	0.468	0.454	0.472

Model 1 = unadjusted. Model 2 = Model 1 + age, gender, and race/ethnicity. Model 3 = Model 2 + BMI, serum fasting glucose, aspartate aminotransferase (AST), and urine creatinine. Model 4 = Model 3 + congestive heart failure, coronary heart disease, angina, heart attack, smoking, caffeine intake, and water intake.

Table 4. Association between urinary caffeine metabolites and urine flow rate as categorized by age.

Variables		Age <60				Age ≥ 60			
		Model 1	Model 2	Model 3	Model 4	Model 1	Model 2	Model 3	Model 4
1-methyluric acid	β(95% CI)	0.102 (0.0538, 0.146)	0.098 (0.053, 0.142)	0.103 (0.058, 0.148)	0.076 (0.025, 0.127)	0.004 (−0.068, 0.075)	0.001 (−0.070, 0.072)	0.006 (−0.066, 0.079)	−0.003 (−0.126, 0.060)
	p value	<0.001	<0.001	<0.001	0.004	0.920	0.987	0.861	0.483
3-methyluric acid	β(95% CI)	3.936 (0.409, 7.462)	3.833 (0.299, 7.368)	4.190 (0.641, 7.740)	2.595 (−1.129, 6.318)	−2.656 (−7.598, 2.286)	−1.480 (−6.431, 3.471)	−1.003 (−6.017, 4.011)	−1.733 (−7.035, 3.569)
	p value	0.029	0.034	0.021	0.172	0.291	0.557	0.694	0.521
7-methyluric acid	β(95% CI)	0.212 (0.033, 0.391)	0.212 (0.033, 0.391)	0.214 (0.035, 0.394)	0.130 (−0.057, 0.011)	−0.134 (−0.384, 0.115)	−0.063 (−0.313, 0.187)	−0.065 (−0.315, 0.185)	−0.156 (−0.423, 0.112)
	p value	0.021	0.021	0.019	0.172	0.290	0.619	0.609	0.253
1,3-dimethyluric acid	β(95% CI)	0.912 (0.428, 1.395)	0.894 (0.401, 1.387)	0.943 (0.447, 1.438)	0.546 (−0.022, 1.114)	−0.056 (−0.233, 0.121)	−0.080 (−0.256, 0.095)	−0.086 (−0.261, 0.089)	−0.100 (−0.276, 0.077)
	p value	<0.001	0.001	<0.001	0.059	0.536	0.369	0.333	0.268
1,7-dimethyluric acid	β(95% CI)	0.220 (0.104, 0.337)	0.224 (0.105, 0.344)	0.229 (0.110, 0.349)	0.132 (−0.003, 0.267)	−0.056 (−0.206, 0.095)	−0.045 (−0.196, 0.106)	−0.044 (−0.196, 0.109)	−0.124 (−0.305, 0.057)
	p value	<0.001	<0.001	<0.001	0.056	0.466	0.554	0.572	0.179
3,7-dimethyluric acid	β(95% CI)	2.883 (0.280, 5.485)	3.333 (0.754, 5.912)	3.317 (0.736, 5.897)	2.314 (−0.299, 4.926)	−0.044 (−5.104, 5.015)	−0.319 (−4.697, 5.335)	−0.350 (−5.344, 4.644)	−1.263 (−6.403, 3.877)
	p value	0.030	0.011	0.012	0.083	0.986	0.900	0.890	0.629
1,3,7-trimethyluric acid	β(95% CI)	2.977 (1.365, 4.589)	3.220 (1.587, 4.853)	3.366 (1.729, 5.002)	2.180 (0.420, 3.939)	−0.146 (−2.565, 2.273)	−0.058 (−2.482, 2.366)	0.294 (−2.149, 2.737)	−0.487 (−3.270, 2.297)
	p value	<0.001	<0.001	<0.001	0.015	0.906	0.962	0.813	0.731
1-methylxanthine	β(95% CI)	0.164 (0.094, 0.233)	0.160 (0.090, 0.229)	0.164 (0.093, 0.235)	0.122 (0.043, 0.201)	0.162 (−0.012, 0.337)	0.144 (−0.030, 0.317)	0.108 (−0.069, 0.285)	0.068 (−0.146, 0.283)
	p value	<0.001	<0.001	<0.001	0.002	0.068	0.105	0.232	0.531
3-methylxanthine	β(95% CI)	0.142 (0.039, 0.244)	0.159 (0.056, 0.262)	0.159 (0.056, 0.263)	0.105 (−0.001, 0.0211)	0.009 (−0.146, 0.164)	0.036 (−0.118, 0.191)	0.004 (−0.151, 0.159)	−0.015 (−0.175, 0.145)
	p value	0.007	0.002	0.003	0.051	0.908	0.643	0.957	0.855

Table 4. Cont.

Variables		Age <60				Age ≥ 60			
		Model 1	Model 2	Model 3	Model 4	Model 1	Model 2	Model 3	Model 4
7-methylxanthine	β(95% CI)	0.086 (0.029,0.143)	0.094 (0.038,0.150)	0.093 (0.036,0.150)	0.068 (0.010,0.127)	0.054 (−0.062,0.170)	0.066 (−0.049,0.181)	0.035 (−0.081,0.152)	0.013 (−0.110,0.135)
	p value	0.003	0.001	0.001	0.022	0.361	0.258	0.549	0.839
1,3-dimethylxanthine (theophylline)	β(95% CI)	5.900 (4.433,7.367)	6.267 (4.792,7.742)	6.401 (4.911,7.891)	5.823 (4.204,7.442)	0.283 (−0.378,0.943)	0.185 (−0.470,0.841)	0.110 (−0.544,0.764)	0.059 (−0.602,0.721)
	p value	<0.001	<0.001	<0.001	<0.001	0.401	0.578	0.741	0.860
1,7-dimethylxanthine (paraxanthine)	β(95% CI)	0.618 (0.487,0.749)	0.627 (0.496,0.759)	0.640 (0.508,0.773)	0.613 (0.469,0.757)	0.536 (0.349,0.724)	0.513 (0.326,0.700)	0.479 (0.287,0.671)	0.532 (0.314,0.750)
	p value	<0.001	<0.001	<0.001	<0.001	<0.001	<0.001	<0.001	<0.001
3,7-dimethylxanthine (theobromine)	β(95% CI)	0.376 (0.245,0.507)	0.407 (0.278,0.537)	0.405 (0.275,0.536)	0.358 (0.227,0.488)	0.340 (0.123,0.557)	0.344 (0.130,0.559)	0.289 (0.071,0.507)	0.260 (0.036,0.484)
	p value	<0.001	<0.001	<0.001	<0.001	0.002	0.002	0.009	0.023
1,3,7-trimethylxanthine (caffeine)	β(95% CI)	1.319 (1.020,1.618)	1.377 (1.078,1.676)	1.398 (1.097,1.698)	1.265 (0.948,1.582)	0.763 (0.374,1.152)	0.791 (0.405,1.176)	0.749 (0.361,1.137)	0.762 (0.338,1.186)
	p value	<0.001	<0.001	<0.001	<0.001	<0.001	<0.001	<0.001	<0.001
5-acetylamino-6-amino-3-methyluracil	β(95% CI)	0.094 (0.048,0.141)	0.088 (0.040,0.135)	0.088 (0.040,0.136)	0.045 (−0.001,0.102)	0.020 (−0.037,0.077)	0.018 (−0.039,0.074)	0.016 (−0.041,0.072)	−0.002 (−0.073,0.068)
	p value	<0.001	<0.001	<0.001	0.117	0.486	0.539	0.591	0.946

Model 1 = unadjusted. Model 2 = Model 1 + age, gender, and race/ethnicity. Model 3 = Model 2 + BMI, serum fasting glucose, aspartate aminotransferase (AST), and urine creatinine. Model 4 = Model 3 + congestive heart failure, coronary heart disease, angina, heart attack, smoking, caffeine intake, and water intake.

Table 3 shows the results for male and female subgroups, respectively. In the male subgroup, caffeine and 14 of its metabolites revealed positive correlations with urine flow rate, in contrast with the female subgroup, with a number of 5. Among them, 1-methyluric acid, 7-methyluric acid, 1,7-dimethyluric acid, 3,7-dimethyluric acid, 1,3,7-trimethyluric acid, 3-methylxanthine, 7-methylxanthine, and 5-acetylamino-6-amino-3-methyluracil presented significance in males but not females. 1,3-Dimethylxanthine (theophylline) was the only one showing a positive correlation in females but marginal significance in males (p-value = 0.067 in males, p-value < 0.001 in females).

Table 4 shows the results in participants aged under and over 60 years old, respectively, referring to the cutoff point of the elderly population agreed on by the United Nations [20]. In the subgroup of age <60 years old, caffeine and 14 of its metabolites all revealed positive correlations. On the contrary, in the elderly subgroup ≥ 60 years old, the number of metabolites presenting significant correlations shrank to 3, namely, paraxanthine (p-value <0.001), theobromine (p-value = 0.011), and caffeine (p-value <0.001).

4. Discussion

In the US population, we found that urine levels of caffeine metabolites were positively associated with urine flow rate. Furthermore, there are more caffeine metabolites showing a flow-dependency in males than females and more in younger participants than older ones. Notably, caffeine and two of its metabolites, paraxanthine and theobromine, revealed significance across all subgroups. They were the main primary metabolites of caffeine, with paraxanthine composing 84% and theobromine composing 12% [18]. Other metabolites were formed by successive demethylations and hydroxylations. The large proportion of caffeine metabolites being flow-dependent across subgroups proves that urine flow rate is a nonnegligible influencing factor in caffeine excretion.

Previous literature discussing caffeine metabolites and urine flow rate focused more on theophylline, which not only belongs to the same methylxanthine family as caffeine but is itself also one of the main urinary metabolites [16,17,21–25]. Previous studies have mentioned the renal clearance of theophylline being highly dependent on urine flow rate [16,17,21–23]. Some pharmacologists have developed a mathematical model that explains the dependence of renal clearance on urine flow rate in drugs such as theophylline, ethanol, and butabarbital [24,25]. Being siblings in the same methylxanthine family, with similar metabolic pathways, caffeine and 14 of its metabolites presenting flow-dependency in our study is plausible.

Other studies focusing directly on caffeine were of limited sample size and did not mention comparisons among gender and age, two unneglectable factors that determine urine flow rate. One early study observed a positive association in 10 elderly men [26], while another proposed a positive relationship in 16 volunteers [27]. Several reports mentioned different flow-dependency of caffeine metabolite ratios (MRs) contributing to different roles in the assessment of cytochrome P450 1A2 (CYP1A2) activity [28,29]. These studies revealed evident results but lacked further comparisons in the subgroups. Our study was composed of 1410 participants from a representative sample, providing highly robust evidence with a much bigger number of participants, and made comparisons in subgroups to investigate whether different tendencies existed.

In the present study, we observed differences in the number of caffeine metabolites showing a relationship with urine flow rate. Males outnumbered females, and younger participants outnumbered older ones. We surveyed the factors affecting caffeine metabolism and urine flow rate and found possible reasons for this difference. The rate of caffeine metabolism primarily depends on the genetic variability of enzymes dominating caffeine breakdown, smoking status, alcohol intake, specific medications, liver diseases, and pregnancy [30–32]. CYP1A2, the main enzyme metabolizing caffeine, is known to show higher activity in men [33]. In contrast, female hormones decrease CYP1A2 activity during pregnancy and with oral contraceptive use [34]. Furthermore, studies have described that males show a significant decline in urinary flow rate with age, whereas females show less variation in urine flow rate with respect to age [35]. In sum, a slower rate of caffeine metabolism and a more constant feature of urine flow rate in females may explain the observation of less metabolites being flow-dependent in this group. In addition, the urine flow rate declines with age due to various reasons aside from the one that was already excluded in our study, benign prostate hyperplasia. Prolapsed bladder after vaginal childbirth and menopause in females are also factors that may influence urine flow rate [35]. In the elderly group, increased factors affecting the urine flow rate may perturb and weaken the flow-dependency of metabolites.

The potential mechanism that links urinary caffeine metabolites and the urine flow rate together might contribute to the physiological interplay in the kidneys. Tang-Liu et al. established a model that explained drugs with a dependence of renal clearance on urine flow rate [24]. Theophylline and caffeine fall into the category of those that are reabsorbed in the renal tubule, but the diffusional rate is less than that of water. This results in a disequilibrium state that causes the renal clearance of these drugs to be dependent on urine flow rates. Other drugs that showed no flow-dependency were either not reabsorbed at all or their diffusional rate was equal to or greater than that of water. In another study, the rate–concentration curve of theophylline was depicted to be convex-ascending but not linear. The clearance of drugs increases markedly with urine flow up to a certain degree and, thereafter, increases only slightly [18].

The clinical application of assessing caffeine and its metabolites in urine is multifaceted. Medical research fields extend physiology, psychology, and pharmacology. The finding in our study illustrates the necessity of controlling urine flow rates in studies relevant to caffeine, especially when subjects are male and with younger participants. Restriction of fluid intake, salt intake, avoidance of diuretic foods, and adjustment of renal function are reasonable means to approach more adequate assessment. Moreover, other practice could be inferred from this observation. Increasing urine flow rate can act as a means of detoxifying in caffeine-overdosed patients. Those who wish to stay awake by caffeine may consider avoiding factors that speed up their urine flow rate. These practices require further studies to validate their effectiveness. However, they are worth a try according to the flow-dependent feature demonstrated in this study.

Several limitations of this study should be mentioned. Firstly, NHANES is a cross-sectional study in which urinary caffeine metabolites and urine flow rate were examined at one particular time point rather than continuously collected for a long period of time. The causal relationship could not be established due to possible biased results by single measurement. Secondly, we put more emphasis on the dataset from NHANES 2011–2012 but less on NHANES 2009–2010, which was another cycle that collected urinary caffeine metabolite data. The official website mentioned the different instruments used in the two cycles, which may cause analytical bias due to the earlier one requiring the specimens to be analyzed twice. Even so, the results of 2009–2010 of 1853 participants in Table A1 still revealed a similar trend of flow-dependency, only that the amount of metabolites is not the same. Thirdly, we measured the average urine flow rate rather than the peak urine flow rate. Combining both certainly offers a more comprehensive view of urodynamic studies, but peak flow rate requires more complicated calculations with uroflowmetry. Previous comparable studies have utilized the average urine flow rate, as shown in Table 5 [17,21–23,25–29], and thus we followed their practice.

Table 5. Summary of the literature review findings on the association between urinary caffeine metabolites and urine flow rate.

Study Details	Study Design	Participants	Caffeine Metabolites	Evaluation of Urine Flow Rate	Findings on Urinary Caffeine Metabolites and Urine Flow Rate
			Caffeine		
Our study	cross-sectional study	N = 1410	Caffeine and 14 of its metabolites	Average flow rate	Positive correlations were shown between several urinary metabolites and urine flow rate. Men showed more correlation than females, and the young (age < 60) showed more correlation than the elderly (age > 60).
Blanchard, J. et al. (1983), Scotland [25]	cross-sectional study	N = 16	Caffeine	Average flow rate	Positive correlation between the renal clearance of both unbound (CLU) and total (CLR) caffeine and the mean urine flow rate.
Trang, J.M. et al. (1985), USA [24]	cross-sectional study	N = 10	Caffeine	Average flow rate	Positive correlations were observed between total body clearance (CL), renal clearance (CL), and nonrenal clearance (CL) and urine flow rate (UFR)
Sinués, B. et al. (1999), Spain [26]	cross-sectional study	N = 125	5 urinary caffeine metabolite ratios (MRs)	Average flow rate	MR1, MR3, and MR4 were the most flow-dependent. MR2 was flow-independent. MR5 was less flow-dependent.
Sinués, B. et al. (2002), Spain [27]	cross-sectional study	N = 152	8 caffeine metabolites and 5 urinary caffeine metabolite ratios (MRs)	Average flow rate	7 caffeine metabolites were flow-dependent. MR1, MR3, and MR4 were flow-dependent. MR2 and MR5 were flow-independent.
			Theophylline		
Our study	cross-sectional study	N = 1410	Theophylline	Average flow rate	Positive correlations were shown between theophylline and urine flow rate in the female subgroup and the young (age <60) subgroup.
Gerhard Levy. et al. (1976), USA [17]	cross-sectional study	N = 6	Theophylline	Average flow rate	Positive correlation was shown between the renal clearance of theophylline and the urine flow rate.
Tang-Liu, D.D.S. et al. (1982), USA [23]	cross-sectional study	N = 14	Theophylline	Average flow rate	Theophylline renal clearance is highly dependent on urine flow rate and is neither concentration- nor dose-related.
St-Pierre, M.V. et al. (1985), USA [19]	cross-sectional study	N = 8	Theophylline and 3 of its major metabolites	Average flow rate	Renal clearance of metabolites was greater after morning dosing, the time with enhanced urine flow rate.
Bonnacker, I. et al. (1989), Germany [20]	cross-sectional study	N = 10	Theophylline and 3 of its metabolites	Average flow rate	The renal clearance of 1,3-DMU, the main metabolite of theophylline, was found to depend both upon urine flow rate and age.
Agbaba, D. et al., (1990), Yugoslavia [21]	cross-sectional study	N = 22	Theophylline	Average flow rate	The dependence of the renal excretion of theophylline on urine flow rate was found after both IV administration and at steady state.

5. Conclusions

A positive association exists between several urinary caffeine metabolites and urine flow rate. The number of metabolites showing certain flow-dependency is higher in males than females and also higher in young participants compared to elderly participants. Further studies are necessary to elucidate the mechanisms underlying the flow-dependency appearance of caffeine metabolites in urine. Our study highlights the importance of considering the urine flow rate as an influencing factor in interpretations of urinary data regarding caffeine.

Author Contributions: Conceptualization, S.E.W. and W.-L.C.; methodology, W.-L.C.; software, W.-L.C.; validation, S.E.W. and W.-L.C.; formal analysis, S.E.W. and W.-L.C.; investigation, S.E.W. and W.-L.C.; resources, W.-L.C.; data curation, S.E.W. and W.-L.C.; writing—original draft preparation, S.E.W.; writing—review and editing, S.E.W. and W.-L.C.; visualization, S.E.W. and W.-L.C.; supervision, W.-L.C. All authors have read and agreed to the published version of the manuscript.

Funding: This research received no external funding.

Conflicts of Interest: The authors declare no conflict of interest.

Appendix A

Table A1. Association between urinary caffeine metabolites and urine flow rate in NHANES 2009–2010.

Variables	Model 1 β(95% CI)	p Value	Model 2 β(95% CI)	p Value	Model 3 β(95% CI)	p Value	Model 4 β(95% CI)	p Value
1-methyluric acid	0.041 (0.011, 0.070)	0.008	0.049 (0.019, 0.079)	0.001	0.050 (0.020, 0.080)	0.001	0.032 (−0.003, 0.066)	0.072
3-methyluric acid	−1.087 (−3.174, 1.000)	0.307	0.096 (−2.045, 2.236)	0.930	0.826 (−0.244, 3.027)	0.073	1.281 (−1.698, 2.282)	0.399
7-methyluric acid	−0.002 (−0.112, 0.228)	0.968	0.061 (−0.052, 0.260)	0.287	0.072 (−0.042, 0.271)	0.215	0.025 (−2.157, 0.192)	0.670
1,3-dimethyluric acid	0.006 (−0.064, 0.065)	0.851	0.015 (−0.045, 0.074)	0.626	0.014 (−0.046, 0.073)	0.630	0.008 (−0.051, 0.067)	0.783
1,7-dimethyluric acid	0.097 (0.025, 0.169)	0.008	0.136 (0.064, 0.209)	<0.001	0.137 (0.064, 0.209)	<0.001	0.088 (0.008, 0.167)	0.031
3,7-dimethyluric acid	0.561 (−1.314, 2.435)	0.557	1.367 (−0.515, 3.249)	0.154	1.323 (−0.561, 3.207)	0.169	0.714 (−1.191, 2.618)	0.462
1,3,7-trimethyluric acid	2.345 (1.405, 3.285)	<0.001	2.759 (1.819, 3.698)	<0.001	2.770 (1.832, 3.709)	<0.001	2.373 (1.383, 3.363)	<0.001
1-methylxanthine	0.124 (0.067, 0.180)	<0.001	0.131 (0.075, 0.187)	<0.001	0.127 (0.071, 0.184)	<0.001	0.101 (0.037, 0.166)	0.002
3-methylxanthine	0.022 (−0.043, 0.090)	0.526	0.064 (−0.005, 0.132)	0.071	0.063 (−0.006, 0.132)	0.073	0.038 (−0.016, 0.108)	0.280
7-methylxanthine	0.037 (−0.010, 0.083)	0.125	0.052 (0.006, 0.099)	0.028	0.050 (0.003, 0.097)	0.037	0.032 (0.010, 0.081)	0.189

Table A1. Cont.

Variables	Model 1 β(95% CI)	p Value	Model 2 β(95% CI)	p Value	Model 3 β(95% CI)	p Value	Model 4 β(95% CI)	p Value
1,3-dimethylxanthine (theophylline)	0.897 (0.494, 1.300)	<0.001	1.004 (0.604, 1.405)	<0.001	0.986 (0.586, 1.387)	<0.001	0.896 (0.496, 1.296)	0.002
1,7-dimethylxanthine (paraxanthine)	0.538 (0.446, 0.631)	<0.001	0.565 (0.473, 0.656)	<0.001	0.558 (0.466, 0.650)	<0.001	0.552 (0.454, 0.650)	<0.001
3,7-dimethylxanthine (theobromine)	0.358 (0.271, 0.445)	<0.001	0.409 (0.323, 0.496)	<0.001	0.403 (0.316, 0.490)	<0.001	0.382 (0.295, 0.469)	<0.001
1,3,7-trimethylxanthine (caffeine)	1.079 (0.910, 1.248)	<0.001	1.153 (0.985, 1.321)	<0.001	1.153 (0.985, 1.321)	<0.001	1.097 (0.924, 1.270)	<0.001
5-acetylamino-6-amino-3-methyluracil	0.036 (0.003, 0.068)	0.031	0.046 (0.013, 0.078)	0.006	0.045 (0.013, 0.078)	0.006	0.024 (−0.014, 0.061)	0.213

Model 1 = unadjusted. Model 2 = Model 1 + age, gender, and race/ethnicity. Model 3 = Model 2 + BMI, serum fasting glucose, aspartate aminotransferase (AST), and urine creatinine. Model 4 = Model 3 + congestive heart failure, coronary heart disease, angina, heart attack, smoking, caffeine intake, and water intake.

References

1. Nehlig, A.; Daval, J.L.; Debry, G. Caffeine and the central nervous system: Mechanisms of action, biochemical, metabolic and psychostimulant effects. *Brain Res. Brain Res. Rev.* **1992**, *17*, 139–170. [CrossRef]
2. Sattin, A.; Rall, T.W. The effect of adenosine and adenine nucleotides on the cyclic adenosine 3′, 5′-phosphate content of guinea pig cerebral cortex slices. *Mol. Pharmacol.* **1970**, *6*, 13–23.
3. Huang, Z.-L.; Qu, W.-M.; Eguchi, N.; Chen, J.-F.; Schwarzschild, M.A.; Fredholm, B.B.; Urade, Y.; Hayaishi, O. Adenosine A 2A, but not A 1, receptors mediate the arousal effect of caffeine. *Nat. Neurosci.* **2005**, *8*, 858–859. [CrossRef]
4. Shi, D.; Nikodijević, O.; Jacobson, K.A.; Daly, J.W. Chronic caffeine alters the density of adenosine, adrenergic, cholinergic, GABA, and serotonin receptors and calcium channels in mouse brain. *Cell. Mol. Neurobiol.* **1993**, *13*, 247–261. [CrossRef] [PubMed]
5. Nawrot, P.; Jordan, S.; Eastwood, J.; Rotstein, J.; Hugenholtz, A.; Feeley, M. Effects of caffeine on human health. *Food Addiv. Contam.* **2003**, *20*, 1–30. [CrossRef] [PubMed]
6. Pelchovitz, D.J.; Goldberger, J.J. Caffeine and cardiac arrhythmias: A review of the evidence. *Am. J. Med.* **2011**, *124*, 284–289. [CrossRef] [PubMed]
7. Rieg, T.; Steigele, H.; Schnermann, J.; Richter, K.; Osswald, H.; Vallon, V. Requirement of intact adenosine A1 receptors for the diuretic and natriuretic action of the methylxanthines theophylline and caffeine. *J. Pharmacol. Exp. Ther.* **2005**, *313*, 403–409. [CrossRef] [PubMed]
8. Ogawa, N.; Ueki, H.J.P.; Neurosciences, C. Clinical importance of caffeine dependence and abuse. *Psychiatry Clin. Neurosci.* **2007**, *61*, 263–268. [CrossRef]
9. Roehrs, T.; Roth, T. Caffeine: Sleep and daytime sleepiness. *Sleep Med. Rev.* **2008**, *12*, 153–162. [CrossRef]
10. Angelucci, M.E.; Vital, M.A.; Cesário, C.; Zadusky, C.R.; Rosalen, P.L.; Da Cunha, C. The effect of caffeine in animal models of learning and memory. *Eur. J. Pharmacol.* **1999**, *373*, 135–140. [CrossRef]
11. Kalow, W.; Tang, B.K. Use of caffeine metabolite ratios to explore CYP1A2 and xanthine oxidase activities. *Clin. Pharmacol. Ther.* **1991**, *50*, 508–519. [CrossRef] [PubMed]
12. Butler, M.; Lang, N.; Young, J.; Caporaso, N.; Vineis, P.; Hayes, R.; Teitel, C.; Massengill, J.; Lawsen, M.; Kadlubar, F.J.P. Determination of CYP1A2 and NAT2 phenotypes in human populations by analysis of caffeine urinary metabolites. *Pharmacogenetics* **1992**, *2*, 116–127. [CrossRef] [PubMed]

13. Fujimaki, M.; Saiki, S.; Li, Y.; Kaga, N.; Taka, H.; Hatano, T.; Ishikawa, K.-I.; Oji, Y.; Mori, A.; Okuzumi, A.J.N. Serum caffeine and metabolites are reliable biomarkers of early Parkinson disease. *Neurology* **2018**, *90*, e404–e411. [CrossRef] [PubMed]
14. Benowitz, N.L. Clinical pharmacology of caffeine. *Ann. Rev. Med.* **1990**, *41*, 277–288. [CrossRef] [PubMed]
15. Faber, M.S.; Jetter, A.; Fuhr, U. Assessment of CYP1A2 activity in clinical practice: Why, how, and when? *Basic Clin. Pharmacol. Toxicol.* **2005**, *97*, 125–134. [CrossRef]
16. Birkett, D.; Dahlqvist, R.; Miners, J.; Lelo, A.; Billing, B. Comparison of theophylline and theobromine metabolism in man. *Drug Metab. Dispos.* **1985**, *13*, 725–728.
17. Levy, G.; Koysooko, R. Renal clearance of theophylline in man. *J. Clin. Pharmacol.* **1976**, *16*, 329–332. [CrossRef]
18. Tang-Liu, D.; Williams, R.; Riegelman, S. Disposition of caffeine and its metabolites in man. *J. Pharmacol. Exp. Ther.* **1983**, *224*, 180–185.
19. Roebuck, J. When does old age begin?: The evolution of the English definition. *J. Soc. Hist.* **1979**, *12*, 416–428. [CrossRef]
20. United Nations. *Department of Economic*; Affairs, S. World Population Ageing, 1950-2050; United Nations Publications: New York, NY, USA, 2002.
21. St-Pierre, M.V.; Spino, M.; Isles, A.F.; Tesoro, A.; MacLeod, S.M. Temporal variation in the disposition of theophylline and its metabolites. *Clin. Pharmacol. Ther.* **1985**, *38*, 89–95. [CrossRef]
22. Bonnacker, I.; Berdel, D.; Süverkrüp, R.; Berg, A.V. Renal clearance of theophylline and its major metabolites: Age and urine flow dependency in paediatric patients. *Eur. J. Clin. Pharmacol.* **1989**, *36*, 145–150. [CrossRef]
23. Agbaba, D.; Pokrajac, M.; Varagić, V.M.; Pešić, V. Dependence of the renal excretion of theophylline on its plasma concentrations and urine flow rate in asthmatic children. *J. Pharm. Pharmacol.* **1990**, *42*, 827–830. [CrossRef] [PubMed]
24. Tang-Liu, D.D.-S.; Tozer, T.N.; Riegelman, S. Dependence of renal clearance on urine flow: A mathematical model and its application. *J. Pharm. Sci.* **1983**, *72*, 154–158. [CrossRef]
25. Tang-Liu, D.D.-S.; Tozer, T.N.; Riegelman, S. Urine flow-dependence of theophylline renal clearance in man. *J. Pharmacokinet. Biopharm.* **1982**, *10*, 351–364. [CrossRef] [PubMed]
26. Trang, J.M.; Blanchard, J.; Conrad, K.A.; Harrison, G.G. Relationship between total body clearance of caffeine and urine flow rate in elderly men. *Biopharm. Drug Dispos.* **1985**, *6*, 51–56. [CrossRef]
27. Blanchard, J.; Sawers, S.J.A. Relationship between urine flow rate and renal clearance of caffeine in man. *J. Clin. Pharmacol.* **1983**, *23*, 134–138. [CrossRef]
28. Sinués, B.; Sáenz, M.A.; Lanuza, J.; Bernal, M.L.; Fanlo, A.; Juste, J.L.; Mayayo, E. Five caffeine metabolite ratios to measure tobacco-induced CYP1A2 activity and their relationships with urinary mutagenicity and urine flow. *Cancer Epidemiol. Prev. Biomark.* **1999**, *8*, 159–166.
29. Sinués, B.; Fanlo, A.; Bernal, M.L.; Mayayo, E.; Soriano, M.A.; Martínez-Ballarin, E. Influence of the urine flow rate on some caffeine metabolite ratios used to assess CYP1A2 activity. *Ther. Drug Monit.* **2002**, *24*, 715–721. [CrossRef]
30. Kalow, W.; Tang, B.K. Caffeine as a metabolic probe: Exploration of the enzyme-inducing effect of cigarette smoking. *Clin. Pharmacol. Ther.* **1991**, *49*, 44–48. [CrossRef]
31. George, J.; Murphy, T.; Roberts, R.; Cooksley, W.G.; Halliday, J.W.; Powell, L.W. Influence of alcohol and caffeine consumption on caffeine elimination. *Clin. Exp. Pharmacol. Physiol.* **1986**, *13*, 731–736. [CrossRef]
32. Carrillo, J.A.; Benitez, J. Clinically significant pharmacokinetic interactions between dietary caffeine and medications. *Clin. Pharmacokinet.* **2000**, *39*, 127–153. [CrossRef] [PubMed]
33. Relling, M.V.; Lin, J.S.; Ayers, G.D.; Evans, W.E. Racial and gender differences in N-acetyltransferase, xanthine oxidase, and CYP1A2 activities. *Clin. Pharmacol. Ther.* **1992**, *52*, 643–658. [CrossRef] [PubMed]
34. Tracy, T.S.; Venkataramanan, R.; Glover, D.D.; Caritis, S.N. Temporal changes in drug metabolism (CYP1A2, CYP2D6 and CYP3A Activity) during pregnancy. *Am. J. Obstet. Gynecol.* **2005**, *192*, 633–639. [CrossRef] [PubMed]
35. Haylen, B.T.; Ashby, D.; Sutherst, J.R.; Frazer, M.I.; West, C.R. Maximum and average urine flow rates in normal male and female populations–the Liverpool nomograms. *Br. J. Urol.* **1989**, *64*, 30–38. [CrossRef]

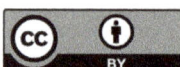

© 2020 by the authors. Licensee MDPI, Basel, Switzerland. This article is an open access article distributed under the terms and conditions of the Creative Commons Attribution (CC BY) license (http://creativecommons.org/licenses/by/4.0/).

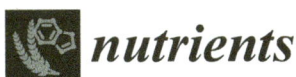

Article

Trait Energy and Fatigue Modify the Effects of Caffeine on Mood, Cognitive and Fine-Motor Task Performance: A Post-Hoc Study

Daniel T. Fuller [1], Matthew Lee Smith [2,3] and Ali Boolani [4,5,*]

1 Department of Mathematics, Clarkson University, Potsdam, NY 13699, USA; fullerdt@clarkson.edu
2 Center for Population Health and Aging, Texas A&M University, College Station, TX 77843, USA; matthew.smith@tamu.edu
3 Department of Environmental and Occupational Health, School of Public Health, Texas A&M University, College Station, TX 77843, USA
4 Department of Physical Therapy, Clarkson University, Potsdam, NY 13699, USA
5 Department of Biology, Clarkson University, Potsdam, NY 13699, USA
* Correspondence: aboolani@clarkson.edu

Abstract: Multiple studies suggest that genetic polymorphisms influence the neurocognitive effects of caffeine. Using data collected from a double-blinded, within-participants, randomized, crossover design, this study examined the effects of trait (long-standing pre-disposition) mental and physical energy and fatigue to changes in moods (Profile of Mood Survey-Short Form (POMS-SF), state mental and physical energy and fatigue survey), cognitive (serial subtractions of 3 (SS3) and 7 (SS7)), and fine-motor task (nine-hole peg test) performance after consuming a caffeinated beverage and a non-caffeinated placebo. Results indicate that trait mental and physical fatigue and mental energy modified the effects of caffeine on vigor, tension-anxiety, physical, and mental fatigue. Additionally, we report that those who were high trait physical and mental fatigue and low-trait mental energy reported the greatest benefit of caffeine on the SS3 and SS7, while those who were high trait mental and physical fatigue reported the greatest benefit of consuming caffeine on fine-motor task performance. The results of our study suggest that trait mental and physical fatigue and mental energy modify the acute effects of caffeine among a group of healthy, young adults and should be measured and controlled for by researchers who choose to study the effects of caffeine on acute moods and cognitive and fine-motor task performance.

Keywords: trait energy; trait fatigue; caffeine; moods; cognitive tasks; psychomotor tasks

Citation: Fuller, D.T; Smith, M.L.; Boolani, A. Trait Energy and Fatigue Modify the Effects of Caffeine on Mood, Cognitive and Fine-Motor Task Performance: A Post-Hoc Study. *Nutrients* **2021**, *13*, 412. https://doi.org/10.3390/nu13020412

Academic Editor: Raquel Abalo
Received: 14 December 2020
Accepted: 25 January 2021
Published: 28 January 2021

Publisher's Note: MDPI stays neutral with regard to jurisdictional claims in published maps and institutional affiliations.

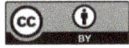

Copyright: © 2021 by the authors. Licensee MDPI, Basel, Switzerland. This article is an open access article distributed under the terms and conditions of the Creative Commons Attribution (CC BY) license (https://creativecommons.org/licenses/by/4.0/).

1. Introduction

Fatigue is a common, costly, and poorly understood problem, which affects approximately 45% of the United States (US) population [1]. It has been estimated that fatigue costs employers over $136 billion per year in lost productivity [2]; however, these estimates do not account for fatigue-related driving and other accidents [3,4], poor medical performance [5], and negative health outcome [6]. Fatigue is also underreported in medical care [7] and has been linked to many diseases and disorders [8]. Despite the high financial and social costs of fatigue, it is a poorly understood problem. For example, until recently, most researchers viewed energy and fatigue on a bipolar continuum (e.g., if an individual is not energetic, then they are fatigued). However, Loy and colleagues [9] recently provided evidence that energy and fatigue are two distinct moods (e.g., an individual can be energetic and fatigued simultaneously), with multiple studies since showing that feelings of energy and fatigue are distinct yet overlapping constructs [10–12], with their own mental and physical components [13,14]. Although we are aware of multiple interventions, such as exercise [15], caffeine [16,17], and sleep [18], that increase feelings of energy and/or decrease feelings of fatigue, evidence regarding the effectiveness of these interventions is mixed. Additional research is needed to better understand the inter- and intra-individual differences in the efficacy of these interventions.

One common acute intervention for feelings of low energy and high fatigue is caffeine [16,17]. Caffeine is consumed in various forms, with coffee and energy beverages being the most prevalent. However, to our knowledge, the release and absorption rates of caffeine from coffee and energy beverages is the same [19]. Multiple studies have reported that there are inter-individual differences in the influence of caffeine on moods [20–24]. These studies [20–24] have reported that ADORA2A gene polymorphism may be primarily responsible for the inter-individual variations in the effects of caffeine on anxiety [21,24] and physical fatigue [22,23]. While substantial evidence exists on the role of the ADORA2A gene in determining the ergogenic effects of caffeine [20–24], identifying gene mutation prior to administering caffeine as an ergogenic aid may be impractical for most nutrition researchers and practitioners. Therefore, finding low-cost validated methods to identify factors that influence the ergogenic effect of caffeine is pragmatic and desirable to both practitioners and researchers.

One such potential measure, is trait (long-standing pre-disposition) mental and physical energy and fatigue, a construct only recently reported in the literature [13,14]. While the authors of this study are aware of only one study that examines the effects of trait mental and physical energy and fatigue on moods [14], that study reports that trait mental and physical energy and fatigue moderates the effects of sleep on state energy and fatigue [14]. These findings raise an interesting question about whether trait mental and physical energy and fatigue may also modify the intensity or effects of other interventions (e.g., caffeine) on changes in self-reported mood and/or objective measures of mental energy during the performance of a common mental test battery [25–29] used in nutritional science research. Based on this premise, we re-examined data from a previously published study [28] that investigated whether an adaptogenic-rich caffeine-containing beverage would modulate the effects of caffeine on self-reported mood and objective measures of energy and fatigue.

Therefore, the aims of our current analyses were to determine whether trait mental and physical energy and fatigue influence the rate of change in (1) state moods, (2) cognitive task performance (objective mental energy measure), and (3) fine motor task performance, when participants perform a commonly used mental energy test battery [25–29] on days when they consumed caffeine compared to the days when they consumed placebo. To address these aims, we performed a post-hoc analysis of our previous study [28] limited to the days when participants consumed placebo and the active comparator (caffeinated) conditions only.

2. Methodology

2.1. Study Design and Study Products

A full description of the methodology has been previously published [28]. In our previous double-blinded, placebo-controlled, within-participants, randomized cross-over study, we examined the effects of three 60 mL interventions: (1) a placebo; (2) an active comparator (caffeine); and (3) e+™ shot (e+ shot, Isagenix International, LLC, Gilbert, AZ, USA). For the purposes of this study, we only examined the placebo and active comparator (caffeine). To ensure effective blinding in the main study, none of the scientists conducting the study or analyzing the data were aware of treatment assignments. All treatments were delivered in identical unmarked white containers with a black top. The placebo and caffeine beverages had the same base components as e+ shot (purified water, apple juice concentrate, glycerin, pomegranate juice concentrate, natural flavors, malic acid, potassium sorbate, and sodium citrate) to which either 0 mg (placebo) or approximately 98 mg synthetic caffeine (caffeine) were added. Quantitation of caffeine in the study products was verified according to Eurofins Scientific Inc. (Des Moines, IA, USA).

2.2. Screening and Participants

After receiving Clarkson University Institutional Review Board (IRB) approval (approval # 16-34.1), participants were recruited from 16 September 2015 to 9 August 2016 from a small private university and local community using in-class announcements, bulletin boards, electronic listservs, flyers at local businesses, and word of mouth. Potential participants were invited to complete a screening questionnaire administered online using SurveyMonkey Inc. (San Mateo, CA, USA).

The exclusion criteria were as follows: under the age of 18 or over the age of 45; self-reported body mass index (BMI) > 30; above-average feelings of energy on the Profile of Mood Survey- Short Form (POMS-SF) (scores > 12); high caffeine consumers (>21 servings of 170.5–341 mL caffeine beverages per week; high consumption of polyphenols (>100 total combined servings per week); self-reported chronic physical or mental health condition requiring prescription or over-the-counter medication (excluding contraception) on a continual basis; pregnant or reported a chance of being pregnant; allergy to caffeine; current smoker; or consumption of nutritional supplements (i.e., herbs, vitamins, or creatine, not including supplementation of protein without caffeine).

Volunteers not excluded by the screening were invited to the testing facility. All participants read and signed the informed consent form. Participants were informed that they would be taking part in a study investigating the effects of caffeine beverages on mental function, blood pressure, heart rate and fine motor control. Thirty (17 women and 13 men) participants completed the original study and were all included in our current post-hoc analysis. Characteristics from the sample (n = 30) are reported in Table 1.

Table 1. Participant Characteristics.

Sex (Males/Females)	13/17
Age (years)	21.8 ± 4.4
Height (cm)	169.6 ± 12.4
Weight (kg)	67.6 ± 11.0
Body Mass Index (kg/m^2)	23.5 ± 2.5
Race	
White	21
Asian	4
Black	4
More than one race	1
Trait Physical Energy	6.5 ± 2.1
Trait Physical Fatigue	3.5 ± 2.0
Trait Mental Energy	5.7 ± 1.7
Trait Mental Fatigue	3.8 ± 1.9
Amount of sleep on a typical night in the past month (hrs)	7.6 ± 0.8
Consumption of High-Flavanol Foods or Beverages during the Past Month	
Caffeine drinks (servings) per week	4.2 ± 3.8
Caffeine drinks (mg caffeine) per day	60 ± 54.3
Cocoa (servings) per month	0.7 ± 1.3
Fruits (servings) per month	12.3 ± 12.4
Vegetables (servings) per month	25.1 ± 14.5

Data are reported as means ± standard deviations.

The average reported nightly sleep during the month prior to the study was 7.6 ± 0.8 h. The number of hours of reported sleep the night before each of the testing sessions did not significantly differ from between conditions (t = 0.38, p = 0.71); placebo (6.5 ± 1.3 h); caffeine (6.4 ± 1.1 h). Participants appeared to be low consumers of caffeine (4.2 ± 3.8 servings per week) and polyphenols (56.74 ± 8.16 servings per month). All participants were asked to refrain from consuming caffeine 24 h prior to testing, and salivary analyses were completed on each testing day to confirm compliance.

2.3. Measures

During the survey to determine eligibility for the study, participants completed a series of assessments. For the purposes of this study, we chose to analyze the influence of trait mental and physical energy and fatigue on the testing day measures. On testing days, participants completed a series of mental energy tests consisting of self-reported motivation and mood measures and computerized cognitive tasks of sustained attention. Additionally, we measured fine motor task performance using the nine-hole peg test.

All testing was performed in a seated position in a thermoneutral (72 ± 0.8 °F/22.2 ± 0.8 °C), private lab setting, with sound attenuation and controlled lighting. Visual stimuli were presented that required a finger response. Participants used the keyboard to respond to information presented on a 17" screen on an Alienware laptop (17 R2 Model #P43F, Roundrock, TX, USA). Prior to each cognitive task, participants were given on-screen instructions about how to perform the task and asked to press the "enter" key if they understood the directions or to get help from a researcher if they were uncertain. All cognitive tests were performed using the Membrain Platform (PsychTechSolutions, Potsdam, NY, USA) using Java-coded software. Results from the cognitive tasks were downloaded into Microsoft Excel and two research assistants independently manually re-arranged data for analysis.

For the purposes of this study, we only describe the measures used in the present analyses. For a full list of pre-testing and testing day measures, the reader may refer to Boolani et al. [13] and Boolani et al. [28], respectively.

2.3.1. Pre-Testing Measure

Trait Mental and physical energy and fatigue: The trait aspect of the mental and physical state and trait energy and fatigue scale was used to collect pre-testing information on trait (long-standing pre-disposition) mental and physical energy and fatigue. The trait component, which references how the respondent usually feels, contains 12 total items with three items for each of the four trait outcomes (physical and mental energy and fatigue). Representative statements include: "I feel I have energy" and "I have feelings of being worn out." Responses were collected on a 5-point scale ranging from "never" to "always". In other studies, the Cronbach's alpha coefficients range from 0.82 to 0.93 [13,14,30]. With the current data, alpha coefficients ranged from 0.73 to 0.88 (trait mental energy = 0.73, trait mental fatigue = 0.88, trait physical energy = 0.75, trait physical fatigue = 0.84).

2.3.2. Testing Day Measures

(1) State Moods: The 30-item Profile of Mood Survey–Short Form (POMS-SF) was used to assess mood states in the moment using a five-point scale ranging from "Not at all" (scored as 0) to "Extremely" (scored as 4). Scores from these questions were used to calculate the different components of tension/anxiety ($\alpha = 0.364$), depression ($\alpha = 0.598$), anger ($\alpha = 0.519$), vigor ($\alpha = 0.922$), fatigue ($\alpha = 0.863$), and confusion ($\alpha = 0.419$). All dimensions were made of five items (i.e., tension= tension + shaky + uneasy + nervous + anxious) [31].

(2) State Mental and Physical Energy and Fatigue: The state aspect of the mental and physical state and trait energy and fatigue scale was used to measure feelings in the immediate moment [29]. Like the trait component, the state component had the same 12 items as the trait scale, but this time a 0 to 100 Visual Analog Scale (VAS). However, due to limitation in data collection techniques, the scale was modified to a 0–10 Likert Scale anchored by "absence of feelings (left end, scored as 0) and the "strongest intensity of feelings" (right end, scored as 10). The modification is the same as Boolani et al. previously used (10,29). The Cronbach's alpha for this current study was between 0.707 and 0.874 (state physical energy = 0.785, state physical fatigue= 0.837, state mental energy = 0.707, and state mental fatigue = 0.874).

(3) Serial Three and Serial Seven subtraction tasks: Participants were asked to silently subtract backwards in three's or seven's from a random starting number between 800 and 999 that was presented on the computer screen (Tahoma Regular font, size 20 pt).

Participants were instructed to type their answers as quickly and as accurately as possible. After each answer was entered by the participant, the number was cleared from the screen. Participants were allowed to complete as many attempts as possible in two minutes [26,27]. For the purposes of this study, we did not analyze the number of correct responses because all tests had >97.5% response accuracy. Therefore, we only analyzed the total number of attempts for these serial subtraction tests. The maintained correct response rate suggests that participants sacrificed speed for accuracy as they became more fatigued.

(4) Fine motor control: The validated nine-hole peg test of finger dexterity was used to measure fine motor control [32]. The 12 × 12 cm wooden pegboard contained nine holes and was placed on the desktop in front of the seated participant. There were nine cylindrical pegs that were placed on the desktop outside of the container on the right or left side of the board for when the participant's right- and left-hand dexterity was tested. Participants were instructed to place one peg into the pegboard holes one at a time and then remove each peg one at a time, as fast as possible. The first test was performed with the dominant hand and the next with their non-dominant hand. Each test was performed twice. For the purposes of this study, we examined the mean scores from the two tests. Results are presented as the average time (measured in seconds) of the two times for the dominant hand (DH) and the average of the results of the two times for the non-dominant hand (NDH).

2.4. Procedure

The study consisted of a familiarization day (~1 h) followed by three testing days (~3 h) scheduled a minimum of 48 h apart. Each day started between 6 and 8 am and was scheduled within ±30 min of the familiarization day to account for diurnal variations [33]. Participants were advised to get their typical amount of sleep and asked to refrain from caffeine and alcohol consumption the night before testing. Additionally, they were asked to refrain caffeine and alcohol consumption the day of testing.

Familiarization Day: To reduce the experimental error that may occur due to learning effect, participants were asked to come to lab for a practice session where they completed a single trial run of all the daily assessments. These data were not included in any of our analyses. On familiarization day, we also measured participants' characteristics. Height was measured using a stadiometer and weight was measured using a digital scale (Tanita TBF-410, Tanita Corporation, Tokyo, Japan).

Testing days 1–3: Using randomizer.org, participants were randomly assigned to the order in which the beverage was administered. Participants came to lab each testing day and completed a series of surveys that asked them about their previous night's sleep, food, beverage, and drug consumption over the prior 24 h. Participants who reported ±2 h of their usual sleep duration (reported during the screening) were not tested that day and rescheduled. Those who reported drug use or the consumption of caffeine-containing foods or beverages the night before were also rescheduled. After screening, participants were instructed to accumulate ~2 mL of saliva in a 10 mL test tube. Baseline measures of sustained attention (cognitive task measures as part of the mental energy test battery), motivation, mood, blood pressure (BP), heart rate (HR), and fine motor task performance were obtained (Figure 1). After baseline testing, participants were administered one of the beverages and instructed to consume it within 2 min. Following the administration of the beverage, participants were given a 28 min break and were not allowed to participate in strenuous physical or mental activity or consume additional snacks or beverages. Three additional 27 min mental energy battery tests were completed, with 10 min rest breaks between each test battery (Figure 2). At the end of the last test battery, participants provided a post-test saliva sample using the same drool-down method described above.

2.5. Data Treatment and Statistics

2.5.1. Data Handling

The medians for each trait variable (Trait Physical Energy = 7.0, Trait Physical Fatigue = 3.5, Trait Mental Energy = 6.0, Trait Mental Fatigue = 3.0) were identified, and then surrogate variables were created to represent these in dichotomous format with their values at 0 up to the 50th percentile and 1 otherwise. All data processing and analyses were done with R version 4.0.0. Scripts for these tasks can be found at Trait-Caffeine study.

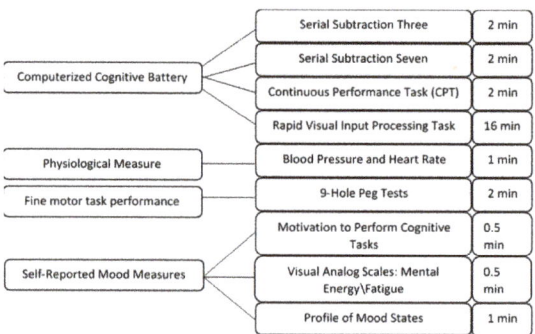

Figure 1. Test battery sequence.

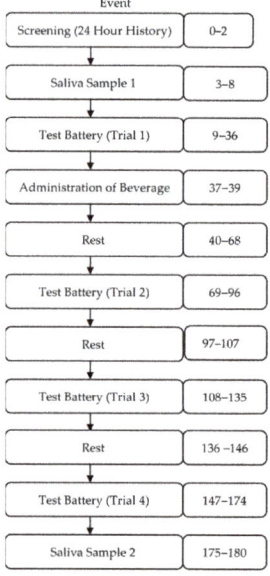

Figure 2. Testing day schedule.

2.5.2. Primary Analysis

Linear mixed-effects regressions were performed on each set of variables to test for significant differences across testing groups before and after they consumed the intervention [34,35]. For one-way effects, this test provides equivalent results to a type III repeated-measures ANOVA, computing and comparing the estimated population marginal means for two time points. For two-way effects, singularly significant mixed-effects results are interpreted in a straightforward manner, unlike those of an ANOVA, which are interpreted as crossover effects. All tests and relevant marginal means figures were computed and generated using the lmerTest package in R. Statistically significant relationships are presented in manuscript tables; however, a table containing values for all statistical relationships can be found in the Supplementary Materials (Table S1).

3. Results

After screening 1035 surveys for eligibility, 43 participants qualified for the study and were randomly allocated to the order in which they would receive the intervention. Due to logistical issues, 13 participants started the study but did not complete it. A total of 30 participants completed both days of the study, and their data were used for our final analysis (Figure 3). Recruitment and data collection lasted from 25 September 2015 to 10 December 2016 until 30 participants had completed both days of treatment. There were no harms or unintended consequences for any of the interventions. No participants pre-testing salivary caffeine levels >0.05 µg/mL, suggesting that all participants followed instructions of abstaining from caffeine prior to testing day. Post-hoc power analysis revealed a calculated power >0.90 for all analyses.

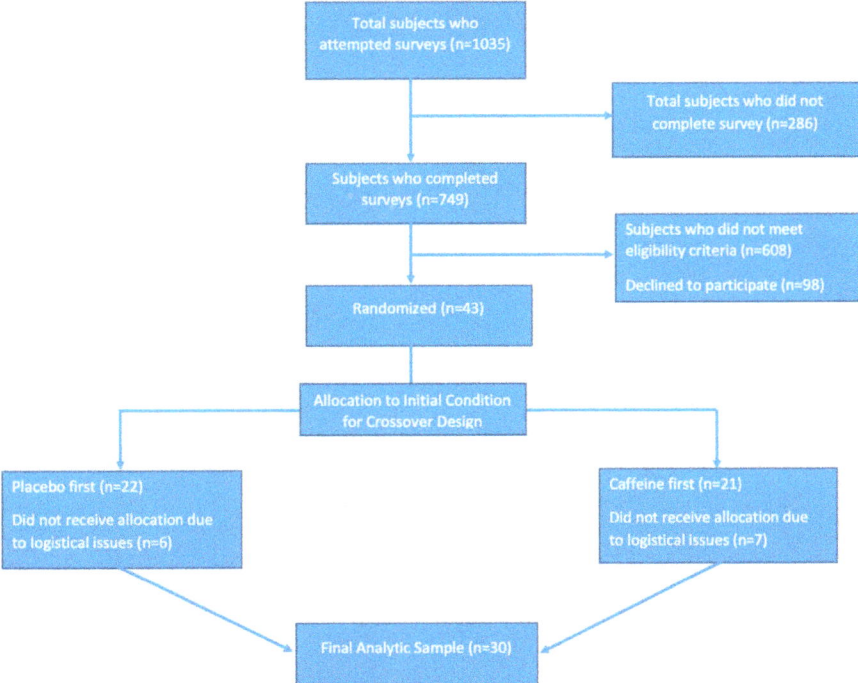

Figure 3. Consolidating Standards of Report Trials (CONSORT) Flow Diagram.

3.1. Trait Influence on State Mood

When testing the caffeinated and placebo conditions together, we report that independent of caffeine, high trait physical energy increased fatigue ($\beta = 1.70$, 95% CI: 0.43, 3.00) and confusion ($\beta = 0.830$, 95% CI: 0.033, 1.628) and decreased POMS vigor ($\beta = -3.20$, 95% CI: -5.43, -1.58) and motivation to perform mental tasks ($\beta = -1.469$, 95% CI: -2.827, -0.111). Low trait physical energy increased state physical fatigue ($\beta = -4.90$, 95% CI: -5.724, -1.33) and state metal fatigue ($\beta = -4.50$, 95% CI: -5.67, -1.33) with performance of the mental test battery (Table 2).

Independently, caffeine was found to increase POMS vigor ($\beta = 1.30$, 95% CI: -0.82, 1.95), POMS tension/anxiety ($\beta = 0.63$, 95% CI: $-0.07, 0.54$), and POMS anger ($\beta = 0.400$, 95% CI: $-0.013, 0.787$). However, low trait physical fatigue and caffeine increased POMS tension/anxiety scores ($\beta = -0.80$, 95% CI: $-0.23, 0.63$), meaning that low trait physical fatigue amplifies the effects of caffeine on POMS tension/anxiety (Figure 4). The interaction between all the trait moods and caffeine were not significant for vigor and anger, suggesting that trait did not modify the effect of caffeine on vigor and anger (Table 2).

Table 2. Trait and caffeine influence on moods, cognitive tasks and fine motor tasks (significant relationships only).

Factor	Measure	Beta	2.5%	97.5%	t stat	p Value
TPE	Vigor	−3.234	−5.686	−0.783	−2.586	0.014
Caffeine	Vigor	1.300	0.211	2.389	2.341	0.022
Caffeine	Vigor	1.437	0.396	2.479	2.706	0.008
TMF × Caffeine	Vigor	−1.866	−3.390	−0.342	−2.400	0.019
Caffeine	Tension	0.633	0.265	1.001	3.372	0.001
TPF × Caffeine	Tension	−0.800	−1.321	−0.279	−3.012	0.003
Caffeine	Anger	0.400	0.013	0.787	2.028	0.046
Caffeine	Anger	0.364	0.045	0.683	2.234	0.028
TMF × Caffeine	Depression	−0.339	−0.632	−0.047	−2.276	0.025
TPE	Confusion	0.830	0.033	1.628	2.040	0.047
TPE	Motivation	−1.469	−2.827	−0.111	−2.121	0.040
Caffeine	Motivation	0.812	0.094	1.531	2.215	0.029
TMF × Caffeine	Motivation	−1.312	−2.365	−0.260	−2.444	0.017
TPE	Physical Fatigue	−4.926	−8.137	−1.715	−3.007	0.004
TME × Caffeine	Physical Fatigue	5.369	1.502	9.237	2.721	0.008
TPE	Mental Fatigue	−4.483	−7.678	−1.289	−2.751	0.008
TME × Caffeine	Mental Fatigue	5.199	1.306	9.092	2.617	0.010
TPF × Caffeine	Sub3total	4.400	0.796	8.004	2.393	0.019
TME	Sub3total	9.222	2.045	16.398	2.519	0.017
TME × Caffeine	Sub3total	−6.244	−10.242	−2.247	−3.062	0.003
Caffeine	Sub3total	−2.875	−5.290	−0.46	−2.334	0.022
TMF × Caffeine	Sub3total	5.661	2.126	9.196	3.139	0.002
Caffeine	Sub7total	2.632	0.518	4.746	2.440	0.017
TME	Sub7total	6.858	1.106	12.61	2.337	0.025
Caffeine	Sub7total	2.886	0.933	4.840	2.896	0.005
TMF × Caffeine	Sub7total	4.964	1.751	8.178	3.028	0.003
TPF × Caffeine	DH	−9.433	−15.295	−3.572	−3.154	0.002
TMF × Caffeine	DH	−8.862	−14.777	−2.947	−2.936	0.004
TPF × Caffeine	NDH	−8.033	−13.744	−2.322	−2.757	0.007
TMF × Caffeine	NDH	−7.978	−13.706	−2.250	−2.730	0.008

TPE = Trait Physical Energy, TPF = Trait Physical Fatigue, TME = Trait Mental Energy, TMF = Trait Mental Fatigue, DH = Dominant Hand, NDH = Non-dominant hand.

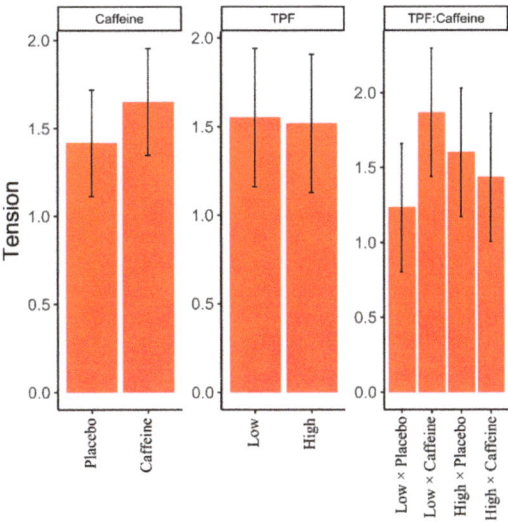

Figure 4. Profile of Mood Survey (POMS) Tension score changes. TPF = Trait Physical Fatigue. Data are presented as means ± standard deviations.

Low trait mental energy and caffeine together decreased state physical fatigue (β = 5.40, 95% CI: −0.23, 6.35) and mental fatigue (β = 5.20, 95% CI: −0.27, 6.27), while alone neither had any statistically significant independent effect. We also found that low trait mental fatigue and caffeine increased feelings of depression (β = −0.339, 95% CI: −0.632, −0.047) and motivation to perform mental tasks (β = −1.312, 95% CI: −2.365, −0.260) (Table 2).

3.2. Trait Influence on Cognitive Task Performance

When testing the caffeinated condition and placebo together, we found that while trait physical fatigue did not independently influence attempts of serial subtraction 3, the interaction between caffeine and trait physical fatigue was positive (β = 4.40, 95% CI: −3.23, 6.50), suggesting that those who reported high trait physical fatigue reported a greater benefit of consuming caffeine. While high trait mental energy increased serial subtraction 3 attempts (β = 9.20, 95% CI: −0.07, 12.27), the interaction between trait mental energy and caffeine was negative (β = −6.20, 95% CI: −1.97, 10.79). This suggests that those with low trait mental energy enjoyed greater benefits of caffeine on serial subtraction 3 attempts. While consuming caffeine reduced subtract 3 attempts (β = −2.9, 95% CI: −1.16, 4.80) independently of trait mental fatigue, caffeine and high trait mental fatigue together increased subtract 3 attempts (β = 5.70, 95% CI: −3.42, 6.66). This suggests that participants with high trait mental fatigue received the most benefit from consuming caffeine on the serial subtract 3 (Table 2).

3.3. Trait Influence on Fine Motor Task Performance

High trait physical fatigue and caffeine together decreased dominant hand average completion time by 9.4 s (β = −9.40, 95% CI: −8.05, 9.25) and nondominant hand average completion time by 8 s (β = −8.00, 95% CI: −13.27, 4.14). High trait mental fatigue and caffeine together decreased dominant hand average completion time by 8.9 s (β = −8.90, 95% CI: −12.11, 5.82) and nondominant hand average completion time by 8.0 s (β = −8.00, 95% CI: −17.75, −0.08) (Figure 5). These results imply that those with high trait mental and physical fatigue reported the most benefit of consuming caffeine on the 9-hole peg test (Table 2).

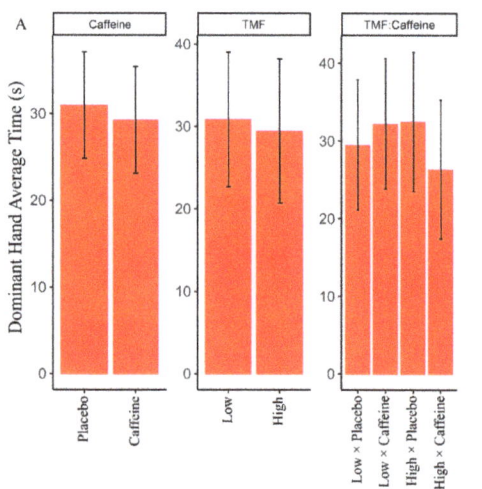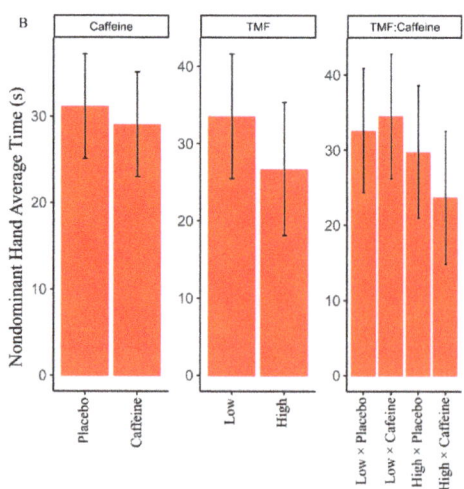

Figure 5. Trait and caffeine influence on nine-hole peg test times for both (**A**) dominant hand and (**B**) nondominant hand average times. TMF = Trait Mental Fatigue.

3.4. Post-Hoc Salivary Analysis

There were no statistically significant effects of Trait Physical Energy ($p = 0.487$), Trait Physical Fatigue ($p = 0.312$), Trait Mental Energy ($p = 0.458$), or Trait Mental Fatigue ($p = 0.837$) on pre-post salivary caffeine composition.

4. Discussion

To our knowledge, this post-hoc analysis is the first study to analyze the influence of trait mental and physical energy and fatigue on the neurocognitive effects of caffeine during the performance of a commonly used mental energy test battery. The results of our study provide new evidence suggesting that trait energy and fatigue may explain the interpersonal differences in the effects of caffeine on mood, cognitive and fine-motor task performance.

4.1. Trait Influence on State Moods

The results of our study indicate that trait physical energy by itself influences mood responses as a result of performing the mental test battery. For example, we found that those who reported being high trait physical energy reported a greater decline in POMS vigor (energy) scores and a greater increase in POMS fatigue and confusion scores and motivation to perform mental tasks. These results suggest that participants who report being normally very physically energetic may respond more negatively to repeatedly performing this mental task battery. However, in our study, when we split fatigue into mental and physical aspects of fatigue, those with low trait physical energy reported greater declines in both physical and mental fatigue during the repeated performance of this mental test battery. This relationship is contrary to their responses to the POMS fatigue scores. While we cannot explain these differences, it raises questions as to the constructs measured by the two surveys. While the POMS-SF and the state mental and physical energy and fatigue surveys are widely used together [16,17,23,28,29], in our study, their results were incongruent. With high alphas (>0.84), the consistency of the item responses within our study is strong, which suggests responses were not biased by measurement error.

As expected, when comparing the caffeine to placebo condition, we found that caffeine increased feelings of vigor [16,17,29], anger [29,36], and anxiety [24,29,37]; however, our findings were unique in that we reported that trait physical fatigue moderated the effects of caffeine on feelings of anxiety. Our findings suggest that those who were low trait physical fatigue reported an increase in feelings of anxiety on days they consumed caffeine compared to days they consumed placebo, as shown in Figure 4. The opposite is true for those who reported high trait physical fatigue, in that these individuals reported reduced feelings of anxiety on days they consumed caffeine compared to days they consumed the placebo beverage. Our findings may explain the results of the study by Childs and colleagues [24], where most, but not all, participants reported increased feelings of anxiety after a high dose of caffeine. Another associated interaction in our results was the fact that individuals with low trait mental energy reported greater decreases in feelings of mental and physical fatigue after the consumption of caffeine. Our results suggest that those who normally report feeling mentally energetic may not receive the same anti-fatiguing benefits of consuming caffeine as those who normally report not feeling mentally energetic. These two findings may be related because we find that the ADORA2A gene, a dopaminergic gene, is associated with both feelings of energy [9] and anxiety [24]. Therefore, we may hypothesize that genetic polymorphisms associated with the fatigue may modify the expression of the ADORA2A gene with caffeine consumption.

We also reported that those who were low trait mental fatigue reported increased feelings of depression after consuming caffeine. These results may explain why some of the participants in a study by Dawkins and colleagues [38] reported an increase in feelings of depression after consuming caffeine. Additionally, we found that those who were low trait mental fatigue reported greater increases in motivation to perform mental tasks, suggesting that those who are normally mentally fatigued may receive a boost in motivation compared to those who are not normally mentally fatigued. The results of our study might explain why cyclists who reported feeling mentally fatigued reported increases in motivation to perform mental tasks after consuming caffeine, while those who were not mentally fatigued at baseline reported no increases in motivation [39]. Other studies that have examined their population as a whole and have not split them up by those who normally feel mentally fatigued compared to those who do not, have reported inconsistent findings for the effects of caffeine on motivation [29,40], including the primary study from this data [28]. All of the aforementioned studies [28,29,40] used very similar protocols and similar amounts of caffeine (66–100 mg), yet they had differing results as it relates to the effects of caffeine on motivation to perform mental tasks. Our results suggest that studies should control for trait mental and physical energy and fatigue as those traits may modify the effects of caffeine on motivation.

4.2. Trait Influence on Cognitive Task Performance

Our results found that overall, those who were high trait physical and mental fatigue or low trait mental energy enjoyed the benefits of caffeine consumption on the serial subtraction 3 task, while caffeine only had an effect on participants who were high trait mental fatigue on the serial subtraction 7 task. These results were intuitive in that those who need the biggest boost to perform cognitive tasks received it when they consumed caffeine. Our results were also in line with previous findings that caffeine by itself increased serial subtraction attempts [29]. An interesting finding from our study was that those who were normally mentally energetic reported improvement in serial subtraction 7 attempts during this protocol even without the benefit of consuming caffeine. Although the protocol in our study has been validated [25] and used in multiple previous studies [16,17,26,27,29], our findings suggest that not everyone may report the intended mental-fatigue-associated decline in mental task performance with this protocol.

4.3. Trait Influence on Fine Motor Task Performance

The findings of our study suggest those who were normally mentally and physically fatigued reported improvement in fine motor task performance with both their dominant and non-dominant hands after consuming caffeine. While caffeine has been known to decrease fine motor task performance [41–43], it seems that those who normally report feeling physically or mentally fatigued report acute motor dexterity benefits of consuming caffeine. We are unaware of literature that reports a group of individuals who report improvements in motor task performance after caffeine consumption. However, from the results of our study, we may argue that there is a subset of the population that may respond counter to expectations with caffeine consumption as it relates to performance on fine motor tasks.

4.4. Implications

This study deepens our understanding of the influence of long-standing predisposition of mental and physical energy and fatigue on acute responses to caffeine consumption. Our results found that trait mental and physical energy and fatigue may explain many of the interpersonal differences in responses to caffeine consumption. These results provide us with an inexpensive measure to control for inter-individual effects of caffeine and help us identify hyper- and non-responders, or, in the case of fine motor task performance, a group that has the opposite response to caffeine consumption than what has been previously reported in the literature. While most caffeine researchers account for prior night's sleep [16,17,29] in their studies, we find that researchers should also account for an individual's trait mental and physical energy and fatigue, as this predisposition may play a role in how individuals respond acutely to caffeine. Additionally, while some researchers utilize random group assignments when performing caffeine research [44,45], our findings suggest that these random group assignments may not control for the inter-individual differences in caffeine response. We recommend the use of a cross-over design where all participants receive all interventions, as it may be best at reducing the risk that individuals who were on one end of one of a trait spectrum are not accidentally assigned to the same group. Therefore, it is the suggestion of the authors that nutrition researchers who are interested in understanding the acute effects of caffeine (1) measure trait mental and physical energy and fatigue in their participants, (2) control for trait mental and physical energy and fatigue in their analyses, and (3) avoid random group assignment when possible and utilize a cross-over design.

4.5. Limitations

Like all studies, this study has several aspects that may limit the generalizability of the findings. First, recruitment was limited to average or lower than average consumers of caffeine (<200 mg/day), fruits, vegetables, and other foods rich in polyphenols and POMS vigor scores of <13. Second, although our models reported adequate power, we had a relatively small number of participants and we also did not control for the timing and composition of the meals preceding testing. Third, although we did not find any significant effect of trait moods on pre–post caffeine differences, we did not obtain saliva samples between completion of beverage consumption, the second, and the third mental energy test battery. Therefore, it is unclear if caffeine's bioavailability between mental energy test batteries varied based on trait. Another limitation of our study is the poor psychometric properties of the POMS survey. While the POMS in healthy populations has been reported to have a Cronbach's $\alpha < 0.90$ [31], the α's for anxiety, depression, anger, and confusion in our study were surprisingly low. Another potential limitation of our study was that we only allowed participants to practice cognitive tasks once prior to administering the protocol, which may have led to learning effects during the study. To mitigate the risk of learning effects, we initially compared all measures by testing days, regardless of the intervention. No significant differences in performance between days were identified. Another possible limitation may have been the carryover effect of one of the beverages on subsequent testing sessions. To mitigate this risk, consistent with prior literature [16,17,26,27,29], we randomized the order of the allocation and scheduled participants a minimum of 48 h after completion of the prior session to allow for a washout period. The average time between treatments was 7.4 ± 2.8 days (i.e., 13.7 ± 3.1 days between the two treatments analyzed in this study). Additionally, some participants may have been more sensitive to the taste of caffeine, thus being able to identify when they were given the placebo versus when they were given the caffeinated beverage.

5. Conclusions

The objective of this study was to determine the influence of trait to mental and physical energy and fatigue on state moods and cognitive and fine-motor task performance when participants consumed caffeine compared to days they consumed a placebo. Our results found that trait mental and physical energy and fatigue modified the effects of caffeine on all three parameters and in the instance of fine motor skill had the opposite of the intended effect on participants who reported being high trait mental and physical fatigue. This analysis helps us better identify hyper- and non-responders to caffeine without performing genetic testing. Our results suggest that nutrition researchers should consider trait mental and physical energy and fatigue when conducting studies on acute responses of caffeine on mood, cognitive and fine-motor tasks. Future research should compare these trends on longer time frames (e.g., chronic caffeine consumption).

Supplementary Materials: The following are available online at https://www.mdpi.com/2072-6643/13/2/412/s1, Table S1: Trait and caffeine influence on moods, cognitive tasks, and fine motor tasks.

Author Contributions: Author D.T.F. was responsible for study conceptualizing, performing and interpreting all statistical analysis, writing of the initial draft, and approving the final draft. Author M.L.S. was responsible for interpreting all statistical analyses, writing the initial draft, and approving the final draft. Author A.B. was responsible for conceptualization, study design, data collection, data interpretation, writing of the first and final draft. All authors have read and agreed to the published version of the manuscript.

Funding: The original study was funded by a grant from Isagenix International, LLC. The funders had no role in study design, data collection and analysis, or the decision to publish the manuscript.

Institutional Review Board Statement: The study was approved by Clarkson University Institutional Review Board (IRB approval #16-34.1).

Informed Consent Statement: All participants read and signed an informed consent form prior to participation.

Data Availability Statement: The dataset supporting the conclusions of this article is available in the Mendley repository. The DOI number for this dataset is 10.17632/3s8sr9zth9.1.

Acknowledgments: The authors would like to acknowledge undergraduate research assistants Stephanie Grobe and Joanne tiRiele for help with data collection.

Conflicts of Interest: The authors declare no conflict of interest.

References

1. Chen, M.K. The epidemiology of self-perceived fatigue among adults. *Prev. Med.* **1986**, *15*, 74–81. [CrossRef]
2. Ricci, J.A.; Chee, E.; Lorandeau, A.L.; Berger, J. Fatigue in the US workforce: Prevalence and implications for lost productive work time. *J. Occup. Environ. Med.* **2007**, *49*, 1–10. [CrossRef] [PubMed]
3. Taylor, A.H.; Dorn, L. Stress, fatigue, health, and risk of road traffic accidents among professional drivers: The contribution of physical inactivity. *Annu. Rev. Publ. Health* **2006**, *27*, 371–391. [CrossRef] [PubMed]
4. Van Drongelen, A.; Boot, C.R.; Hlobil, H.; Smid, T.; van der Beek, A.J. Risk factors for fatigue among airline pilots. *Int. Archiv. Occup. Environ. Health* **2017**, *90*, 39–47. [CrossRef] [PubMed]
5. Samkoff, J.S.; Jacques, C.H. A review of studies concerning effects of sleep deprivation and fatigue on residents' performance. *Acad. Med.* **1991**, *66*, 687–693. [CrossRef] [PubMed]
6. Fukuda, S.; Yamano, E.; Joudoi, T.; Mizuno, K.; Tanaka, M.; Kawatani, J.; Takano, M.; Tomoda, A.; Imai-Matsumura, K.; Miike, T.; et al. Effort-reward imbalance for learning is associated with fatigue in school children. *Behav. Med.* **2010**, *36*, 53–62. [CrossRef]
7. Verbrugge, L.M.; Ascione, F.J. Exploring the iceberg: Common symptoms and how people care for them. *Med. Care* **1987**, *25*, 539–569. [CrossRef]
8. Lewis, G.; Wessely, S. The epidemiology of fatigue: More questions than answers. *J. Epidemiol. Commun. Health* **1992**, *46*, 92. [CrossRef]
9. Loy, B.D.; Cameron, M.H.; O'Connor, P.J. Perceived fatigue and energy are independent unipolar states: Supporting evidence. *Med. Hypotheses* **2018**, *113*, 46–51. [CrossRef]
10. Boolani, A.; O'Connor, P.J.; Reid, J.; Ma, S.; Mondal, S. Predictors of feelings of energy differ from predictors of fatigue. *Fatigue Biomed. Health Behav.* **2019**, *7*, 12–28. [CrossRef]
11. Dupree, E.J.; Goodwin, A.; Darie, C.C.; Boolani, A. A Pilot exploratory proteomics investigation of mental fatigue and mental energy. In *Advancements of Mass Spectrometry in Biomedical Research*; Springer: Berlin, Germany, 2019; pp. 601–611.
12. Boolani, A.; Ryan, J.; Vo, T.; Wong, B.; Banerjee, N.; Banerjee, S.; Fulk, G.; Smith, L.M.; Martin, R. Do changes in mental energy and fatigue impact functional assessments associated with fall risks? An exploratory study using machine learning. *Phys. Occup. Ther. Geriatr.* **2020**, *38*, 283–301. [CrossRef]
13. Boolani, A.; Manierre, M. An exploratory multivariate study examining correlates of trait mental and physical fatigue and energy. *Fatigue Biomed. Health Behav.* **2019**, *7*, 29–40. [CrossRef]
14. Manierre, M.; Jansen, E.; Boolani, A. Sleep quality and sex modify the relationships between trait energy and fatigue on state energy and fatigue. *PLoS ONE* **2020**, *15*, e0227511. [CrossRef] [PubMed]
15. Loy, B.D.; O'Connor, P.J.; Dishman, R.K. The effect of a single bout of exercise on energy and fatigue states: A systematic review and meta-analysis. *Fatigue Biomed. Health Behav.* **2013**, *1*, 223–242. [CrossRef]
16. Maridakis, V.; O'Connor, P.J.; Tomporowski, P.D. Sensitivity to change in cognitive performance and mood measures of energy and fatigue in response to morning caffeine alone or in combination with carbohydrate. *Int. J. Neurosci.* **2009**, *119*, 1239–1258. [CrossRef] [PubMed]
17. Maridakis, V.; Herring, M.P.; O'Connor, P.J. Sensitivity to change in cognitive performance and mood measures of energy and fatigue in response to differing doses of caffeine or breakfast. *Int. J. Neurosci.* **2009**, *119*, 975–994. [CrossRef]
18. Herring, M.P.; Monroe, D.C.; Kline, C.E.; O'Connor, P.J.; MacDonncha, C. Sleep quality moderates the association between physical activity frequency and feelings of energy and fatigue in adolescents. *Eur. Child Adolesc. Psych.* **2018**, *27*, 1425–1432. [CrossRef]

19. White, J.R., Jr.; Padowski, J.M.; Zhong, Y.; Chen, G.; Luo, S.; Lazarus, P.; McPherson, S. Pharmacokinetic analysis and comparison of caffeine administered rapidly or slowly in coffee chilled or hot versus chilled energy drink in healthy young adults. *Clin. Toxic.* **2016**, *54*, 308–312. [CrossRef]
20. Childs, E.; de Wit, H. Subjective, behavioral, and physiological effects of acute caffeine in light, nondependent caffeine users. *Psychopharmacology* **2006**, *185*, 514. [CrossRef]
21. Rogers, P.J.; Hohoff, C.; Heatherley, S.V.; Mullings, E.L.; Maxfield, P.J.; Evershed, R.P.; Deckert, J.; Nutt, D.J. Association of the anxiogenic and alerting effects of caffeine with ADORA2A and ADORA1 polymorphisms and habitual level of caffeine consumption. *Neuropsychopharmacology* **2010**, *35*, 1973–1983. [CrossRef]
22. Davis, J.M.; Zhao, Z.; Stock, H.S.; Mehl, K.A.; Buggy, J.; Hand, G.A. Central nervous system effects of caffeine and adenosine on fatigue. *Am. J. Phys. Regul. Int. Comp. Phys.* **2003**. [CrossRef] [PubMed]
23. Loy, B.D.; O'Connor, P.J.; Lindheimer, J.B.; Covert, S.F. Caffeine is ergogenic for adenosine A2A receptor gene (ADORA2A) T allele homozygotes: A pilot study. *J. Caffeine Res.* **2015**, *5*, 73–81. [CrossRef]
24. Childs, E.; Hohoff, C.; Deckert, J.; Xu, K.; Badner, J.; De Wit, H. Association between ADORA2A and DRD2 polymorphisms and caffeine-induced anxiety. *Neuropsychopharmacology* **2008**, *33*, 2791–2800. [CrossRef] [PubMed]
25. O'Connor, P.J. Mental energy: Developing a model for examining nutrition-related claims. *Nutr. Rev.* **2006**, *6*, 2–6. [CrossRef]
26. Scholey, A.B.; French, S.J.; Morris, P.J.; Kennedy, D.O.; Milne, A.L.; Haskell, C.F. Consumption of cocoa flavanols results in acute improvements in mood and cognitive performance during sustained mental effort. *J. Psychopharm.* **2010**, *24*, 1505–1514. [CrossRef] [PubMed]
27. Haskell, C.F.; Kennedy, D.O.; Wesnes, K.A.; Scholey, A.B. Cognitive and mood improvements of caffeine in habitual consumers and habitual non-consumers of caffeine. *Psychopharmacology* **2005**, *179*, 813–825. [CrossRef]
28. Boolani, A.; Fuller, D.T.; Mondal, S.; Wilkinson, T.; Darie, C.C.; Gumpricht, E. Caffeine-containing, adaptogenic-rich drink Modulates the effects of caffeine on mental performance and cognitive parameters: A double-blinded, placebo-controlled, randomized trial. *Nutrients* **2020**, *12*, 1922. [CrossRef]
29. Boolani, A.; Lindheimer, J.B.; Loy, B.D.; Crozier, S.; O'Connor, P.J. Acute effects of brewed cocoa consumption on attention, motivation to perform cognitive work and feelings of anxiety, energy and fatigue: A randomized, placebo-controlled crossover experiment. *BMC Nutr.* **2017**, *3*, 8. [CrossRef]
30. O'Connor, P. *Mental and Physical State and Trait Energy and Fatigue Scales*; University of Georgia: Athens, GA, USA, 2006.
31. Curran, S.L.; Andrykowski, M.A.; Studts, J.L. Short form of the profile of mood states (POMS-SF): Psychometric information. *Psychol. Assess.* **1995**, *7*, 80. [CrossRef]
32. Mathiowetz, V.; Weber, K.; Kashman, N.; Volland, G. Adult norms for the nine hole peg test of finger dexterity. *Occup. Ther. J. Res.* **1985**, *5*, 24–38. [CrossRef]
33. Pilcher, J.J.; Huffcutt, A.I. Effects of sleep deprivation on performance: A meta-analysis. *Sleep* **1996**, *19*, 318–326. [CrossRef] [PubMed]
34. Kuznetsova, A.; Brockhoff, P.B.; Christensen, R.H. lmerTest package: Tests in linear mixed effects models. *J. Stat. Softw.* **2017**, *82*, 1–26. [CrossRef]
35. Kuznetsova, A.; Christensen, R.H.; Bavay, C.; Brockhoff, P.B. Automated mixed ANOVA modeling of sensory and consumer data. *Food Qual. Pref.* **2015**, *40*, 31–38. [CrossRef]
36. Lieberman, H.R.; Tharion, W.J.; Shukitt-Hale, B.; Speckman, K.L.; Tulley, R. Effects of caffeine, sleep loss, and stress on cognitive performance and mood during US Navy SEAL training. *Psychopharmacology* **2002**, *164*, 250–261. [CrossRef]
37. Smith, A. Effects of caffeine on human behavior. *Food Chem. Toxicol.* **2002**, *40*, 1243–1255. [CrossRef]
38. Dawkins, L.; Shahzad, F.-Z.; Ahmed, S.S.; Edmonds, C.J. Expectation of having consumed caffeine can improve performance and mood. *Appetite* **2011**, *57*, 597–600. [CrossRef]
39. Franco-Alvarenga, P.E.; Brietzke, C.; Canestri, R.; Goethel, M.F.; Hettinga, F.; Santos, T.M.; Pires, F.O. Caffeine improved cycling trial performance in mentally fatigued cyclists, regardless of alterations in prefrontal cortex activation. *Physiol. Behav.* **2019**, *204*, 41–48. [CrossRef]
40. Shields, K.A.; Silva, J.E.; Rauch, J.T.; Lowery, R.P.; Ormes, J.A.; Sharp, M.H.; McCleary, S.A.; Georges, J.; Joy, J.M.; Purpura, M.; et al. The effects of a multi-ingredient cognitive formula on alertness, focus, motivation, calmness and psychomotor performance in comparison to caffeine and placebo. *J. Int. Soc. Sports Nutr.* **2014**, *11*, 1–2. [CrossRef]
41. Jacobson, B.H.; Thurman-Lacey, S.R. Effect of caffeine on motor performance by caffeine-naive and -familiar subjects. *Percept. Motor Skills* **1992**, *74*, 151–157. [CrossRef]
42. Jacobson, B.H.; Winter-Roberts, K.; Gemmell, H.A. Influence of caffeine on selected manual manipulation skills. *Percept. Motor Skills* **1991**, *72* (Suppl. 3), 1175–1181. [CrossRef]
43. Mednick, S.C.; Cai, D.J.; Kanady, J.; Drummond, S.P. Comparing the benefits of caffeine, naps and placebo on verbal, motor and perceptual memory. *Behav. Brain Res.* **2008**, *193*, 79–86. [CrossRef] [PubMed]
44. Fillmore, M.; Vogel-Sprott, M. Expected effect of caffeine on motor performance predicts the type of response to placebo. *Psychopharmacology* **1992**, *106*, 209–214. [CrossRef] [PubMed]
45. Jacobson, B.H.; Edgley, B.M. Effects of caffeine in simple reaction time and movement time. *Aviat. Space Environ. Med.* **1987**, *58*, 1153–1156. [PubMed]

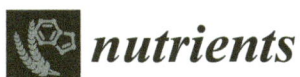 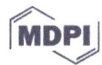

Article

Acute Caffeine Intake Enhances Mean Power Output and Bar Velocity during the Bench Press Throw in Athletes Habituated to Caffeine

Michal Wilk [1],*, Aleksandra Filip [1], Michal Krzysztofik [1], Mariola Gepfert [1], Adam Zajac [1] and Juan Del Coso [2]

1. Institute of Sport Sciences, The Jerzy Kukuczka Academy of Physical Education, 40-065 Katowice, Poland; a.filip@awf.katowice.pl (A.F.); m.krzysztofik@awf.katowice.pl (M.K.); m.gepfert@awf.katowice.pl (M.G.); a.zajac@awf.katowice.pl (A.Z.)
2. Centre for Sport Studies, Rey Juan Carlos University, 28942 Fuenlabrada, Spain; juan.delcoso@urjc.es
* Correspondence: m.wilk@awf.katowice.pl

Received: 3 January 2020; Accepted: 3 February 2020; Published: 4 February 2020

Abstract: Background: The main objective of the current investigation was to evaluate the effects of caffeine on power output and bar velocity during an explosive bench press throw in athletes habituated to caffeine. Methods: Twelve resistance trained individuals habituated to caffeine ingestion participated in a randomized double-blind experimental design. Each participant performed three identical experimental sessions 60 min after the intake of a placebo, 3, and 6 mg/kg/b.m. of caffeine. In each experimental session, the participants performed 5 sets of 2 repetitions of the bench press throw (with a load equivalent to 30% repetition maximum (RM), measured in a familiarization trial) on a Smith machine, while bar velocity and power output were registered with a rotatory encoder. Results: In comparison to the placebo, the intake of caffeine increased mean bar velocity during 5 sets of the bench press throw (1.37 ± 0.05 vs. 1.41 ± 0.05 and 1.41 ± 0.06 m/s for placebo, 3, and 6 mg/kg/b.m., respectively; $p < 0.01$), as well as mean power output (545 ± 117 vs. 562 ± 118 and 560 ± 107 W; $p < 0.01$). However, caffeine was not effective at increasing peak velocity ($p = 0.09$) nor peak power output ($p = 0.07$) during the explosive exercise. Conclusion: The acute doses of caffeine before resistance exercise may increase mean power output and mean bar velocity during the bench press throw training session in a group of habitual caffeine users. Thus, caffeine prior to ballistic exercises enhances performance during a power-specific resistance training session.

Keywords: ballistic exercise; upper limbs; resistance exercise; ergogenic substances; sport performance

1. Introduction

Caffeine (CAF) is one of the most common substances used in sport which enhances physical performance [1]. Although CAF may affect various body tissues [2,3], there is a growing body of evidence in animal [4] and human models [5] sustaining the ability of CAF to act as an adenosine antagonist, as the main mechanism behind CAF ergogenic effect. Current research recommends doses of CAF ranging from 3 to 6 mg/kg body mass to elicit ergogenic benefits, while the time of ingestion (from 30 to 90 min before exercise) and the form of ingestion (pills, liquid, chewing gum) are less significant as CAF is rapidly absorbed after ingestion [6]. However, the optimal protocol of CAF supplementation may differ based on the type and duration of exercise, previous habituation to CAF and the type of muscle contraction [6–10].

Acute CAF intake causes a slightly different response to upper and lower body exercise [10], despite the lack of a mechanisms explaining this phenomenon. A recent meta-analysis about the effects of CAF on muscle strength and power output found that CAF significantly improved upper but not lower body strength [7]. Although the outcomes of the first investigations were contradictory [11–13], more recent studies have found a clear effect of CAF on several forms of upper body muscle performance [14–16], when the used dose was at least 3 mg/kg/b.m. [17]. Interestingly, the effect of CAF on upper body muscle performance may be partially dampened in athletes habituated to CAF because the regular use of CAF-containing products [18] may develop tolerance to this substance. It must be noticed that this decreased ergogenic effect of CAF is not removed even with the ingestion of doses >9 mg/kg/b.m. [19,20].

Most studies on the acute effects of CAF on upper body muscle performance used the bench press exercise. The bench press exercise is widely used as a means of developing strength and power of the upper limbs [21,22]. However, other authors, recommend the use of ballistic exercises for the development of upper body power, such as the bench press throw (BPT) [23,24]. Specifically, to increase power output, the loads ranging from 0% to 50% of one-repetition maximum (1 RM) moved at maximal speed are recommended as the most potent loading stimuli for improving power output [23]. However, this type of routine can only be performed on a Smith machine while using the BPT exercise (i.e., maximal bar velocity is obtained at the moment of throw). The traditional free-weight bench press exercise does not allow for the attainment of maximal velocity of execution (i.e., velocity equals 0 m/s at maximal arm extension). Thus, ballistic exercises could be an optimal choice for power training as they allow for greater velocity, and muscle activation in comparison to similar traditional resistance training routines [21]. Perhaps, the main asset of the BPT is the maximum acceleration of a given load, which ultimately produces high movement velocity in a short time [25]. In this respect, the loads applied in ballistic exercises during training will depend on the specific requirements of particular sport disciplines and will determine success in numerous power-based competitions [23]. Furthermore, the BPT performance has been associated with overall performance in different sport-specific tasks [26–29]. Therefore, it seems reasonable to use the BPT as a means of testing upper-body ballistic performance. Although the BPT is indicated as the most effective exercise for developing power of the upper limbs [30], previous studies have not determined the acute effects of CAF on power output and bar velocity during this type of exercise.

Burke [31] has suggested that, in the current literature, there is a lack of data about the practical use of supplements in competitive sports because experimental protocols are often different from sports practice. In case of CAF, most studies considering the acute effects of this supplement were assessed on the basis of only a single set of an exercise [7,8,32], while real resistance training sessions in trained individuals rarely contain only one set of a particular exercise [31]. On the other hand, the investigations analyzing the acute effects of CAF on performance during successive sets of resistance exercises are scarce. Bowtell et al. [3] showed that pre-exercise CAF (6 mg/kg/b.m.) intake improved total exercise time during 5 sets of one-legged knee extensions performed to failure in comparison to a placebo (PLAC). It is worth noting that this ergogenic effect was achieved despite significantly lower muscle phosphocreatine concentration (PCr) and pH in the latter sets of an exercise in the CAF trial. Further, CAF ingestion (6 mg/kg/b.m.) attenuated the increase in interstitial potassium during one-legged knee extensions at 20 W (10 min) and 50 W (3 × 3 min) measured using microdialysis [33], which resulted in a 16% improvement in high-intensity exercise capacity.

Most studies related to the acute impact of CAF intake on power output and bar velocity have used participants unhabituated to CAF or individuals with low-to-moderate daily consumption of this stimulant [11,16,34]. However, the analysis of urinary CAF concentrations after official competitions suggests that CAF is widely employed before or during exercise to enhance performance [35,36]. This would mean that it is highly likely that some athletes are habituated to CAF due to daily consumption of caffeine-containing products. The existence of athletes habituated to CAF may be particularly common in sports such as cycling, rowing, triathlon, athletics, and weightlifting, sport disciplines that benefit from the use of ballistic exercises during training to increase power output. Habitual CAF intake modifies physiological responses to acute ingestion of this stimulant by the up-regulation of adenosine receptors [37,38]. This effect would produce a progressive reduction of CAF ergogenicity in those athletes consuming CAF on a regular basis, because the newly created adenosine receptors may bind to adenosine and induce fatigue. However, the fact of habituation to the ergogenic benefits of CAF is still inconclusive. The studies by Dodd et al. [39] and de Souza [40] showed similar responses to endurance exercise after acute CAF intake between low and habitual CAF consumers, although this is not always the case [41]. Considering the above, the use of cross-sectional investigations including participants with different degrees of habituation to CAF may explain the lack of consistency when concluding about tolerance to the ergogenic effect of CAF. Lara's et al. [42] crossover design showed that the ergogenicity of CAF was reduced when the substance was consumed daily for 20 days, yet afterwards the ergogenic properties of CAF were maintained. On the contrary, tolerance to some of the side-effects associated to CAF has been observed in habitual consumers of CAF [43]. However, only two previous studies analyzed the impact of CAF intake in habitual CAF consumers using resistance exercise test protocols [18–20]. These investigations indicate that CAF ergogenicity to power output is mostly reduced in individuals habituated to CAF, while only high doses (>9 mg/kg/b.m.) may exert some benefit in maximal strength [19,20]. However, to date, there is no available data regarding the influence of acute CAF intake on power output and bar velocity during ballistic exercises in athletes habitually consuming CAF.

Given the widespread use of the BPT exercise as a mean of developing power output in the upper limbs [44,45] and the widespread use of CAF in sport, it would be interesting to investigate whether acute CAF intake affects power output and bar velocity in athletes habituated to CAF. For this reason, the aim of the present study was to evaluate the effects of the acute intake of 3 and 6 mg/kg/b.m. of CAF on power output and bar velocity during five sets of the BPT in participants habituated to CAF. It was hypothesized that acute CAF intake would increase power output and bar velocity during the BPT training session when compared to a control situation, even in participants habituated to CAF.

2. Materials and Methods

A randomized, double-blind, PLAC-controlled crossover design was used for this investigation. Initially, the participants performed a familiarization session with the experimental protocols that included a 1 RM measurement for the bench press exercise. Afterwards, they performed 3 different experimental sessions with a one-week interval between sessions to allow for complete recovery and a wash-out of ingested substances (Figure 1). During the 3 experimental sessions, the study participants either ingested a PLAC, 3 mg/kg/b.m. of CAF (CAF-3) or 6 mg/kg/b.m. of CAF (CAF-6). One hour after ingestion of CAF or PLAC, they performed 5 sets of 2 repetitions of the BPT exercise at 30% 1 RM. Both CAF and PLAC were administered orally to allow for peak blood CAF concentration during the training session and at least 2 h after the last meal to avoid any interference of the diet with the absorption of the experimental substances. CAF supplementation was provided to participants in the form of unidentifiable capsules (Caffeine Kick®, Olimp Laboratories, Debica, Poland). The manufacturer of the CAF capsules also provided identical PLAC capsules filled with all-purpose flour. Participants refrained from strenuous physical activity the day before the experimental trials but they maintained their training routines during the duration of the experiment to avoid any performance decrement due to inactivity. Additionally, the participants maintained their dietary habits during the study period, including daily CAF intake. They received a list of products containing CAF which could not be consumed within 12 h of each experimental trial. Compliance was tested verbally and by using dietary records. Additionally, the participants were required to refrain from alcohol and tobacco, medications or dietary supplements for two weeks prior to the experiment. All subjects registered their calorie intake using the "Myfitness pal" software [46] (Under Armour, Baltimore, MD, USA) every 24 h before the testing procedure, to ensure that the caloric intake was similar between experimental sessions.

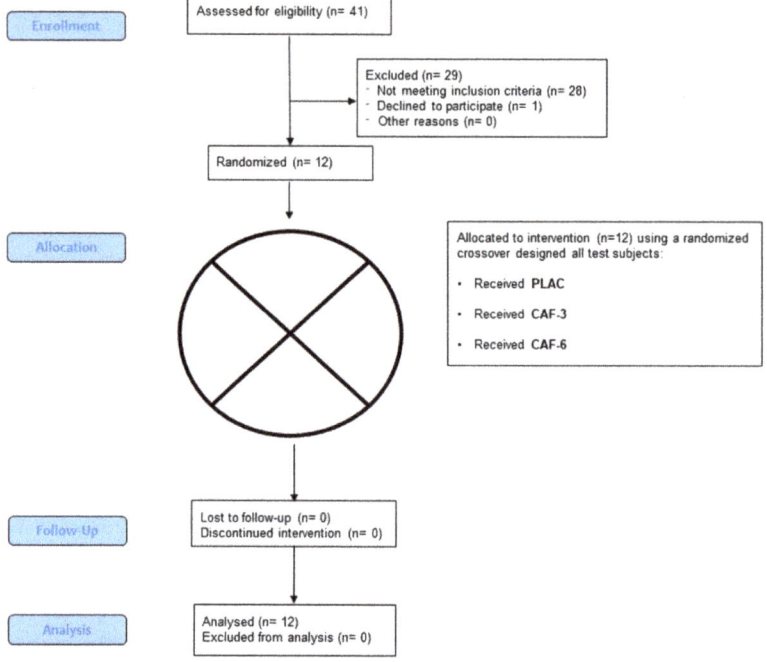

Figure 1. CONSORT flow diagram. n—number of participants; PLAC—placebo; CAF-3—caffeine 3mg/kg/b.m; CAF-6—caffeine 6mg/kg/b.m.

2.1. Participants

Twelve healthy strength-trained male athletes (age: 25.3 ± 1.7 years., body mass: 88.4 ± 16.5 kg, body mass index (BMI): 26.5 ± 4.7, bench press 1 RM: 128.6 ± 36.0 kg; mean ± SD) volunteered to participate in the study. All participants completed a written consent form after they had been informed of the risks and benefits of the study protocols. The participants had a minimum of 3 years of strength training experience (4.4 ± 1.6 years). All of them were classified as high habitual CAF consumers according to the classification recently proposed by de Souza Gonçalves et al. [40]. They self-reported their daily ingestion of CAF (5.0 ± 0.95 mg/kg/b.m./day, 443 ± 142 mg/day) based on a Food Frequency Questionnaire (FFQ). The inclusion criteria were as follows: (a) free from neuromuscular and musculoskeletal disorders, (b) 1 RM bench press performance with a load of at least 120% body mass, (c) habitual CAF intake in the range of 4–6 mg/day/kg/b.m. The athletes were excluded from the study when they suffered from any pathology or injury or when they were unable to perform the exercise protocol at the maximum effort. The investigation protocols were approved by the Bioethics Committee for Scientific Research at the Academy of Physical Education in Katowice (March 2019), Poland, according to the ethical standards of the latest version of the Declaration of Helsinki, 2013.

2.2. Habitual Caffeine Intake Assessment

Daily CAF intake was measured by an adapted version of the Food Frequency Questionnaire (FFQ) proposed by Bühler et al. [47]. Household measures were employed to individually assess the amount of food consumed during a day, week and month. The list was composed of dietary products with moderate-to-high CAF content including different types of coffee, tea, energy drinks, cocoa products, popular beverages, medications, and CAF supplements. Nutritional tables were used for database construction [48–50] and an experienced nutritionist calculated the daily CAF intake for each participant.

2.3. Familiarization Session and One Repetition Maximum Test

A familiarization session with the experimental procedures preceded 1 RM testing in the bench press exercise. In this session, the athletes arrived at the laboratory between 9:00 and 10:00 am. and cycled on an ergometer for 5 min. Afterwards, they performed 15 repetitions at 20% of their estimated 1 RM in the barbell bench press exercise followed by 10 repetitions at 40% 1 RM, 5 repetitions at 60% 1 RM and 3 repetitions at 80% 1 RM. Then they executed single repetitions of the bench press exercise with a 5 min rest interval between successful attempts. The load for each subsequent attempt was increased by 2.5 to 10 kg, and the process was repeated until failure. Hand placement on the barbell was individually selected grip width (~150% individual bi-acromial distance). After completing the 1 RM test in the bench press exercise, the participants performed a maximal BPT on a Smith machine with a load of 30% 1 RM from 1 RM bench press test result, with a maximal tempo of movement.

2.4. Experimental Sessions

During experimental sessions, the athletes participated in three identical training trials. All trials took place between 9.00 and 11.00 am. to avoid the effect of circadian variations on the outcomes of the investigation. After replicating the warm-up procedures of the familiarization trial, the athletes performed 5 sets of the 2 BPT repetitions at 30% 1 RM on the Smith machine. The repetitions were performed without rest to produce a ballistic movement while the rest interval between sets was 3 min. The participants were encouraged to produce maximal velocity during both the eccentric and concentric phase of the BPT movement. Two spotters were present on each side of the bar during the exercise protocol to ensure safety. To standardize the exercise protocol for all trials, each BPT was performed without bouncing the barbell off the chest, with the lower back in contact with the bench and without any pause between the eccentric and concentric phases of the movement. A rotatory encoder (Tendo Power Analyzer, Tendo Sport Machines, Trencin, Slovakia) was used for instantaneous recording of bar velocity during the whole range of motion, as in previous investigations [51]. During each BPT, peak power output (PP, in W) mean power output (MP, in W); peak bar velocity (PV, in m/s); and mean bar velocity (MV, in m/s) were registered. MP and MV were obtained as the mean of the two repetitions while PP and PV were obtained from the best repetition.

2.5. Statistical Analysis

Data are presented as the mean ± SD. All variables presented a normal distribution according to the Shapiro-Wilk test. Verification of differences in peak power output (PP), mean power output (MP), peak bar velocity (PV), and mean bar velocity (MV) was performed using a two-way (substance × set) analysis of variance (ANOVA) with repeated measures. In the event of a significant main effect, post-hoc comparisons were conducted using the Tukey's test. Percent changes and 95% confidence intervals were also calculated. Effect sizes (Cohen's d) were reported where appropriate and interpreted as large ($d \geq 0.80$); moderate (d between 0.79 and 0.50); small (d between 0.49 and 0.20); and trivial ($d < 0.20$); [52].

3. Results

The two-way repeated measures ANOVA indicated no significant substance × set main interaction effect for MP (F = 1.19; $p = 0.32$); MV (F = 1.18; $p = 0.32$); PP (F = 1.05; $p = 0.40$); PV (F = 1.09; $p = 0.38$). However, there was a significant main effect of substance in MP (F = 7.27; $p < 0.01$) and MV (F = 6.75; $p < 0.01$). No statistically significant main effect of substance was revealed in PP (F = 2.91; $p = 0.07$) and PV (F = 2.63; $p = 0.09$; Table 1).

Table 1. The main effect for substance on performance variables measured during 5 sets of the bench press throw with the ingestion of 3 and 6 mg/kg/b.m. of caffeine or a placebo.

Bench Press Throw (Mean of the 5 Sets)	Conditions			p
	PLAC	CAF-3	CAF-6	
Mean Power (W)	545 ± 117	562 ± 118	560 ± 107	0.01 *
Peak Power (W)	1250 ± 274	1261 ± 220	1297 ± 293	0.07
Mean Velocity (m/s)	1.37 ± 0.05	1.41 ± 0.05	1.41 ± 0.06	0.01 *
Peak Velocity (m/s)	2.14 ± 0.10	2.16 ± 0.07	2.17 ± 0.13	0.09

These data represent the mean values of the 5 sets. All data are presented as mean ± standard deviation. * significant main substance effect. PLAC: placebo; CAF-3: caffeine 3mg/kg/b.m; CAF-6: caffeine 6mg/kg/b.m.

Post hoc analyses for main effect of substance indicated significant increases in MP ($p < 0.01$; ES = 0.14) and MV ($p = 0.01$; ES = 0.78) in BPT (mean of the 5 sets) after the intake of CAF-3 compared to PLAC as well as significant increases in MP ($p = 0.01$; ES = 0.13) and MV ($p = 0.01$; ES = 0.72) in the BPT (mean of the 5 sets) after the intake of CAF-6 compared to PLAC. There were no significant differences in MP and MV between the two doses of CAF (CAF-3 vs. CAF-6). The results of particular sets in MP, MV, PP, and PV as well ES between PLAC and CAF-3, CAF-6 in each set are presented in Table 2.

Table 2. Power output and bar velocity during 5 sets of the bench press throw with the ingestion of 3 and 6 mg/kg/b.m. of caffeine or with a placebo.

	Conditions	Set 1	Set 2	Set 3	Set 4	Set 5
			Mean Power (W)			
	PLAC	542 ± 126	548 ± 119	551 ± 117	543 ± 115	540 ± 114
	(95%CI)	(462 to 622)	(472 to 623)	(477 to 626)	(470 to 616)	(468 to 613)
	CAF-3	552 ± 124	564 ± 115	567 ± 116	557 ± 112	570 ± 124
	(95%CI)	(473 to 631)	(490 to 637)	(493 to 640)	(486 to 628)	(492 to 649)
	CAF-6	559 ± 109	563 ± 107	562 ± 113	556 ± 103	562 ± 105
	(95%CI)	(489 to 628)	(495 to 631)	(489 to 634)	(491 to 621)	(496 to 629)
ES	PLAC vs. CAF-3	0.07	0.14	0.14	0.12	0.25
	PLAC vs. CAF-6	0.14	0.13	0.09	0.12	0.20
			Peak Power (W)			
	PLAC	1245 ± 248	1252 ± 291	1286 ± 378	1244 ± 252	1222 ± 250
	(95%CI)	(1088 to 1402)	(1067 to 1437)	(1045 to 1526)	(1083 to 1404)	(1063 to 1381)
	CAF-3	1243 ± 218	1252 ± 265	1285 ± 216	1241 ± 199	1283 ± 224
	(95%CI)	(1105 to 1382)	(1084 to 1420)	(1147 to 1422)	(1114 to 1368)	(1141 to 1425)
	CAF-6	1253 ± 294	1338 ± 362	1338 ± 344	1278 ± 255	1278 ± 250
	(95%CI)	(1066 to 1440)	(1107 to 1568)	(1119 to 1556)	(1116 to 1440)	(1119 to 1437)
ES	PLAC vs. CAF-3	0.01	0.00	0.01	0.01	0.26
	PLAC vs. CAF-6	0.03	0.26	0.14	0.13	0.22
			Mean Velocity (m/s)			
	PLAC	1.36 ± 0.06	1.38 ± 0.08	1.38 ± 0.05	1.37 ± 0.04	1.36 ± 0.07
	(95%CI)	(1.32 to 1.40)	(1.33 to 1.43)	(1.35 to 1.41)	(1.35 to 1.41)	(1.32 to 1.40)
	CAF-3	1.39 ± 0.07	1.42 ± 0.05	1.43 ± 0.05	1.40 ± 0.05	1.43 ± 0.05
	(95%CI)	(1.34 to 1.43)	(1.39 to 1.45)	(1.40 to 1.46)	(1.37 to 1.43)	(1.40 to 1.46)
	CAF-6	1.41 ± 0.07	1.42 ± 0.07	1.41 ± 0.05	1.40 ± 0.07	1.42 ± 0.09
	(95%CI)	(1.36 to 1.45)	(1.37 to 1.47)	(1.38 to 1.45)	(1.35 to 1.44)	(1.37 to 1.47)
ES	PLAC vs. CAF-3	0.46	0.60	1.0	0.40	1.15
	PLAC vs. CAF-6	0.77	0.60	0.6	0.33	0.77
			Peak Velocity (m/s)			
	PLAC	2.13 ± 0.08	2.15 ± 0.11	2.17 ± 0.13	2.15 ± 0.12	2.10 ± 0.14
	(95%CI)	(2.08 to 2.18)	(2.08 to 2.22)	(2.09 to 2.26)	(2.07 to 2.22)	(2.01 to 2.19)
	CAF-3	2.14 ± 0.08	2.17 ± 0.07	2.18 ± 0.09	2.14 ± 0.05	2.19 ± 0.08
	(95%CI)	(2.09 to 2.18)	(2.12 to 2.22)	(2.12 to 2.24)	(2.11 to 2.17)	(2.14 to 2.25)
	CAF-6	2.16 ± 0.12	2.18 ± 0.13	2.19 ± 0.14	2.17 ± 0.14	2.17 ± 0.17
	(95%CI)	(2.08 to 2.23)	(2.10 to 2.26)	(2.10 to 2.28)	(2.09 to 2.26)	(2.06 to 2.28)
ES	PLAC vs. CAF-3	0.13	0.22	0.09	0.11	0.79
	PLAC vs. CAF-6	0.29	0.25	0.15	0.15	0.45

All data are presented as mean ± standard deviation. CI: confidence interval. ES: effect size.

Figures 2 and 3 represent the individual responses induced by CAF-3 and CAF-6, in comparison to the placebo, for MP and MV. The 11 out of 12 participants showed an increase in MP and MV after the ingestion of CAF-3, while CAF-6 produced higher values for MP and MV in 10 out of 12 participants.

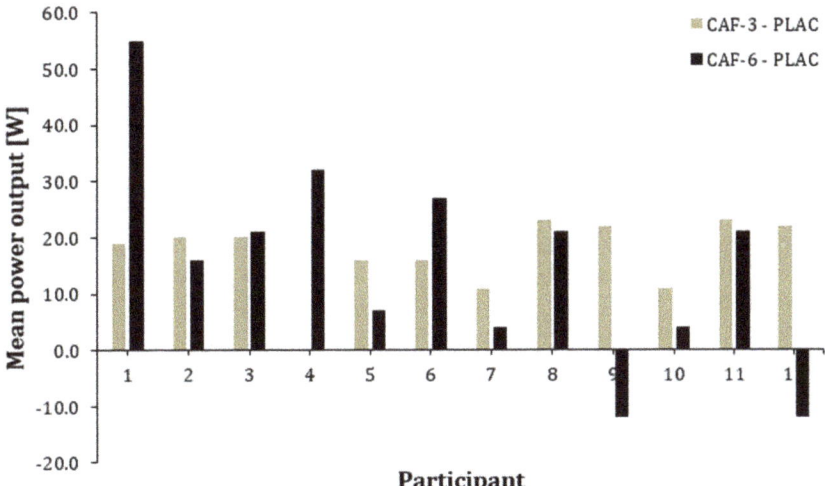

Figure 2. Individual differences in mean power output during 5 sets of bench press throw (BPT) between caffeine and placebo conditions.

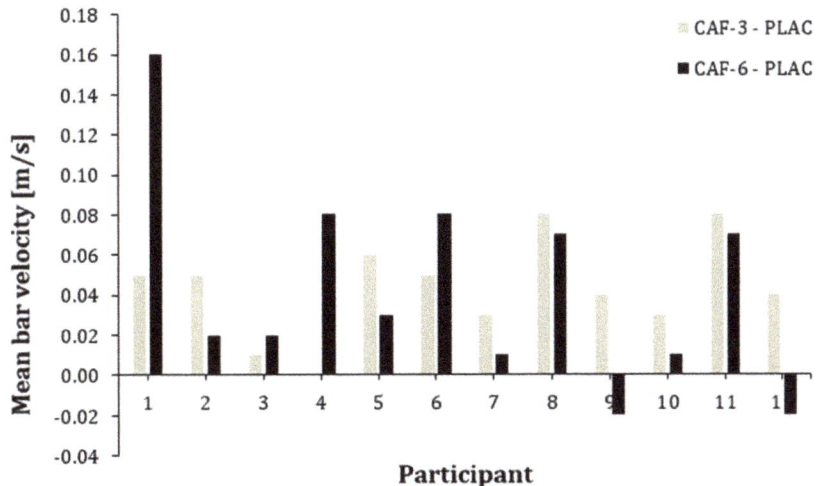

Figure 3. Individual differences in mean bar velocity during 5 sets of bench press throw (BPT) between caffeine and placebo conditions.

The y-axis represents the difference in mean bar velocity output during the 5 sets of BPT between PLAC–CAF-3; PLAC–CAF-6 for each individual.

4. Discussion

The main finding of this study was that acute CAF intake has a positive effect on MP and MV during a training session of the BPT performed at 30% 1 RM. Interestingly, both 3 and 6 mg/kg/b.m. doses of

CAF had similar effectiveness in enhancing performance when compared to PLAC. Additionally, the ergogenic effect of CAF on MP and MV was evident in most of participants, as all of them responded by improving performance with either CAF-3 or CAF-6, even when they were catalogued as individuals habituated to CAF (Figures 2 and 3). However, the study did not show significant changes in PP and PV after CAF intake with either dose of CAF (3 and 6 mg/kg/b.m.) compared to PLAC. These outcomes suggest that acute CAF intake in a moderate dose (from 3 to 6 mg/kg/b.m.) is effective in increasing mean power and bar velocity during the BPT without a significant influence on peak values of these variables. These results suggest that CAF can be effectively used to acutely improve this power-specific training routine even with individuals habituated to CAF, although the long-term training effects with CAF should be further investigated.

The y-axis represents the difference in mean power output during the 5 sets of BPT between PLAC–CAF-3; PLAC–CAF-6 for each individual.

Previous research showed that acute CAF intake increases power output during the bench press exercise [8,14–16]. However, most of these studies included only one set of the exercise which is not the habitual practice during sports training, where several sets of a particular exercise are performed in order to obtain significant adaptations derived from training. In presented study, the main effect of increase in MP and MV after the intake of CAF-3 and CAF-6 over the placebo has occurred for training session consisting several sets (Table 2). The ergogenic effect of CAF observed during the BPT is partly consistent with the results of previous findings [8,16]. However, it should be emphasized that this is the first study investigating the effects of CAF during a training session that includes several sets of a ballistic exercise. Experimental procedures with the use of CAF in which more than one set of an upper body exercise are used are scarce [18,53,54]. The study of Lane and Byrd [53] showed that the intake of 300 mg of CAF, representing 3.5 mg/kg/b.m. increased peak velocity during 10 sets of the bench press exercise at 80% 1 RM compared to PLAC. Wilk et al. [18] did not show significant changes after the intake of different doses of CAF (3, 6, and 9 mg/kg/b.m.) in both, mean and peak power output and bar velocity during the BP exercise at 50% 1 RM (3 sets of 5 repetitions), although this investigation was carried out in athletes habituated to CAF. No changes in mean and peak bar velocity after CAF intake of 150 mg, representing 1.74 mg/kg/b.m. were observed in a study by Lane et al. [54] where 10 sets of 3 repetitions of the bench press exercise were performed at 80% 1 RM. The current study is quite innovative because it is the first investigation geared to assess the effects of CAF intake on power output by using a ballistic upper body exercise with a low external load (30% 1 RM), geared for power training of athletes [55]. The current state of the literature, indicates that CAF is useful in increasing power during one or multiple sets of the bench press exercise when the dose ingested is >3 mg/kg/b.m., but it seems particularly effective when using low and moderate loads during an explosive exercise, such as the BPT.

The overall increase of MP and MV during the training session of the BPT after ingestion of CAF-3 and CAF-6 can be also attributed to increased pre-exercise central excitability. Specifically, the pre-exercise ingestion of CAF would allow the athletes to maintain a certain amount of force even in the presence of biochemical changes within the working muscle that lead to fatigue [3]. Under this theory, CAF intake would allow a higher physical performance because it would help to maintain the neural response even in the presence of metabolic perturbations such as low muscle pH. This effect may be accompanied by reductions in interstitial potassium accumulation found after CAF intake [2], that ultimately leads to the maintenance of excitability during exercise [33,56]. In the central nervous system (CNS), CAF binds to adenosine receptors that influence the release of neurotransmitters, such as noradrenaline and acetylcholine [4,57–59] and consequently, increase muscle tension [60]. However, in the current investigation, this purported effect of CAF on CNS was not sufficient to enhance PP and PV during the BPT at 30% 1 RM. Thus, reduced fatigue through CAF-induced modulation of both peripheral and central neural processes may explain the obtained results and higher MP and MV of the bar during the BPT training session. Nevertheless, the association of the ergogenic effect with the mechanisms that allowed this ergogenic effect is speculative at this moment because no measurements were carried out to test the origin of caffeine's ergogenic effects.

It should be taken into consideration that the study participants in the current study were habitual CAF users. In contrast, most of the investigations aimed at determination of the ergogenic effect of CAF on muscle performance have selected individuals unhabituated to this stimulant or with low-to-moderate daily consumption of CAF (e.g., from 58 to 250 mg/day), [11,16,34], to avoid the effects that tolerance to CAF may. However, CAF is an ergogenic aid frequently used in training and competition and it is likely that some athletes seeking for ergogenic benefits of CAF are already habituated to this substance due to the chronic use of caffeine-containing supplements during training and competition. In fact, previous investigations have suggested that between 75% and 90% of athletes use CAF in competitive and training settings [35,36,61], suggesting that studies on the effect of acute CAF intake on physical performance during real training and competition settings are particularly important in athletes habituated to CAF. In this respect, previous research using well-controlled CAF treatments has suggested that the habitual intake of this stimulant may progressively reduce its ergogenic effect on exercise performance [42,62] and then, it has been speculated that the ergogenic effect of CAF could be dampened in habitual CAF users.

To the authors' knowledge, only three previous studies analyzed power output of the upper limbs in a group of participants habituated to CAF [9,18–20]. The study of Sabol et al. [9] showed an increase in medicine ball throwing distance after the acute intake of 6 mg/kg/b.m. of CAF but the doses of 2 and 4 mg/kg/b.m. did not show any differences with the PLAC. The study by Wilk et al. [18] did not show increases in power output and bar velocity during the bench press exercise in high habitual CAF users that ingested from 3 to 9 mg/kg/b.m. Although it has been theorized that the reduction in the ergogenic effects of CAF in habitual users can be modified using doses greater than the daily habitual intake [63], previous investigations indicate that athletes habituated to CAF do not benefit from the acute ingestion of CAF in doses above their habitual intake while the prevalence of side effects is greatly increased [19,20]. Interestingly, participants in the presented study self-reported their daily ingestion of CAF, which amounted to 5.0 ± 0.95 mg/kg/b.m., (443 ± 142 mg of CAF per day), and the acute CAF doses (especially CAF-3) and some performance enhancements were obtained even when de dose of CAF did not exceed the value of habitual consumption. In any case, although the current investigation found a positive effect of CAF on mean power output and mean bar velocity during the BPT in athletes habituated to CAF, it is still possible that the effect of this substance is higher in unhabituated individuals.

In addition to its strengths, the current study presents limitations that should be addressed. Although the results showed a significant main effect on MP and MV after CAF intake, the direct causes of these changes cannot be determined and explained. The study did not include biochemical analysis which could explain the obtained results. In addition, blood samples were not obtained and thus, we have no data about serum CAF concentrations with each of the dosages of CAF employed in this investigation. Further, we did not analyze the genetic intolerance on CAF in the tested subjects. However, the participants of this study did not report any side effects after consuming CAF in the six months prior to the experiment. Due to the fact that the response to CAF is related to the individual tolerance of this substance [42], the dose [19,20], and gender [64] therefore the results of this study should only be translated to males habituated to CAF who use low to moderate CAF doses to enhance performance. Another limitation of the study was that the 1 RM test was performed using the barbell bench press exercise while the BPT was performed on a Smith machine during the experimental trials to increase the security of participants and investigators. Although there is a high transfer between the results obtained in both types of exercise, the calculation of loading would be more reliable if both evaluations were performed on the same resistance exercise. In any case, this limitation did not affect the outcomes of the investigation because the load was the same for all experimental trials.

5. Conclusions

The results of the present study indicate that acute doses of CAF, between 3 and 6 mg/kg/b.m., ingested before the onset of an explosive resistance exercise produced an overall effect on mean power output and mean bar velocity during a BPT training session in a group of habitual CAF users. The main effect in mean power and bar velocity was found in several sets during the trial which may indicate that the use of CAF was effective in increasing performance in the whole training session. In contrast, no significant changes were observed for peak power output and peak bar velocity. These results suggest that the ingestion of CAF prior to ballistic exercise can enhance the outcomes of resistance training. However, the results of our study refer only to power output and bar velocity of the upper limbs during the BPT with an external load of 30% 1 RM and further investigations should consider the effect of CAF with different loads or the use of lower-body exercises.

Author Contributions: Data curation, M.W., A.F., M.K., and M.G.; formal analysis, M.W., A.F.; investigation, M.W., A.F., M.K., and M.G.; methodology, M.W. and A.F.; project administration, A.F., M.K., and M.G.; software, A.F., M.K., and M.G.; supervision, M.W., A.Z., and J.D.C.; writing—original draft, M.W., A.F., M.K., and J.D.C.; writing—review and editing, M.W., A.Z., and J.D.C. All authors have read and agreed to the published version of the manuscript.

Funding: This study would not have been possible without our participants' commitment, time and effort. The study was supported and funded by the statutory research of the Jerzy Kukuczka Academy of Physical Education in Katowice, Poland.

Conflicts of Interest: The authors declare that they have no conflicts of interest.

References

1. Maughan, R.J.; Burke, L.M.; Dvorak, J.; Larson-Meyer, D.E.; Peeling, P.; Phillips, S.M.; Rawson, E.S.; Walsh, N.P.; Garthe, I.; Geyer, H.; et al. IOC Consensus Statement: Dietary Supplements and the High-Performance Athlete. *Int. J. Sport Nutr. Exerc. Metab.* **2018**, *28*, 104–125. [CrossRef] [PubMed]
2. Shushakov, V.; Stubbe, C.; Peuckert, A.; Endeward, V.; Maassen, N. The relationships between plasma potassium, muscle excitability and fatigue during voluntary exercise in humans: Plasma potassium, muscle excitability and fatigue in humans. *Exp. Physiol.* **2007**, *92*, 705–715. [CrossRef] [PubMed]
3. Bowtell, J.L.; Mohr, M.; Fulford, J.; Jackman, S.R.; Ermidis, G.; Krustrup, P.; Mileva, K.N. Improved Exercise Tolerance with Caffeine Is Associated with Modulation of both Peripheral and Central Neural Processes in Human Participants. *Front. Nutr.* **2018**, *5*, 6. [CrossRef] [PubMed]
4. Davis, J.M.; Zhao, Z.; Stock, H.S.; Mehl, K.A.; Buggy, J.; Hand, G.A. Central nervous system effects of caffeine and adenosine on fatigue. *Am. J. Physiol. Regul. Integr. Comp. Physiol.* **2003**, *284*, R399–R404. [CrossRef]
5. Elmenhorst, D.; Meyer, P.T.; Matusch, A.; Winz, O.H.; Bauer, A. Caffeine occupancy of human cerebral A1 adenosine receptors: In vivo quantification with 18F-CPFPX and PET. *J. Nucl. Med.* **2012**, *53*, 1723–1729. [CrossRef]
6. Grgic, J.; Grgic, I.; Pickering, C.; Schoenfeld, B.J.; Bishop, D.J.; Pedisic, Z. Wake up and smell the coffee: Caffeine supplementation and exercise performance—An umbrella review of 21 published meta-analyses. *Br. J. Sports Med..* in press. [CrossRef]
7. Grgic, J.; Trexler, E.T.; Lazinica, B.; Pedisic, Z. Effects of caffeine intake on muscle strength and power: A systematic review and meta-analysis. *J. Int. Soc. Sports Nutr.* **2018**, *15*, 11. [CrossRef]
8. Pallarés, J.G.; Fernández-Elías, V.E.; Ortega, J.F.; Muñoz, G.; Muñoz-Guerra, J.; Mora-Rodríguez, R. Neuromuscular Responses to Incremental Caffeine Doses: Performance and Side Effects. *Med. Sci. Sport Exer.* **2013**, *45*, 2184–2192. [CrossRef]
9. Sabol, F.; Grgic, J.; Mikulic, P. The Effects of 3 Different Doses of Caffeine on Jumping and Throwing Performance: A Randomized, Double-Blind, Crossover Study. *Int. J. Sports Physiol. Perform.* **2019**, *14*, 1170–1177. [CrossRef]
10. Tallis, J.; Yavuz, H.C.M. The effects of low and moderate doses of caffeine supplementation on upper and lower body maximal voluntary concentric and eccentric muscle force. *Appl. Physiol. Nutr. Metab.* **2018**, *43*, 274–281. [CrossRef]

11. Astorino, T.A.; Rohmann, R.L.; Firth, K. Effect of caffeine ingestion on one-repetition maximum muscular strength. *Eur. J. Appl. Physiol.* **2007**, *102*, 127–132. [CrossRef] [PubMed]
12. Forbes, S.C.; Candow, D.G.; Little, J.P.; Magnus, C.; Chilibeck, P.D. Effect of Red Bull energy drink on repeated Wingate cycle performance and bench-press muscle endurance. *Int. J. Sport Nutr. Exerc. Metab.* **2007**, *17*, 433–444. [CrossRef] [PubMed]
13. Williams, A.D.; Cribb, P.J.; Cooke, M.B.; Hayes, A. The effect of ephedra and caffeine on maximal strength and power in resistance-trained athletes. *J. Strength Cond. Res.* **2008**, *22*, 464–470. [CrossRef] [PubMed]
14. Venier, S.; Grgic, J.; Mikulic, P. Caffeinated Gel Ingestion Enhances Jump Performance, Muscle Strength, and Power in Trained Men. *Nutrients* **2019**, *11*, 937. [CrossRef] [PubMed]
15. Astley, C.; Souza, D.B.; Polito, M.D. Acute Specific Effects of Caffeine-containing Energy Drink on Different Physical Performances in Resistance-trained Men. *Int. J. Exerc. Sci.* **2018**, *11*, 260–268. [PubMed]
16. Grgic, J.; Mikulic, P. Caffeine ingestion acutely enhances muscular strength and power but not muscular endurance in resistance-trained men. *Eur. J. Sport Sci.* **2017**, *17*, 1029–1036. [CrossRef] [PubMed]
17. Del Coso, J.; Salinero, J.J.; González-Millán, C.; Abián-Vicén, J.; Pérez-González, B. Dose response effects of a caffeine-containing energy drink on muscle performance: A repeated measures design. *J. Int. Soc. Sports Nutr.* **2012**, *9*, 21. [CrossRef]
18. Wilk, M.; Filip, A.; Krzysztofik, M.; Maszczyk, A.; Zajac, A. The Acute Effect of Various Doses of Caffeine on Power Output and Velocity during the Bench Press Exercise among Athletes Habitually Using Caffeine. *Nutrients* **2019**, *11*, 1465. [CrossRef]
19. Wilk, M.; Krzysztofik, M.; Filip, A.; Zajac, A.; Del Coso, J. The Effects of High Doses of Caffeine on Maximal Strength and Muscular Endurance in Athletes Habituated to Caffeine. *Nutrients* **2019**, *11*, 1912. [CrossRef]
20. Wilk, M.; Krzysztofik, M.; Filip, A.; Zajac, A.; Del Coso, J. Correction: Wilk et al. "The Effects of High Doses of Caffeine on Maximal Strength and Muscular Endurance in Athletes Habituated to Caffeine." *Nutrients* **2019**, *11*, 1912. *Nutrients* **2019**, *11*, 2660. [CrossRef]
21. Stastny, P.; Golas, A.; Blazek, D.; Maszczyk, A.; Wilk, M.; Pietraszewski, P.; Petr, M.; Uhlir, P.; Zajac, A. A systematic review of surface electromyography analyses of the bench press movement task. *PLoS ONE* **2017**, *12*, e0171632. [CrossRef]
22. Wilk, M.; Golas, A.; Stastny, P.; Nawrocka, M.; Krzysztofik, M.; Zajac, A. Does Tempo of Resistance Exercise Impact Training Volume? *J. Hum. Kinet.* **2018**, *62*, 241–250. [CrossRef]
23. Cormie, P.; McGuigan, M.R.; Newton, R.U. Developing Maximal Neuromuscular Power: Part 1—Biological Basis of Maximal Power Production. *Sports Med.* **2011**, *41*, 17–38. [CrossRef]
24. Newton, R.U.; Kraemer, W.J.; Häkkinen, K.; Humphries, B.J.; Murphy, A.J. Kinematics, Kinetics, and Muscle Activation during Explosive Upper Body Movements. *J. Appl. Biomech.* **1996**, *12*, 31–43. [CrossRef]
25. Samozino, P.; Rejc, E.; Di Prampero, P.E.; Belli, A.; Morin, J.-B. Optimal Force–Velocity Profile in Ballistic Movements—Altius. *Med. Sci. Sport Exer.* **2012**, *44*, 313–322. [CrossRef]
26. Baker, D. Comparison of upper-body strength and power between professional and college-aged rugby league players. *J. Strength Cond. Res.* **2001**, *15*, 30–35.
27. Cronin, J.B.; Owen, G.J. Upper-Body Strength and Power Assessment in Women Using a Chest Pass. *J. Strength Cond. Res.* **2004**, *18*, 401.
28. Liossis, L.D.; Forsyth, J.; Liossis, C.; Tsolakis, C. The Acute Effect of Upper-Body Complex Training on Power Output of Martial Art Athletes as Measured by the Bench Press Throw Exercise. *J. Hum. Kinet.* **2013**, *39*, 167–175. [CrossRef]
29. Terzis, G.; Georgiadis, G.; Vassiliadou, E.; Manta, P. Relationship between shot put performance and triceps brachii fiber type composition and power production. *Eur. J. Appl. Physiol.* **2003**, *90*, 10–15. [CrossRef]
30. Sarabia, J.M.; Moya-Ramón, M.; Hernández-Davó, J.L.; Fernandez-Fernandez, J.; Sabido, R. The effects of training with loads that maximise power output and individualised repetitions vs. traditional power training. *PLoS ONE* **2017**, *12*, e0186601. [CrossRef]
31. Burke, L.M. Practical Issues in Evidence-Based Use of Performance Supplements: Supplement Interactions, Repeated Use and Individual Responses. *Sports Med.* **2017**, *47*, 79–100. [CrossRef]
32. Wilk, M.; Krzysztofik, M.; Maszczyk, A.; Chycki, J.; Zajac, A. The acute effects of caffeine intake on time under tension and power generated during the bench press movement. *J. Int. Soc. Sports Nutr.* **2019**, *16*, 8. [CrossRef]

33. Mohr, M.; Nielsen, J.J.; Bangsbo, J. Caffeine intake improves intense intermittent exercise performance and reduces muscle interstitial potassium accumulation. *J. Appl. Physiol.* **2011**, *111*, 1372–1379. [CrossRef]
34. Duncan, M.J.; Oxford, S.W. The Effect of Caffeine Ingestion on Mood State and Bench Press Performance to Failure. *J. Strength Cond. Res.* **2011**, *25*, 178–185. [CrossRef]
35. Del Coso, J.; Muñoz, G.; Muñoz-Guerra, J. Prevalence of caffeine use in elite athletes following its removal from the World Anti-Doping Agency list of banned substances. *Appl. Physiol. Nutr. Metab.* **2011**, *36*, 555–561. [CrossRef]
36. Aguilar-Navarro, M.; Muñoz, G.; Salinero, J.; Muñoz-Guerra, J.; Fernández-Álvarez, M.; Plata, M.; Del Coso, J. Urine Caffeine Concentration in Doping Control Samples from 2004 to 2015. *Nutrients* **2019**, *11*, 286. [CrossRef]
37. Svenningsson, P.; Nomikos, G.G.; Fredholm, B.B. The stimulatory action and the development of tolerance to caffeine is associated with alterations in gene expression in specific brain regions. *J. Neurosci.* **1999**, *19*, 4011–4022. [CrossRef]
38. Fredholm, B.B.; Bäättig, K.; Holmén, J.; Nehlig, A.; Zvartau, E.E. Actions of caffeine in the brain with special reference to factors that contribute to its widespread use. *Pharmacol. Rev.* **1999**, *51*, 83–133.
39. Dodd, S.L.; Brooks, E.; Powers, S.K.; Tulley, R. The effects of caffeine on graded exercise performance in caffeine naive versus habituated subjects. *Eur. J. Appl. Physiol. Occup. Physiol.* **1991**, *62*, 424–429. [CrossRef]
40. de Souza Gonçalves, L.; de Salles Painelli, V.; Yamaguchi, G.; de Oliveira, L.F.; Saunders, B.; da Silva, R.P.; Maciel, E.; Artioli, G.G.; Roschel, H.; Gualano, B. Dispelling the myth that habitual caffeine consumption influences the performance response to acute caffeine supplementation. *J. Appl. Physiol.* **2017**, *123*, 213–220. [CrossRef]
41. Bell, D.G.; McLellan, T.M. Exercise endurance 1, 3, and 6 h after caffeine ingestion in caffeine users and nonusers. *J. Appl. Physiol.* **2002**, *93*, 1227–1234. [CrossRef] [PubMed]
42. Lara, B.; Ruiz-Moreno, C.; Salinero, J.J.; Del Coso, J. Time course of tolerance to the performance benefits of caffeine. *PLoS ONE* **2019**, *14*, e0210275. [CrossRef] [PubMed]
43. Ruiz-Moreno, C.; Lara, B.; Salinero, J.J.; Brito de Souza, D.; Ordovás, J.M.; Del Coso, J. Time course of tolerance to adverse effects associated with the ingestion of a moderate dose of caffeine. *Eur. J. Nutr.* **2020**, *2010*, 1–10. [CrossRef]
44. García-Ramos, A.; Padial, P.; García-Ramos, M.; Conde-Pipó, J.; Argüelles-Cienfuegos, J.; Štirn, I.; Feriche, B. Reliability Analysis of Traditional and Ballistic Bench Press Exercises at Different Loads. *J. Hum. Kinet.* **2015**, *47*, 51–59. [CrossRef]
45. Marques, M.C.; van den Tillaar, R.; Vescovi, J.D.; González-Badillo, J.J. Relationship Between Throwing Velocity, Muscle Power, and Bar Velocity During Bench Press in Elite Handball Players. *Int. J. Sports Physiol. Perform.* **2007**, *2*, 414–422. [CrossRef]
46. Teixeira, V.; Voci, S.M.; Mendes-Netto, R.S.; da Silva, D.G. The relative validity of a food record using the smartphone application MyFitnessPal: Relative validity of a smartphone dietary record. *Nutr. Diet.* **2018**, *75*, 219–225. [CrossRef]
47. Bühler, E.; Lachenmeier, D.W.; Winkler, G. Development of a tool to assess caffeine intake among teenagers and young adults. *Ernahrungs. Umschau.* **2014**, *61*, 58–63.
48. Frankowski, M.; Kowalski, A.; Ociepa, A.; Siepak, J.; Niedzielski, P. Caffeine levels in various caffeine-rich and decaffeinated coffee grades and coffee extracts marketed in Poland. *Bromat. Chem. Toksykol.* **2008**, *1*, 21–27.
49. Burke, L.M. Caffeine and sports performance. *Appl. Physiol. Nutr. Metab.* **2008**, *33*, 1319–1334. [CrossRef]
50. SELF Nutrition Data. Available online: https://nutritiondata.self.com/ (accessed on 2 April 2019).
51. García-Ramos, A.; Pestaña-Melero, F.L.; Pérez-Castilla, A.; Rojas, F.J.; Haff, G.G. Differences in the Load–Velocity Profile Between 4 Bench-Press Variants. *Int. J. Sports Physiol. Perform.* **2018**, *13*, 326–331. [CrossRef]
52. Cohen, J. *Statistical Power Analysis for the Behavioral Sciences*, 2nd ed.; Routledge: New York, NY, USA, 2013.
53. Lane, M.; Byrd, M. Effects of Pre-Workout Supplements on Power Maintenance in Lower Body and Upper Body Tasks. *JFMK* **2018**, *3*, 11. [CrossRef]
54. Lane, M.T.; Byrd, M.T.; Bell, Z.; Hurley, T. Effects of Supplementation of a Pre-workout on Power Maintenance in Lower Body and Upper Body Tasks in Women. *JFMK* **2019**, *4*, 18. [CrossRef]

55. Cormie, P.; McGuigan, M.R.; Newton, R.U. Developing maximal neuromuscular power: Part 2—training considerations for improving maximal power production. *Sports Med.* **2011**, *41*, 125–146. [CrossRef]
56. Fortune, E.; Lowery, M.M. Effect of Extracellular Potassium Accumulation on Muscle Fiber Conduction Velocity: A Simulation Study. *Ann. Biomed. Eng.* **2009**, *37*, 2105–2117. [CrossRef]
57. Daly, J.W.; Shi, D.; Nikodijevic, O.; Jacobson, K.A. The role of adenosine receptors in the central action of caffeine. *Pharmacopsychoecologia* **1994**, *7*, 201–213.
58. Goldstein, E.R.; Ziegenfuss, T.; Kalman, D.; Kreider, R.; Campbell, B.; Wilborn, C.; Taylor, L.; Willoughby, D.; Stout, J.; Graves, B.S.; et al. International society of sports nutrition position stand: Caffeine and performance. *J. Int. Soc. Sports Nutr.* **2010**, *7*, 5. [CrossRef]
59. Ferré, S. Mechanisms of the psychostimulant effects of caffeine: Implications for substance use disorders. *Psychopharmacology* **2016**, *233*, 1963–1979. [CrossRef]
60. Behrens, M.; Mau-Moeller, A.; Weippert, M.; Fuhrmann, J.; Wegner, K.; Skripitz, R.; Bader, R.; Bruhn, S. Caffeine-induced increase in voluntary activation and strength of the quadriceps muscle during isometric, concentric and eccentric contractions. *Sci. Rep.* **2015**, *5*, 10209. [CrossRef]
61. Desbrow, B.; Leveritt, M. Awareness and Use of Caffeine by Athletes Competing at the 2005 Ironman Triathlon World Championships. *Int. J. Sport Nutr. Exerc. Metab.* **2006**, *16*, 545–558. [CrossRef]
62. Beaumont, R.; Cordery, P.; Funnell, M.; Mears, S.; James, L.; Watson, P. Chronic ingestion of a low dose of caffeine induces tolerance to the performance benefits of caffeine. *J. Sports Sci.* **2017**, *35*, 1920–1927. [CrossRef]
63. Pickering, C.; Kiely, J. Are the Current Guidelines on Caffeine Use in Sport Optimal for Everyone? Inter-individual Variation in Caffeine Ergogenicity, and a Move Towards Personalised Sports Nutrition. *Sports Med.* **2018**, *48*, 7–16. [CrossRef] [PubMed]
64. Mielgo-Ayuso, J.; Marques-Jiménez, D.; Refoyo, I.; Del Coso, J.; León-Guereño, P.; Calleja-González, J. Effect of Caffeine Supplementation on Sports Performance Based on Differences Between Sexes: A Systematic Review. *Nutrients* **2019**, *11*, 2313. [CrossRef] [PubMed]

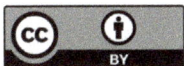

© 2020 by the authors. Licensee MDPI, Basel, Switzerland. This article is an open access article distributed under the terms and conditions of the Creative Commons Attribution (CC BY) license (http://creativecommons.org/licenses/by/4.0/).

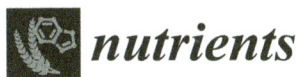 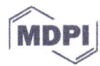

Article

Eurycoma longifolia—Infused Coffee—An Oral Toxicity Study

Norzahirah Ahmad *, Bee Ping Teh, Siti Zaleha Halim, Nor Azlina Zolkifli, Nurulfariza Ramli and Hussin Muhammad

Herbal Medicine Research Centre, Institute for Medical Research, National Institutes of Health, Ministry of Health Malaysia, Setia Alam, Shah Alam 40170, Malaysia; bpteh_km@yahoo.com (B.P.T.); ctzaleha.h2@gmail.com (S.Z.H.); azlina.zolkifli@moh.gov.my (N.A.Z.); nurulfariza.r@moh.gov.my (N.R.); hussin.m@moh.gov.my (H.M.)
* Correspondence: norzahirah.a@moh.gov.my

Received: 10 August 2020; Accepted: 31 August 2020; Published: 13 October 2020

Abstract: Coffee infused with the additive *Eurycoma longifolia*, also known as Tongkat ali (TA), has become widely available in the Malaysian market. Safety evaluations for consumption of the products have been called for due to the herbal addition. This study investigates the acute, subacute and chronic effects of a commercial TA coffee in Sprague Dawley rats when given in a single, repeated and prolonged dosage. The dosages of 0.005, 0.05, 0.30 and 2 g/kg body weight (BW) were used in the acute study and 0.14, 0.29 and 1 g/kg BW were used in the repeated dose studies. The in-life parameters measured were food and water intake, body weight and clinical observations. Blood were collected for hematology and clinical biochemistry analyses. All animals were subjected to full necropsies. Non-toxicity-related changes were observed in the food and water consumption parameters. Body weight showed normal increments and none of the animals had any clinical signs of toxicity. Microscopically assessed organ tissues did not reveal any abnormalities. There was significant decrease of platelet count in all the chronic study male treated groups. Significant elevation of renal profile parameters in both gender groups given 0.29 g/kg BW, along with liver and lipid profile elevation in some female groups of the chronic study were noted. No dose-dependent relationship was apparent in the dosage range tested, though these changes may suggest an initial safety indication to the TA coffee. The study concludes that the no observed adverse effect level (NOAEL) for this commercial TA coffee was 1 g/kg BW.

Keywords: *Eurycoma longifolia*; Tongkat ali; toxicity; infused coffee; herbal additives

1. Introduction

Eurycoma longifolia, also known as Tongkat ali (TA), is a native plant to Southeast Asian rain forests. The roots are believed to boost wellness while having aphrodisiac, anti-malarial and other therapeutic properties, such as anti-inflammatory and anti-osteoporosis [1–8]. TA has received considerable attention among Malaysian consumers and is traditionally processed into a drink, although coffee makers also tout it as a healthy additive in coffee drinks. Safety information such as the no observed adverse effect level (NOAEL) for *E. longifolia* in its aqueous extract form has been previously reported to be more than 3 g/kg in mice [9] and more than 1 g/kg and 5 g/kg in rats in two separate studies [10,11], while the powdered form of the root was reported to have an acute limit dose of more than 6 g/kg [12]. Although these studies reported a high tolerance of the highest dose used, they also reported hydropic liver histology indicating hepatotoxicity [11] and minor yet significant hematology and clinical biochemistry changes [10,12]. Additionally, information for TA extract long-term consumption is limited and its use as an herbal additive in food products has never been evaluated and warrants further investigation.

Worldwide, the legislation with regards to beverages with herbal additives varies between countries [13], whereas currently in Malaysia, safety testing for food products in this category has not been accounted under the Food Act (1983), Ministry of Health, Malaysia and Food Regulation (1985), Ministry of Health, Malaysia [14,15]. While there have been no claims of ill health and the existing legislation in Malaysia does not require safety testing for using *E. longifolia* extracts in coffee, the World Health Organization (2004) recommends herbal medicinal ingredients in products to be assessed for its safety [16]. Furthermore, the addition of therapeutically claimed traditional ingredients have clouded the definitions between the food and drug regulations. It is often unclear which testing standards are required and the sets of regulations to abide by for the herbal additives in food products [17–19]. Consequently, without safety testing, marketing of such coffee outside of Malaysia is restricted due to strict import regulations with various levels of evidence requirements.

Safety testing adds value to the product, elevates the product safety information, improve consumer trust and may prevent potential incidents such as interaction between pharmaceutical drugs and herbal-incorporated food products, where occurrence may have gone unnoticed [17,18,20,21]. The aim of this paper is to investigate the safety of a commercial TA coffee, with reference to the Organization for Economic Cooperation and Development (OECD) testing guidelines 420, 407 and 452 [22–24]. The TA coffee was administered to Sprague Dawley rats in a single-dose 14-day acute study and as a repeated daily dose for 28 days and 6 months in the subacute and chronic toxicity studies, respectively.

2. Materials and Methods

2.1. Test and Reference Item Preparation

The commercial GTHerb Gold Coffee *E. longifolia*-mixed coffee was provided by GTHerb Industries Sdn. Bhd. Analysis of the content was done by Als Technician and Technology Park Malaysia, Biotech Sdn. Bhd. (Kuala Lumpur, Malaysia). The TA coffee (test item) was physically in powdered form and dark brown in color. Prior to the daily preparation, the test item was kept at temperatures between 25 and 28 °C. The test item prepared was calculated based on the individual rat's body weight and according to the required dosage. The test item for rats weighing less than 100 g was dissolved in 1 mL hot distilled water, whereas for rats weighing 200 g and above, 2 mL of hot distilled water was used. The reference item (distilled water) was administered in the same manner. The administered amount of test item was adjusted weekly to correspond with the weekly change in the body weights.

2.2. Care and Handling of Experimental Animal

The three oral toxicity studies used a total of 208 Sprague Dawley rats purchased from BioLASCO Taiwan Co. Ltd. (Taipei City, Taiwan). The rats, hereafter referred to as the test system (TS), arrived at four weeks of age and were quarantined for two weeks under the care of the veterinarian. Following quarantine, the TS were housed individually in the Individual Ventilated Cage (IVC) and acclimatized to the experimental environment for seven days. The room had a 12 h light and dark cycle where the lights were switched on from 7 a.m. to 7 p.m.; the temperature was kept at 22 ± 3 °C and relative humidity was maintained at $57.5 \pm 7.5\%$. The cages and bedding were changed every two weeks. Food (200 g) was placed in each cage weekly and replenished if inadequate. The amount of food left weekly was measured and used to calculate the week's food consumption. Reverse osmosis water was provided ad libitum and the water intake was also measured in a similar approach. This study followed the Principle and Guide to Ethical Use of Laboratory Animals prepared by the Ministry of Health Malaysia (2000) [25]. Approval from the Animal Care and Use Committee (ACUC) at the Institute for Medical Research, Malaysia was obtained; ACUC number ACUC/KKM/02(5/2008).

2.3. Single Dose Acute Oral Toxicity Study

The acute oral toxicity was done following the OECD Guideline No. 420 [22], where the sighting study was done using single dosages of 0.005, 0.05, 0.30 and 2 g/kg BW of test item and administered orally to female TS. First, one of the TS was orally administered with the lowest dose and observed for any signs of acute toxicity 24 h post-dosing. As the first TS showed no signs of toxicity, a second TS was administered the second lowest dose (0.05 g/kg BW) and observed in the same manner. This procedure was repeated until the highest dose (2 g/kg BW) was administered. The highest dose did not trigger any acute effects; thus 2 g/kg BW was used in the main study. Four new TS were given 2 g/kg BW of the test item and monitored for 14 days. The TS were monitored for any signs of acute toxicity, including morbidity and mortality, at 0.5, 1, 2 and 4 h after treatment, then twice daily until day 14. The BW, food and water consumption were measured weekly. The TS were sacrificed following the 14-day observation period and gross observations of all organs were recorded.

2.4. Subacute 28-Day and Chronic 6-Month Oral Toxicity Studies

2.4.1. Subacute 28-Day Experimental Design

The subacute oral toxicity study was based on the OECD Guideline No. 407 [23], with modifications. Male and female TS were grouped into four groups of five TS, where each group received doses of 0.14, 0.29 and 1 g/kg BW of test item, orally administered in 2 mL volumes. The control group received distilled water. The TS were observed twice daily for any clinical signs, morbidity and mortality. Individual TS's dosage was corrected each week to correspond with the TS's body weight. Detailed clinical observations and food intake measurements were performed, while water was given ad libitum. The TS were anaesthetized and blood samples were collected by cardiac puncture. Blood samples were sent for hematology analysis (2.5 mL) in EDTA tubes. The TS were then sacrificed with an overdose of diethyl ether and necropsies were performed. At necropsy, gross pathology was conducted and the internal organs; lung, heart, liver, kidneys, adrenals, ovaries, testes, spleen, stomach and intestinal tract were collected. All organs were cleaned of excess fat and absolute weights were taken immediately. The organs were then placed in 10% formalin for histopathology evaluations.

2.4.2. Chronic 6-Month Experimental Design

The chronic 6-month oral toxicity study was carried out in accordance with OECD Guideline No. 452 [24], with modifications, where 20 rats per group per sex were used in the same dosage group (0.14 g/kg BW, 0.29 g/kg BW, 1 g/kg BW and Control) as in the subacute study. The test item (2 mL) was orally administered daily. During the in-life phase, the TS were observed daily for mortality, morbidity and clinical observations. Their food and water intake were monitored weekly, while detailed clinical observations by the attending veterinarian was conducted monthly. At necropsy, gross observation was conducted and blood was collected for hematology and serum clinical biochemistry analysis. The absolute weights of the internal organs were recorded, then treated with 10% formalin for histopathology investigation. The list of organs was as in the subacute study.

2.4.3. Hematology Analysis

Blood was analyzed using Medonic CA620 Vet Analyzer (Boule Diagnostics AB, Stockholm, Sweden) for white blood cells (WBC), red blood cells (RBC), hemoglobin (HGB), hematocrit (HCT), mean corpuscular hemoglobin concentration (MCHC) and platelets (PLT) for the subacute study. In the chronic study, the RBC, HGB, HCT and PLT levels were determined.

2.4.4. Clinical Biochemistry Analysis

Serum in the chronic study was analyzed using the biochemistry analyzer (Vitalab Selectra E-series, Vital Scientific N.V., Spankeren/Dieren, Netherlands). Liver function profile—total protein, albumin, enzymes; alkaline phosphatase (ALP), alanine amino-transferase (ALT) and aspartate amino-transferase (AST), lactate dehydrogenase (LDH), creatine kinase (CK); renal profile—creatinine, urea and uric acid; lipid profile—cholesterol and triglycerides; and glucose and calcium were determined.

2.4.5. Relative Organ Weight

The weight of the organs relative to 100 g BW of the TS were calculated based on the TS body weights recorded prior to necropsy and their absolute internal organ weights.

2.4.6. Histopathological Examination

All organs collected (lung, heart, liver, kidneys, adrenals, ovaries, testes, spleen, stomach and intestinal tract) were fixed in 10% formalin, sectioned and stained using hematoxylin and eosin (H&E) before microscopically observed for any pathological abnormalities.

2.5. Statistical Analysis

The data for body and organ weights, food and water consumptions, as well as hematology and clinical biochemistry results, was checked for normality using Kolmogorov-Smirnov and Shapiro-Wilk tests. Normally distributed data were analyzed using the one-way analysis of variance (ANOVA), while in not normally distributed cases, Kruskal-Wallis test was used. In cases where statistically significant differences were noted, Post-Hoc tests were used to elucidate the differences between the control and treated groups. Male and female data were analyzed separately. When there was any death during the study period, the data for body weight, food intake and water intake were included up until the last recorded weekly data and then excluded thereafter. Consequently, the hematology, clinical biochemistry and organ weight data were excluded for animals that died in the group. The actual sample size is denoted in the result figures and tables. Statistical analyses were performed using SPSS 18.0 statistical software (SPSS Inc., Chicago, IL, USA) and GraphPad Prism 7.0 software (GraphPad Software, La Jolla, CA, USA). Statistically significant differences were considered when $p < 0.05$.

3. Results

3.1. Single Dose Acute Oral Toxicity Study

No mortality was recorded during the 14-day observation period and the TS showed no sign of toxicity. No major findings were detected in the body weight and food intake parameters of the TS (Table A1). Internal and external examination of the TS and organs revealed no abnormalities. It was concluded that the test item exerted no acute toxicity in the TS.

3.2. Subacute 28-Day and Chronic 6-Month Oral Toxicity Studies

3.2.1. Clinical Signs and Mortality

The TS did not produce any mortality or toxicology-related clinical signs due to the consumption of the test item in either study. However, in the subacute study, one female TS in the medium dosage group on day 18 died due to a gavage accident. While in the chronic study, five females given 0 g/kg BW (day 56), 0.14 g/kg BW (day 121), 0.29 g/kg BW (two TS; day 44 and day 126) and 1 g/kg BW (day 158) and 2 males given 0 g/kg BW (day 158) and 1 g/kg BW (day 76) died also due to gavage accidents. Autopsy revealed no treatment-related alteration in the dead TS.

3.2.2. Body Weights, Food and Water Intake

The subacute study showed that the mean body weights for both males and females did not depict any significant difference between the control and the treated groups. The weekly mean body weight also increased gradually over the dosing period (Figure 1a,b). The food consumption (Table A2) was noted to be normal for growing TS and no significant increase or decrease was evident.

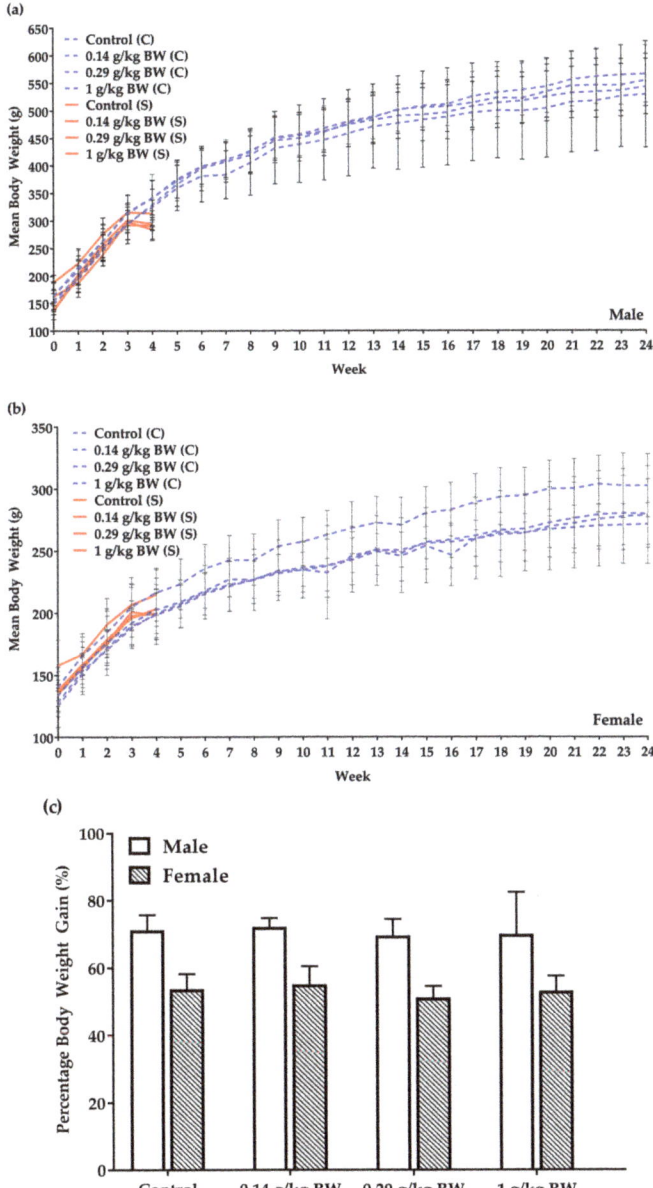

Figure 1. In-life parameters monitored in male and female test systems: (**a**) Mean body weight (BW) of male test systems in the 28-day subacute toxicity study (red line) and the 6-month chronic toxicity study (dotted blue line). (**b**) Mean body weight of female test systems in the 28-day subacute toxicity study (red line) and the 6-month chronic toxicity study (dotted blue line). (**c**) No difference in the body weight (BW) gain in male and female test systems of the 6-month chronic toxicity study. (Group 0.29 g/kg BW female (S): n = 5, week 1–2; n = 4, week 3–4. Group 0 g/kg BW male (C): n = 20, week 1–22; n = 19, week 23–24. Group 1 g/kg BW male (C): n = 20, week 1–11; n = 19, week 12–24. Group 0 g/kg BW female (C): n = 20, week 1–8; n = 19, week 9–24. Group 0.14 g/kg BW female (C): n = 20, week 1–17; n = 19, week 18–24. Group 0.29 g/kg BW female (C): n = 20, week 1–6; n = 19, week 7–18; n = 18, week 19–24. Group 1 g/kg BW female (C): n = 20, week 1–22; n = 19, week 23–24). S = subacute, C = chronic.

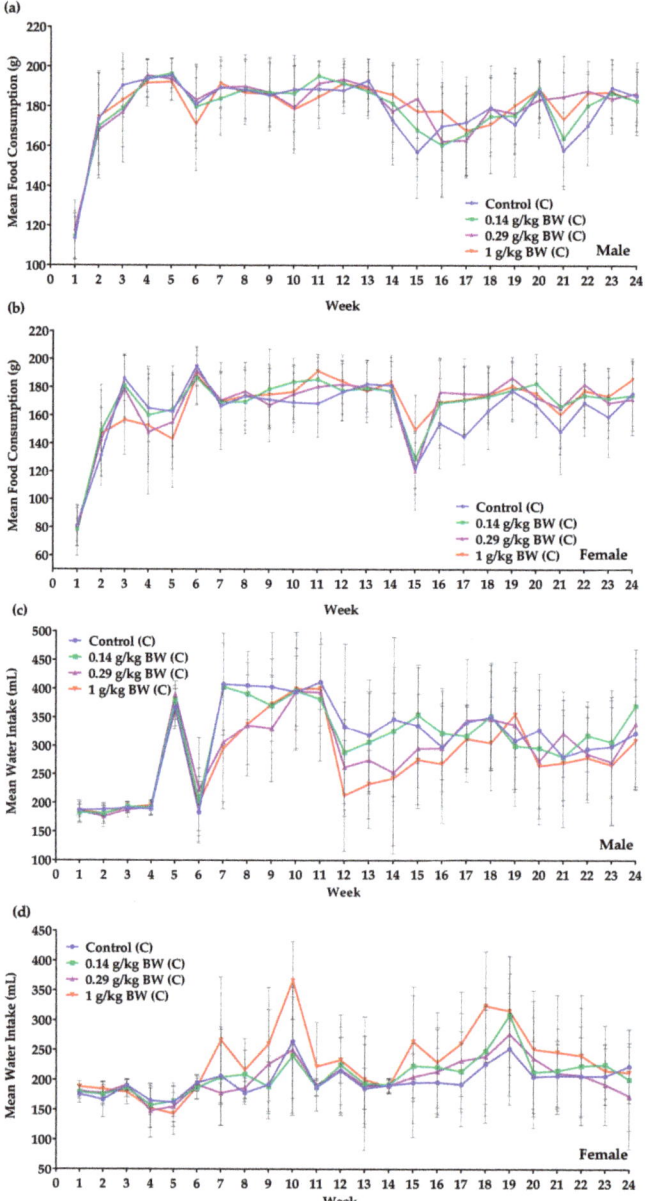

Figure 2. In-life parameters monitored in male and female test systems: (**a**) Mean food consumption of male test systems in the 6-month chronic toxicity study. (**b**) Mean food consumption of female test systems in the 6-month chronic toxicity study. (**c**) Mean water intake of male test systems in the 6-month chronic toxicity study. (**d**) Mean water intake of female test systems in the 6-month chronic toxicity study. Each graph is expressed as mean ± SD (Group 0 g/kg BW male: n = 20, week 1–22; n = 19, week 23–24. Group 1 g/kg BW male: n = 20, week 1–11; n = 19, week 12–24. Group 0 g/kg BW female: n = 20, week 1–8; n = 19, week 9–24. Group 0.14 g/kg BW female: n = 20, week 1–17; n = 19, week 18–24. Group 0.29 g/kg BW female: n = 20, week 1–6; n = 19, week 7–18; n = 18, week 19–24. Group 1 g/kg BW female: n = 20, week 1–22; n = 19, week 23–24).

In the 6 months chronic study, female rats administered 1 g/kg BW dosage of the test item had a significant ($p < 0.05$) increase in body weight each week (Figure 1a,b). However, there was no significant difference in the percentage body weight gain throughout the study of TS administered 1 g/kg BW as compared to the control group in either gender (Figure 1c). Overall, elevating trends in body weight was observed weekly. Looking at food consumption (Figure 2a) in males, a significant increase was observed in weeks 15, 21 and 22 in the 0.29 g/kg BW dosage group when compared to the control group. A significant increase in food intake was seen in females (Figure 2b) given 1 g/kg BW dosage in weeks 11 and 15 when compared to the control group. In week 17, a significant increase in food intake was recorded for all the treated groups. Female TS given 1 g/kg BW showed a significant decrease in food consumption in week 3.

The water consumption trend (Figure 2c) in male TS showed that TS administered 1 g/kg BW consumed less water in weeks 7, 8, 12 and 13, while those given 0.29 g/kg BW only showed a decrease in week 8. Female TS given high doses of the test item (1 g/kg BW dosage) had a significant increase in water intake in weeks 1, 8–10 and 18 (Figure 2d). A significant increase in water intake of female rats given low and medium dosage test item occurred in week 8 and week 22, respectively.

3.2.3. Hematology Analysis

No abnormal levels were detected in the hematological analysis of the blood samples for the subacute study (Table 1). After the 6-month prolonged exposure, the hematologic profile (Table 2) showed a decrease in the platelet (PLT) count in all treated male dosage groups, while other parameters did not show any significant difference. Females given 1 g/kg showed a significant increase in HGB levels when compared to the control group.

Table 1. Hematology values of male and female test systems in the 28-day subacute study.

Sex	Dosage (g/kg BW)	WBC ($10^3/\mu L$)	RBC ($10^6/\mu L$)	HGB (g/dL)	HCT (%)	MCHC (g/dL)	PLT ($10^5/\mu L$)
Male	0.00	5.18 ± 2.01	8.05 ± 0.48	16.40 ± 0.82	49.10 ± 2.53	33.40 ± 0.39	11.17 ± 1.97
	0.14	4.06 ± 2.52	8.44 ± 0.31	16.70 ± 0.74	50.74 ± 2.40	32.92 ± 0.40	10.64 ± 0.90
	0.29	5.40 ± 1.66	8.09 ± 0.55	16.34 ± 0.84	48.62 ± 2.92	33.64 ± 0.53	11.77 ± 1.57
	1.00	4.22 ± 1.43	8.03 ± 0.63	16.36 ± 0.82	48.22 ± 2.91	33.94 ± 0.48	11.48 ± 1.04
Female	0.00	6.52 ± 3.29	6.92 ± 0.19	14.42 ± 0.54	40.46 ± 1.42	35.64 ± 0.46	10.82 ± 0.91
	0.14	4.66 ± 2.84	6.63 ± 0.79	13.50 ± 1.90	38.56 ± 5.04	34.98 ± 0.87	10.21 ± 3.30
	0.29	5.30 ± 1.48	6.76 ± 0.36	14.13 ± 0.34	39.38 ± 1.79	35.90 ± 1.23	9.16 ± 4.68
	1.00	3.00 ± 1.78	6.88 ± 0.57	14.34 ± 0.72	40.38 ± 2.17	35.50 ± 0.32	12.51 ± 1.44

Values expressed as mean ± SD (n = 5 for all groups, except n = 4 for group 0.29 g/kg BW female). No significant changes were found ($p > 0.05$). Body weight, BW; white blood cells, WBC; red blood cells, RBC; hemoglobin, HGB; hematocrit, HCT; mean corpuscular hemoglobin concentration, MCHC; platelets, PLT.

Table 2. Hematology values of male and female test systems in the 6-month chronic study.

Sex	Dosage (g/kg BW)	RBC ($10^6/\mu L$)	HGB (g/dL)	HCT (%)	PLT ($10^5/\mu L$)
Male	0.00 (n = 19)	8.41 ± 0.57	72.99 ±3.76	44.92 ± 2.96	6.87 ± 1.42
	0.14 (n = 20)	8.03 ± 0.92	71.99 ± 8.0	43.39 ± 5.27	5.51 ± 1.12 *
	0.29 (n = 20)	8.10 ± 0.39	73.25 ± 3.03	44.78 ± 2.07	5.57 ± 0.95 *
	1.00 (n = 19)	8.06 ± 0.52	72.99 ± 3.49	44.66 ± 3.26	5.35 ± 0.74 *
Female	0.00 (n = 19)	7.11 ± 0.77	65.02 ± 6.58	39.38 ± 4.25	7.81 ± 1.39
	0.14 (n = 19)	6.92 ± 1.43	63.49 ± 14.44	37.81 ± 7.81	8.70 ± 2.44
	0.29 (n = 18)	7.21 ± 0.35	66.68 ± 2.45	39.76 ± 1.65	7.88 ± 1.06
	1.00 (n = 19)	7.67 ± 0.61	71.41 ± 5.46*	42.79 ± 4.06	7.38 ± 0.93

Values expressed as mean ± SD. BW = body weight. * Significantly different from control group at $p < 0.05$.

3.2.4. Clinical Biochemistry Analysis

The liver and enzyme parameters showed reduced levels of albumin, alkaline phosphatase (ALP), alanine amino-transferase (ALT) and triglyceride in males administered 0.14 g/kg BW (Table 3). Significantly elevated total protein, creatinine and urea levels in males administered 0.29 g/kg BW was observed. There was also a significant increase in creatine kinase level in males given 1.0 g/kg BW dosage. In female test groups, elevated albumin, ALT, aspartate amino-transferase (AST), creatinine, urea, cholesterol and calcium levels were observed in the 0.29 g/kg BW group. The 1 g/kg BW group had a significant increase in lactate dehydrogenase (LDH), cholesterol and calcium levels, while there was a significant decrease in the triglyceride level.

3.2.5. Organ Weights

In the subacute study, there was no significant difference in the relative organ weights (ROW) of any organs in males. Some ROW in females were significantly decreased, including stomachs in the 0.14 g/kg BW group and spleens for the 0.14 and 0.29 g/kg BW groups (Table 4). In the 6-month chronic study, no significant differences in the ROW was observed in any of the collected organs for all the tested groups (Table 5).

3.2.6. Gross Necropsy and Histopathology Examination

No abnormalities were visually detected when gross pathological examination was carried out postmortem. Microscopic histopathology revealed no abnormalities.

Table 3. Clinical biochemistry values of male and female test systems in the 6-month chronic study.

Parameters	Male Dosage (g/kg BW)				Female Dosage (g/kg BW)			
	0 (n = 19)	0.14 (n = 20)	0.29 (n = 20)	1.00 (n = 19)	0 (n = 19)	0.14 (n = 19)	0.29 (n = 18)	1.00 (n = 19)
Liver Function Profile								
Total protein (g/L)	49.66 ± 12.42	43.80 ± 17.07	60.49 ± 10.67 *	56.97 ± 7.49	63.42 ± 16.47	58.49 ± 5.64	66.94 ± 8.18	72.30 ± 6.11
Albumin (g/L)	34.19 ± 10.72	24.97 ± 9.61 *	37.25 ± 7.25	32.45 ± 5.08	39.72 ± 10.60	43.39 ± 5.17	53.53 ± 5.94 *	40.46 ± 2.57
Enzymes								
ALP (U/L)	123.32 ± 115.61	46.18 ± 26.25 *	118.39 ± 42.71	88.95 ± 38.77	25.79 ± 32.79	24.34 ± 43.78	33.07 ± 22.50	18.44 ± 42.67
ALT (U/L)	63.69 ± 31.90	34.03 ± 21.37 *	65.75 ± 25.36	50.49 ± 14.19	54.29 ± 15.50	50.29 ± 10.10	68.96 ± 17.57 *	57.94 ± 12.06
AST (U/L)	155.73 ± 54.04	137.55 ± 68.31	194.22 ± 54.69	171.56 ± 36.13	195.82 ± 75.82	205.78 ± 59.05	270.29 ± 50.25*	229.72 ± 47.78
LDH (U/L)	1993.46 ± 904.07	1671.46 ± 772.76	1430 ± 726.58	1690 ± 819.68	2053.36 ± 793.69	2363.14 ± 721.41	2367.04 ± 763.32	2615.74 ± 491.17 *
CK (U/L)	408.07 ± 253.91	392.64 ± 174.86	562.87 ± 342.05	701.64 ± 292.43 *	653.74 ± 422.37	537.59 ± 372.26	682.9 ± 277.82	756.82 ± 443.50
Renal Profile								
Creatinine (µmol/L)	47.08 ± 13.48	44.27 ± 22.79	61.77 ± 11.69 *	54.83 ± 6.76	55.31 ± 12.92	56.18 ± 6.51	66.91 ± 8.90 *	59.86 ± 6.85
Urea (mmol/L)	5.88 ± 1.33	5.02 ± 2.18	7.11 ± 1.12 *	7.00 ± 1.15	7.02 ± 1.61	7.10 ± 0.81	8.65 ± 1.91 *	8.17 ± 0.87
Uric Acid (µmol/L)	283.07 ± 140.43	247.44 ± 137.08	286.70 ± 129.19	334.95 ± 131.69	379.23 ± 125.43	328.01 ± 142.28	449.77 ± 161.52	382.73 ± 142.01
Lipid Profile								
Cholesterol (mmol/L)	1.59 ± 0.52	3.73 ± 11.12	1.52 ± 0.36	1.2 ± 0.40	1.72 ± 0.50	1.94 ± 0.46	2.28 ± 0.44 *	2.21 ± 0.31 *
Triglyceride (mmol/L)	1.29 ± 0.64	0.58 ± 0.37 *	1.06 ± 0.59	0.92 ± 0.36	0.89 ± 0.55	0.69 ± 0.45	0.92 ± 0.55	0.46 ± 0.32 *
Glucose (mmol/L)	5.33 ± 4.38	3.83 ± 2.88	6.12 ± 4.22	6.81 ± 5.45	5.27 ± 4.59	3.34 ± 3.43	5.29 ± 5.98	5.60 ± 4.24
Calcium (mmol/L)	1.91 ± 0.62	1.60 ± 0.60	2.12 ± 0.39	1.64 ± 0.25	1.93 ± 0.57	2.22 ± 0.24	2.62 ± 0.32 *	2.36 ± 0.29 *

Values expressed as mean. BW = body weight. * Significantly different from control group at $p < 0.05$. Alkaline phosphatase, ALP; alanine amino-transferase, ALT; aspartate amino-transferase, AST; lactate dehydrogenase, LDH; creatine kinase, CK.

Table 4. Relative organ weights of male and female test systems in the 28-day subacute study.

Parameters	Male Dosage (g/kg BW)				Female Dosage (g/kg BW)			
	0 (n = 5)	0.14 (n = 5)	0.29 (n = 5)	1.00 (n = 5)	0 (n = 5)	0.14 (n = 5)	0.29 (n = 4)	1.00 (n = 5)
BW [a]	295.00 ± 11.73	285.00 ± 17.68	292.00 ± 27.06	314.00 ± 24.08	200.00 ± 16.20	215.00 ± 21.21	203.75 ± 24.62	199.00 ± 24.08
Lung [b]	0.41 ± 0.04	0.43 ± 0.06	0.45 ± 0.02	0.43 ± 0.04	0.57 ± 0.11	0.51 ± 0.08	0.57 ± 0.08	0.55 ± 0.12
Heart [b]	0.35 ± 0.02	0.35 ± 0.02	0.33 ± 0.03	0.32 ± 0.04	0.36 ± 0.05	0.35 ± 0.03	0.34 ± 0.01	0.37 ± 0.05
Spleen [b]	0.18 ± 0.03	0.15 ± 0.03	0.16 ± 0.02	0.15 ± 0.01	0.23 ± 0.02	0.19 ± 0.02 *	0.19 ± 0.01 *	0.21 ± 0.03
Stomach [b]	0.47 ± 0.05	0.46 ± 0.04	0.53 ± 0.02	0.51 ± 0.07	0.64 ± 0.03	0.56 ± 0.05 *	0.66 ± 0.02	0.65 ± 0.05
Intestinal tract [b]	0.49 ± 0.08	0.41 ± 0.05	0.52 ± 0.12	0.47 ± 0.09	0.48 ± 0.20	0.65 ± 0.21	0.57 ± 0.10	0.69 ± 0.10
Liver [b]	3.09 ± 0.24	3.21 ± 0.41	2.91 ± 0.21	2.89 ± 0.15	3.23 ± 0.14	3.29 ± 0.36	3.25 ± 0.30	3.21 ± 0.46
Kidney R [b]	0.39 ± 0.02	0.41 ± 0.03	0.37 ± 0.03	0.38 ± 0.03	0.38 ± 0.02	0.36 ± 0.05	0.38 ± 0.04	0.39 ± 0.02
Kidney L [b]	0.39 ± 0.02	0.40 ± 0.03	0.37 ± 0.02	0.38 ± 0.04	0.38 ± 0.03	0.35 ± 0.04	0.37 ± 0.03	0.38 ± 0.02
Adrenal R [b]	0.01 ± 0.00	0.01 ± 0.00	0.01 ± 0.01	0.01 ± 0.01	0.01 ± 0.01	0.01 ± 0.00	0.02 ± 0.01	0.01 ± 0.01
Adrenal L [b]	0.01 ± 0.00	0.01 ± 0.01	0.01 ± 0.00	0.01 ± 0.00	0.02 ± 0.00	0.01 ± 0.00	0.02 ± 0.01	0.01 ± 0.00
Testes R [b]	0.51 ± 0.05	0.51 ± 0.03	0.49 ± 0.06	0.46 ± 0.05				
Testes L [b]	0.50 ± 0.09	0.50 ± 0.03	0.48 ± 0.04	0.48 ± 0.04				
Ovary R [b]					0.03 ± 0.01	0.03 ± 0.01	0.03 ± 0.01	0.04 ± 0.02
Ovary L [b]					0.04 ± 0.01	0.04 ± 0.01	0.03 ± 0.00	0.04 ± 0.01

Values expressed as mean ± SD (n = 5 for all groups, except n = 4 for group 0.29 g/kg BW female). BW = body weight, R = right, L = left, [a] Unit: g; [b] Unit: % body weights. * Significantly different from control group at $p < 0.05$.

Table 5. Relative organ weights of male and female test systems in the 6-month chronic study.

Parameters	Male Dose (g/kg BW)				Female Dosage (g/kg BW)			
	0 (n = 19)	0.14 (n = 20)	0.29 (n = 20)	1.00 (n = 19)	0 (n = 19)	0.14 (n = 19)	0.29 (n = 18)	1.00 (n = 19)
BW [a]	578.95 ± 57.82	568.00 ± 50.22	557.75 ± 51.75	543.42 ± 100.90	286.32 ± 41.36	291.84 ± 30.70	281.94 ± 19.56	314.17 ± 26.91
Lung [b]	0.36 ± 0.09	0.37 ± 0.11	0.38 ± 0.07	0.39 ± 0.15	0.53 ± 0.12	0.51 ± 0.12	0.57 ± 0.08	0.48 ± 0.14
Heart [b]	0.26 ± 0.02	0.25 ± 0.02	0.25 ± 0.02	0.25 ± 0.05	0.30 ± 0.03	0.30 ± 0.04	0.31 ± 0.03	0.30 ± 0.03
Spleen [b]	0.13 ± 0.02	0.13 ± 0.03	0.13 ± 0.02	0.14 ± 0.05	0.16 ± 0.02	0.17 ± 0.02	0.18 ± 0.04	0.17 ± 0.02
Stomach [b]	0.50 ± 0.06	0.46 ± 0.04	0.44 ± 0.05	0.49 ± 0.17	0.70 ± 0.09	0.71 ± 0.11	0.74 ± 0.08	0.67 ± 0.09
Intestinal tract [b]	0.40 ± 0.08	0.36 ± 0.08	0.36 ± 0.08	0.41 ± 0.10	0.51 ± 0.17	0.49 ± 0.15	0.51 ± 0.10	0.50 ± 0.12
Liver [b]	2.77 ± 0.39	2.63 ± 0.29	2.80 ± 0.28	2.70 ± 0.29	3.01 ± 0.26	2.94 ± 0.25	3.01 ± 0.28	2.85 ± 0.24
Kidney R [b]	0.28 ± 0.02	0.27 ± 0.02	0.27 ± 0.02	0.28 ± 0.04	0.31 ± 0.07	0.31 ± 0.06	0.33 ± 0.05	0.32 ± 0.02
Kidney L [b]	0.28 ± 0.02	0.27 ± 0.02	0.27 ± 0.03	0.28 ± 0.04	0.32 ± 0.03	0.32 ± 0.04	0.33 ± 0.03	0.32 ± 0.03
Adrenal R [b]	0.004 ± 0.002	0.004 ± 0.002	0.004 ± 0.002	0.005 ± 0.002	0.009 ± 0.005	0.014 ± 0.015	0.011 ± 0.007	0.015 ± 0.022
Adrenal L [b]	0.004 ± 0.001	0.005 ± 0.002	0.003 ± 0.001	0.005 ± 0.002	0.010 ± 0.005	0.011 ± 0.006	0.011 ± 0.005	0.011 ± 0.004
Testes R [b]	0.31 ± 0.04	0.31 ± 0.05	0.33 ± 0.03	0.32 ± 0.07				
Testes L [b]	0.34 ± 0.06	0.32 ± 0.03	0.33 ± 0.03	0.33 ± 0.09				
Ovary R [b]					0.02 ± 0.01	0.02 ± 0.01	0.03 ± 0.01	0.02 ± 0.01
Ovary L [b]					0.03 ± 0.01	0.03 ± 0.01	0.03 ± 0.01	0.02 ± 0.01

Values expressed as mean ± SD. BW = body weight, R = right, L = left. [a] Unit: g; [b] Unit: % body weights. No significant changes were found ($p > 0.05$).

4. Discussion

Herbal-infused beverages have been introduced into the market where countless other beverages are marketed. With the extra edge of having herbal concoctions incorporated, herbal additives in beverages have gained popularity and are widely consumed in Malaysia. A rat model was used to investigate the acute and prolonged repeated consumption of such product to establish its safety profile and infer its effects at its expected exposure dose in humans.

The test item did not exert any acute toxicity and no mortality was observed at any of the tested doses. In both the subacute and chronic studies, there were no significant clinical signs of toxicity, body weight changes were normal and gross and histopathology investigations did not reveal any significant toxicity effect. There was a total of seven incidental deaths in the repeated dose studies due to technical error by personnel. The gavage error may have led to gavage-assisted reflux in the TS causing these deaths [26]. We report the following findings, namely fluctuations in the food and water intake measurements, the relative organ weights (ROW) in two organs in the subacute study and platelet changes observed in the chronic study with some alterations to the clinical biochemical parameters.

The statistically significant reduction in food consumption which only occurred in the female high dose group in week 3 of the chronic study and the increased water intake in some female treated groups may indicate natural physiological changes. It has been reported that female TS consume less food and become active during their estrus cycle which may incur responses as manifested in the amount of food and water consumed, as seen in this study [27,28]. On the other hand, males in the chronic studies consumed significantly less water, where coffee consumption itself may have caused the TS to drink less water [29]. Despite the fluctuating food and water intake, the body weight measurements showed elevating trends, indicating normal development of the TS. Similar body weight trends were also reported by other authors [30–32]. Hence, it is concluded that the fluctuations observed in the food and water intake did not cause any treatment-related effects in the TS.

In the subacute female group, there was a reduction in ROW for the stomach (0.14 g/kg BW group) and spleen in the 0.14 and 0.29 g/kg BW dosage groups. There was no clear dose-relationship in reduction of ROW as the highest dose group did not produce any changes. Further microscopic examination of these two organs did not show any correlation to the decrease in size. As the changes were only observed in the subacute female group and prolonged exposure of six months revealed no effect on any of the organs inspected in either gender, these two observations are not considered treatment-related.

No significant differences were seen in the hematology profile of the 28-day study of the treated groups when compared to the control group. The hematology parameter findings for the subacute and chronic studies were similar to published control data, except for the WBC, HGB, MCHC and PLT counts, where slight differences were found between the two reference intervals [31,33]. After prolonged exposure of the test item over a substantial lifetime of the TS, some changes in the blood investigations were observed, where platelet numbers of males from all the treated groups significantly decreased. A drop in the platelet reading may be a cause of concern as they are primarily involved in blood coagulation and hemostasis [34]. Coffee by itself has been shown to reduce platelet activation resulting in reduced platelet aggregation though platelet aggregate formation was not evaluated in the current study [35]. The decreased platelet levels recorded were lower than the average platelet levels in males when compared to the reference interval by He et al. (2017) but were comparable to the reference values from Delwatta et al. (2018) [31,36]. However, the decrease was not dose-dependent, as the highest dose did not further reduce the platelet reading compared with the lowest dose.

Creatinine, urea, cholesterol, triglyceride and glucose levels were similar to published control data [31,36]. It was noted that there were large differences in the control data range published. Hence, the control group data in this study were used for all statistical analysis as the control group TS were subjected to the same environment as the treated groups. Elevated renal profile (creatinine and urea), total protein and creatine kinase in the male treated groups (0.29 and 1 g/kg BW dosage) and elevation of the liver, renal and lipid profiles in the female treated groups (0.29 and 1 g/kg BW dosage) may indicate the TS early response to the test item. A recent study by Riza & Andina Putri et al. (2019)

also found an increase in creatinine levels in rats administered coffee [37]. However, in our current study, no further correlation in liver nor kidney histopathology were apparent. No dose-dependent conclusion can be drawn from the changes observed in the 0.29 g/kg BW group, as the highest dose did not exacerbate the parameters measured. Contrarily, the consumption of coffee has been reported to decrease liver enzymes associated with liver damage and has shown protective effects attributed to its polyphenol content [38–43]. There were favorable significant reductions in liver enzymes (ALP and ALT) and lipid profile indicator (triglyceride) in the low male dose group but no trend was evident in the higher dose groups except in the female triglyceride level when given the high dose.

The interactions between the different components present in both coffee and TA and additionally with food may have exerted their effects on the parameters measured in this study. Both coffee and TA are made up of various phytochemicals, such as caffeine and polyphenols, found in coffee, and eurycomanone, a major compound found in TA [1,39,40]. Caffeine has been well studied and is reported to have a high tolerance dose of 400 mg/day in human [44–46]. Although eurycomanone has been reported to have low bioavailability in rats [47,48], its pharmacokinetic behavior may be modified when incorporated with coffee. A recent study reported coffee's potential to alter acetaminophen drug pharmacokinetic profile when consumed together [49]. Due to this multi-component nature and interactions, safety evaluation of herbal incorporated food products is crucial.

In this study, the toxicity was assessed in one mammalian rodent model, whereas regulatory submissions may require the safety tests to be conducted in more than one species, typically in either rats, mice or rabbits and in dogs to compare the effect and rate of severity of the toxicity [50]. Despite this limitation, the study was conducted for three different durations that covers the acute response of the administered product, as well as the repeated exposure. The studies covered a substantial duration of the rodents' lifetimes. Therefore, conclusions drawn from this study are exhaustive.

Considering an average consumption of 2 cups (2.5 g test item per cup) per person per day, an average adult (70 kg body weight), ingests on average 0.07 g/kg body weight of the test item daily. The calculated human equivalent dose (HED) for 1 g/kg BW in rats is 0.16 g/kg BW in humans. As the calculated HED is twice the predicted average daily consumption dosage, the present study suggests that the highest dose tested in the prolonged toxicity study (1 g/kg BW per day) of *E. longifolia* infused coffee, may be well tolerated for human consumption.

5. Conclusions

In conclusion, the highest single dose administration of TA coffee (2 g/kg of body weight) did not show acute oral toxicity in Sprague Dawley rats in the present study. The 28-day subacute toxicity study reported no toxic change in any observed parameters. No dose-dependent nor morphological changes were attributed to the consumption of TA coffee in the 6-month chronic toxicity study and consumption of TA coffee at a dose of 1 g/kg/day in male and female rats was identified as the no observed adverse effect level (NOAEL).

Author Contributions: Conceptualization, N.A., B.P.T. and H.M.; Methodology, S.Z.H., N.A.Z. and N.R.; Software, N.A., S.Z.H. and N.R.; Validation, N.A., B.P.T. and S.Z.H.; Formal Analysis, N.A. and S.Z.H.; Investigation, S.Z.H., N.A.Z. and N.R.; Resources, N.A. and H.M.; Data Curation, N.A. and S.Z.H.; Writing—Original Draft Preparation, N.A. and B.P.T.; Writing—Review and Editing, N.A., B.P.T. and H.M.; Visualization, N.A., B.P.T. and H.M.; Supervision, H.M.; Project Administration, N.A. and H.M.; Funding Acquisition, N.A. and H.M. All authors have read and agreed to the published version of the manuscript.

Funding: This research was funded by the Ministry of Agriculture, Malaysia under the ScienceFund Grant (05-03-20-SF1001) and the Ministry of Health, Malaysia.

Acknowledgments: We would like to thank the Director General of Health Malaysia for his permission to publish this article. We thank GTHerb Industries Sdn. Bhd. for providing the TA coffee. The authors would also like to thank Zakiah Ismail and Noor Rain Abdullah for their perceptive guidance in this research.

Conflicts of Interest: The authors declare no conflict of interest.

Appendix A

Table A1. Summary of 14-day acute study findings.

Test System	Dosage (g/kg BW)	Mortality	Clinical Signs of Toxicity	Body Weight (g)			Body Weight Gain (%)	Food Intake (g)		Organs Gross Pathology Findings
				Initial	Week 1	Week 2		Week 1	Week 2	
1	0.005	0/1	NAD	219.87	234.52	246.07	10.60	86.05	69.45	NAD
2	0.050	0/1	NAD	216.90	254.89	292.81	25.90	87.35	112.47	NAD
3	0.300	0/1	NAD	216.94	246.34	278.95	22.20	93.79	113.47	NAD
4	2.000	0/1	NAD	234.14	260.60	274.50	14.70	106.92	82.80	NAD
5	2.000	0/1	NAD	243.15	275.31	291.17	16.50	132.83	76.80	NAD
6	2.000	0/1	NAD	202.05	219.19	222.79	9.31	92.12	62.31	NAD
7	2.000	0/1	NAD	211.36	244.51	250.01	15.50	113.11	76.19	NAD
8	2.000	0/1	NAD	218.59	268.09	253.17	13.70	125.38	67.20	NAD
				221.90 ± 16.71	253.50 ± 22.34	258.30 ± 25.98	13.92 ± 2.78	114.10 ± 15.92	73.06 ± 8.19	

The body weight, food intake and percentage body weight gain values are expressed as mean ± SD of 5 test systems given the 2 g/kg dosage in the acute study. No statistical comparison was made as the method used was fixed dose procedure with emphasis on the acute clinical response and no acute death was observed. BW = body weight, NAD = no abnormality detected.

Table A2. Food consumption of male and female test systems in the 28-day subacute study.

Weekly Food Consumption	Male Dosage (g/kg BW)				Female Dosage (g/kg BW)			
	0 (n = 5)	0.14 (n = 5)	0.29 (n = 5)	1.00 (n = 5)	0 (n = 5)	0.14 (n = 5)	0.29 (n = 4)	1.00 (n = 5)
Week 1	117.00 ± 11.51	123.00 ± 17.89	109.00 ± 12.94	117.00 ± 16.43	85.00 ± 7.91	91.00 ± 15.17	108.00 ± 28.64	84.00 ± 11.94
Week 2	134.00 ± 17.10	116.40 ± 14.74	130.00 ± 9.35	135.00 ± 12.75	91.00 ± 6.52	99.00 ± 8.94	109.00 ± 38.63	81.00 ± 14.32
Week 3	160.00 ± 20.92	160.00 ± 12.75	145.00 ± 14.14	157.00 ± 17.18	98.00 ± 13.51	116.00 ± 39.91	111.25 ± 49.56	108.00 ± 33.28
Week 4	173.00 ± 8.37	136.00 ± 30.50	148.00 ± 22.80	162.00 ± 13.04	128.00 ± 21.68	166.00 ± 28.81	147.50 ± 22.17	126.00 ± 27.02

Values expressed as mean ± SD (n = 5 for all groups, except n = 4 for group 0.29 g/kg BW female). BW = body weight. No significant changes were found ($p > 0.05$).

References

1. Rehman, S.U.; Choe, K.; Yoo, H.H. Review on a traditional herbal medicine, *Eurycoma longifolia* Jack (Tongkat Ali): Its traditional uses, chemistry, evidence-based pharmacology and toxicology. *Molecules* **2016**, *21*, 331. [CrossRef]
2. Kotirum, S.; Ismail, S.B.; Chaiyakunapruk, N. Efficacy of Tongkat Ali (*Eurycoma longifolia*) on erectile function improvement: Systematic review and meta-analysis of randomized controlled trials. *Complement. Ther. Med.* **2015**, *23*, 693–698. [CrossRef]
3. Henkel, R.R.; Wang, R.; Bassett, S.H.; Chen, T.; Liu, N.; Zhu, Y.; Tambi, M.I. Tongkat Ali as a potential herbal supplement for physically active male and female seniors—A pilot study. *Phytother. Res. PTR* **2014**, *28*, 544–550. [CrossRef]
4. Solomon, M.C.; Erasmus, N.; Henkel, R.R. In vivo effects of *Eurycoma longifolia* Jack (Tongkat Ali) extract on reproductive functions in the rat. *Andrologia* **2014**, *46*, 339–348. [CrossRef]
5. Abdul Razak, H.S.; Shuid, A.N.; Naina Mohamed, I. Combined effects of *Eurycoma longifolia* and testosterone on androgen-deficient osteoporosis in a male rat model. *Evid. Based Complement. Altern. Med.* **2012**, *2012*, 872406.
6. Shuid, A.N.; El-arabi, E.; Effendy, N.M.; Abdul Razak, H.M.; Muhammad, N.; Mohamed, N.; Soelaiman, I.M. *Eurycoma longifolia* upregulates osteoprotegerin gene expression in androgen-deficient osteoporosis rat model. *BMC Complement. Altern. Med.* **2012**, *12*, 152. [CrossRef]
7. Low, B.S.; Teh, C.H.; Yuen, K.H.; Chan, K.L. Physico-chemical effects of the major quassinoids in a standardized *Eurycoma longifolia* extract (Fr 2) on the bioavailability and pharmacokinetic properties, and their implications for oral antimalarial activity. *Nat. Prod. Commun.* **2011**, *6*, 337–341.
8. Mohd Abdul Razak, M.R.; Abdullah, N.R.; Ismail, Z.; Ismail, Z. Effect of *Eurycoma longifolia* extract on the glutathione level in *Plasmodium falciparum* infected erythrocytes in vitro. *Trop. Biomed.* **2005**, *22*, 155–163.
9. Satayavivad, J.; Noppamas, S.; Aimon, S.; Yodhathai, T. Toxicological and antimalaria activity of *Eurycoma longifolia* Jack extracts in mice. *Thai. J. Phytopharm.* **1998**, *5*, 14–27.
10. Choudhary, Y.K.; Bommu, P.; Ming, Y.K. Acute, subacute and subchronic 90-days toxicity of *Eurycoma longifolia* aqueous extract (Physta) in Wistar rats. *Int. J. Pharm. Pharm. Sci.* **2012**, *4*, 232–238.
11. Shuid, A.N.; Siang, L.K.; Chin, T.G.; Muhammad, N.; Mohamed, N.; Soelaiman, I.N. Acute and subacute toxicity studies of *Eurycoma longifolia* in male rats. *Int. J. Pharmacol.* **2011**, *7*, 641–646. [CrossRef]
12. Li, C.H.; Liao, J.W.; Liao, P.L.; Huang, W.K.; Tse, L.S.; Lin, C.H.; Kang, J.J.; Cheng, Y.W. Evaluation of acute 13-week subchronic toxicity and genotoxicity of the powdered root of Tongkat Ali (*Eurycoma longifolia* jack). *Evid. Based Complement. Altern. Med.* **2013**, *2013*, 102987.
13. Lenssen, K.G.M.; Bast, A.; de Boer, A. International perspectives on substantiating the efficacy of herbal dietary supplements and herbal medicines through evidence on traditional use. *Compr. Rev. Food Sci. Food Saf.* **2019**, *18*, 910–922. [CrossRef]
14. Ministry of Health. *Food Act*; Ministry of Health: Putrajaya, Malaysia, 1983.
15. Ministry of Health. *Food Regulation*; Ministry of Health: Putrajaya, Malaysia, 1985.
16. World Health Organization. *WHO Guidelines on Safety Monitoring of Herbal Medicines in Pharmacovigilance Systems*; World Health Organization: Geneva, Switzerland, 2004.
17. Abdel-Tawab, M. Do we need plant food supplements? A critical examination of quality, safety, efficacy, and necessity for a new regulatory framework. *Planta Med.* **2018**, *84*, 372–393. [CrossRef]
18. Khedkar, S.; Carraresi, L.; Bröring, S. Food or pharmaceuticals? Consumers' perception of health-related borderline products. *PharmaNutrition* **2017**, *5*, 133–140. [CrossRef]
19. de Boer, A.; van Hunsel, F.; Bast, A. Adverse food-drug interactions. *Regul. Toxicol. Pharmacol. RTP* **2015**, *73*, 859–865. [CrossRef]
20. Quintus, C.; Schweim, H.G. European regulation of herbal medicinal products on the border area to the food sector. *Phytomedicine* **2012**, *19*, 378–381. [CrossRef]
21. Jordan, S.A.; Cunningham, D.G.; Marles, R.J. Assessment of herbal medicinal products: Challenges, and opportunities to increase the knowledge base for safety assessment. *Toxicol. Appl. Pharmacol.* **2010**, *243*, 198–216. [CrossRef]
22. OECD. *OECD Guideline for Testing of Chemicals No. 420: Acute Oral Toxicity—Fixed Dose Procedure*; OECD: Paris, France, 2001.

23. OECD. *OECD Guideline for Testing of Chemicals No. 407: Repeated Dose 28-Day Oral Toxicity Study in Rodents*; OECD: Paris, France, 1995.
24. OECD. *OECD Guideline for Testing of Chemicals No. 452: Chronic Toxcity Studies*; OECD: Paris, France, 2009.
25. Ministry of Health. *Principles and Guide to Ethical Use of Laboratory Animals*; Ministry of Health: Putrajaya, Malaysia, 2002.
26. Damsch, S.; Eichenbaum, G.; Tonelli, A.; Lammens, L.; Van den Bulck, K.; Feyen, B.; Vandenberghe, J.; Megens, A.; Knight, E.; Kelley, M. Gavage-related reflux in rats: Identification, pathogenesis, and toxicological implications. *Toxicol. Pathol.* **2011**, *39*, 348–360. [CrossRef]
27. Clifton, P.G. Eating. In *The Behaviour of the Laboratory Rat. A Handbook with Tests*; Whishaw, I.Q., Kolb, B., Eds.; Oxford University Press: Oxford, UK, 2004; pp. 214–223.
28. Rowland, N.E. Drinking. In *The Behaviour of the Laboratory Rat. A Handbook with Tests*; Whishaw, I.Q., Kolb, B., Eds.; Oxford University Press: Oxford, UK, 2004; pp. 224–233.
29. Nolen, G.A. The effect of brewed and instant coffee on reproduction and teratogenesis in the rat. *Toxicol. Appl. Pharmacol.* **1981**, *58*, 171–183. [CrossRef]
30. Jacob Filho, W.; Lima, C.C.; Paunksnis, M.R.R.; Silva, A.A.; Perilhão, M.S.; Caldeira, M.; Bocalini, D.; de Souza, R.R. Reference database of hematological parameters for growing and aging rats. *Aging Male* **2018**, *21*, 145–148. [CrossRef]
31. He, Q.; Su, G.; Liu, K.; Zhang, F.; Jiang, Y.; Gao, J.; Liu, L.; Jiang, Z.; Jin, M.; Xie, H. Sex-specific reference intervals of hematologic and biochemical analytes in Sprague-Dawley rats using the nonparametric rank percentile method. *PLoS ONE* **2017**, *12*, e0189837. [CrossRef]
32. Lillie, L.E.; Temple, N.J.; Florence, L.Z. Reference values for young normal Sprague-Dawley rats: Weight gain, hematology and clinical chemistry. *Hum. Exp. Toxicol.* **1996**, *15*, 612–616. [CrossRef]
33. Petterino, C.; Argentino-Storino, A. Clinical chemistry and haematology historical data in control Sprague-Dawley rats from pre-clinical toxicity studies. *Exp. Toxicol. Pathol.* **2006**, *57*, 213–219. [CrossRef]
34. Takahashi, O. Characteristics of rat platelets and relative contributions of platelets and blood coagulation to haemostasis. *Food Chem. Toxicol.* **2000**, *38*, 203–218. [CrossRef]
35. Olas, B.; Bryś, M. Effects of coffee, energy drinks and their components on hemostasis: The hypothetical mechanisms of their action. *Food Chem. Toxicol.* **2019**, *127*, 31–41. [CrossRef]
36. Delwatta, S.L.; Gunatilake, M.; Baumans, V.; Seneviratne, M.D.; Dissanayaka, M.; Batagoda, S.S.; Udagedara, A.H.; Walpola, P.B. Reference values for selected hematological, biochemical and physiological parameters of Sprague-Dawley rats at the animal house, Faculty of Medicine, University of Colombo, Sri Lanka. *Anim. Models Exp. Med.* **2018**, *1*, 250–254. [CrossRef]
37. Riza, M.; Andina Putri, A. The comparison effect of energy drinks and coffee on creatinin level in rats. *Int. J. Hum. Health Sci.* **2019**, *3*, 231–234. [CrossRef]
38. Curti, V.; Verri, M.; Baldi, A.; Dacrema, M.; Masiello, I.; Dossena, M.; Daglia, M. In vivo modulatory effect of coffee (*Coffea canephora* var. Robusta) on the expression levels of murine microRNA-124-3p associated with antioxidant defenses. *eFood* **2020**, *1*, 140–146. [CrossRef]
39. Kolb, H.; Kempf, K.; Martin, S. Health effects of coffee: Mechanism unraveled? *Nutrients* **2020**, *12*, 1842. [CrossRef]
40. Chen, Y.P.; Lu, F.B.; Hu, Y.B.; Xu, L.M.; Zheng, M.H.; Hu, E.D. A systematic review and a dose-response meta-analysis of coffee dose and nonalcoholic fatty liver disease. *Clin. Nutr.* **2019**, *38*, 2552–2557. [CrossRef]
41. Feyisa, T.O.; Melka, D.S.; Menon, M.; Labisso, W.L.; Habte, M.L. Investigation of the effect of coffee on body weight, serum glucose, uric acid and lipid profile levels in male albino Wistar rats feeding on high-fructose diet. *Lab. Anim. Res.* **2019**, *35*, 29. [CrossRef]
42. Sedaghat, G.; Mirshekar, M.A.; Amirpour, M.; Montazerifar, F.; Miri, S.; Shourestani, S. Sub-chronic administration of brewed coffee on rat behavior and cognition and oxidative stress Alzheimer's disease model. *Clin. Nutr. Exp.* **2019**, *28*, 62–73. [CrossRef]
43. Hasegawa, R.; Ogiso, T.; Imaida, K.; Shirai, T.; Ito, N. Analysis of the potential carcinogenicity of coffee and its related compounds in a medium-term liver bioassay of rats. *Food Chem. Toxicol.* **1995**, *33*, 15–20. [CrossRef]
44. Lee, C.H.; George, O.; Kimbrough, A. Chronic voluntary caffeine intake in male Wistar rats reveals individual differences in addiction-like behavior. *Pharmacol. Biochem. Behav.* **2020**, *191*, 172880. [CrossRef]

45. Wikoff, D.; Welsh, B.T.; Henderson, R.; Brorby, G.P.; Britt, J.; Myers, E.; Goldberger, J.; Lieberman, H.R.; O'Brien, C.; Peck, J.; et al. Systematic review of the potential adverse effects of caffeine consumption in healthy adults, pregnant women, adolescents, and children. *Food Chem. Toxicol.* **2017**, *109*, 585–648. [CrossRef]
46. Adamson, R.H. The acute lethal dose 50 (LD50) of caffeine in albino rats. *Regul. Toxicol. Pharmacol. RTP* **2016**, *80*, 274–276. [CrossRef]
47. Ahmad, N.; Samiulla, D.S.; Teh, B.P.; Zainol, M.; Zolkifli, N.A.; Muhammad, A.; Matom, E.; Zulkapli, A.; Abdullah, N.R.; Ismail, Z.; et al. Bioavailability of eurycomanone in its pure form and in a standardised *Eurycoma longifolia* water extract. *Pharmaceutics* **2018**, *10*, 90. [CrossRef]
48. Low, B.S.; Ng, B.H.; Choy, W.P.; Yuen, K.H.; Chan, K.L. Bioavailability and pharmacokinetic studies of eurycomanone from *Eurycoma longifolia*. *Planta Med.* **2005**, *71*, 803–807. [CrossRef]
49. Win, M.; Das, S.; Deborah, S.; Latt, S.; Soe, T. Coffee modify pharmacokinetics of acetaminophen. *EC Pharmacol. Toxicol.* **2019**, *7*, 1091–1098.
50. Hayes, A.W.; Wang, T.; Dixon, D. Chapter 13—Toxicologic testing methods. In *Loomis's Essentials of Toxicology*, 5th ed.; Academic Press: London, UK, 2020; pp. 189–222.

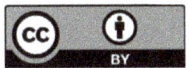

© 2020 by the authors. Licensee MDPI, Basel, Switzerland. This article is an open access article distributed under the terms and conditions of the Creative Commons Attribution (CC BY) license (http://creativecommons.org/licenses/by/4.0/).

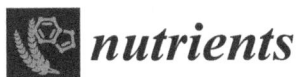

Article

Effects of a Low Dose of Caffeine Alone or as Part of a Green Coffee Extract, in a Rat Dietary Model of Lean Non-Alcoholic Fatty Liver Disease without Inflammation

Ana Magdalena Velázquez [1,†], Núria Roglans [1,2,3,†], Roger Bentanachs [1], Maria Gené [1], Aleix Sala-Vila [4,5], Iolanda Lázaro [4], Jose Rodríguez-Morató [3,4,6], Rosa María Sánchez [1,2,3], Juan Carlos Laguna [1,2,3,*] and Marta Alegret [1,2,3,*]

[1] Department of Pharmacology, Toxicology and Therapeutic Chemistry, School of Pharmacy and Food Science, University of Barcelona, Avda Joan XXIII 27-31, 08028 Barcelona, Spain; avelazquezpy@gmail.com (A.M.V.); roglans@ub.edu (N.R.); bentanachs96@gmail.com (R.B.); mariagene_15@hotmail.com (M.G.); rmsanchez@ub.edu (R.M.S.)
[2] Institute of Biomedicine, University of Barcelona, 08028 Barcelona, Spain
[3] Spanish Biomedical Research Centre in Physiopathology of Obesity and Nutrition (CIBEROBN), Instituto de Salud Carlos III (ISCIII), 28029 Madrid, Spain; jose.rodriguez@upf.edu
[4] IMIM-Hospital del Mar Medical Research Institute, 08003 Barcelona, Spain; asala@barcelonabeta.org (A.S.-V.); iolan.lazaro@gmail.com (I.L.)
[5] Barcelonaβeta Brain Research Center, Pasqual Maragall Foundation, 08005 Barcelona, Spain
[6] Department of Experimental and Health Sciences, Universitat Pompeu Fabra (CEXS-UPF), 08003 Barcelona, Spain
* Correspondence: jclagunae@ub.edu (J.C.L.); alegret@ub.edu (M.A.); Tel.: +34-93-4024531 (M.A.)
† These authors contributed equally to this work.

Received: 21 September 2020; Accepted: 21 October 2020; Published: 23 October 2020

Abstract: Non-alcoholic fatty liver disease is a highly prevalent condition without specific pharmacological treatment, characterized in the initial stages by hepatic steatosis. It was suggested that lipid infiltration in the liver might be reduced by caffeine through anti-inflammatory, antioxidative, and fatty acid metabolism-related mechanisms. We investigated the effects of caffeine (CAF) and green coffee extract (GCE) on hepatic lipids in lean female rats with steatosis. For three months, female Sprague-Dawley rats were fed a standard diet or a cocoa butter-based high-fat diet plus 10% liquid fructose. In the last month, the high-fat diet was supplemented or not with CAF or a GCE, providing 5 mg/kg of CAF. Plasma lipid levels and the hepatic expression of molecules involved in lipid metabolism were determined. Lipidomic analysis was performed in liver samples. The diet caused hepatic steatosis without obesity, inflammation, endoplasmic reticulum stress, or hepatic insulin resistance. Neither CAF nor GCE alleviated hepatic steatosis, but GCE-treated rats showed lower hepatic triglyceride levels compared to the CAF group. The GCE effects could be related to reductions of hepatic (i) mTOR phosphorylation, leading to higher nuclear lipin-1 levels and limiting lipogenic gene expression; (ii) diacylglycerol levels; (iii) hexosylceramide/ceramide ratios; and (iv) very-low-density lipoprotein receptor expression. In conclusion, a low dose of CAF did not reduce hepatic steatosis in lean female rats, but the same dose provided as a green coffee extract led to lower liver triglyceride levels.

Keywords: caffeine; coffee; dietary supplements; hepatic steatosis; non-alcoholic fatty liver disease

1. Introduction

Non-alcoholic fatty liver disease (NAFLD) is a spectrum of alterations ranging from simple hepatic steatosis to non-alcoholic steatohepatitis (NASH), cirrhosis, and hepatocellular carcinoma. Hepatic steatosis, defined as the accumulation of triglycerides (TGs) in lipid droplets in at least 5% of the hepatocytes, is the initial reversible phase of NAFLD, affecting around 33% of adults in the US [1]. Although NAFLD is usually associated with obesity, this condition might also be present in individuals with a body mass index in the normal range, which is referred to as lean or non-obese NAFLD [2]. Compared to obese NAFLD, lean individuals with NAFLD are more commonly female and exhibit a lower prevalence of insulin resistance [2,3].

Consumption of sweetened beverages with a high fructose content is one of the main dietary triggers of NAFLD [4]. Despite the implementation of public policies that aim to reduce their consumption, a recent study on diet population trends showed that 42% of energy intake in US adults still comes from low-quality carbohydrates, including fruit juices and added sugars in beverages [5]. Moreover, the consumption of saturated fats, another dietary factor associated with NAFLD, still remains above the recommended maximal intake of 10% of the energy intake [5].

Given the difficulty to avoid excessive consumption of simple sugars and fats in the population, one strategy to fight NAFLD is the inclusion in the usual diet of functional foods or dietary supplements that could be effective to prevent or reduce hepatic lipid accumulation. Several meta-analysis of randomized clinical trials showed that compounds such as resveratrol, silymarin, vitamin E or D, and curcumin, exert positive effects on NAFLD, which might be attributed to their antioxidant or anti-inflammatory properties [4]. However, not all evidences showed clinical efficacy, which could be related to the different doses, formulation issues, or duration of studies [6–8]. Coffee was reported to exert beneficial effects on liver-related disorders [9], including a reduced risk of NAFLD and of liver fibrosis in NAFLD patients, as revealed by a recent meta-analysis [10]. Effects of coffee on NAFLD development were mainly ascribed to its caffeine content. Several studies indicated that caffeine reduces intrahepatic fat accumulation in mice and rats, however, these studies did not specify the dose of caffeine based on animal weight or they used a dose close to the maximal one admitted in humans after interspecies conversion [11–13]. Moreover, coffee contains more than one hundred compounds besides caffeine, and it is especially rich in polyphenols such as chlorogenic acids [14], which might also be responsible for its beneficial effects.

In the present study, we investigated the effects of a moderate dose of caffeine (5 mg/kg/day, alone or as part of a green coffee extract) in a model of hepatic steatosis without obesity and without inflammation, induced in female rats by feeding a cocoa butter-rich, high-fat diet, together with liquid fructose. Female rats were used, as non-obese steatosis is more frequent in females than in males [3]. The aims of the study were to determine whether caffeine at this low dose reversed hepatic steatosis in this model, whether there were different effects when the same dose of caffeine was administered in the form of a coffee extract, and to explore the mechanisms involved.

2. Materials and Methods

2.1. Animals

Female Sprague Dawley rats were purchased from Envigo (Barcelona, Spain). Animals were maintained under conditions of constant humidity (40–60%) and temperature (20–24°C), with a light/dark cycle of 12 h (2 rats/cage). Studies were conducted in accordance with the principles and procedures outlined in the guidelines established by the Bioethics Committee of the University of Barcelona (Autonomous Government of Catalonia Act 5/21 July 1995). The Animal Experimentation Ethics Committee of the University of Barcelona approved all experimental procedures involving animals (approval no. 10106).

2.2. Dosage Regimen

Forty-eight female rats aged 8 weeks were randomly assigned into 4 groups ($n = 12$ in each), which received: (1) standard rodent chow (control group, CT); (2) high-fat diet, and 10% w/v fructose in the drinking water (high-fat-high-fructose group, HF-HFr); (3) high-fat diet containing caffeine (from Sigma–Aldrich, St. Louis, MO, USA, 0.18 g/kg of diet) and 10% w/v fructose in drinking water (caffeine group, CAF); or (4) high-fat diet containing a green coffee extract providing 0.18 g of caffeine/kg of diet, and 10% w/v fructose in the drinking water (green coffee extract group, GCE). Groups 1 and 2 received their respective diets for 3 months. Groups 3 and 4 received the HF-HFr diet for 2 months, with the caffeine or green coffee extract supplied to the rats incorporated in the high-fat diet pellets during the third month of the protocol. The green coffee extract (a generous gift from Applied Food Science Inc., Austin, TX, USA) was obtained by extraction with 70:30 ethanol: water mixture, and then the extract was filtered, evaporated, and spray dried. The compositions of the control diet (2018 Teklad Global 18% protein) and the high-fat diet (Teklad Custom Diet TD.180456) are detailed in Supplementary material Table S1. Diets containing caffeine and green coffee extract were prepared by Envigo (Madison, WI, USA), by mixing the compounds with the different ingredients of the high-fat diet and pelleting. Fructose solutions were changed every two days. Throughout the treatment, solid food and liquid consumption was controlled three times a week, and body weight was recorded once a week. Based on the amount of diet consumed and the body weight of each rat, the amount of caffeine ingested in both the CAF and GCE groups was 5.0 ± 0.8 mg/kg/day. The human equivalent dose based on body surface area (K_m value for humans = 37 and for rats weighing 250 g = 7) was 0.95 mg/kg/day [15].

2.3. Open Field Test

In the last week of the treatment, an open field test (OFT) was performed to study locomotor activity in the control and treated rats. Rats were placed in the middle of a black box ($40 \times 40 \times 40$ cm), under a low illumination of 12 lux. Rats underwent habituation sessions for two consecutive days. On the third day, the distance traveled by each rat was monitored during 60 min (SMART® version 3.0 software, Panlab SL, Barcelona, Spain). The OFT apparatus was cleaned with 10% ethanol solution, before using it with another rat.

2.4. Oral Glucose Tolerance Test

An oral glucose tolerance test (OGTT) was performed in the last week of the treatment, one day after the OFT test. Rats were fasted for 6 h, and a sample of blood was collected from the tail vein (time 0). A glucose solution of 2 g/kg of body weight was then administered by oral gavage, and blood samples were collected from the tail vein at 15, 30, 60, and 120 min after glucose administration. Glucose levels were determined in all blood samples using a hand-held glucometer (Accutrend® Plus System, Cobas, Roche Farma, Barcelona, Spain). Plasma was obtained from blood samples collected at 0, 15, and 120 min, and insulin levels were measured using a rat insulin enzyme-linked immunosorbent assay (ELISA) kit (Millipore, Billerica, MA, USA).

2.5. Sample Preparation

At the end of the treatment, rats were fasted for 2 h and blood samples were obtained from the tail vein to measure TG, cholesterol, and glucose levels, using an Accutrend® Plus system glucometer (Cobas, Roche Farma, Barcelona, Spain). The rats were then immediately anesthetized with ketamine/xylazine (9 mg/40 µg per 100 g of body weight, respectively) and blood was collected into micro-tubes (Sarstedt AG & Co., Nümbrecht, Germany) through cardiac puncture and centrifuged at $10{,}000\times g$ for 5 min, at room temperature. Rats were euthanized by exsanguination, and the liver and visceral white adipose tissue (vWAT) were collected and weighed. For the histological studies, samples of the liver of each animal were fixed in buffered formalin or were embedded in OCT, frozen quickly in liquid nitrogen, and stored at −80 °C. The remaining liver tissues were immediately frozen in liquid nitrogen and stored at −80 °C until needed for biomolecular assays.

2.6. Plasma Analysis

Plasma samples were assayed in duplicates. Insulin and adiponectin concentrations were determined using specific ELISA kits (Millipore, Billerica, MA, USA). Alanine aminotransferase (ALT) activity was determined using an ALT/GPT enzymatic assay kit (Spinreact, Girona, Spain). Insulin sensitivity index (ISI) was calculated as 2/[plasma insulin (nM) × blood glucose (μM) + 1].

2.7. Histological Studies

Liver samples were dehydrated and paraffin embedded using a Leica TP1020 automatic tissue processor and a Leica EG1150 H Paraffin Embedding Module (Leica Microsistemas, Barcelona, Spain). Samples were cut to 5 microns and stained with hematoxylin and eosin (H&E). Lipid accumulation was analyzed in OCT-embedded liver sections stained with Oil-Red O (ORO). Images were acquired with a Leica DMSL microscope equipped with a DP72 camera (Leica Microsistemas, Barcelona, Spain) and analyzed using Image J 1.49 software (National Institutes of Health, Bethesda, MD, USA). The area of positive ORO staining was calculated as the positively stained area per total area. All procedures were carried out in the Animal Histopathology Laboratory at the University of Barcelona.

2.8. Liver Assays

Liver TGs were extracted as described by Qu et al. [16] and determined using a TG colorimetric assay kit (Spinreact, Girona, Spain). Total hepatic fatty acid β-oxidation was determined in rat livers, as described by Lazarow [17], using 30 μg of postnuclear supernatant.

2.8.1. Measurement of Fatty Acid Methyl Esters in Liver TGs

Fatty acid methyl esters (FAMEs) from liver TGs were determined by gas chromatography/electron ionization mass spectrometry as described in the Supplementary Methods and Table S3.

2.8.2. Lipidomic Analysis in Rat Liver Homogenates

Levels of diacylglycerols [DAG], ceramides [Cer], and hexosylceramides [HexCer] in rat livers were determined by liquid chromatography-tandem mass spectrometry (LC–MS/MS) system, as described in Supplementary Methods and Table S4.

2.9. RNA Preparation and Analysis

Total RNA was isolated from the liver samples using Trizol® (Invitrogen, Carlsbad, CA, USA), cDNA was synthesized by reverse transcription and specific mRNAs were assessed by real-time reverse transcription polymerase chain reaction (RT-PCR), as described previously [18]. TBP (TATA-box-binding protein) was used as an internal control. The primer sequences and PCR product lengths are listed in Supplementary Material (Table S2).

2.10. Preparation of Protein Extracts

Liver samples were homogenized with a Polytron PT 1200E in lysis buffer containing proteases, phosphatases, and deacetylase inhibitors, and incubated for 1.5 h at 4 °C. Samples were then centrifuged at 15,000× g for 15 min at 4 °C, and the supernatants were collected. To obtain hepatic nuclear extracts, samples were homogenized with a homogenization buffer, kept on ice for 10 min, and centrifuged at 1000× g for 10 min at 4 °C. Lysis buffer was added to the obtained pellet and samples were incubated for 1.5 h at 4 °C, before being centrifuged at 25,000× g for 30 min at 4 °C. The resulting supernatants were then collected. Protein concentrations were determined by the Bradford method [19].

2.11. Western Blot Analysis

Western blots were performed using three samples per group, each sample was pooled from two animals. A total of 20–30 μg of protein extracts were subjected to SDS-polyacrylamide gel electrophoresis. Proteins were then transferred onto Immobilon polyvinylidene difluoride transfer membranes (Millipore, Billerica, MA, USA), and blocked for 1 h at room temperature, with 5% non-fat milk solution in Tris-buffered saline (TBS) containing 0.1% Tween-20. Membranes were then incubated with specific primary antibodies. Detection was performed using the Immobilion Western HRP substrate Peroxide Solution® (Millipore, Billerica, MA, USA). To confirm the uniformity of protein loading, blots were incubated with anti-β-actin or anti-β-tubulin antibody (Sigma–Aldrich, St. Louis, MO, USA) as a control for total protein extracts, and with anti-TBP antibody (AbCam, Cambridge, UK) for nuclear protein extracts.

2.12. Statistical Analysis

The results are expressed as mean ± standard deviation (SD). Significant differences between the groups were established by one-way ANOVA and Šidák's post-hoc test for selected comparisons (GraphPad Software version 8, San Diego, CA, USA). When the SD of the groups was different according to Bartlett's test, the data were transformed into their logarithms and ANOVA was rerun, or the corresponding non-parametric test was applied. The OGTT curves for glucose and insulin were analyzed by two-way ANOVA. The level of statistical significance was set at $p \leq 0.05$.

3. Results

3.1. The HF-HFr Diet Does Not Induce Obesity or Gluconeogenic Gene Expression

As shown in Table 1, although the HF-HFr diet induced a 1.8-fold increase in total caloric intake, the final body weight and vWAT weight were not significantly modified. Only the liver weight/body weight ratio showed a significant increase in response to the HF-HFr diet. Locomotor activity (measured as the total distance travelled in the open field test) was not significantly affected by the diet or treatments.

Table 1. Zoometric parameters, blood analytes, and open field test results.

	CT ($n = 12$)	HF-HFr ($n = 10$)	CAF ($n = 12$)	GCE ($n = 12$)
Final body weight (g)	270 ± 13	271 ± 13	280 ± 10	270 ± 12
Liver weight/body weight	2.9 ± 0.2	3.5 ± 0.4 **	3.8 ± 0.4 ***	3.6 ± 0.3 ***
vWAT weight/body weight	2.5 ± 0.7	3.1 ± 0.8	3.0 ± 0.6	2.9 ± 0.7
AUC consumed diet (Kcal/90 days/rat)	3884 ± 122	2728 ± 511 ***	2821 ± 352 ***	2710 ± 438 ***
AUC ingested liquid (Kcal/90 days/rat)	0	4098 ± 1201 ***	4330 ± 565 ***	4093 ± 750 ***
Total calorie intake (kcal/animal/90 days)	3884 ± 122	6827 ± 744 ***	7151 ± 141 ***	6803 ± 401 ***
Blood insulin (ng/mL)	1.2 ± 1.1	2.3 ± 1.0	3.3 ± 1.0	2.9 ± 1.4
Blood glucose (mg/dL)	117.2 ± 19.1	111.9 ± 12.7	120.2 ± 11.9	121.4 ± 15.3
ISI	1.1 ± 0.4	0.5 ± 0.2 *	0.5 ± 0.1 ***	0.6 ± 0.3 **
ALT (U/L)	19.9 ± 5.2	23.4 ± 5.2	19.8 ± 6.0	22.1 ± 5.8
Distance travelled in the OFT (cm)	8537 ± 1523	8429 ± 2110	8429 ± 1454	8316 ± 1985

Values are expressed as mean ± SD ($n = 10$–12). ALT: alanine aminotransferase; AUC: area under the curve; CAF: caffeine; CT: control; GCE: green coffee extract; HF-HFr: high-fat-high-fructose; ISI: insulin sensitivity index, calculated as 2/(plasma insulin (nM) × blood glucose (μM) + 1); OFT: open field test; vWAT: visceral white adipose tissue. * $p < 0.05$; ** $p < 0.01$; *** $p < 0.001$ vs. control.

Basal blood glucose and insulin levels were similar across the different groups (Table 1). After a glucose challenge in the OGTT, all groups on the HF-HFr diet exhibited higher glucose levels than the CT group at the shortest time points (Figure 1A). However, no differences were observed in the integrated glucose concentration, which was calculated as the area under the curve (AUC) (Figure 1B). Both the insulin levels (Figure 1C) and the corresponding AUC (Figure 1D) were significantly increased by the HF-HFr diet, with neither CAF nor GCE attenuating this increase. Accordingly, the ISI was significantly reduced in the HF-HFr group and none of the treatments reversed this decrease (Table 1). The mRNA levels of the insulin-responsive gluconeogenic genes phosphoenolpyruvate carboxykinase (*Pepck*) and glucose-6 phosphatase (*G6Pase*) decreased in the rats fed the HF-HFr diet (Figure 1E–F).

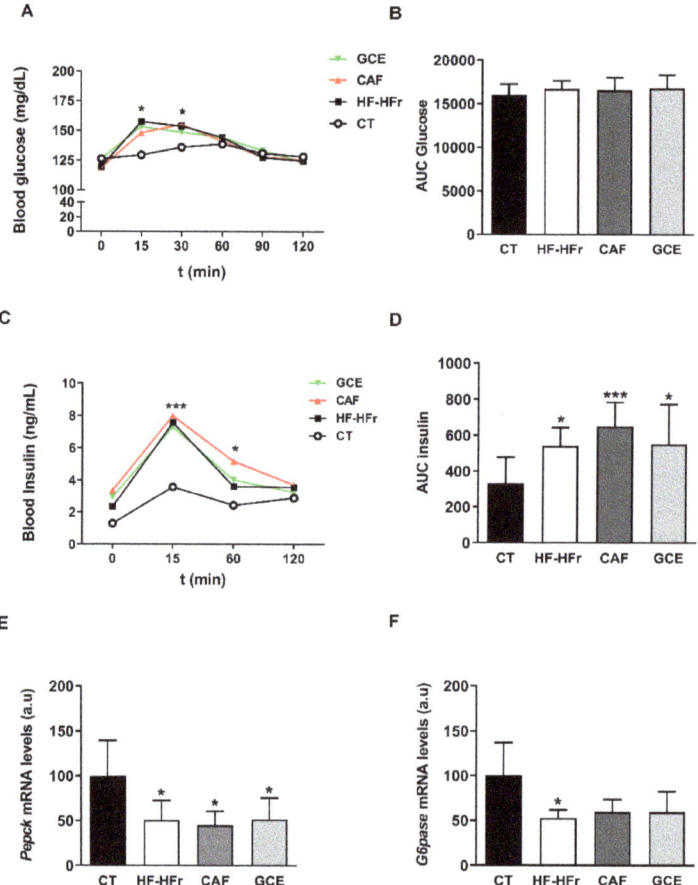

Figure 1. Blood glucose (**A**), area under the curve (AUC) for glucose (**B**), plasma insulin (**C**), and AUC for insulin (**D**) at different times after oral administration of a glucose solution (2 g/kg body weight). Results are the mean ± SD of values from 10–12 animals/group. Bar plots representing the mean ± SD mRNA levels corresponding to liver *Pepck* (**E**) and *G6Pase* (**F**) genes from CT ($n = 5$), HF-HFr ($n = 6$), CAF ($n = 6$) and GCE ($n = 6$) experimental groups. * $p < 0.05$; *** $p < 0.001$ vs. control.

3.2. GCE Exerts Different Effects Compared to CAF on Hepatic TG Amount and Composition

Blood cholesterol was unaffected by the diet or treatments, whereas blood TG levels were similarly increased in the HF-HFr, CAF, and GCE groups, compared to the control rats (Figure 2A,B).

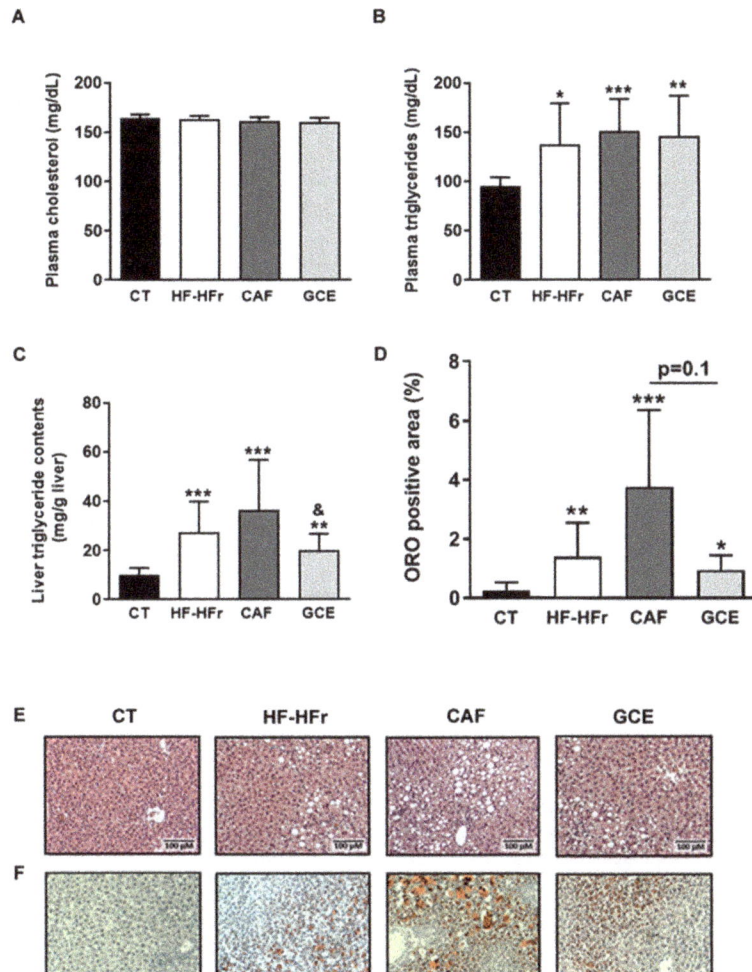

Figure 2. Blood cholesterol (**A**), blood triglyceride (**B**), and liver triglyceride (**C**) levels. Results are the mean ± SD of values from 10–12 animals/group. (**D**) Bar plot representing the mean ± SD percentage of area of positive Oil Red O staining calculated as positive stained area per total area section in CT, HF-HFr, CAF, and GCE experimental groups ($n = 10$–12/group). Representative hematoxylin and eosin (**E**) and Oil Red O (**F**) stained liver sections from the four experimental groups. * $p < 0.05$; ** $p < 0.01$; *** $p < 0.0001$ vs. control. & $p < 0.05$ vs. CAF group.

The hepatic TG concentration was also increased in the HF-HFr group versus the CT group, and neither CAF or GCE attenuated this increase. Interestingly, hepatic TG levels were significantly lower in the GCE group than in the CAF group (Figure 2C). The same trend was observed in the liver sections stained with H&E and ORO, although the difference between the GCE and CAF groups was only marginally significant ($p = 0.1$) (Figure 2D–F).

We also aimed to determine the fatty acid profile of the hepatic TGs. As shown in Figure 3A, the amount of SFAs [palmitic acid (16:0) and stearic acid (18:0)] and MUFAs [palmitoleic acid (16:1 n-7) and oleic acid (18:1 n-9)] in the hepatic TG fraction was strikingly increased by the HF-HFr diet. The addition of CAF or GCE did not significantly affect the levels of these SFAs compared to the

HF-HFr group. Interestingly, the levels of both MUFAs were lower in the GCE group than in the CAF group, although the difference was significant only for palmitoleic acid. We also analyzed the levels of a less abundant MUFA in the TG fraction, 20:1 n-9, which showed also a significant increase in response to the HF-HFr diet and a decrease in the GCE group, compared to the CAF group (Figure 3A). Regarding PUFAs 20:4 n-6, 20:5 n-3, and 22:6 n-3, all showed lower levels in the GCE group than in the HF-HFr and the CT groups. The amount of linoleic acid (18:2 n-6) was not significantly altered by the diet or treatments (Figure 3B).

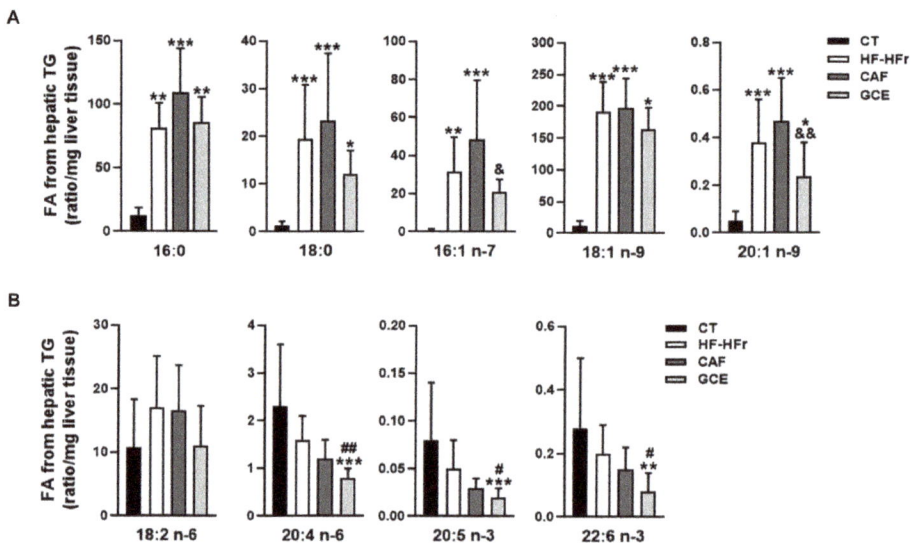

Figure 3. Fatty acid composition of hepatic triglycerides. (**A**) Saturated and monounsaturated fatty acids and (**B**) polyunsaturated fatty acids in the hepatic triglyceride fraction from CT, HF-HFr, CAF, and GCE experimental groups. Results are the mean ± SD of values from 9–10 animals/group. * $p < 0.05$; ** $p < 0.01$; *** $p < 0.001$ vs. control. # $p < 0.05$; ## $p < 0.01$ vs. HF-HFr group. & $p < 0.05$; && $p < 0.01$ vs. CAF group.

3.3. Liver Lipidomic Signatures Induced by the HF-HFr Diet and Effects of CAF and GCE

Analysis of hepatic DAGs showed a striking effect of the HF-HFr diet, which increased the amount of SFA-, and MUFA-containing DAGs (Figure 4A). The addition of GCE to the HF-HFr diet significantly attenuated the increase in DAG 18:0/18:0 whereas CAF supplementation had no effect on this species. By contrast, the HF-HFr diet did not significantly increase the levels of PUFA-containing DAG (Figure 4B) and caused a large reduction in DAG 18:2/18:2. GCE treatment reduced the amount of DAG 16:0/18:2 and DAG 18:0/20:4.

We also analyzed the effect of diet and treatments on the amount of hepatic Cer and HexCer (Figure 4C,D). The HF-HFr diet significantly reduced the levels of Cer 14:0 and Cer 16:0. By contrast, the amount of Cer 18:1 was increased by the HF-HFr diet, with CAF significantly attenuating this increase. Similarly, HexCer 18:0 and HexCer 20:0 levels were increased in the HF-HFr group, with GCE attenuating the increases. Moreover, GCE exerted specific effects on several species that were not modified by the HF-HFr diet, such as the reduction of Cer 20:0 and HexCer 16:0, 22:0, and 24:1 levels.

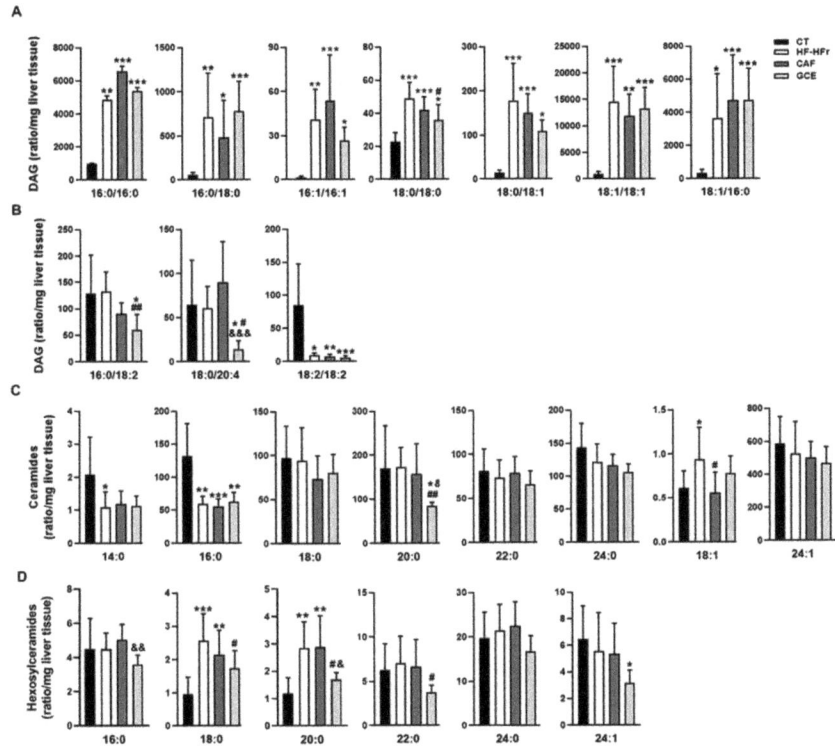

Figure 4. Lipidomic analysis in rat liver homogenates. Levels of diacylglycerols (DAG) (**A**,**B**), ceramides (Cer) (**C**), and hexosylceramides (HexCer) (**D**) in CT, HF-HFr, CAF, and GCE experimental groups. Results are the mean ± SD of values from 9–10 animals/group. * $p < 0.05$; ** $p < 0.01$; *** $p < 0.001$ vs. control. # $p < 0.05$, ## $p < 0.01$ vs. HF-HFr group. & $p < 0.05$; && $p < 0.01$; &&& $p < 0.001$ vs. CAF group.

As shown in Table 2, the ratio of HexCer 16:0, 18:0, 20:0, and 24:0 to the corresponding Cer was very low in the CT group and was increased by the HF-HFr diet. Again, we observed a differential effect of GCE, as this group showed lower HexCer/Cer ratios for 16:0 and 18:0 than the HF-HFr group, whereas CAF did not cause this effect.

Table 2. Ratio hexosylceramide/ceramide.

	CT	HF-HFr	CAF	GCE
16_0	0.038 ± 0.017	0.076 ± 0.009 ***	0.093 ± 0.022 ***	0.059 ± 0.014 *** #
18_0	0.010 ± 0.004	0.028 ± 0.004 ***	0.030 ± 0.007 ***	0.021 ± 0.003 *** # &&
20_0	0.007 ± 0.002	0.016 ± 0.004 ***	0.019 ± 0.004 ***	0.019 ± 0.003 ***
22_0	0.076 ± 0.026	0.104 ± 0.049	0.082 ± 0.025	0.060 ± 0.015
24_0	0.139 ± 0.033	0.178 ± 0.040 *	0.191 ± 0.025 **	0.157 ± 0.024

Values are expressed as mean ± SD ($n = 9$–10). * $p < 0.05$; ** $p < 0.01$; *** $p < 0.001$ vs. CT. # $p < 0.05$ vs. HF-HFr; && $p < 0.01$ vs. CAF.

3.4. Effects of the Diet and Treatments on the Fatty Acid Biosynthetic Pathway

We determined the hepatic expression of sterol regulatory element-binding protein-1c (SREBP-1c), a transcription factor that controls the expression of enzymes involved in fatty acid synthesis. Both the precursor (125 kD) and the active form of SREBP-1c (68 kD) remained unaltered in the hepatic protein samples of all groups (Figure 5A). By contrast, the hepatic protein level of fatty acid synthase (FAS), a lipogenic enzyme controlled by this transcription factor, was increased significantly by the HF-HFr diet, with GCE partially preventing this increase (Figure 5B). The mRNA levels of another lipogenic enzyme controlled by SREBP-1c, stearoyl-CoA desaturase (*Scd1*), followed the same pattern of an increase in the HF-HFr group (Figure 5C). Interestingly, CAF increased *Scd1* expression even more than the HF-HFr diet, whereas GCE did not.

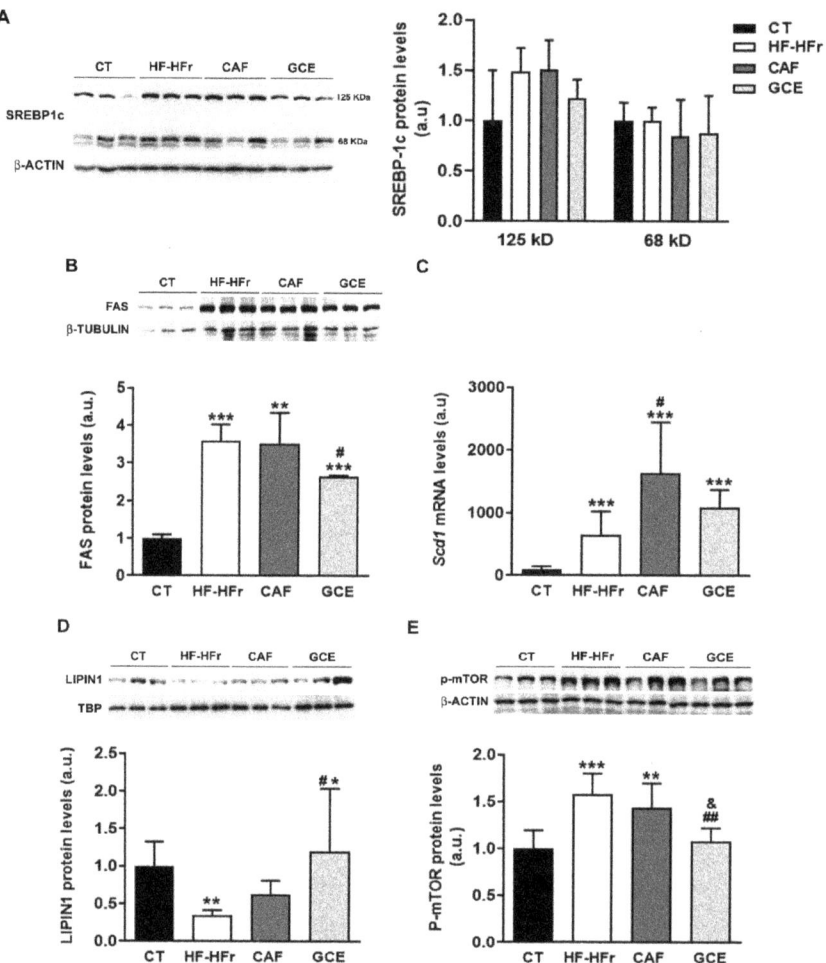

Figure 5. Western Blot of precursor (125 kD) and mature (68 kD) SREBP-1c (**A**) FAS: fatty acid synthase (**B**) lipin-1 (**D**) and phospho-mTOR proteins (**E**) in liver samples. Bar plots represent the mean ± SD band intensity of the proteins obtained from three samples per group, each one pooled from two animals. Bands are shown in the upper part of the figures. (**C**) Bar plot representing the mean ± SD mRNA levels corresponding to liver *Scd1* from CT ($n = 5$), HF-HFr ($n = 6$), CAF ($n = 6$), and GCE ($n = 6$) experimental groups. * $p < 0.05$; ** $p < 0.01$; *** $p < 0.001$ vs. CT. # $p < 0.05$; ## $p < 0.01$ vs. HF-HFr. & $p < 0.05$ vs. CAF.

The observed effects of the diet on FAS and SCD1 expression suggested increased SREBP-1c transcriptional activity despite no changes in the amount of the active form of the protein. As shown in Figure 5D, the HF-HFr group showed a significant decrease in hepatic nuclear levels of lipin-1, which could modulate the transcriptional activity of SREBP-1c. Accordingly, the expression of phosphorylated mammalian target of rapamycin (P-mTOR), which phosphorylates lipin-1 and causes its nuclear exclusion, was increased in the livers of the rats from the HF-HFr group (Figure 5E). Interestingly, GCE relieved the reduction in lipin-1 levels caused by the diet, increasing the amount of this protein in nuclear extracts above CT levels (Figure 5D). Moreover, the GCE group returned P-mTOR levels to the control values, showing a significant reduction compared to the HF-HFr and CAF groups, which was in accordance with the increase in nuclear lipin-1 levels (Figure 5E).

3.5. CAF or GCE Does Not Affect Lipid Catabolic Pathways

To explore other mechanisms potentially involved in the observed effects on hepatic TGs, we determined the β-oxidation activity in liver samples. The results showed a significant decrease in response to the HF-HFr diet, with CAF or GCE addition having no effect on this decrease (Figure 6A). The mRNA levels of peroxisome proliferator-activated receptor α (*Pparα*), and the PPARα target genes acyl-CoA oxidase (*Aco*) and very-low density lipoprotein receptor (*Vldlr*) were not modified by the diet or treatments (Figure 6B–D). However, the protein levels of VLDLR despite not being increased by the HF-HFr diet were significantly lower in the CAF and GCE groups, and GCE even lowered the amount of this protein compared to the CAF group (Figure 6E).

The autophagy of lipid droplets was described as another form of lipid catabolism. As shown in Figure 6F, the ratio of the microtubule-associated protein 1A/1B-light chain 3 (LC3) B-II/I was significantly reduced in the HF-HFr group, with CAF or GCE treatment not reversing this decrease. However, neither diet nor treatments reduced the levels of the autophagy substrate p62 (Figure 6G), while beclin-1 levels showed a small but significant increase in the CAF group (Figure 6H).

3.6. Endoplasmic Reticulum Stress, Inflammation, and Oxidative Stress Markers

We also explored other cell signaling pathways that could modulate hepatic lipid levels, such as endoplasmic reticulum (ER) stress. The HF-HFr diet significantly increased inositol-requiring enzyme-1α (IRE1α) phosphorylation, with neither CAF nor GCE reversing this increase (Figure 7A). However, levels of the active/spliced form of X-box-binding protein 1 (XBP-1s) protein in nuclear extracts were not significantly modified by any treatment, and mRNA levels of the XBP-1s target gene ER degradation-enhancing α-mannosidase-like 1 (*Edem1*) were not altered by HF-HFr diet and showed reduced expression in the CAF group (Figure 7B,C). Levels of the precursor (90 kD) and mature form (50 kD) of activating transcription factor 6 (ATF6) and phosphorylation of protein kinase RNA-like ER kinase (PERK) were not altered in any group (Figure 7D,E).

Finally, we assessed the expression of several inflammation and oxidative stress markers. The experimental diet used did not induce an inflammatory response in the liver. In fact, the mRNA expression of several inflammation-related genes was reduced, with the treatments showing negligible effect (Figure 8A). In line with these results, the plasma levels of the inflammation marker ALT were not increased by the diet or treatments (Table 1). Similarly, the HF-HFr diet did not induce hepatic oxidative stress, and even reduced glutathione peroxidase 1 (*Gpx1*) expression. The GCE group showed lower mRNA levels of superoxide dismutase 2 (*Sod2*) compared to the CAF group (Figure 8B).

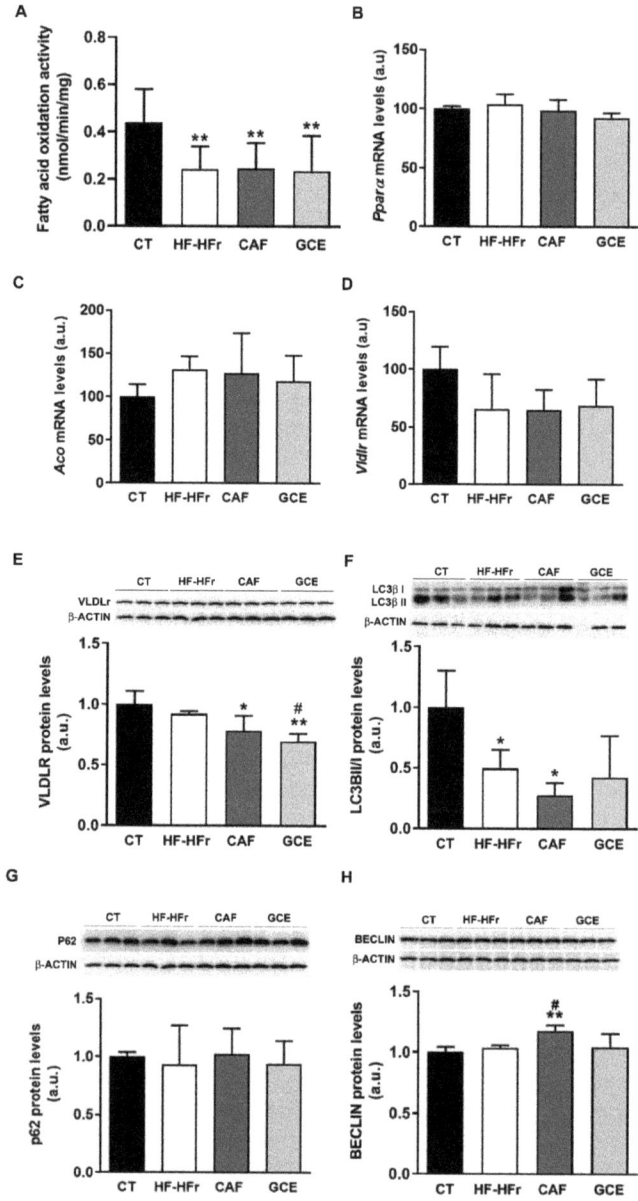

Figure 6. (**A**) β-oxidation activity in liver samples. Bars represent the mean ± SD of 10–12 samples per group. Bar plots representing the mean ± SD mRNA levels corresponding to liver *Pparα* (**B**), *Aco* (**C**), and *Vldlr* (**D**) genes from CT (*n* = 5), HF-HFr (*n* = 6), CAF (*n* = 6), and GCE (*n* = 6) experimental groups. Western Blot of VLDLR (**E**), LCII/I ratio (**F**), p62 (**G**), and beclin-1 (**H**) proteins, in liver samples obtained from CT, HF-HFr, CAF, and GCE experimental groups. Bar plots represent the mean ± SD band intensity of the proteins obtained from three samples per group, each one pooled from two animals. Bands are shown in the upper part of the figures. * $p < 0.05$; ** $p < 0.01$ vs. CT. # $p < 0.05$ vs. HF-HFr group.

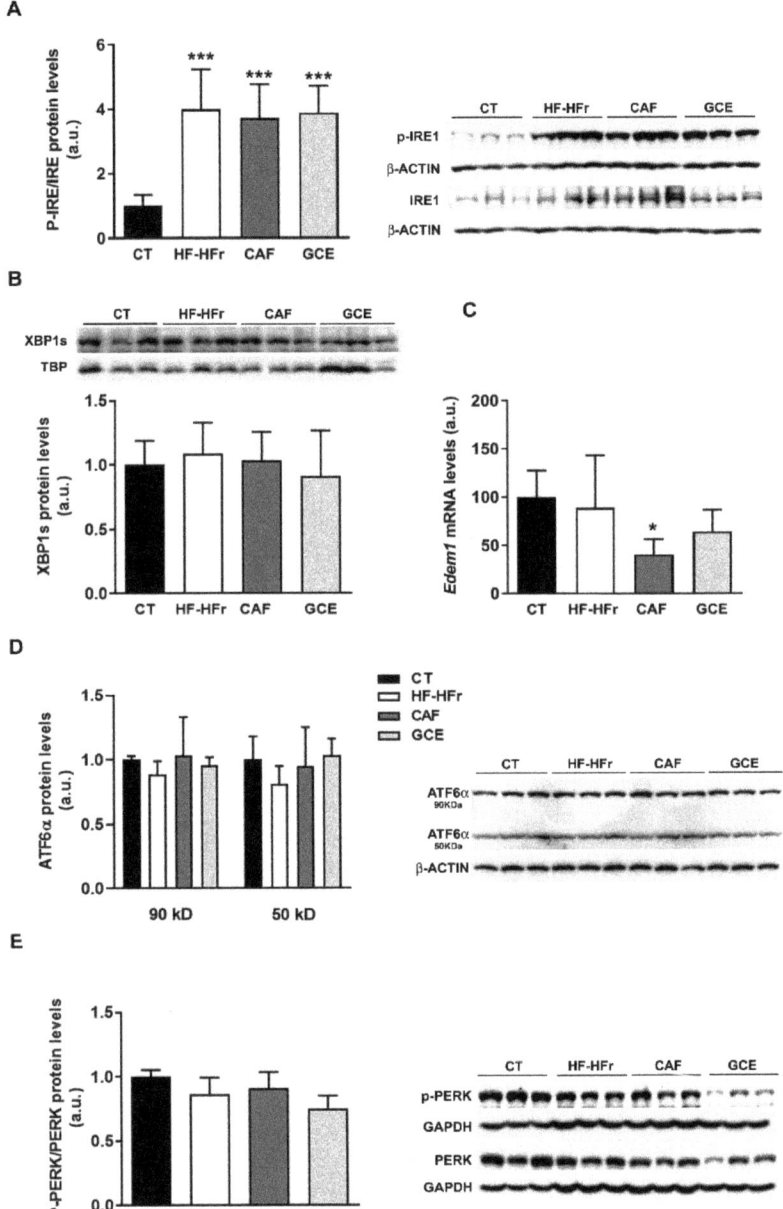

Figure 7. Western Blot of phosphorylated and total IRE1 (**A**), nuclear XBP1S (**B**), precursor (90 kD) and mature (50 kD) ATF6 (**D**), and phosphorylated and total PERK (**E**) in liver samples. Bar plots represent the mean ± SD band intensity of the proteins obtained from three samples per group, each one pooled from two animals. Bands are shown in the upper part of the figures. (**C**) mRNA levels of *Edem1* in the livers from CT ($n = 5$), HF-HFr ($n = 6$), CAF ($n = 6$), and GCE ($n = 6$) experimental groups. * $p < 0.05$; *** $p < 0.001$ vs. CT.

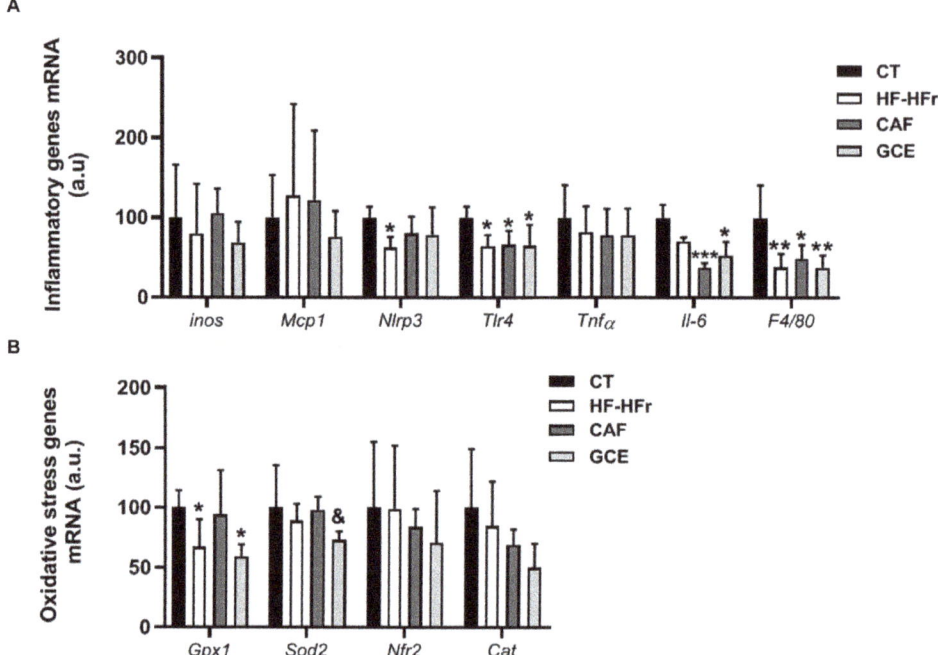

Figure 8. Bar plots showing the mean ± SD of specific mRNAs of pro-inflammatory molecules *iNos*, *Mcp1*, *Nlrp3*, *Tlr4*, *Tnfα*, *Il-6*, and *F4/80* (**A**) and oxidative stress genes *Gpx1*, *Sod2*, *Nrf2*, and *Cat* (**B**) in the livers from CT ($n = 5$), HF-HFr ($n = 6$), CAF ($n = 6$), and GCE ($n = 6$) experimental groups. * $p < 0.05$; ** $p < 0.01$; *** $p < 0.001$ vs. control. & $p < 0.05$ vs. CAF group.

4. Discussion

Although nearly all rodent models on a high-fat diet rich in saturated fatty acids are characterized by obesity and insulin resistance [20], it is increasingly being recognized that a substantial proportion of individuals present NAFLD without obesity [2]. To obtain a model of NAFLD in its initial phase of simple hepatic steatosis, we fed female Sprague-Dawley rats a high-fat diet, which provides an exogenous source of fatty acids, and added liquid fructose (10% w/v) to their drinking water to promote de novo lipogenesis (DNL) [21]. To avoid the dietary intake of cholesterol, which is thought to activate Kupffer cells and stellate cells, and induce inflammation and fibrosis characteristic of NASH [22], we used cocoa butter instead of milk, as the source of saturated fatty acids in the high-fat diet.

Administration of the HF-HFr diet for three months caused hypertriglyceridemia and hepatic lipid deposition in the female Sprague-Dawley rats, but not inflammation, ER stress, or oxidative stress. Moreover, the rats fed the HF-HFr diet did not show an increase in body weight and adiposity, despite receiving around 1.8-times more calories than the control rats, which could not be ascribed to increased energy expenditure through spontaneous locomotor activity. Furthermore, although the rats on the HF-HFr diet responded to a glucose challenge with a higher insulin secretion, the increased insulin levels successfully controlled blood glucose levels and reduced the expression of hepatic gluconeogenic genes. This suggests that despite a decrease in the ISI, the hepatic glucose output was reduced, whereas in a typical situation of hepatic insulin resistance it would be increased [23].

The lipidomic analysis of liver samples from the rats offered some clues to explain these features of the HF-HFr diet. One of the most important bioactive lipids are ceramides, a class of sphingolipids involved in insulin resistance, inflammation, oxidative stress, and NAFLD development [24]. It was suggested that saturated fat derived from DNL or from the diet induces ceramide synthesis and insulin resistance [25]. However, we found that the hepatic levels of most ceramide species were not increased by the diet, which could be attributed to the absence of inflammation, as liver ceramides were reported to be increased in NASH, but not in simple steatosis in humans [26]. Remarkably, mice deficient in ceramide synthase 5 (CerS5), which exhibit lower hepatic levels of Cer 16:0, were protected from developing obesity and insulin resistance when fed a high-fat diet [27]. Therefore, the 50% reduction in hepatic Cer 16:0 levels in the HF-HFr group might help explain the absence of liver insulin resistance and obesity in rats fed this diet.

Having obtained a model of lean NAFLD with simple hepatic steatosis, we aimed to determine whether a moderate dose of caffeine, or a green coffee extract providing the same dose of caffeine, was effective in reducing the liver lipid burden. One of the major sources of caffeine in the human diet is coffee, which was reported to have beneficial effects on liver health [9]. However, a positive effect of coffee on NAFLD was not clearly established in human studies. Thus, a lower prevalence of NAFLD was associated with higher coffee intake in the NHANES study [28] and in some meta-analyses [10], but this association was not confirmed in other studies [29,30]. However, studies in animal models of diet-induced steatosis showed that several components of coffee, including caffeine, might be effective in reducing liver fat deposition [31]. The different outcomes from the human and animal studies might be due to the high doses of caffeine administered to laboratory animals, which in some studies were equivalent to 6 cups of coffee a day, much higher than the usual consumption in humans [32]. To provide a more realistic scenario, we treated rats with a low dose of caffeine (5 mg/kg/day), which after conversion based on body surface area was equivalent to 66 mg of caffeine for a 70-kg human being [15]. This amount roughly corresponded to 1 cup (20–25 mL) of espresso coffee per day, which was reported to contain 2.4 to 4.5 mg/mL of caffeine [33].

We observed that neither CAF nor GCE alleviated the hypertriglyceridemia and hepatic steatosis caused by the HF-HFr diet. However, rats treated with GCE exhibited lower levels of hepatic TG than those treated with CAF. When we analyzed the fatty acid composition of these TGs, we found that the amounts of palmitoleic acid and 20:1 *n*-9 were increased by the HF-HFr diet but were lower in the GCE group than in the CAF group. Palmitoleic acid is generated from palmitic acid through SCD1, which, together with FAS, are lipogenic enzymes regulated by SREBP-1c. The HF-HFr diet, despite not affecting the SREBP-1c levels, increased mTOR phosphorylation, which is known to phosphorylate and exclude lipin-1 from the nucleus [34]. This might lead to increased SREBP-1 transcriptional activity and, consequently, to FAS and SCD1 induction. Interestingly, the livers of the HF-HFr rats showed reduced nuclear levels of lipin-1 together with increased FAS and *Scd1* expression. These changes were not reversed neither by CAF nor by GCE. In fact, the expression of *Scd1* was higher in the CAF group than in the HF-HFr group, suggesting that CAF could further increase hepatic lipogenesis and worsen hepatic lipid deposition. However, neither the amount of hepatic TG nor lipin-1 or p-mTOR protein levels were different between the CAF and HF-HFr groups. In contrast, the GCE-treated rats showed lower mTOR phosphorylation and higher nuclear levels of lipin-1 than those of the rats from the HF-HFr group, suggesting lower SREBP-1 transcriptional activity. This might explain why FAS and SCD1 expression were induced to a lesser extent by GCE than CAF, and was in accordance with the lower levels of palmitoleic acid and total TGs observed in the livers of the GCE-treated rats.

The different effects of GCE compared to CAF were also observed with several DAG species, namely 18:0/18:0, 16:0/18:2, and 18:0/20:4, whose levels were reduced by GCE treatment compared to the HF-HFr group, but not by CAF treatment. Although there is a paucity of information about the effects of specific DAG species, it is generally assumed that DAGs play a role not only in insulin resistance but also in hepatic steatosis [35]. Therefore, the reduction of at least some of the DAGs accumulated in the liver might be regarded as a positive effect of other compounds contained in the GCE, given that caffeine alone did not cause such a reduction.

The hepatic levels of HexCer, which are formed from Cer by the enzyme glucosylceramide synthase (GCS), were reduced in the GCE group, as well as the 16_0 and 18_0 HexCer/Cer ratio. The HexCer/Cer ratio was considered to be an indicator of GCS activity. Interestingly, treatment of ob/ob mice with an inhibitor of GCS was reported to reduce TG accumulation in the liver [36]. Thus, the lower HexCer/Cer ratios observed in the GCE group might also be associated with reduced GCS activity and lower levels of liver triglycerides in this group, suggesting beneficial effects of GCE on hepatic steatosis.

To gain more insight into the mechanisms involved in the regulation of hepatic TG accumulation, we also examined several pathways linked to fatty acid catabolism. The reduced hepatic activity of β-oxidation could contribute to increased liver TG accumulation in the HF-HFr group. However, none of the treatments reversed this decrease, suggesting that reduced catabolism of fatty acids also occurred in the CAF and GCE groups. By contrast, the hepatic protein levels of VLDLR, which were reported to increase in animal models and humans with hepatic steatosis [37], were significantly reduced by GCE, compared to the CAF group, although they were not significantly modified by the HF-HFr diet. Reduced VLDLR levels could contribute, at least partly, to the lower hepatic TG accumulation observed in the GCE group.

Due to its role in lipid droplet degradation, autophagy is another mechanism that can lead to liver fat removal [38]. Our group previously showed that liquid fructose supplementation in female rats inhibit liver autophagy, as shown by the lower LC3II/I ratio, which leads to increased liver TG levels [39]. In the current study, we also observed a reduced LC3II/I ratio and TG accumulation in the livers of rats receiving the HF-HFr diet, suggesting inhibition of hepatic autophagy. CAF-treated rats showed the lowest LC3II/I ratio and the highest TG levels in the liver, which despite a slight increase in the beclin-1 protein levels indicated that CAF did not activate autophagy in our model. Other studies suggest that CAF induced autophagy in the liver [11], but they used higher doses of CAF (30 mg/kg/day compared to 5 mg/kg/day in our study).

In conclusion, a moderate dose of caffeine, equivalent to 1 cup of coffee a day in humans, did not alleviate liver lipid deposition in a model of diet-induced hepatic steatosis, without obesity and inflammation. One limitation of our study was that we did not treat rats fed a control diet, so we cannot rule out that caffeine could have exerted some effects in rats not exposed to HF-HFr. However, our goal was to investigate whether caffeine could reverse the hepatic steatosis induced by the HF-HFr diet. The lack of effect of caffeine in our study could be attributed to the duration of treatment, to the fact that treatment was initiated two months after the introduction of the HF-HFr diet or to the low dose used. However, when the same dose of caffeine was administered through a coffee extract, despite not normalizing the hepatic TG levels, these were lower than when the caffeine was administered alone. The coffee extract was rich in other compounds such as polyphenols, which might be responsible for the different effects observed. Vitaglione et al. showed that decaffeinated coffee reduced lipid droplet accumulation in hepatocytes, in a model of NASH, suggesting that caffeine was not essential for the anti-steatotic effect of coffee [40]. However, few studies compared the effects of caffeine with other coffee compounds on hepatic steatosis. A study conducted in mice concluded that only treatment with chlorogenic acid significantly reduced hepatic TG levels, whereas administration of pure caffeine did not [41]. Similarly, female mice treated with catechines or with catechines combined with caffeine, reduced liver TG levels, whereas caffeine alone did not [42]. In mice fed an HFD, administration of chlorogenic acid or caffeine alone did not reduce hepatic TG, but a combination of both compounds was effective [43]. Although the molecular mechanisms involved are not clearly established, this study suggest a synergistic effect on several pathways controlling fatty acid metabolism, including SREBP1c and lipogenic enzymes, such as SCD1 and FAS. Along the same lines, our results suggest that GCE components, either independently or in combination with CAF, might lead to: (i) less lipogenesis due to lower mTOR phosphorylation and higher nuclear levels of lipin-1, affecting FAS and SCD1 expression; (ii) a reduced amount of several DAG species; (iii) a lower HexCer/Cer ratio, which is a marker of GCS activity; and (iv) reduced expression of hepatic VLDLR. Although these changes are subtle, their combination might contribute to the different effects of the extract when compared to caffeine alone.

Supplementary Materials: The following are available online at http://www.mdpi.com/2072-6643/12/11/3240/s1, Supplemental Methods: Measurement of fatty acid methyl esters in liver TGs, Lipidomic analysis in rat liver homogenates. Table S1: Composition of the diets used in the study. Table S2: Primers used for RT-PCR. Table S3: GC-MS parameters for detection of fatty acid methyl esters using single ion monitoring. Table S4: Retention times and transitions for detection of lipids using LC-MS/MS.

Author Contributions: A.M.V. and N.R. were in charge of all experiments and prepared the figures; R.B. and M.G. contributed to the PCR/Western blot experiments; A.S.-V. and I.L. performed FAME analysis; J.R.-M. Performed lipidomic analysis; R.M.S. helped in data interpretation and reviewed the manuscript; J.C.L. and M.A. designed the experiments, analyzed the data and wrote the manuscript. All authors have read and agreed to the published version of the manuscript.

Funding: This research was funded by the Spanish Ministry of Economy, Industry, and Competitiveness (SAF2017-82369-R), Generalitat de Catalunya (2017 SGR 38), and European Commission FEDER funds. A.M.V. is a predoctoral fellow, BECAL grant program BCAL04-327, from the Government of Paraguay. A.S.-V. is recipient of the Instituto de Salud Carlos III Miguel Servet fellowship (grant CP II 17/00029).

Conflicts of Interest: The authors declare no conflict of interest.

References

1. Than, N.N.; Newsome, P.N. A concise review of non-alcoholic fatty liver disease. *Atherosclerosis* **2015**, *239*, 192–202. [CrossRef] [PubMed]
2. Ye, Q.; Zou, B.; Yeo, Y.H.; Li, J.; Huang, D.Q.; Wu, Y.; Yang, H.; Liu, C.; Kam, L.Y.; Tan, X.X.E.; et al. Global prevalence, incidence, and outcomes of non-obese or lean non-alcoholic fatty liver disease: A systematic review and meta-analysis. *Lancet Gastroenterol. Hepatol.* **2020**, *1253*, 1–14. [CrossRef]
3. Younossi, Z.M.; Stepanova, M.; Negro, F.; Hallaji, S.; Younossi, Y.; Lam, B.; Srishord, M. Nonalcoholic fatty liver disease in lean individuals in the United States. *Medicine* **2012**, *91*, 319–327. [CrossRef]
4. Cicero, A.F.G.; Colletti, A.; Bellentani, S. Nutraceutical approach to non-alcoholic fatty liver disease (NAFLD): The available clinical evidence. *Nutrients* **2018**, *10*, 1153. [CrossRef]
5. Shan, Z.; Rehm, C.D.; Rogers, G.; Ruan, M.; Wang, D.D.; Hu, F.B.; Mozaffarian, D.; Zhang, F.F.; Bhupathiraju, S.N. Trends in dietary carbohydrate, protein, and fat intake and diet quality among US adults, 1999–2016. *JAMA J. Am. Med. Assoc.* **2019**, *322*, 1178–1187. [CrossRef]
6. Jafarirad, S.; Mansoori, A.; Adineh, A.; Panahi, Y.; Hadi, A.; Goodarzi, R. Does Turmeric/curcumin Supplementation Change Anthropometric Indices in Patients with Non-alcoholic Fatty Liver Disease? A Systematic Review and Meta-analysis of Randomized Controlled Trials. *Clin. Nutr. Res.* **2019**, *8*, 196–208. [CrossRef]
7. Jalali, M.; Mahmoodi, M.; Mosallanezhad, Z.; Jalali, R.; Imanieh, M.H.; Moosavian, S.P. The effects of curcumin supplementation on liver function, metabolic profile and body composition in patients with non-alcoholic fatty liver disease: A systematic review and meta-analysis of randomized controlled trials. *Complement. Ther. Med.* **2020**, *48*, 102283. [CrossRef]
8. Baziar, N.; Parohan, M. The effects of curcumin supplementation on body mass index, body weight, and waist circumference in patients with nonalcoholic fatty liver disease: A systematic review and dose-response meta-analysis of randomized controlled trials. *Phytother. Res.* **2020**, *34*, 464–474. [CrossRef]
9. Poole, R.; Kennedy, O.J.; Roderick, P.; Fallowfield, J.A.; Hayes, P.C.; Parkes, J. Coffee consumption and health: Umbrella review of meta-analyses of multiple health outcomes. *BMJ* **2017**, *359*, j5024. [CrossRef]
10. Hayat, U.; Siddiqui, A.A.; Okut, H.; Afroz, S.; Tasleem, S.; Haris, A. The effect of coffee consumption on the non-alcoholic fatty liver disease and liver fibrosis: A meta-analysis of 11 epidemiological studies. *Ann. Hepatol.* **2020**. [CrossRef]
11. Sinha, R.A.; Farah, B.L.; Singh, B.K.; Siddique, M.M.; Li, Y.; Wu, Y.; Ilkayeva, O.R.; Gooding, J.; Ching, J.; Zhou, J.; et al. Caffeine stimulates hepatic lipid metabolism by the autophagy-lysosomal pathway in mice. *Hepatology* **2014**, *59*, 1366–1380. [CrossRef] [PubMed]
12. Helal, M.G.; Ayoub, S.E.; Elkashefand, W.F.; Ibrahim, T.M. Caffeine affects HFD-induced hepatic steatosis by multifactorial intervention. *Hum. Exp. Toxicol.* **2018**, *37*, 983–990. [CrossRef] [PubMed]
13. Fang, C.; Cai, X.; Hayashi, S.; Hao, S.; Sakiyama, H.; Wang, X.; Yang, Q.; Akira, S.; Nishiguchi, S.; Fujiwara, N.; et al. Caffeine-stimulated muscle IL-6 mediates alleviation of non-alcoholic fatty liver disease. *Biochim. Biophys. Acta—Mol. Cell Biol. Lipids* **2019**, *1864*, 271–280. [CrossRef] [PubMed]

14. Gressner, O.A. Less Smad2 is good for you! A scientific update on coffee's liver benefits. *Hepatology* **2009**, *50*, 970–978. [CrossRef]
15. Nair, A.; Jacob, S. A simple practice guide for dose conversion between animals and human. *J. Basic Clin. Pharm.* **2016**, *7*, 27. [CrossRef]
16. Qu, S.; Su, D.; Altomonte, J.; Kamagate, A.; He, J.; Perdomo, G.; Tse, T.; Jiang, Y.; Dong, H.H. PPAR{alpha} mediates the hypolipidemic action of fibrates by antagonizing FoxO1. *Am. J. Physiol. Endocrinol. Metab.* **2007**, *292*, E421–E434. [CrossRef]
17. Lazarow, P.B. Assay of peroxisomal ß-oxidation of fatty acids. *Methods Enzymol.* **1981**, *72*, 315–319.
18. Sangüesa, G.; Roglans, N.; Montañés, J.C.; Baena, M.; Velázquez, A.M.; Sánchez, R.M.; Alegret, M.; Laguna, J.C. Chronic Liquid Fructose, but not Glucose, Supplementation Selectively Induces Visceral Adipose Tissue Leptin Resistance and Hypertrophy in Female Sprague-Dawley Rats. *Mol. Nutr. Food Res.* **2018**, *62*, 1800777. [CrossRef]
19. Bradford, M.M. A rapid and sensitive method for the quantitation of microgram quantities of protein utilizing the principle of protein-dye binding. *Anal. Biochem.* **1976**, *72*, 248–254. [CrossRef]
20. Small, L.; Brandon, A.E.; Turner, N.; Cooney, G.J. Modeling insulin resistance in rodents by alterations in diet: What have high-fat and high-calorie diets revealed? *Am. J. Physiol.-Endocrinol. Metab.* **2018**, *314*, E251–E265. [CrossRef]
21. Rebollo, A.; Roglans, N.; Alegret, M.; Laguna, J.C.C. Way back for fructose and liver metabolism: Bench side to molecular insights. *World J. Gastroenterol.* **2012**, *18*, 6552–6559. [CrossRef]
22. Arguello, G.; Balboa, E.; Arrese, M.; Zanlungo, S. Recent insights on the role of cholesterol in non-alcoholic fatty liver disease. *Biochim. Biophys. Acta—Mol. Basis Dis.* **2015**, *1852*, 1765–1778. [CrossRef]
23. Biddinger, S.B.; Kahn, C.R. From mice to men: Insights into the insulin resistance syndromes. *Annu. Rev. Physiol.* **2006**, *68*, 123–158. [CrossRef] [PubMed]
24. Kasumov, T.; Li, L.; Li, M.; Gulshan, K.; Kirwan, J.P.; Liu, X.; Previs, S.; Willard, B.; Smith, J.D.; McCullough, A. Ceramide as a mediator of non-alcoholic fatty liver disease and associated atherosclerosis. *PLoS ONE* **2015**, *10*, 1–26. [CrossRef]
25. Chavez, J.A.; Summers, S.A. A ceramide-centric view of insulin resistance. *Cell Metab.* **2012**, *15*, 585–594. [CrossRef] [PubMed]
26. Apostolopoulou, M.; Gordillo, R.; Koliaki, C.; Gancheva, S.; Jelenik, T.; De Filippo, E.; Herder, C.; Markgraf, D.; Jankowiak, F.; Esposito, I.; et al. Specific hepatic sphingolipids relate to insulin resistance, oxidative stress, and inflammation in nonalcoholic steato hepatitis. *Diabetes Care* **2018**, *41*, 1235–1243. [CrossRef]
27. Gosejacob, D.; Jäger, P.S.; Dorp, K.V.; Frejno, M.; Carstensen, A.C.; Köhnke, M.; Degen, J.; Dörmann, P.; Hoch, M. Ceramide synthase 5 is essential to maintain C16:0-Ceramide pools and contributes to the development of diet-induced obesity. *J. Biol. Chem.* **2016**, *291*, 6989–7003. [CrossRef] [PubMed]
28. Birerdinc, A.; Stepanova, M.; Pawloski, L.; Younossi, Z.M. Caffeine is protective in patients with non-alcoholic fatty liver disease. *Aliment. Pharmacol. Ther.* **2012**, *35*, 76–82. [CrossRef]
29. Veronese, N.; Notarnicola, M.; Cisternino, A.M.; Reddavide, R.; Inguaggiato, R.; Guerra, V.; Rotolo, O.; Zinzi, I.; Leandro, G.; Correale, M.; et al. Coffee intake and liver steatosis: A population study in a mediterranean area. *Nutrients* **2018**, *10*, 89. [CrossRef]
30. Shen, H.; Rodriguez, A.C.; Shiani, A.; Lipka, S.; Shahzad, G.; Mustacchia, P.; Kumar, A. Association between caffeine consumption and nonalcoholic fatty liver disease: A systemic review and meta-analysis. *Ther. Adv. Gastroenterol.* **2016**, *9*, 113–120. [CrossRef]
31. Alferink, L.J.M.; Kiefte-De Jong, J.C.; Darwish Murad, S. Potential Mechanisms Underlying the Role of Coffee in Liver Health. *Semin. Liver Dis.* **2018**, *38*, 193–214. [CrossRef] [PubMed]
32. Chen, S.; Teoh, N.C.; Chitturi, S.; Farrell, G.C. Coffee and non-alcoholic fatty liver disease: Brewing evidence for hepatoprotection? *J. Gastroenterol. Hepatol.* **2014**, *29*, 435–441. [CrossRef] [PubMed]
33. Angeloni, G.; Guerrini, L.; Masella, P.; Bellumori, M.; Daluiso, S.; Parenti, A.; Innocenti, M. What kind of coffee do you drink? An investigation on effects of eight different extraction methods. *Food Res. Int.* **2019**, *116*, 1327–1335. [CrossRef]
34. Peterson, T.R.; Sengupta, S.S.; Harris, T.E.; Carmack, A.E.; Kang, S.A.; Balderas, E.; Guertin, D.A.; Madden, K.L.; Carpenter, A.E.; Finck, B.N.; et al. MTOR complex 1 regulates lipin 1 localization to control the srebp pathway. *Cell* **2011**, *146*, 408–420. [CrossRef] [PubMed]

35. Gorden, D.L.; Ivanova, P.T.; Myers, D.S.; McIntyre, J.O.; VanSaun, M.N.; Wright, J.K.; Matrisian, L.M.; Brown, H.A. Increased diacylglycerols characterize hepatic lipid changes in progression of human nonalcoholic fatty liver disease; comparison to a murine model. *PLoS ONE* **2011**, *6*, e22775. [CrossRef]
36. Zhao, H.; Przybylska, M.; Wu, I.H.; Zhang, J.; Maniatis, P.; Pacheco, J.; Piepenhagen, P.; Copeland, D.; Arbeeny, C.; Shayman, J.A.; et al. Inhibiting glycosphingolipid synthesis ameliorates hepatic steatosis in obese mice. *Hepatology* **2009**, *50*, 85–93. [CrossRef]
37. Zarei, M.; Barroso, E.; Palomer, X.; Dai, J.; Rada, P.; Quesada-López, T.; Escolà-Gil, J.C.; Cedó, L.; Zali, M.R.; Molaei, M.; et al. Hepatic regulation of VLDL receptor by PPARβ/δ and FGF21 modulates non-alcoholic fatty liver disease. *Mol. Metab.* **2018**, *8*, 117–131. [CrossRef]
38. Schulze, R.J.; Drižytė, K.; Casey, C.A.; McNiven, M.A. Hepatic lipophagy: New insights into autophagic catabolism of lipid droplets in the liver. *Hepatol. Commun.* **2017**, *1*, 359–369. [CrossRef]
39. Baena, M.; Sanguesa, G.; Hutter, N.; Sanchez, R.M.; Roglans, N.; Laguna, J.C.; Alegret, M. Fructose supplementation impairs rat liver autophagy through mTORC activation without inducing endoplasmic reticulum stress. *Biochim. Biophys. Acta—Mol. Cell Biol. Lipids* **2015**, *1851*, 107–116. [CrossRef]
40. Vitaglione, P.; Morisco, F.; Mazzone, G.; Amoruso, D.C.; Ribecco, M.T.; Romano, A.; Fogliano, V.; Caporaso, N.; D'Argenio, G. Coffee reduces liver damage in a rat model of steatohepatitis: The underlying mechanisms and the role of polyphenols and melanoidins. *Hepatology* **2010**, *52*, 1652–1661. [CrossRef]
41. Shimoda, H.; Seki, E.; Aitani, M. Inhibitory effect of green coffee bean extract on fat accumulation and body weight gain in mice. *BMC Complement. Altern. Med.* **2006**, *6*, 9. [CrossRef] [PubMed]
42. Zhao, Y.; Yang, L.; Huang, Z.; Lin, L.; Zheng, G. Synergistic effects of caffeine and catechins on lipid metabolism in chronically fed mice via the AMP-activated protein kinase signaling pathway. *Eur. J. Nutr.* **2017**, *56*, 2309–2318. [CrossRef]
43. Xu, M.; Yang, L.; Zhu, Y.; Liao, M.; Chu, L.; Li, X.; Lin, L.; Zheng, G. Collaborative effects of chlorogenic acid and caffeine on lipid metabolism via the AMPKα-LXRα/SREBP-1c pathway in high-fat diet-induced obese mice. *Food Funct.* **2019**, *10*, 7489–7497. [CrossRef]

Publisher's Note: MDPI stays neutral with regard to jurisdictional claims in published maps and institutional affiliations.

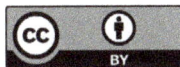 © 2020 by the authors. Licensee MDPI, Basel, Switzerland. This article is an open access article distributed under the terms and conditions of the Creative Commons Attribution (CC BY) license (http://creativecommons.org/licenses/by/4.0/).

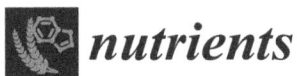

Article

Red Bull Increases Heart Rate at Near Sea Level and Pulmonary Shunt Fraction at High Altitude in a Porcine Model

Benedikt Treml [1], Elisabeth Schöpf [2], Ralf Geiger [3], Christian Niederwanger [4], Alexander Löckinger [5], Axel Kleinsasser [2] and Mirjam Bachler [6],*

[1] Department of General and Surgical Intensive Care, Medical University Innsbruck, 6020 Innsbruck, Austria; benedikt.treml@tirol-kliniken.at
[2] Department of Anesthesiology and Critical Care Medicine, Medical University Innsbruck, 6020 Innsbruck, Austria; elisabeth.schoepf@kssg.ch (E.S.); axel.kleinsasser@tirol-kliniken.at (A.K.)
[3] Department for Pediatrics, Pediatrics III, Medical University Innsbruck, 6020 Innsbruck, Austria; ralf.geiger@tirol-kliniken.at
[4] Department for Pediatrics, Pediatrics I, Intensive Care Unit, Medical University Innsbruck, 6020 Innsbruck, Austria; christian.niederwanger@tirol-kliniken.at
[5] Hanusch Hospital, 1140 Vienna, Austria; alexander.loeckinger@oegk.at
[6] Institute for Sports, Alpine Medicine and Health Tourism, Private University for Health Sciences, Medical Informatics and Technology GmbH, 6060 Hall in Tirol, Austria
* Correspondence: mirjam.bachler@tirol-kliniken.at; Tel.: +43-050504-80451

Received: 18 May 2020; Accepted: 8 June 2020; Published: 10 June 2020

Abstract: Red Bull energy drink is popular among athletes, students and drivers for stimulating effects or enhancing physical performance. In previous work, Red Bull has been shown to exert manifold cardiovascular effects at rest and during exercise. Red Bull with caffeine as the main ingredient increases blood pressure in resting individuals, probably due to an increased release of (nor)-epinephrine. Red Bull has been shown to alter heart rate or leaving it unchanged. Little is known about possible effects of caffeinated energy drinks on pulmonary ventilation/perfusion distribution at sea level or at altitude. Here, we hypothesized a possible alteration of pulmonary blood flow in ambient air and in hypoxia after Red Bull consumption. We subjected eight anesthetized piglets in normoxia ($FiO_2 = 0.21$) and in hypoxia ($FiO_2 = 0.13$), respectively, to 10 mL/kg Red Bull ingestion. Another eight animals served as controls receiving an equivalent amount of saline. In addition to cardiovascular data, ventilation/perfusion distribution of the lung was assessed by using the multiple inert gas elimination technique (MIGET). Heart rate increased in normoxic conditions but was not different from controls in acute short-term hypoxia after oral Red Bull ingestion in piglets. For the first time, we demonstrate an increased fraction of pulmonary shunt with unchanged distribution of pulmonary blood flow after Red Bull administration in acute short-term hypoxia. In summary, these findings do not oppose moderate consumption of caffeinated energy drinks even at altitude at rest and during exercise.

Keywords: Red Bull energy drink; caffeine; taurine; hypoxia; ventilation/perfusion distribution; multiple inert gas elimination technique; piglets

1. Introduction

After market release of Red Bull energy drink in April 1987 in Austria, caffeinated energy drinks have become increasingly popular. During leisure time and in training, these energy drinks are popular among athletes, students and drivers for stimulating effects or enhancing physical performance.

Beyond caffeine, one of the most popular beverages worldwide, these sugary drinks are enriched with additives like taurine and glucuronolactone to a variable amount. Vitamins and minerals are contained to a smaller amount. These ingredients account for a manifold of effects [1]. In previous work, Red Bull has been shown to exert cardiovascular effects at rest and during exercise [2–11].

Plenty of data demonstrate a change of heart rate to a minor extent. Already one century ago, the earliest studies in regards to the effect of caffeine on heart rate were reviewed [12]. Two decade ago, Alford et al. demonstrated a rise of heart rate after ingestion of a 250 mL can of Red Bull [2]. This is in line with work of Grasser et al., who demonstrated an increased heart rate and cardiac output after 355 mL of Red Bull at rest in 25 young healthy adults [3]. Moreover, such an increased heart rate has been shown during a mental arithmetic task in 20 young healthy adults [7]. A current randomized, crossover trial subjecting 38 healthy adults to several caffeinated energy drinks showed an increased mean arterial blood pressure (MAP), QTc interval and heart rate [13]. These findings are supported by other studies [4,5,11]. Aside of that data two studies reported an unchanged heart rate [8,9]. A larger trial examining 68 young adults at rest demonstrated even a small drop in heart rate [10].

In regards to 24-h blood pressure, a study demonstrated an increased 24-h blood pressure in nine healthy normotensive adults after 250 mL Red Bull compared to an equivalent amount of caffeine [4]. This is in line with a larger study demonstrating an increased heart rate and systolic blood pressure (SBP) and diastolic blood pressure (DBP) in 50 subjects early after 355 mL RB ingestion [5]. Furthermore, this group could exclude any acute effects on ventricular repolarization or conventional electrocardiographic parameters, such as the PR-, QRS-, QT-, and QTc-intervals [5]. Earlier work by Ragsdale, showing an unchanged blood pressure after 250 mL Red Bull ingestion, further impedes interpretation of data [6].

In addition to the reported cardiovascular effects at rest, Alford demonstrated an improved aerobic endurance and an improved anaerobic endurance during cycling after use of Red Bull [2]. In triathletes, an increased stroke volume and left ventricular end diastolic diameter after exercise has been shown. The researchers of this small-scale study (with 13 subjects) concluded that taurine, either alone or in combination with caffeine, is responsible for this increased contractility of the left atrium [11]. More recently, Doerner and co-workers demonstrated an increased left ventricular contractility assessed by cardiac magnetic resonance in 32 healthy resting volunteers [8].

Given those cardiovascular influences after energy drink consumption, sojourning to high altitude may further amplify physiologic responses to hypoxia. At high altitude the reduced inspired paO_2 leads to hypoxia-mediated smooth muscle contraction in the pulmonary vasculature. This hypoxic pulmonary vasoconstriction (HPV) occurs without impairment in gas exchange. If caffeinated energy drinks lead to ventilation/perfusion mismatching, it could further aggravate hypoxemia. Moreover, hypoxic induced demand tachycardia may further rise after Red Bull consumption. The current knowledge concerning effects of caffeine consumption at altitude is limited to four small studies. Those trials show an increased endurance performance in hypoxic conditions [14–17]. However, no data exist about possible effects of caffeinated energy drinks on pulmonary ventilation/perfusion distribution at altitude. The scarcity of literature encountered when designing the study led us to believe that this porcine model would be suitable for such a first pilot trial. Here, we hypothesized a possible effect of Red Bull in regards to ventilation/perfusion distribution in hypoxia. We subjected eight anesthetized piglets in normoxia (FiO_2 = 0.21) and in hypoxia (FiO_2 = 0.13) to 10 mL/kg Red Bull ingestion, whereas another eight served as controls. In addition to standard cardiovascular data, ventilation/perfusion distribution of the lung assessed by using the multiple inert gas elimination technique (MIGET) was measured.

2. Materials and Methods

2.1. Subjects

All experiments conformed to the guidelines of the National Institute of Health and were approved on 27.09.2006 by the Austrian Federal Animal Investigational Committee (# GZ66.011/127-BrGT/2006).

Sixteen healthy, 4-week-old cross breed piglets (German land-race x Pietrain) of either sex were selected from a local stock regularly used for experimental research. Prior to the experiment, all animals were examined in the barn by a veterinarian to affirm healthy piglets. Acute sickness of piglets would have led to exclusion. After arrival at the animal research facility, they were housed in a quiet and dark barn. Thereafter, premedication was administered intramuscularly (im.) using Ketamine (20 mg/kg) and Azaperon (4 mg/kg). Additionally, Atropine im. (0.01 mg/kg) was used to oppose a possible ketamine-induced hypersalivation. After venepuncture of an ear, anaesthesia was inducted with Propofol (4 mg/kg iv.) followed by tracheal intubation. Anaesthesia was maintained using Propofol iv. (1–1.5 mg/kg/h; Perfusor, B. Braun Melsungen AG, Melsungen, Germany) and several boluses of 15 mg Piritramide in order to keep all piglets deeply anesthetized.

All piglets were mechanically ventilated in a volume-controlled mode (Evita 2, Dräger, 23,558 Lübeck, Germany) with a fraction of inspired oxygen (FiO_2) of 0.21 and a positive end-expiratory pressure (PEEP) set at 5 mmHg. Tidal volumes (TV) were adjusted to values of 10 mL/kg at 15 breaths/min.

Throughout the procedure, Ringer's solution (6 mL/kg/h) and a 3% gelatine solution (4 mL/kg/h) served as compensation for any loss of blood and fluid. However, blood loss was less than 100 mL during instrumentation. A standard lead II ECG was used to monitor cardiac rhythm. Body temperature was maintained between 38 and 39 °C by using an electric heating blanket.

An 8.5 French pulmonary artery catheter was advanced from the internal jugular vein into the pulmonary artery to measure mean pulmonary arterial pressure (mPAP), pulmonary capillary wedge pressure (PCWP), central venous pressure (CVP) and cardiac output by the thermodilution technique (10 mL saline in triplicate) and to withdraw mixed venous blood. A 6.0 French arterial catheter introduced into the femoral artery was used to monitor systemic blood pressure and to take blood samples. All catheters were filled with saline and connected to pressure transducers zeroed to ambient pressure at the level of the right atrium.

2.2. Experimental Protocol

After surgical preparation, the animals were moved into prone position and left for a stabilization phase of 30 min. Thereafter the first baseline measurements (i.e., 0 min) including hemodynamics, blood gases, ventilation and MIGET were taken.

Sixteen animals were randomly assigned into two groups. Eight animals received Red Bull (10 mL/kg) over a stomach tube (Charriere 10, length 125 cm, Maersk Medical A/S, Roskilde, Denmark), whereas another eight were sham-tested with an equivalent volume of saline. All animals were mechanically ventilated, spontaneous breathing efforts were not observed. Thirty min after baseline, the first experimental leg started exposing all animals to ambient air (i.e., normobaric normoxia). After 120 min, the second experimental leg started with taking a second baseline. Thereafter, all animals were exposed to normobaric hypoxia with an FiO2 of 0.13 simulating an altitude of 14.000 feet (equivalent to 4.267 m). After 150 min, animals assigned to the Red Bull group received another bolus of Red Bull (5 mL/kg), whereas the remaining six received the corresponding amount of saline. Hemodynamics and blood gas samples were performed every 30 min. MIGET was performed at 0, 30, 90, 120, 150 and 240 min.

We used a standard 250 mL can of Red Bull energy drink, containing 80 mg caffeine, 1.000 mg taurine, 0.6 g glucuronolactone, 27 g carbohydrate (glucose, sucrose), 20 mg niacin (vitamin B3), 5 mg pantothenic acid (vitamin B5), 5 mg vitamin B6, 5 µg vitamin B1 and 2 µg vitamin B12, respectively [18].

Given the weight of the piglets (23.59 +/− 3.33 kg), 250 mL Red Bull resulted in a 3-fold higher dose compared to the same volume in adults.

Respirator settings were not changed during the observation period in none of the animals. After 240 min, the study ended with killing the animals using pentobarbital and potassium chloride. No adverse events in the animals were observed.

Thereafter, the heart and the proximal parts of the great arteries were removed and inspected to rule out any anatomical intra- or extracardial shunt connection.

The multiple inert gas technique was applied in the usual manner as described by [19–21]. In brief, six inert gases, prepared in sterile 0.9% saline, were infused continuously. After obtaining a steady state after 30 min, the six gas concentrations in expired gas, arterial and venous blood samples were assessed by gas chromatography (Hewlett-Packard 5890, series II). Using the ratios of excretion and retention allows to calculate ventilation/perfusion distribution using a least squares best fit regression analysis.

2.3. Statistical Analysis

A two-way ANOVA was used to determine inter- and intragroup differences. Significant results were analysed post hoc with the Newman–Keuls and Fisher's exact tests. Results are given as mean and standard deviation, values of $p \leq 0.05$ were considered significant.

3. Results

Eight anesthetized piglets were subjected to Red Bull in ambient air followed by normobaric hypoxia. Another eight animals were sham-tested with an equivalent amount of saline in normoxia followed by hypoxia.

Baseline data showed no differences between the two groups.

3.1. Hemodynamic Changes

Red Bull administration increased heart rate after 30 min in normoxia. In contrast, heart rate remained unchanged in normoxic controls. After induction of hypoxia, heart rate increased in the Red Bull group but remained unchanged after the second ingestion of Red Bull. In hypoxic controls, heart rate showed a somewhat delayed course with a lesser increase after induction of hypoxia compared to the verum group. Moreover, placebo treatment showed a trend towards heart rate increase reaching comparable values of the Red Bull group until the end of hypoxia (Figure 1).

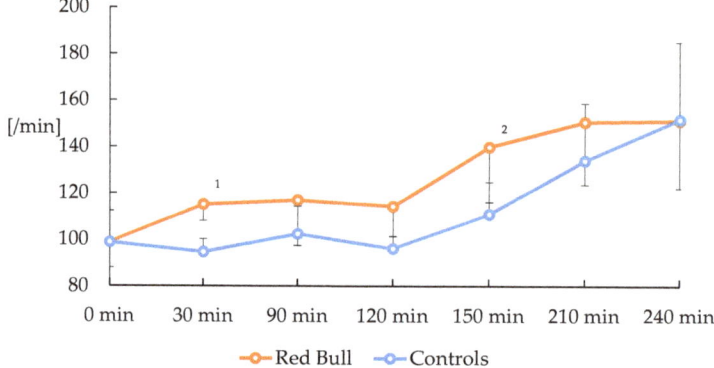

Figure 1. Course of heart rate after consumption of Red Bull or placebo in normoxic and hypoxic piglets (n = 16). [1] $p < 0.01$ versus control, [2] $p < 0.05$ versus control. Normoxia (F_iO_2 = 0.21) 0–120 min, Hypoxia (F_iO_2 = 0.13) 120–240 min. Piglets (n = 8) received 10 mL/kg Red Bull at 0 min and 5 mL/kg at 150 min, respectively. Values are mean ± standard deviation.

MPAP increased nearly 1.5-fold after start of hypoxia in both groups with a further increase in the Red Bull group after the second dose of Red Bull at 210 and 240 min (in intragroup comparison). Placebo treatment did not change mPAP in controls. Cardiac output (CO) remained unchanged during normoxia in both groups. 30 min after induction of hypoxia CO increased in the Red Bull group only. Thereafter, these verum animals showed lower values until the end of the experiment. CO in controls showed a trend towards higher values after 210 min compared to the Red Bull group, but this failed to reach significance (Table 1).

Table 1. Hemodynamic measurements ($n = 16$).

Time Point		0 min	30 min	90 min	120 min	150 min	210 min	240 min
		Normoxia (FiO$_2$ = 0.21)				Hypoxia (FiO$_2$ = 0.13)		
MAP (torr)	RB	87 ± 14	92 ± 12	97 ± 16	89 ± 12	86 ± 15	77 ± 9	82 ± 10
	control	89 ± 9	101 ± 17	98 ± 6	94 ± 12	83 ± 8	83 ± 9	86 ± 16
mPAP (torr)	RB	23 ± 3	24 ± 3	24 ± 2	24 ± 3	37 ± 4	40 ± 2 [1]	41 ± 3 [1]
	control	23 ± 1	24 ± 2	24 ± 2	24 ± 2	38 ± 1	38 ± 5	39 ± 4
CO (l/min)	RB	4.5 ± 0.7	4.3 ± 0.5	4.0 ± 1.0	4.2 ± 0.7	5.4 ± 0.6 [2]	4.8 ± 0.7	4.5 ± 1.1
	control	4.5 ± 0.7	4.0 ± 0.6	4.0 ± 0.7	4.2 ± 1.2	4.3 ± 0.8	5.2 ± 1.3	4.6 ± 2.1
PCWP (torr)	RB	13 ± 0	13 ± 1	12 ± 1	10 ± 2	9 ± 3	9 ± 3	10 ± 4
	control	15 ± 2	15 ± 3	14 ± 2	12 ± 1	11 ± 1	10 ± 2	10 ± 2
CVD (torr)	RB	9 ± 1	10 ± 2	10 ± 1	9 ± 3	9 ± 3	10 ± 1	10 ± 2
	Control	10 ± 1	9 ± 1	9 ± 1	10 ± 1	11 ± 1	10 ± 2	10 ± 1

[1] $p < 0.05$ versus 150 min, [2] $p < 0.05$ versus control. MAP reflects mean arterial blood pressure; mPAP reflects mean pulmonary arterial blood pressure; CO reflects cardiac output; PCWP reflects pulmonary capillary wedge pressure; CVD reflects central venous pressure. RB reflects Red Bull energy drink. Piglets ($n = 8$) received 10 mL/kg Red Bull at 0 min and 5 mL/kg at 150 min, respectively. Values are mean ± standard deviation.

3.2. Bloodgas Changes

Arterial partial pressure of oxygen (paO$_2$) and mixed venous partial pressure of oxygen (pvO$_2$) remained unchanged after oral Red Bull ingestion in normoxia. Shortly after exposure to hypoxia arterial partial pressure of oxygen (paO$_2$) and mixed venous partial pressure of oxygen (pvO$_2$) decreased in both groups. The second administration of Red Bull or placebo did not change paO$_2$. However, PvO$_2$ was smaller at the end of the experiment after 240 min in the Red Bull group.

The first administration of Red Bull increased arterial partial pressure of carbon dioxide (paCO$_2$) after 30 min in normoxia. During the rest of the experiment, paCO$_2$ in animals subjected to Red Bull was higher than in the placebo group without reaching significance. In the Red Bull group, mixed venous partial pressure of carbon dioxide (pvCO$_2$) was greater after 30 min in normoxia compared to controls and baseline values. Thereafter, pvCO$_2$ in the verum group was greater after 90 min in normoxia and after 210 and 240 min in hypoxia, respectively (Table 2).

Table 2. Blood gas measurements ($n = 16$).

Time Point		0 min	30 min	90 min	120 min	150 min	210 min	240 min
		Normoxia (FiO$_2$ = 0.21)				Hypoxia (FiO$_2$ = 0.13)		
paO$_2$ (torr)	RB	98 ± 5	88 ± 4	88 ± 6	93 ± 4	35 ± 4	33 ± 2	33 ± 2
	control	98 ± 6	90 ± 5	87 ± 3	93 ± 3	35 ± 5	33 ± 3	34 ± 4
paCO$_2$ (torr)	RB	37 ± 2	40 ± 3 [1]	39 ± 2	37 ± 1	38 ± 4	39 ± 5	39 ± 5
	control	35 ± 2	35 ± 3	35 ± 3	36 ± 2	34 ± 5	36 ± 3	37 ± 3
pH	RB	7.44 ± 0.03	7.40 ± 0.01 [1]	7.40 ± 0.02	7.43 ± 0.03	7.44 ± 0.04	7.33 ± 0.09	7.29 ± 0.10
	control	7.46 ± 0.02	7.46 ± 0.03	7.43 ± 0.06	7.51 ± 0.02	7.48 ± 0.04	7.43 ± 0.04	7.39 ± 0.05
pvO$_2$ (torr)	RB	37 ± 2	35 ± 2	34 ± 2	34 ± 3	22 ± 1	17 ± 2	14 ± 2 [1]
	control	36 ± 0	33 ± 2	33 ± 2	35 ± 3	22 ± 3	19 ± 2	21 ± 4
pvCO$_2$ (torr)	RB	41 ± 2	46 ± 3 [1,2]	46 ± 2 [1,2]	43 ± 2	43 ± 4	47 ± 6 [3]	48 ± 6 [3]
	control	41 ± 3	40 ± 5	41 ± 4	41 ± 4	39 ± 4	40 ± 3	42 ± 3

[1] $p < 0.05$ versus control, [2] $p < 0.05$ versus 0 min, [3] $p < 0.05$ versus 150 min. PaO$_2$ reflects arterial partial pressure of oxygen; paCO$_2$ reflects arterial partial pressure of carbon dioxide; pH reflects arterial pH; pvO$_2$ reflects mixed venous partial pressure of oxygen; pvCO$_2$ reflects mixed venous partial pressure of carbon dioxide. RB reflects Red Bull energy drink. Piglets ($n = 8$) received 10 mL/kg Red Bull at 0 min and 5 mL/kg at 150 min, respectively. Values are mean ± standard deviation.

3.3. Ventilation/Perfusion Changes

In normoxic conditions, ingestion of Red Bull or placebo did not change ventilation/perfusion distribution. Furthermore, induction of hypoxia did not change these variables. After the second Red Bull dose, blood flow to unventilated lung units (i.e., the fraction of shunt) increased after 240 min (Figure 2).

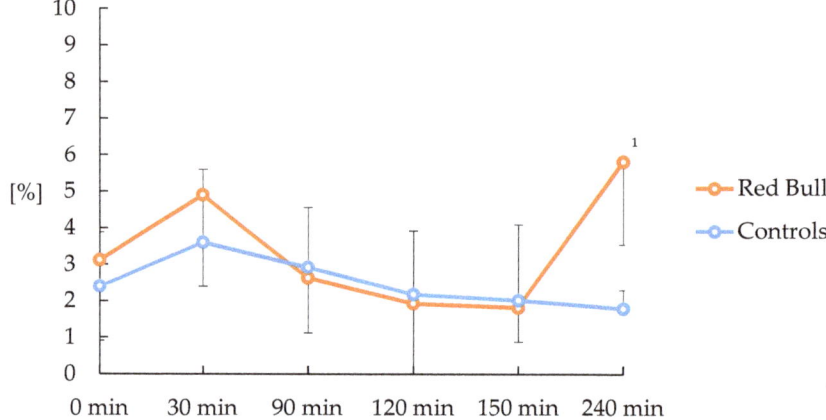

Figure 2. Course of shunt fraction after consumption of Red Bull or placebo in normoxic and hypoxic piglets ($n = 16$). [1] $p < 0.05$ versus control. Shunt reflects unventilated lung units. Normoxia ($F_iO_2 = 0.21$) 0–120 min; Hypoxia ($F_iO_2 = 0.13$) 120–240 min. Piglets ($n = 8$) received 10 mL/kg Red Bull at 0 min and 5 mL/kg at 150 min, respectively. Values are mean ± standard deviation.

Moreover, in these verum animals, blood flow to normally ventilated units (normal V_A/Q of Q) showed a trend towards decrease after 240 min without reaching significance. The mean of the distribution of perfusion (mean of Q) showed a trend towards a small increase, but this also did not reach significance. The distribution of pulmonary blood flow (expressed as the logarithmic deviation of the standard of the mean of the distribution of perfusion, i.e., LogSDQ) remained unchanged (Table 3).

Table 3. Inert gas data ($n = 16$).

Time Point		0 min	30 min	90 min	120 min	150 min	240 min
		Normoxia ($FiO_2 = 0.21$)				Hypoxia ($FiO_2 = 0.13$)	
Low V_A/Q of Q (%)	RB	0 ± 0	0 ± 0	0 ± 0	0 ± 0	0 ± 0	0 ± 0
	control	0 ± 0	0 ± 0	0 ± 0	0 ± 0	1.2 ± 1.8	0.7 ± 1.1
Norm V_A/Q of Q (%)	RB	96.8 ± 2.2	95.0 ± 2.5	97.3 ± 1.5	98.0 ± 2.5	98.1 ± 0.9	93.3 ± 2.2
	control	99.1 ± 1.4	99.2 ± 1.9	98.8 ± 1.5	97.8 ± 1.7	96.7 ± 1.7	97.0 ± 1.7
High V_A/Q of Q (%)	RB	0 ± 0	0 ± 0	0 ± 0	0 ± 0	0 ± 0	0.5 ± 0.9
	control	0 ± 0	0 ± 0	0 ± 0	0 ± 0	0 ± 0	0 ± 0
Mean of Q	RB	0.62 ± 0.18	0.60 ± 0.16	0.62 ± 0.11	0.73 ± 0.26	0.75 ± 0.32	1.26 ± 0.54
	control	0.86 ± 0.19	0.88 ± 0.31	0.86 ± 0.20	0.63 ± 0.14	0.59 ± 0.21	0.67 ± 0.29
LogSDQ	RB	0.39 ± 0.08	0.45 ± 0.16	0.43 ± 0.06	0.36 ± 0.05	0.43 ± 0.15	0.68 ± 0.27
	control	0.45 ± 0.14	0.52 ± 0.12	0.47 ± 0.12	0.63 ± 0.20	0.57 ± 0.13	0.54 ± 0.06

Low V_A/Q reflects lung units with a low V_A/Q ratio; norm V_A/Q reflects normal V_A/Q lung units; high V_A/Q reflects high V_A/Q lung units; mean of Q reflects mean of the distribution of perfusion; logSDQ reflects logarithmic deviation of standard of the mean of the distribution of perfusion; RB reflects red Bull energy drink. Piglets ($n = 8$) received 10 mL/kg Red Bull at 0 min and 5 mL/kg at 150 min, respectively. Values are mean ± standard deviation.

In the MIGET, adequacy of fit of the data to the model is assessed by the remaining sum of squares (RSS). RSS was ≥ 10.6 in 91.2% of all MIGET analysis, thereby indicating good data quality.

4. Discussion

The salient finding of this study is that, in a controlled laboratory trial, Red Bull significantly increased pulmonary shunt fraction with unchanged distribution of pulmonary blood flow after Red Bull consumption during short-term exposure to acute hypoxia. Moreover, we could demonstrate an increased heart rate after high dose Red Bull ingestion at near sea level in piglets.

The increased heart rate after Red Bull ingestion is in line with previous work performed in man [2–5,7,11,13,22]. We observed a larger increase of heart rate as we chose a threefold higher amount of Red Bull compared to studies conducted in adults. In contrast to those studies, two recent trials reported an unchanged heart rate [8,9]. In total, 67 adults received Red Bull doses of 168 mL/m^2 body surface area (BSA) corresponding to a volume of about 350 mL.

Ten years ago, Ragsdale and co-workers reported a trend towards drop of heart rate after 250 mL Red Bull ingestion in 68 undergraduate students [6].

Recent work examining 44 young Iranians at rest demonstrated a small drop in heart rate after Red Bull administration [10]. However, Hajsadeghi et al. used 250 mL but did not report the weight of the subjects. A study conducted over two decades ago reported a drop in heart rate in 10 endurance athletes after consumption of half a litre of Red Bull during submaximal exercise [23]. Bichler et al. observed a decreased heart rate shortly after administration of pills containing caffeine and taurine in college-students [24].

In summary, a comparison of trials reporting changes in heart rate still remains difficult given the different approaches used, variable volumes of Red Bull or any potential influences of sex category or age. Moreover, the extent of common caffeine consumption plays a pivotal role. As early as 1981, frequent caffeine consumers have been shown to respond less to acute administration than caffeine-naive individuals [25]. However, since piglets are life-long caffeine abstinent, we did not take regular caffeine consumption into account.

Acute hypoxia induces demand tachycardia as one mechanism of short-term adaption in preserving convective oxygen transport [26]. Here, we observed an accelerated heart rate at once in acute hypoxic exposure in the verum group only. Moreover, cardiac output at this time point was also higher, most likely due to the tachycardic response and a preserved stroke volume [27]. One could guess that consumption of Red Bull at high altitude may further accelerate tachycardia. Thus, maximum heart rate could be reached earlier being detrimental for oxygen delivery at high altitude. However, after the second dose of Red Bull, heart rate showed a trend to rise without any significance. Moreover, it remained nearly unchanged thereafter. In contrast, placebo treated piglets showed a smaller increase of heart rate at commencement of hypoxia. Until the end of the experiment, this group reached nearly the same heart rate as the verum group. In summary, our findings demonstrate that a high dose of Red Bull does not worsen tachycardia at high altitude.

Staying at high altitude exposes to reduced inspired paO$_2$ without impairment in gas exchange. Whether energy drink consumption at high altitude impairs pulmonary blood flow and thus may limit hypoxic exercise performance is still not answered. Up to date, only four small studies reporting caffeine consumption in hypoxic conditions exist, all of them reporting an increased endurance performance [14–17]. Nearly twenty years ago, researchers Berglund and Hemmingsson reported an improved exercise performance at 2900 m. They subjected fourteen well-trained cross-country skiers to 6 mg/kg caffeine during competition in a time trial over 21 km [14]. Later on, Fulco and co-workers used a smaller caffeine dose (4 mg/kg) in eight adults cycling at 4300 m. These researchers demonstrated a prolonged time to exhaustion at 80% of the altitude-specific maximal oxygen consumption (VO$_{2max}$) [15]. A small controlled study investigated the ergogenic effect of ingestion of 4 mg/kg caffeine in seven male adults in moderate hypoxia. At simulated 2500 m, caffeine prolonged time to exhaustion and increased the heart rate to a greater extent during high-intensity cycling than in controls. Moreover, the authors excluded a caffeine-associated reduction in neuromuscular fatigue during performance at moderate altitude [16]. Stadheim and colleagues demonstrated a prolonged time to exhaustion during double poling at sub-maximal exercise in 2000 m. However, the 13 cross-country skiers consumed half as much caffeine (4.5 mg/kg) as used in our study [17].

Those four studies used caffeine only and focused on exercise performance. In the present study, we were interested to know if Red Bull, a caffeinated energy drink, impacts pulmonary blood flow or HPV. We observed an increased shunt fraction after Red Bull consumption during acute exposure to short-term hypoxia. Furthermore, we observed increased $pvCO_2$ values shortly after Red Bull ingestion in hypoxia. A possible explanation could be a decreased pulmonary CO_2 elimination due to shunt which can be excluded here as arterial gas exchange appeared to be unchanged. The 20-fold higher diffusion capacity of CO_2 compared to O_2 makes this even more unlikely. In addition to that, the increased shunt did not correspond with a decreased normal V_A/Q (only a trend) as one could expect. Moreover, we did not observe a further worsening of gas exchange or ventilation/perfusion distribution in hypoxia. In summary, Red Bull consumption did not alter gas exchange at high altitude in piglets. However, careful transfer of our findings to humans is coercible.

The respiratory stimulant nature of caffeine is long known. Before World War I, Cushney showed an increased respiratory rate to carbon dioxide after caffeine [28]. These data have been confirmed some decades later [29,30]. Moderate caffeine doses (around 3 mg/kg) have been demonstrated to increase alveolar ventilation while exercising moderately [31]. Another group showed a rise of hypoxic ventilatory response (HVR) using high doses (nearly 10 mg/kg) [32].

Recently, Cavka and co-workers were able to demonstrate an increased respiratory rate and flow rate, respectively, at rest and during moderate exercise after ingestion of half a litre of Red Bull in 38 college students. These researchers showed an activation of the sympathetic nervous system and hypothesized a notable dilation of bronchioles [33]. Recent data from Spanish colleagues showed an increased cycling performance in ambient air as well as enhanced muscle oxygen saturation assessed at the thigh at moderate workloads (30–60% of VO_{2max}) after caffeine intake (3 mg/kg). Moreover, peak pulmonary ventilation during exercise and blood lactate after exercise were higher [34]. The most likely candidate for these effects is caffeine without any certain evidence up to date. Here, we did not observe an influence of Red Bull on respiratory drive as $paCO_2$ and ventilation of the anesthetized piglets remained unchanged until termination of the experiment.

From a physiological point of view the intake of an ample amount of sugar (here around 40 g of sugars in about 375 mL Red Bull per piglet) has to be taken into account when interpreting our results. In the present study, $paCO_2$ was higher after Red Bull ingestion (i.e., after 27 g of sugars) in ambient air. Such a glucose load may have led to an increased carbon dioxide production (VCO_2) and consequently, given our fixed minute ventilation, an increased $PaCO_2$ with a successive depression of pH. Moreover, it is known that combined consumption of caffeine and glucose causes a state of hyperinsulinemia and hyperlipidemia [35].

Beside the actions of caffeine and glucose, taurine needs to be considered when interpreting our results. Hypotensive effects were demonstrated in several studies using different hypertensive animal models (for reviews see [36,37]). Nearly 40 years ago, Bousquet et al. showed a drop in heart rate and blood pressure after taurine injection directly into a ventricle of the brain in cats [38]. Data in man showed a modulation in myocardial myofibrillar proteins with an inotropic effect in the failing heart secondary to cardiomyopathy in seventeen patients [39]. Recently, the first randomized, double-blind, placebo-controlled clinical trial showed a blood pressure drop after a twelve-week lasting oral taurine supplementation in prehypertensive adults. In regards to exercise performance, taurine has been shown to increase left atrial contractility after exercise in endurance-trained subjects [11]. This was demonstrated in comparison of Red Bull and a drink containing only caffeine. Those aforementioned beneficial effects of taurine may counterbalance the cardiovascular effects of the remaining ingredients of Red Bull. We can only hypothesize that taurine attenuated a possible caffeine induced blood pressure rise.

Limits

A few limits have to be taken into account in interpretation of our results. First, the small sample size is clearly a limitation. However, we sought to reduce the number of animals needed as far as possible without curtailing statistical power. Clearly, using a murine model would allow for a greater sample size and deeper statistical analyses. Here we used this porcine model to obtain values resembling those in men (e.g., pulmonary blood pressures) and for giving us the possibility to perform the MIGET method. Second, this data recorded in piglets has to be transferred cautiously into any recommendations regarding humane consumption of caffeinated energy drinks. Third, we did not obtain blood glucose levels, which hampers interpretation of a possible glucose effect in Red Bull.

Lastly, further research, even in a murine or a humane setting, needs to differentiate between effects of caffeine and taurine alone, respectively, either at sea level or at high altitude.

5. Conclusions

In summary, high dose Red Bull consumption raised heart rate at near sea level in piglets. During acute exposure to short-term hypoxia, it did not worsen tachycardia. In regards to pulmonary blood flow, we demonstrated an increased pulmonary shunt fraction with unchanged distribution of pulmonary blood flow. We conclude that Red Bull did not alter gas exchange at high altitude in a porcine model of acute short-term hypoxia.

Author Contributions: Conceptualization, R.G., A.L. and A.K.; Data curation, B.T. and A.L.; formal analysis, B.T. and E.S.; funding acquisition, A.L.; investigation, B.T., E.S., R.G., A.L. and A.K.; methodology, B.T., R.G., A.L. and A.K.; project administration, B.T. and A.L.; resources, A.L.; supervision, R.G., A.L. and A.K.; validation, B.T., C.N. and M.B.; visualization, C.N. and M.B.; writing—original draft, B.T.; writing—review and editing, B.T. and A.K. All authors have read and agreed to the published version of the manuscript.

Funding: This research received no external funding.

Acknowledgments: We are deeply indebted to Christian Gritsch for his invaluable support in conducting these experiments. Unfortunately, he could not live to see this publication as he passed away too early.

Conflicts of Interest: The authors declare no conflict of interest.

Abbreviations

CO	cardiac output
CO_2	carbon dioxide
CVD	central venous pressure
DBP	diastolic blood pressure
HPV	hypoxic pulmonary vasoconstriction
MAP	mean arterial blood pressure
LogSDQ	logarithmic deviation of standard of the mean of the distribution of perfusion
Mean of Q	mean of the distribution of perfusion
MIGET	multiple inert gas elimination technique
MPAP	mean pulmonary arterial blood pressure
MR	magnetic resonance
O_2	oxygen
PaO_2	arterial partial pressure of oxygen
$PaCO_2$	arterial partial pressure of carbon dioxide
PCWP	pulmonary capillary wedge pressure
PEEP	positive end-expiratory pressure
pH	arterial pH
PvO_2	mixed venous partial pressure of oxygen
$PvCO_2$	mixed venous partial pressure of carbon dioxide
RSS	remaining sum of squares
SBP	systolic blood pressure

TV   Tidal volumes
V_A/Q Ventilation/perfusion
VO_{2max} maximal oxygen consumption

References

1. Higgins, J.P.; Tuttle, T.D.; Higgins, C.L. Energy beverages: Content and safety. *Mayo Clin. Proc.* **2010**, *85*, 1033–1041. [CrossRef] [PubMed]
2. Alford, C.; Cox, H.; Wescott, R. The effects of Red Bull Energy Drink on human performance and mood. *Amino Acids* **2001**, *21*, 139–150. [CrossRef]
3. Grasser, E.K.; Yepuri, G.; Dulloo, A.G.; Montani, J.-P. Cardio- and cerebrovascular responses to the energy drink Red Bull in young adults: A randomized cross-over study. *Eur. J. Nutr.* **2014**, *53*, 1561–1571. [CrossRef]
4. Franks, A.M.; Schmidt, J.M.; McCain, K.R.; Fraer, M. Comparison of the Effects of Energy Drink Versus Caffeine Supplementation on Indices of 24-Hour Ambulatory Blood Pressure. *Ann. Pharmacother.* **2012**, *46*, 192–199. [CrossRef] [PubMed]
5. Elitok, A.; Oz, F.; Panc, C.; Sarikaya, R.; Sezikli, S.; Pala, Y.; Bugan, O.S.; Ates, M.; Parildar, H.; Ayaz, M.B.; et al. Acute effects of Red Bull energy drink on ventricular repolarization in healthy young volunteers: A prospective study. *Anatol. J. Cardiol.* **2015**, *15*, 919–922. [CrossRef] [PubMed]
6. Ragsdale, F.R.; Gronli, T.D.; Batool, N.; Haight, N.; Mehaffey, A.; McMahon, E.C.; Nalli, T.W.; Mannello, C.M.; Sell, C.J.; McCann, P.J.; et al. Effect of Red Bull energy drink on cardiovascular and renal function. *Amino Acids* **2010**, *38*, 1193–1200. [CrossRef] [PubMed]
7. Grasser, E.K.; Dulloo, A.G.; Montani, J.-P. Cardiovascular and Cerebrovascular Effects in Response to Red Bull Consumption Combined With Mental Stress. *Am. J. Cardiol.* **2015**, *115*, 183–189. [CrossRef]
8. Doerner, J.M.; Kuetting, D.L.; Luetkens, J.A.; Naehle, C.P.; Dabir, D.; Homsi, R.; Nadal, J.; Schild, H.H.; Thomas, D.K. Caffeine and taurine containing energy drink increases left ventricular contractility in healthy volunteers. *Int. J. Cardiovasc. Imaging* **2015**, *31*, 595–601. [CrossRef] [PubMed]
9. Menci, D.; Righini, F.M.; Cameli, M.; Lisi, M.; Benincasa, S.; Focardi, M.; Mondillo, S. Acute Effects of an Energy Drink on Myocardial Function Assessed by Conventional Echo-Doppler Analysis and by Speckle Tracking Echocardiography on Young Healthy Subjects. *J. Amino Acids* **2013**, *2013*, 1–7. [CrossRef] [PubMed]
10. Hajsadeghi, S.; Mohammadpour, F.; Manteghi, M.J.; Kordshakeri, K.; Tokazebani, M.; Rahmani, E.; Hassanzadeh, M. Effects of energy drinks on blood pressure, heart rate, and electrocardiographic parameters: An experimental study on healthy young adults. *Anatol. J. Cardiol.* **2015**, *16*, 94–99. [CrossRef] [PubMed]
11. Baum, M.; Weiß, M. The influence of a taurine containing drink on cardiac parameters before and after exercise measured by echocardiography. *Amino Acids* **2001**, *20*, 75–82. [CrossRef] [PubMed]
12. Bock, J.; Buchholtz, J. Über das Minutenvolum des Herzens beim Hunde und über den Einfluss des Coffeins auf die Grösse des Minutenvolums. *Arch. Exp. Pathol. Pharmakol.* **1920**, *88*, 192–215. [CrossRef]
13. Basrai, M.; Schweinlin, A.; Menzel, J.; Mielke, H.; Weikert, C.; Dusemund, B.; Putze, K.; Watzl, B.; Lampen, A.; Bischoff, S.C. Energy Drinks Induce Acute Cardiovascular and Metabolic Changes Pointing to Potential Risks for Young Adults: A Randomized Controlled Trial. *J. Nutr.* **2019**, *149*, 441–450. [CrossRef] [PubMed]
14. Berglund, B.; Hemmingsson, P. Effects of Caffeine Ingestion on Exercise Performance at Low and High Altitudes in Cross-Country Skiers. *Int. J. Sports Med.* **1982**, *3*, 234–236. [CrossRef] [PubMed]
15. Fulco, C.S.; Rock, P.B.; Trad, L.A.; Rose, M.S.; Forte, V.A.; Young, P.M.; Cymerman, A. Effect of caffeine on submaximal exercise performance at altitude. *Aviat. Space Environ. Med.* **1994**, *65*, 539–545. [PubMed]
16. Smirmaul, B.P.C.; de Moraes, A.C.; Angius, L.; Marcora, S.M. Effects of caffeine on neuromuscular fatigue and performance during high-intensity cycling exercise in moderate hypoxia. *Eur. J. Appl. Physiol.* **2017**, *117*, 27–38. [CrossRef] [PubMed]
17. Stadheim, H.K.; Nossum, E.M.; Olsen, R.; Spencer, M.; Jensen, J. Caffeine improves performance in double poling during acute exposure to 2000-m altitude. *J. Appl. Physiol.* **2015**, *119*, 1501–1509. [CrossRef] [PubMed]
18. Miles-Chan, J.L.; Charrière, N.; Grasser, E.K.; Montani, J.-P.; Dulloo, A.G. The blood pressure-elevating effect of Red Bull energy drink is mimicked by caffeine but through different hemodynamic pathways. *Physiol. Rep.* **2015**, *3*, e12290. [CrossRef] [PubMed]
19. Wagner, P.D.; Naumann, P.F.; Laravuso, R.B. Simultaneous measurement of eight foreign gases in blood by gas chromatography. *J. Appl. Physiol.* **1974**, *36*, 600–605. [CrossRef] [PubMed]

20. Wagner, P.D.; Saltzman, H.A.; West, J.B. Measurement of continuous distributions of ventilation-perfusion ratios: Theory. *J. Appl. Physiol.* **1974**, *36*, 588–599. [CrossRef] [PubMed]
21. Farhi, L.E.; Olszowka, A.J. Analysis of alveolar gas exchange in the presence of soluble inert gases. *Respir. Physiol.* **1968**, *5*, 53–67. [CrossRef]
22. Steinke, L.; Lanfear, D.E.; Dhanapal, V.; Kalus, J.S. Effect of "energy drink" consumption on hemodynamic and electrocardiographic parameters in healthy young adults. *Ann. Pharmacother.* **2009**, *43*, 596–602. [CrossRef] [PubMed]
23. Geiß, K.R.; Jester, I.; Falke, W.; Hamm, M.; Waag, K.L. The effect of a taurine-containing drink on performance in 10 endurance-athletes. *Amino Acids* **1994**, *7*, 45–56. [CrossRef] [PubMed]
24. Bichler, A.; Swenson, A.; Harris, M.A. A combination of caffeine and taurine has no effect on short term memory but induces changes in heart rate and mean arterial blood pressure. *Amino Acids* **2006**, *31*, 471–476. [CrossRef]
25. Robertson, D.; Wade, D.; Workman, R.; Woosley, R.L.; Oates, J.A. Tolerance to the humoral and hemodynamic effects of caffeine in man. *J. Clin. Investig.* **1981**, *67*, 1111–1117. [CrossRef]
26. Siebenmann, C.; Lundby, C. Regulation of cardiac output in hypoxia. *Scand. J. Med. Sci. Sports* **2015**, *25* (Suppl. S4), 53–59. [CrossRef]
27. Siebenmann, C.; Rasmussen, P.; Sørensen, H.; Bonne, T.C.; Zaar, M.; Aachmann-Andersen, N.J.; Nordsborg, N.B.; Secher, N.H.; Lundby, C. Hypoxia increases exercise heart rate despite combined inhibition of β-adrenergic and muscarinic receptors. *Am. J. Physiol. Heart Circ. Physiol.* **2015**, *308*, H1540–H1546. [CrossRef] [PubMed]
28. Cushney, A.R.J. On the pharmacology of the respiratory center. *Pharmacol. Exper. Ther.* **1913**, *4*, 363.
29. Le Messurier, D.H. The site of action of caffeine as a respiratory stimulant. *J. Pharmacol. Exp. Ther.* **1936**, *57*, 458–463.
30. Richmond, G.H. Action of caffeine and aminophylline as respiratory stimulants in man. *J. Appl. Physiol.* **1949**, *2*, 16–23. [CrossRef]
31. Brown, D.D.; Knowlton, R.G.; Sullivan, J.J.; Sanjabi, P.B. Effect of caffeine ingestion on alveolar ventilation during moderate exercise. *Aviat. Space Environ. Med.* **1991**, *62*, 860–864. [PubMed]
32. D'Urzo, A.D.; Jhirad, R.; Jenne, H.; Avendano, M.A.; Rubinstein, I.; D'Costa, M.; Goldstein, R.S.; Rubenstein, I. Effect of caffeine on ventilatory responses to hypercapnia, hypoxia, and exercise in humans. *J. Appl. Physiol.* **1990**, *68*, 322–328. [CrossRef] [PubMed]
33. Cavka, A.; Stupin, M.; Panduric, A.; Plazibat, A.; Cosic, A.; Rasic, L.; Debeljak, Z.; Martinovic, G.; Drenjancevic, I. Adrenergic System Activation Mediates Changes in Cardiovascular and Psychomotoric Reactions in Young Individuals after Red Bull (©) Energy Drink Consumption. *Int. J. Endocrinol.* **2015**, *2015*, 751530. [CrossRef] [PubMed]
34. Ruíz-Moreno, C.; Lara, B.; Brito de Souza, D.; Gutiérrez-Hellín, J.; Romero-Moraleda, B.; Cuéllar-Rayo, Á.; Del Coso, J. Acute caffeine intake increases muscle oxygen saturation during a maximal incremental exercise test. *Br. J. Clin. Pharmacol.* **2020**, *86*, 861–867. [CrossRef] [PubMed]
35. Shearer, J.; Graham, T.E. Performance effects and metabolic consequences of caffeine and caffeinated energy drink consumption on glucose disposal. *Nutr. Rev.* **2014**, *72* (Suppl. S1), 121–136. [CrossRef] [PubMed]
36. Abebe, W.; Mozaffari, M.S. Role of taurine in the vasculature: An overview of experimental and human studies. *Am. J. Cardiovasc. Dis.* **2011**, *1*, 293–311. [PubMed]
37. Ehlers, A.; Marakis, G.; Lampen, A.; Hirsch-Ernst, K.I. Risk assessment of energy drinks with focus on cardiovascular parameters and energy drink consumption in Europe. *Food Chem. Toxicol.* **2019**, *130*, 109–121. [CrossRef] [PubMed]
38. Bousquet, P.; Feldman, J.; Bloch, R.; Schwartz, J. Central cardiovascular effects of taurine: Comparison with homotaurine and muscimol. *J. Pharmacol. Exp. Ther.* **1981**, *219*, 213–218. [PubMed]
39. Azuma, J.; Sawamura, A.; Awata, N. Usefulness of Taurine in Chronic Congestive Heart Failure and Its Prospective Application. *Jpn. Circ. J.* **1992**, *56*, 95–99. [CrossRef] [PubMed]

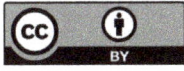

© 2020 by the authors. Licensee MDPI, Basel, Switzerland. This article is an open access article distributed under the terms and conditions of the Creative Commons Attribution (CC BY) license (http://creativecommons.org/licenses/by/4.0/).

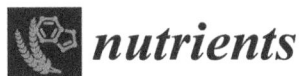

Review

Saccharomyces cerevisiae and Caffeine Implications on the Eukaryotic Cell

Lavinia Liliana Ruta and Ileana Cornelia Farcasanu *

Department of Organic Chemistry, Biochemistry and Catalysis, Faculty of Chemistry, University of Bucharest, Sos. Panduri 90-92, 050663 Bucharest, Romania; lavinia.ruta@chimie.unibuc.ro
* Correspondence: ileana.farcasanu@chimie.unibuc.ro; Tel.: +40-721-067-169

Received: 7 July 2020; Accepted: 10 August 2020; Published: 13 August 2020

Abstract: Caffeine–a methylxanthine analogue of the purine bases adenine and guanine–is by far the most consumed neuro-stimulant, being the active principle of widely consumed beverages such as coffee, tea, hot chocolate, and cola. While the best-known action of caffeine is to prevent sleepiness by blocking the adenosine receptors, caffeine exerts a pleiotropic effect on cells, which lead to the activation or inhibition of various cell integrity pathways. The aim of this review is to present the main studies set to investigate the effects of caffeine on cells using the model eukaryotic microorganism *Saccharomyces cerevisiae*, highlighting the caffeine synergy with external cell stressors, such as irradiation or exposure to various chemical hazards, including cigarette smoke or chemical carcinogens. The review also focuses on the importance of caffeine-related yeast phenotypes used to resolve molecular mechanisms involved in cell signaling through conserved pathways, such as target of rapamycin (TOR) signaling, Pkc1-Mpk1 mitogen activated protein kinase (MAPK) cascade, or Ras/cAMP protein kinase A (PKA) pathway.

Keywords: caffeine; *Saccharomyces cerevisiae*; irradiation; DNA damage; TOR; signaling; lifespan

1. Introduction

Caffeine (1,3,7-trimethylxanthine) is the best-known chemical constituent of coffee and one of the most widely consumed and socially accepted natural stimulants. As an important constituent of coffee, but also of other largely-consumed beverages such as tea, chocolate, and cola-like drinks, caffeine is by far the most ingested methylxanthine, along with the less representative theophylline (1,3-dimethylxanthine, encountered in tea) and theobromine (1,7-dimethylxanthine, mostly found in cocoa). Caffeine is also widely used as an important ingredient of various medicine and non-prescription drugs (used against headaches, common cold, or as appetite suppressants), sports and energy drinks, nutritional supplements, and cosmetics. The scientific literature dealing with the biological effects of caffeine is vast, revealing a large amount of evidence on both the beneficial and deleterious effects, on indications and contraindications, on adverse effects and toxicity, etc. The action of caffeine at the cellular level has been intensively investigated, and there are three fundamental mechanisms which are universally recognized: intracellular mobilization of calcium, inhibition of phosphodiesterases, and antagonism at the level of adenosine receptors [1].

Caffeine belongs to the purine alkaloid family closely linked with the bases adenine and guanine (Figure 1), which are fundamental components of nucleosides, nucleotides, and the nucleic acids [2]. Caffeine is a low-affinity adenosine and ATP analogue which interacts with a number of cellular processes, including cell growth, DNA metabolism, and cell cycle progression [3].

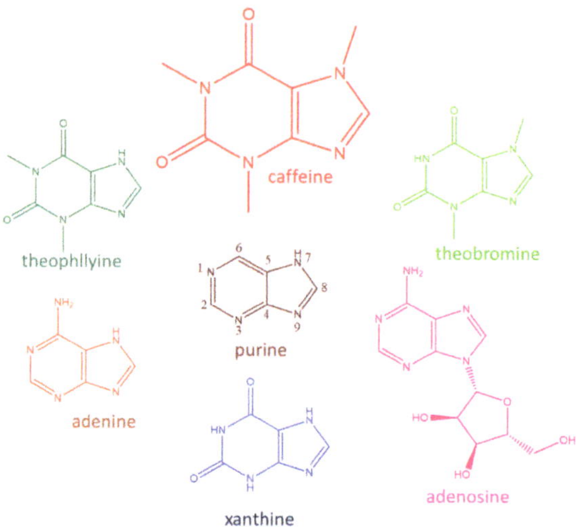

Figure 1. Chemical structures of some purines chemically related to caffeine.

In this review, we present some of the studies set to unravel the caffeine mechanisms of action using *Saccharomyces cerevisiae* as a model for the eukaryotic cell. A model organism is used in scientific research for various reasons: simplification of the biological context, overcoming ethical and experimental constraints, elimination of redundancies, the establishment of a framework for development and optimization of analytical methods, etc. Importantly, a model organism has to be representative of a larger class of living beings [4]. *S. cerevisiae*, a relatively simple unicellular eukaryote, has emerged as a versatile and robust model organism to study the fundamental factors that determine eukaryotic cell biology [5]. *S. cerevisiae* is most utilized by the research community due to its amenability to genetic studies, comprehensive genome annotation [6], and a high degree of homology of essential cellular organization and metabolism with higher eukaryotes [7]. Additionally, *S. cerevisiae* is an invaluable tool in genomic studies, resistance profiling, metabolome studies, and metabolic engineering [8–12]. *S. cerevisiae* offers insights into the complex mechanisms underlying the sensing and response to the external conditions, including exposure to a plethora of synthetic and natural chemical compounds, such as caffeine. *S. cerevisiae* is generally responsive to caffeine, as it was uncovered that this substance affects yeast cell growth and morphology, DNA repair mechanisms, intracellular calcium homeostasis, and cell cycle progression [13].

This paper provides an overview on the studies that used *S. cerevisiae* to unravel some potential effects of caffeine on the eukaryotic cells, with a focus on caffeine transport in yeast cells, caffeine influence on cells exposed to irradiation, caffeine interaction with target of rapamycin (TOR) and cell wall integrity pathways, and caffeine influence on the lifespan of the cells.

2. Caffeine: Transport and Toxicity in *S. cerevisiae*

The effects of caffeine on cells are pleiotropic, causing delays to cell cycle progression; changes in cell morphology; and in high doses, cytotoxicity. Due to structural similarity to nucleotides (Figure 1), it has been considered that caffeine taken up by the cells could affect DNA replication and/or transcription [13]. Caffeine uptake by *S. cerevisiae* cells has not been investigated in detail. Being non-essential, it is expected that caffeine would be carried into the cell by a non-specific transporter, such as purine permease. In *S. cerevisiae*, *FCY2* encodes for a purine-cytosine permease, which mediates purine (adenine, guanine, and hypoxanthine) and cytosine accumulation [14]. Fcy2 may also translocate caffeine into the yeast cell, as it was shown that *fcy2Δ* knock-out strain cannot accumulate caffeine from the medium [15]. In the yeast genome, two more purine-cytosine permease encoding genes are annotated, *FCY21* and *FCY22*, which belong to the same family as *FCY2*. Nevertheless, despite of the nucleotide sequence similarity, neither *FCY21* nor *FCY22* can complement *FCY2* absence [16], and the role of Fcy21 or Fcy22 in the eventual caffeine accumulation has not been specifically investigated.

Caffeine efflux into the extracellular space is better understood, and it is ensured by two ATP-binding cassette (ABC)-transporters responsible for the multidrug resistance in yeast, i.e., Snq2 and Pdr5. In fact, Snq2 was firstly described as the transporter responsible for caffeine detoxification, when *SNQ2* was identified as a caffeine-resistance gene by screening a genomic library of *S. cerevisiae* in a multicopy vector. Multicopy of *PDR5* also conferred resistance to caffeine but to a lower extent compared to *SNQ2* [17]. Pdr5 is also a plasma membrane ABC transporter and a functional homolog of Snq2. Investigation of the functional roles of Snq2 and Pdr5 demonstrated that Snq2 and Pdr5 mediate caffeine efflux (and subsequently caffeine resistance) in *S. cerevisiae* cells [17]. Using evolutionary engineering and molecular characterization of a caffeine-resistant *S. cerevisiae* strain, it was found that caffeine resistance could be gained generally by overexpression of pleiotropic drug resistance genes. The study identified a mutation in *PDR5* but also in *PRD1*, which encodes the transcription factor which regulates *PDR5* and *SNQ2* expression, indicating that resistance to caffeine can be correlated with an efficient and active system of extrusion from the cell [18]. An ABC-transporter gene *BFR1* from *Schizosaccharomyces pombe* was expressed into *S. cerevisiae*, resulting in enhanced caffeine resistance, suggesting that ABC-transporters can be an efficient way to reduce caffeine toxicity in heterologous systems [19]. In mammals, caffeine detoxification is mediated by P450 enzyme [20] and while no specific transporter has been associated with caffeine cellular export, multidrug resistance transporters cannot be excluded. In this line of evidence, caffeine was often used as a pharmacological substrate when studying ABC drug transport characteristics of mammalian cell lines, especially in cocktail approaches [21–24].

Caffeine resistance was also acquired in *S. cerevisiae* by overexpression of *HSE1* (encoding a subunit of the endosomal Vps27p-Hse1p complex required for sorting of ubiquitinated membrane proteins into intralumenal vesicles prior to vacuolar degradation, as well as for recycling of Golgi proteins and formation of lumenal membranes [25]), *RTS3* (encoding a putative component of the protein phosphatase type 2A complex, [26]), and *SDS23* and *SDS24* (both encoding proteins involved in cell separation during budding [27,28]). None of these genes encodes a transporter, and the deletion of any one of these genes resulted only in mild caffeine sensitivity; nevertheless, the combination of multiple deletions strongly sensitized the yeast cells to caffeine, suggesting the multiple effects that caffeine exerts on yeast cells [29].

The pleiotropic effect of caffeine on *S. cerevisiae* can be used to develop a model to study the toxic effects of various substances [30]. It was found that caffeine toxicity is enhanced in yeast cells following exposure to cigarette smoke and that yeast efflux transporters are targets of cigarette smoke chemicals, suggesting once more that associating caffeine-rich products with smoking is not recommended [31]. In line with habitual behavior studies and considering that most of the caffeine beverages are consumed hot (tea, coffee, chocolate), it was revealed that associating caffeine exposure with hyperthermia had an increased mutagenic effect on *S. cerevisiae* cells when pure caffeine was used [32]. Caffeine was also shown to reduce the ozone-survival of the wild-type and the *rad1* and *rad6* mutants of *S. cerevisiae*, whereas no effect was observed in the *rad52* mutant [33]. The interaction between caffeine and *S. cerevisiae* has been also used as a model system to explore the toxicity of the antitumoral agent 1,3-bis(2-chloroethyl)-1-nitrosourea (BCNU), when caffeine showed some effect in enhancing BCNU toxicity by decreasing both the mutagenic and the recombinogenic potential of the drug [34]. A similar system was used to explore the potency of the Topoisomerase II poison N-[2-dimethylamino)ethyl]acridine-4-carboxamide (DACA), whose toxicity on yeast cells was slightly decreased by caffeine [35].

An exogenous substance with biological activity is expected to exert some effect at the plasma membrane level, and the ability of caffeine to block calcium entry into the yeast cell is one of such effects [36]. Caffeine was found to act upon the yeast plasma membrane by effectively inhibiting the uptake of extracellular calcium induced by amiodarone but to be only moderately effective in inhibiting the amiodarone-induced release of calcium from intracellular stores, indicating that caffeine effectively blocks the uptake of extracellular calcium but does not completely eliminate the release of calcium from intracellular stores [37].

3. Caffeine: Between Radio-Protector and Radio-Sensitizer

S. cerevisiae cells is a suitable organism to study the effect of radiation upon the eukaryotic cell and also a convenient platform to identify chemicals that alter this interaction. Some early studies suggested that caffeine potentiates the biological effects of radiation and chemical mutagens in a variety of organisms, including *S. cerevisiae* [38].

3.1. UV Irradiation

S. cerevisiae cells treated with caffeine show a significant increase in radio-sensitivity to various UV doses [39], and it was reported that caffeine had a synergic effect on sensitizing the UV irradiated cells in both haploid and diploid strains [40]. These early studies incriminated caffeine as an inhibitor of DNA repair mechanisms but without relating the caffeine sensitivity with the DNA repair pathways. In subsequent studies, a pronounced inhibitory effect of caffeine on the Rad54-dependent repair of UV-irradiation damage was reported, an inhibition that was strongly dependent on the concentration of caffeine [41]. Later, other research groups confirmed the dose-dependent inhibitory effect of caffeine on the Rad54-dependent repair of UV-irradiation damage [42,43].

Caffeine was also shown to inhibit some DNA repair mechanisms, reducing the generation of cdc^+ colonies under UV irradiation. In *S. cerevisiae*, the *CDC8* gene encodes for a thymidylate kinase involved in DNA replication, also required when UV irradiation induces gene conversion and gene mutation events and induction of cdc^+ colonies. Inhibition of DNA replication by caffeine diminishes the formation of cdc^+ colonies, indicating that the latter arises as a result of errors in DNA replication [44].

3.2. γ-Irradiation

The effect of caffeine on irradiated *S. cerevisiae* cells was also studied for γ-irradiation. A slight caffeine-sensitizing effect was found for the *rad51* and *rad54* mutants, which show defects in the repair of X-ray induced damage [45]. The results suggested that caffeine enhanced radiation-induced cell killing and that the caffeine-sensitive process involved in the repair of γ-ray-induced lesions interfered with a recombinational repair mechanism occurring in cells in S or G2 phase [41].

The DNA damage induced by γ-irradiation of *S. cerevisiae* cells was also analyzed by a single-cell gel electrophoresis of spheroplasts. By monitoring the γ-radiation-induced DNA damage, repair, and radioprotection, this study indicated a radioprotective effect of caffeine in a dose-dependent manner [46].

The *S. cerevisiae* cells have two different physiological states, aerobic and anaerobic. Cells anaerobically grown do not have functionally active mitochondria, and the energy is generated only through glycolysis. It was shown that caffeine acted like a radioprotector against γ-radiation only in the case of yeast cells grown aerobically, in the presence of oxygen. The radioprotection offered to aerobically-grown cells did not influence the recovery process through biosynthetic reparatory ways, as caffeine did not influence the DNA repair process directly. Rather, the caffeine radioprotective phenotype observed involved scavenging of the reactive oxygen species produced by irradiation [47]. In contrast, caffeine acted as a radio-sensitizer for anaerobically grown cells [47].

The effect of caffeine was also monitored in relation with the mutagenic action of ^{60}Co-generated γ-radiation or of 4-nitroquinoline 1-oxide (4-NQO) exposure. The results indicated that caffeine decreased γ-radiation-induced gene conversion frequencies. In contrast, caffeine was found to increase the induced gene conversion frequency in cells treated with 4-NQO, suggesting that the repair processes following γ-irradiation or 4-NQO treatment involve different pathways [48].

4. Caffeine and Cell Response to DNA Damage

Irradiation is often linked to DNA damage events; therefore, it was natural to investigate the effect of caffeine on cell response to DNA damage. In yeast cells, caffeine was shown to inhibit some checkpoint kinases involved in DNA double-strand breaks (DSB) repair. DSB are highly deleterious events that may lead to chromosomal abnormalities, cell death, and cancer, and repair of chromosome breaks occurs by several highly conserved pathways [49]. In *S. cerevisiae*, the response to DSB is controlled by DNA damage checkpoint signal-transduction pathways, which include the redundant protein kinases Mec1 and Tel1, members of the family of phosphatidyl inositol 3 (PI3) kinases [50–52], which are targets of caffeine-induced inhibition. To cope with DNA damage, Mec1/Tel1 and their downstream target kinase Rad53 regulate various cell cycle events (Figure 2). These responses allow enough time for DSB repair and ultimately for mitosis prevention in the presence of a broken chromosome.

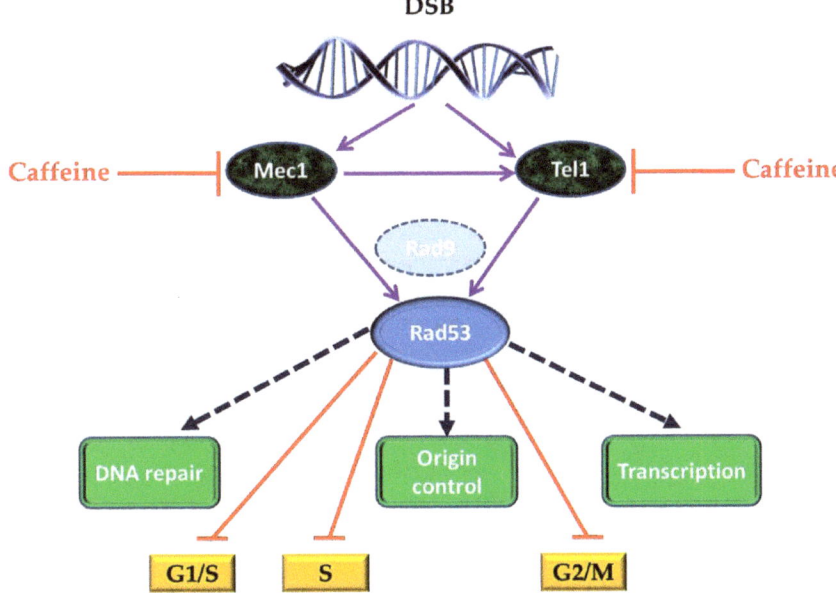

Figure 2. Activation of effector kinases by DNA damage in *Saccharomyces cerevisiae* cells. The central components are two redundant kinases: Mec1 (Mitosis entry checkpoint 1; ATR in mammals) and Tel1. (Telomere maintenance 1; ATM in mammals). Mec1 is hyperactivated in response to different DNA injuries and is essential for cell viability; Tel1 is activated primarily by double-strand breaks (DSBs), and its loss is not lethal in yeast. Mec1/Tel1 activate the effector kinase Rad53. In G2 phase, Rad53 activation is mediated by Rad9, in response to DNA damage. Crosstalk between Mec1 and Tel1 can occur if stalled replication forks collapse since they can generate DSBs. Rad53 inhibits G1/S, Sphase and G2/M cell cycle transitions. Adapted after [51,52].

Interaction between yeast cells and caffeine was used to demonstrate that Mec1/Tel1-dependent intra-S-phase checkpoint activation inhibits Rad52 foci formation, which occurs as a response to replication forks collapsing [53]. Induction of the intra-S-phase checkpoint by hydroxyurea (HU) inhibits Rad52 focus formation in response to ionizing radiation. This inhibition is dependent upon Mec1/Tel1 kinase activity, as HU-treated cells form Rad52 foci in the presence of the PI3 kinase inhibitor caffeine [54].

Upon activation, Mec1 and Tel1 also act directly on chromatin by phosphorylating histone H2A on seryl-129 residue to yield H2A-S129 [55]. When caffeine was used to inhibit Mec1 and Tel1 after DSB induction, it was observed that prolonged phosphorylation of H2A-S129 did not require continuous Mec1 and Tel1 activity and that caffeine treatment could affect homologous recombination also independently of Mec1 and Tel1 inhibition, by interfering with the 5′ to 3′ end resection of the DSB [56]. As similar effects of caffeine treatment were observed on irradiated HeLa cells, the potential of caffeine as a DNA damage-sensitizing agent in cancer cells is considered high, because the caffeine treatment targets one of the earliest steps in homologous recombination, independently of ATM/ATR inhibition (the PI3 kinase in mammalian cells corresponding to Mec1 and Tel1 kinases from the budding yeast) [57].

In eukaryotes, DNA damage triggers the DNA damage checkpoint, causing cells to become blocked in cell cycle progression (Figure 2). In *S. cerevisiae*, even the presence of a single DSB produces G2/M arrest, before anaphase [56]. Sometimes cells with irreparable DNA damage can escape arrest, by adaptation after a long checkpoint-mediated delay; this adaptation depends on the extent of DNA damage [57]. Srs2 is a DNA helicase and a DNA-dependent ATPase with a role in DNA repair and checkpoint recovery, and it was reported that caffeine can reverse the permanent pre-anaphase arrest of *srs2Δ* cells, supporting the idea that caffeine has the ability to override DNA damage checkpoints. Even though the cells lacking Srs2p helicase apparently completed DNA repair after caffeine treatment, the cells failed to recover, proving that Srs2p is required to turn off the DNA damage checkpoint. It was observed that inactivation of the checkpoint restores the viability of most *srs2Δ* cells, indicating that the cause of lethality of these mutant cells is the incapacity to turn off the checkpoint after the completion of DNA repair [58].

Another kinase targeted by caffeine in yeast is Kin3 kinase. In *S. cerevisiae*, *KIN3* was identified as a gene that encodes for a structural homolog of NIMA serine-threonine kinase required in *Aspergillus nidulans* for DNA damage response and in the regulation of G2/M phase progression [59,60]. *S. cerevisiae* cells that were either deleted for *KIN3* or were overexpressing it had no detectable growth phenotypes, but it was noticed that caffeine abolished *KIN3* expression induced by genotoxic agents, such as methyl methanesulfonate (MMS), cisplatin and doxorubicin, indicating that Kin3-activating signal is mediated by the caffeine-sensitive pathways. As caffeine can inhibit the DNA damage checkpoint transducers Mec1 and Tel1 [54,61], it was concluded that Kin3 can play a role in Tel1/Mec1-dependent pathway activation induced after the genotoxic stress [62].

Topoisomerases are highly conserved proteins, required for many aspects of DNA metabolism. In yeast, DNA Topoisomerase III is encoded by gene *TOP3*, whose deletion in *S. cerevisiae* causes hyperrecombination, meiotic defects, sensitivity to genotoxic agents, and poor growth due to accumulation of S/G2 DNA [63]. In a comparative analysis over the effects of caffeine on a cell culture overexpressing *TOP3* after exposure to mutagen MMS, it was observed that caffeine-treated cells successfully traverse S phase, while caffeine non-treated cells failed to show any significant recovery and remained with a mid-S DNA content, suggesting that a persistent checkpoint-mediated cell cycle delay leads to the impaired S-phase progression that can be overridden by the addition of caffeine [64].

Interaction of caffeine with *S. cerevisiae* cells was also used for studies on Ribonucleases H [65]. Ribonucleases H are capable of recognizing RNA-DNA duplexes, degrading only the RNA strand, being of high importance in maintaining the genome stability in the eukaryotic cell. RNases H are classified into type 1 and type 2, encoded in yeast by the *RNH1* and *RNH2* genes, respectively [66]. The effects of caffeine were studied in yeast strains carrying deletions of *RNH1*, *RNH2*, or both, and it was noticed that the absence of RNase H1 in a strain that has an active RNase H2 diminishes the deleterious effects of caffeine and that in caffeine-treated cells, the un-degraded RNA-DNA hybrids influence DNA synthesis by damaging or perturbing the cell cycle [67].

5. The Target-of-Rapamycin (TOR) Pathway is also the Target-of-Caffeine

Evolutionarily conserved target of rapamycin (TOR) kinase is a major regulator of cell growth and metabolism in response to a broad set of environmental signals and stress conditions. Because its defects were noted to be involved in disorders such as cancer, neurological, metabolic, inflammatory, and autoimmune diseases, as well as in ageing [45,68,69], TOR kinase became a target for many clinical research studies, and investigation of TOR signaling regulators is particularly important for developing effective therapeutic strategies [70–72]. The TOR kinase is a member of the phosphatidylinositol 3 (PI3) kinase family, and therefore, it is susceptible to caffeine. In yeast and in higher eukaryotes, the TOR kinase is part of two protein complexes, named TOR Complex 1 (TORC1) and TOR Complex 2 (TORC2) [73].

The TOR pathways regulate the cellular growth under normal conditions, by stimulating ribosome biogenesis and by controlling the precursors for amino acids and other nitrogenous molecules' synthesis (Figure 3a). Under harsh environment conditions, such as starvation or excess, the cell metabolic reprogramming is induced via signal transduction pathways involving Tor1 and Tor2, two homologous TOR kinases found in TORC1 and TORC2 [74]. Either Tor1 or Tor2 can function in TORC1, whereas only Tor2 supports TORC2 function (Figure 3b). *S. cerevisiae* has been very useful as model organism for understanding the role of TOR signaling in the regulation of cell growth and aging [75,76], and for this purpose, yeast cells are usually grown under nitrogen starvation or in the presence of inhibitors such as rapamycin [77]. Rapamycin has many natural analogs termed "rapalogs"; one such rapalog is caffeine [78].

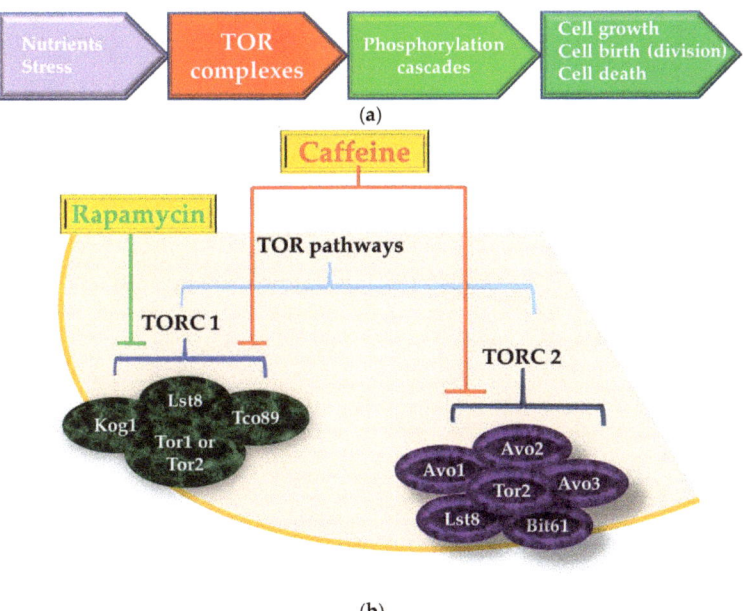

Figure 3. Schematic representation of target of rapamycin (TOR) complexes. (**a**) The main elements up- and downstream of TOR complexes. The TOR complexes are activated by nutrient status or by various stresses. Activated TORCs then initiate phosphorylation cascades involved in regulating fundamental aspects of life such as cell growth, cell birth, and cell death. Adapted after [73,79,80]. (**b**) Caffeine and the TORC in *Saccharomyces cerevisiae* cells. The TOR pathways involve two multiprotein complexes termed TOR complex 1 (TORC1) and TOR complex 2 (TORC2), which are structurally similar but not functionally identical. TORC1 is concentrated at the cell membrane or at the vacuolar membrane and contains Tco89, Lst8, and either Tor1 or Tor2 caffeine-sensitive kinases that act as scaffold to couple TOR and its effectors. The TORC1 is sensitive to rapamycin. TORC2 is rapamycin insensitive, and it contains Tor2 (but not Tor1) Avo1, Avo2, Avo3, Bit61 (and/or its paralog Bit2), Lst8. TORC2 is found in multiple cellular locations, including the plasma membrane. A plasma membrane location is consistent with the role of TORC2 in controlling the actin cytoskeleton and endocytosis. Adapted after [73,79,80].

The macrolide drug rapamycin is a macrocyclic lactone used as immunosuppressive and anti-proliferative antibiotic which inhibits TORC1 [81]. In the presence of rapamycin, the downstream processes regulated by TORC1 (e.g., stress responses, control of gene expression, protein and ribosome synthesis, amino acid biosynthesis, nitrogen assimilation pathways, protein trafficking and stability, starvation and quiescence, autophagy) are consequently inhibited [82]. While TORC1 is involved in activities related to cell growth, TORC2 is required for polarized cell growth and cytoskeleton organization [73,79]. Rapamycin does not interact with TORC2, nor does it inhibit downstream processes, and therefore, its applications are limited in studying TORC2-related processes [58,64].

In yeast, TORC1 contains kinases Tor1 or Tor2, as well as several additional proteins, including Kog1, Lst8, and Tco89; TORC2 contains Tor2 as well as Lst8, Avo1-Avo3, and Bit61 [79] (Figure 3b). In mammalian cells, TORC1 consists of Tor (mTor), mLST8/GβL (the ortholog of Lst8), and Raptor (the ortholog of Kog1), whereas TORC2 consists of mTor, mLST8/GβL, and mAVO3/Rictor (the ortholog of Avo3p) [81]. Caffeine affects TOR signaling by directly inhibiting TORC1 in many organisms, including yeast, plants, and mammals [83]. It is possible that caffeine also inhibits TORC2 but indirectly, at higher concentrations or upon prolonged treatment [77].

Reinke et al. 2006 [81] were among the first researchers that presented evidence that TORC1 is indeed a significant target for caffeine in yeast by identifying mutations within the FRB (rapamycin binding) and kinase domains of Tor1 that revealed important levels of caffeine resistance that were correlated to highly conserved amino acids within TOR proteins from across the phylogenetic spectrum [81]. Especially in mammals, caffeine was shown to affect cells by direct interaction with components of the TOR pathway [84]. On laboratory animals, rapamycin inhibition of TORC1 leads to delays in ageing, increasing healthy longevity. In human beings, rapamycin is used for preventing organ transplant rejection and to treat some forms of cancer, albeit clinical use is associated with important side effects; this is why the scientific community is in continuous search for TORC1 inhibitors with fewer side effects [85]. Although rapamycin and caffeine induce similar profiles of global gene expression [81,83], it was shown that rapamycin is a partial inhibitor of TORC1 [86], while caffeine is a selective inhibitor of TORC1, acting by a different mechanism from rapamycin [81,87]. Rapamycin binds to the FK506 binding protein FKPB12, and the FKBP12-rapamycin complex inhibits the activity of mTORC1 by destroying the physical interaction between the TOR protein and a second TORC1 component, raptor (Kog1 in yeast) [88,89].

The yeast cells treated with caffeine or rapamycin have a transcriptional profiling that proves the inhibition effect of TOR signaling on a broad array of genes associated with a wide range of cellular growth-related functions and also with stress and autophagy-related genes [83,90]. Notably, similar effects that rapamycin and caffeine display on global gene expression prompted the hypothesis that TOR signaling is mediated through common upstream and downstream regulators, that is, a common intracellular signal transduction pathway, in response to rapamycin and caffeine [83]. The direct target of caffeine in yeast cells is Tor1 kinase, whose inhibition triggers the activation of the Pkc1p-Mpk1p cascade; nevertheless, this activation is not essential for cell survival in the presence of caffeine [13]. In order to investigate if caffeine interferes with the TOR pathway, the transcriptomic responses induced by caffeine and rapamycin were compared [91,92], and it was observed that both compounds trigger down-regulation of the genes involved in transcription, protein synthesis, and ribosome assembly, at the same time activating gene expression in the Krebs cycle, the Gln3p/Gat1p-controlled nitrogen catabolite repression (NCR), and the Rtg1/3p-controlled retrograde pathway [13,91,92]. Gln3 is a major transcription activator that regulates transcription of nitrogen catabolite repression (NCR)-sensitive genes, having high similarity to the DNA binding domain of mammalian GATA factors which induce transcription of target genes [93]. S. cerevisiae uses a broad spectrum of compounds as nitrogen sources, and NCR is a physiological response when cells are grown under normal conditions, and preferred nitrogen sources are used (e.g., glutamine) [93]. In cells grown on preferred nitrogen sources, Gln3 is phosphorylated in a TOR-dependent manner, and the transcription of NCR-sensitive genes is repressed. If the cells are grown in the presence of non-preferred nitrogen medium (e.g., proline) or treated with caffeine, Gln3 is dephosphorylated and translocated from the cytoplasm to the nucleus, thereby activating the transcription of NCR-sensitive genes [94]. In this regard, both the intracellular localization and activity of Gln3 are regulated by TORC1 kinase, and caffeine treatment leads to the induction of transcription of NCR-sensitive genes in a similar manner as rapamycin treatment [95].

Rho-family GTPases are key regulators involved in many eukaryotic cell functions (organelle development, cytoskeleton dynamics, cell movement, etc.) and represent a core component of the TORC1 pathway [96–101]. In *S. cerevisiae*, the Rho family has six members, Rho1 to Rho5 and Cdc42. Mutants with *RHO5* gene deleted (*rho5Δ*) had a higher resistance to caffeine, in contrast to the Slt2 mitogen activated pathway kinase (MAPK) mutants, which were highly sensitive to caffeine, indicating a role for *RHO5* in the down regulation of the Slt2-MAPK pathway. This special behavior was explained by the fact that Rho5 acts as an off-switch for the MAPK cascade, which differentiates between MAPK-dependent and independent functions of Pkc1, a prototypic member of the protein kinase C superfamily and the main effector of Rho1 [102]. Rho1 is activated by Rom2, its guanine nucleotide exchange factor (GEF), and several integrin-like cell surface proteins, such as Wsc1 and Mid2 [103]. In stress conditions for the cell wall, these cell surface proteins act as stress sensors and activate Rom2 [99,104]. Upon activation, Rho1 binds directly to Kog1, a component of TORC1, leading to a decrease of activity of TORC1. Consequently, the binding also induced dephosphorylation of Gln3 triggering the release and activation of the Tap42-2A phosphatase (Figure 4), a major effector of TORC1 [100,105]. It was demonstrated that caffeine, just like rapamycin, calcofluor white (a cell wall damage agent), nitrogen starvation, and heat, induces Rho1 activation and directly inhibits TORC1, acting both upstream and downstream of Rho1 GTPase [100].

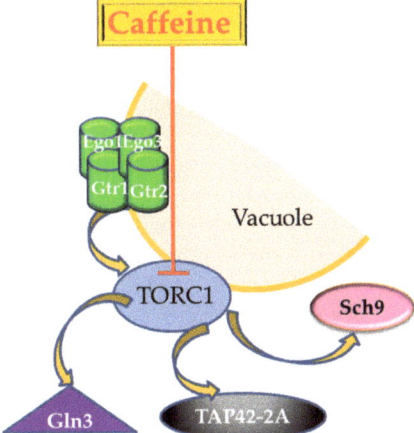

Figure 4. Upstream and downstream components of TORC1 regulation. EGO complex (localized on the vacuolar membrane), which consist in four proteins, Ego1 (a palmitoylated/myristolated protein); Ego3 (a transmembrane protein); and two Ras-family GTPases, Gtr1 and Gtr2, is a major regulator of TORC1 activity, via Tco89. The best characterized substrate of TORC1 is Sch9, a member of AGC family of kinases. When cells are stressed by caffeine, TORC1 is inhibited directly, and the Sch9 phosphorylation is reduced dramatically. TORC1 also regulates the 2A (Pph21, Pph22, and Pph3—generically PP2Ac) and 2A-related phosphatases, including the Tap42-PP2A effector. Inactivation of TORC1 by caffeine results in Tap42 dephosphorylation and TORC1 directly phosphorylate other substrates including Gln3. Adapted from [13,80,81,106].

The Ras-family-GTPase and its homologs [107] mediate the growth factor-dependent or stress-induced signal transduction. In yeasts, the Ras-GTPase is a group of enzymes that comprise Ras1, Ypt1, Cdc42, Gtr2, Arf1, Gtr1, and Gsp1; Gtr1 can form a heterodimer with Gtr2 [108]. These proteins switch between an active GTP-bound form and an inactive GDP-bound form and act as molecular switches for various signaling pathways [109]. In yeast, the Gtr1 and Gtr2 (Figure 4) are proteins involved in response to heat shock and in the pathways that are activated during nitrogen starvation and caffeine treatment, suggesting that they have roles in the TOR kinase pathway [110]. It was shown that Δgtr1 and Δgtr2 have the similar caffeine-sensitive phenotype [110], in concordance with the previous findings of the inhibitory activity of caffeine on the TOR kinase activity [81,91]. Moreover, Gtr1 and Gtr2 were shown to be involved in the response to oxidative stress and caffeine treatment, acting at Ego1 and Ego3 levels (Figure 4), which genetically interact with components of the TOR signaling pathway [111], the EGO complex being a non-essential activator of TORC1 [80,112]. The guanine nucleotide region of Gtr1p situated at the N-terminus is required for Gtr1p–Gtr2p heterodimer formation but not for complex formation with Ego1p, a vacuolar membrane protein. Upon caffeine treatment, the amount of free Gtr1p increases, while it decreases in the protein complexes. Likewise, free Gtr2p is increased by caffeine but the amount form bound in the high molecular weight complexes remains unaffected, indicating that Gtr1p and Gtr2p are necessary for caffeine resistance and that caffeine treatment released Gtr1p from the Gtr1p–Gtr2p complex [110].

In a study over the sensitivity of TORC1 during the rapamycin treatment, it was revealed that the cells recovered efficiently from treatment with saturating concentration of rapamycin alone, as well as with the caffeine alone, and that caffeine is a selective inhibitor of rapamycin-insensitive proliferation; at the same time, the rapamycin-caffeine co-treatment followed by recovery in the presence of caffeine, induced a strong recovery defect [86]. These observations suggested that rapamycin-insensitive TORC1 activity is sensitive to caffeine and is required for residual proliferation rate in the presence of rapamycin and for recovery from the drug [86].

Some new components of TOR signaling were recently identified following direct and specific inhibition of TOR signaling by caffeine and rapamycin using a network-based multi-omics integrative analysis that employed data from transcriptomics, interactomics, and regulomics sources in yeast [80,111–113]. The analysis identified seven previously unannotated proteins, Atg14, Rim20, Ret2, Spt21, Ylr257W, Ymr295c, and Ygr017w, as potential components of TOR-mediated rapamycin and caffeine signaling in *S. cerevisiae*. Study of Ylr257w would be particularly informative since it was the only protein whose removal from the constructed network blocked the signal transduction to the TORC1 effector kinase Npr1 [80,111].

A functional link between Ptc1 and the TOR pathway was established due to the rapamycin and caffeine sensitivity of yeast *ptc1* mutants. Ptc1 is a 2C phosphatase isoform, member of the 2C phosphatase family; a connection with TOR pathways is not shared by most members of the family. Ptc1 is required for normal Gln3 and Msn2-mediated transcriptional responses and nuclear localization [91]. In yeast *ptc1* mutants exposed to rapamycin and caffeine, the translocation of Gln3 and Msn2 to the nucleus is prevented and also the dephosphorylation of the Npr1 kinase. At the same time, the overexpression of other isoforms (such as *PTC2* or *PTC3*) did not confer tolerance to rapamycin, and *ptc1 ptc6* double mutant were more sensitive to both rapamycin and caffeine, suggesting the role of both phosphatases in the signaling of TOR pathway [114].

At the level of the general amino acid control (GAAC) and TOR pathways, the cellular stress response is regulated by the amino acylation status of the cellular tRNA pool, which directs the transcriptional regulation of gene expression in response to nutritional stresses [115]. Under normal nutrient conditions, the TOR pathway regulates the cellular growth in a positive manner, by stimulating ribosome biogenesis and utilization of precursors for the synthesis of amino acids and other nitrogenous macromolecules. Under starvation conditions, yeast cells start metabolic reprogramming via signal transduction pathways involving the two homologous protein kinases, Tor1 and Tor2. The cells with a deficient quality control were more tolerant to caffeine than the wild type cells, due to altered interactions between caffeine and the TOR and GAAC pathways components; the increased caffeine tolerance was correlated with a decreased activity of Gln3 [76].

In yeast, twelve lysine methyltransferases that modify translational elongation factors and ribosomal proteins were identified. Among them, five (Efm1, Efm4, Efm5, Efm6, and Efm7) are specific to elongation factor 1A (EF1A), the protein responsible for bringing aminoacyl-tRNAs to the ribosome. It was demonstrated that loss of EF1A methylation is not essential to cell viability but leads to a decrease in growth rates under caffeine and rapamycin treatment. These findings suggested that EF1A interacts with the TORC1 pathway and that Efm methyltransferases are devoted to the modification of EF1A, finding no evidence for the methylation of other substrates in the yeast cell [116].

The mammalian lysosome has an analogue in yeast, the vacuole, a membrane-bounded organelle. The yeast vacuole contains an acidic environment due to vacuolar hydrolases that degrade structural debris macromolecules and waste products [117]. In a genomic screen of 4828 yeasts haploid deletion strains for growth hypersensitivity to hygromycin B (*hhy* mutants), all the *hhy* mutants revealed severe sensitivities to caffeine and rapamycin, suggesting an interaction between the identified genes in TOR kinase pathway [118,119].

6. Caffeine and the Yeast Cell Wall Integrity Pathway

Investigations regarding the interaction between caffeine and yeast cells demonstrated the existence of additional caffeine targets, including components of cell wall integrity (CWI) pathways [120]. The cell wall of *S. cerevisiae* confers cell shape and protection against harsh environments [121]. It is formed by different types of molecules, including mannoproteins, glucans, and chitin, closely interconnected. For defense against external insults or for adaptation to cell wall defects, cells use a complex CWI signaling pathways. Inhibition of the synthesis of any structural compounds leads to cell death, making the yeast cell wall an attractive target for antifungal therapy against invasive fungi such as *Candida* spp., *Cryptococcus neoformans*, *Aspergillus* spp., *Pneumocystis carinii*, or *Histoplasma capsulatum* [122]. The CWI involves the MAPK cascade downstream of PKC (protein kinase C) signal transduction pathway [123]. Rho1p GTPase controls the CWI, functions in actin polarization [124], and activates the MAPK pathway [123]. A plethora of studies and biochemical evidence suggested links between TOR and CWI pathways, and caffeine was often used as a phenotypic criterion to evaluate the function of the Mpk1-mediated CWI pathway [123]. In *S. cerevisiae*, it was observed that sensitivity to caffeine can be correlated with defects in the CWI pathway and that caffeine activates CWI signaling, when the stability of the cell wall can be monitored in terms of response to osmotic or thermal stress [123]. It was shown that caffeine is not a typical activator of CWI signaling, because it induces phosphorylation of the Mpk1 C-terminus at Ser423 and Ser428 residues independently of the standard dual phosphorylation associated with MAPK activation; nevertheless, these phosphorylations are dependent on the DNA damage checkpoint kinases, Mec1/Tel1 and Rad53 [124]. Other studies also confirmed that yeast strains with altered CWI are caffeine sensitive, including strains lacking one or more of the five *PRS* (phospho ribosylpyrophosphate synthetase) genes, in particular those lacking the Prs1/Prs3 minimal functional unit [125]. In altered versions of *PRS1*, there is a correlation between caffeine sensitivity and increased basal expression of Rlm1, the transcription factor which is an important component of the PKC-mediated MAPK pathway involved in the maintenance of CWI [126].

The loss of function of other proteins involved in CWI can also be related to caffeine sensitive phenotypes. For example, there are six proteins that have the tetratricopeptide repeat (TPR) domain (mediates protein–protein interaction), which are encoded by six essential genes in the *S. cerevisiae* genome. Among these, YNL313c, renamed *EMW1* (essential for the maintenance of the cell wall), proved to be essential for the maintenance of CWI, and the mutants lacking *EMW1* showed sensitivity to diverse stressor compounds, including caffeine [127]. Moreover, the newly described mutant *rim21Δ* (*ynl294c*) showed a moderate hypersensitivity to caffeine owed to a low compensatory response of the cell wall, indicated by the almost complete absence of Slt2 phosphorylation and the modest increase in chitin synthesis after calcofluor treatment [128].

Cell signaling, gene expression and mitosis but also CWI are cellular processes regulated by phosphorylation/dephosphorylation [129]. Based on sequence analysis of *S. cerevisiae* genes (approximately 6000 genes), the yeast has 117 protein kinase (PKase) and 32 protein phosphatases (PPase) genes [130]. As defects in MAPK pathway are often associated with sensitivity to caffeine, a systematic analysis of caffeine-related phenotype in relation with phosphorylation/dephosphorylation and CWI is still a desiderate [106,130,131].

Caffeine, as a CWI pathway activator, was used to show that Puf5 has a role in response to DNA replication stress and does not involve Pop2. Puf5 is a prototypical PUF protein, a family of RNA binding proteins conserved in eukaryotes, with roles in cell growth, division, differentiation, and development [132]. In *S. cerevisiae* cells treated with caffeine, *PUF5* and *POP2* have the same genetic pathway, leading to the conclusion that the CWI functions are mediated by Puf5 or Pop2-mediated gene repression mechanisms [133].

7. Other Pathways Susceptible to Caffeine

Inositol hexakisphosphate (IP6) is the most abundant inositol polyphosphate present in eukaryotes. IP6 is phosphorylated by IP6 kinases (IP6K-s) yielding inositol pyrophosphates, which are important signaling molecules in the eukaryotic cell [134]. Yeast lacking the IP6K known as *Kcs1* display defective vesicular endocytosis, showing a decrease in cell growth [134], sensitivity to environmental stresses [135], and abnormal ribosomal functions [136]. Inositol pyrophosphates are involved in signaling cascades that mediate cell death and telomere length, and they physiologically inhibit signaling by Tel1 and possibly Mec1. Caffeine inhibits the PI3K-related protein kinases Tel1 and Mec1, and therefore, it is expected that *kcs1Δ* mutants are resistant to its lethal effects. Indeed, the lethal action of caffeine is suppressed in mutants that cannot synthesize inositol pyrophosphates because they physiologically antagonize the actions of Tel1 and Mec1 kinases [137].

Other examples of using the pleiotropic action of caffeine on *S. cerevisiae* to understand different molecular mechanism highly conserved in superior eukaryotes and to elucidate the way of action of compounds with potential as human drugs are presented below.

The major component of Lewis Bodies (protein aggregates present in the cytoplasm of neuronal cells in PD (Parkinson Disease)) is the natively disordered protein, α-synuclein [138]. A *S. cerevisiae* proteotoxicity model of PD was employed to evaluate the role of caffeine in the aggregation of α-synuclein. On caffeine treatment, the toxicity of aggregates decreased, the intracellular oxidative stress was diminished, and the survival of the cell increased. It is supposed that caffeine alters the aggregation pathway of α-synuclein by introducing species with reduced proteotoxicity, leading to a decrease of the lag time and an increase in the apparent rate of fibrillation of α-synuclein. α-Synuclein has the ability to assume alternate aggregation pathways more than any other protein that apparently is misfolded in neurodegenerative disorders, because of its natively disordered structure. This effect apparently is heightened by the presence of caffeine, supporting the epidemiological studies that showed that coffee consumption is inversely related to the risk of onset of PD [139,140].

Early studies also introduced caffeine as an activator of the cAMP-dependent protein kinase pathway, based on the in vitro potency of this compound to inhibit the mammalian cAMP phosphodiesterase [141]. In yeast, this hypothesis is still controversial, as some researchers reported an increase of cAMP levels [142], others mentioned no effect on levels of cAMP [143] while other authors showed that caffeine antagonizes the glucose-induced cAMP synthesis [91,144]. Caffeine modifies the metabolic effects produced in the *S. cerevisiae* cell by exposure to glucose, acting on a crossover point at the level of the phosphofructokinase/fructose-bisphosphatase cycle, increasing the ATP levels. Following glucose entry into the cell, caffeine reduces the concentration of intracellular cAMP in a dose-dependent manner, an effect that can be explained by the interference with catabolic inactivation of enzymes [144].

Mitochondria play a fundamental role in eukaryotic cell physiology by integrating numerous death signals, being involved in the control of apoptosis. Mitochondrial genome integrity is essential for the viability of most species. Two mutants of *S. cerevisiae* defective in genes involved in the biosynthesis of mitochondrial phosphatidylglycerol and cardiolipin, *pel1* and *crd1*, were analyzed in the presence of different cell wall perturbing agents. The mutants containing dysfunctional mitochondria revealed a modified sensitivity to metabolic inhibitors. The *S. cerevisiae pell* mutant showed increased sensitivity to the cell-wall perturbing agents such as caffeine, caspofungin, and hygromycin [145].

8. Caffeine and Lifespan

The ageing biology is a new field that emerged since researchers have been attempting to extent the organisms' lifespan (LS), and caloric restriction is a critical method used to understand the mechanism of LS. Because caloric restriction is usually accompanied by a reduction in food consumption over a long period of time, chemical food substitutes called caloric restriction mimetics have been the topic of intense research, and they can be used as starting materials in developing drugs that prevent or ameliorate the ageing-associated illnesses. Such compounds have shown their ability to extend the LS in different model organisms, e.g., rapamycin in mice [146] and yeasts [147]. *S. cerevisiae* is an excellent model to study LS as it has conserved ageing pathways, and the study of new molecules' effect on LS is greatly facilitated by yeast studies which yield significant information before proceeding to animal studies [148].

Physical exercise, caloric restriction, and consumption of moderate amounts of substances such as selenium, zinc, omega 3 unsaturated fatty acids, vitamins E and C, antioxidants, caffeine, or alcohol were proposed as factors essential to extend the human LS or to reduce age-associated diseases. Often, these studies show only correlative (not causative) effects between a compound and longevity. The conservation of most ageing pathways in yeast and their facile genetic manipulation represents a premise to distinguish between the correlative and causative effects of nutrition on ageing [149].

The extent of the LS was studied on *S. cerevisiae* for identifying conserved genetic and pharmacological interventions [150]. The TOR pathway, for example, was first described as genetically involved in aging using experiments made on yeast [151]. Among the many nutraceuticals tested, caffeine was the only compound that induced growth kinetics consistent with a TOR inhibitory effect, increasing doubling time specifically in the *tor1Δ* mutant cells. Studies correlating caffeine, TOR pathway, and LS have since been done on budding yeast [81,87] and fission yeast [83], invertebrate models [152,153] and humans [85,154].

Caffeine treatment of yeast cells releases Rim15 from TORC1-Sch9-mediated inhibition and as a result, it increases LS. Therefore, it is highly probable that an analogous mTORC1/S6K/LATS kinase cascade also has influence on longevity in higher eukaryotes, including humans [155,156]. It was shown that low doses of caffeine significantly extended chronological LS, and partial loss of TORC1 activity increased chronological LS via TORC1–Sch9–Rim15 kinase cascade. Moreover, it was shown that moderate coffee consumption is expected to cause a 4–8% inhibition of mTORC1 activity, suggesting causality explanations for correlation between coffee consumption and longevity [87].

The effect of a polyphenol-rich extract from cocoa on the chronological LS of *S. cerevisiae* was studied under two settings: in the stationary phase reached after glucose depletion and under severe caloric restriction. It was observed that cocoa polyphenol-rich extracts increased the chronological LS of *S. cerevisiae* during the stationary phase in a dose-dependent manner and also extended yeast LS under severe caloric restriction conditions. The cocoa extracts increased the lifespan of wild type cells and also of the *sod2Δ* cells, proving that the mechanism is Mn-SOD2-independent. Nevertheless, this effect was detected only for the polyphenol-rich cocoa extract and not for its individual components, including caffeine [148].

Caffeine (along with curcumin, dapsone, metformin, rapamycin, resveratrol, and spermidine) was evaluated as a LS extender in *S. cerevisiae* under conditions of caloric restriction. In contrast with other studies, caffeine has been claimed to increase the LS of yeast [87], while other groups showed that caffeine, even at higher concentrations, had no effect on LS [157]. Haploid strains of yeast are sometimes unstable in respect to respiratory competence and spontaneously produce the respiration-deficient (RD) mutants with very high frequencies. It was shown that the addition of caffeine to the culture media considerably reduced the production of RD mutants, albeit temporarily [158].

Pathologic endogenous DNA double-strand breaks (EDSB) can occur spontaneously even without exposure to radiation or DNA damaging agents [159]. EDSB can be detected in excess when non-dividing cells have functional DSB repair defects produced independently of replication, a reason why they were named pathologic replication-independent EDSBs (Path-RIND-EDSB) [160]. In chronological aging yeast, reduction of physiologic replication-independent endogenous DNA double strand breaks (Phy-RIND-EDSB) lead to an increase of pathologic RIND-EDSBs (Path-RIND-EDSB); the latter must be repaired instantly as their accumulation can lead to senescence and death [161] or at least a decrease in the cell's viability [162]. In DSB repair-defective cells, the retention of Path-RIND-EDSBs can occur, a phenomenon that is normally encountered in chronological aging yeast. In caffeine-treated cells, significant accumulation of Path-RIND-EDSB was recorded as quantitatively similar to aging cells with defects in DSB repair, making caffeine an invaluable tool in mimicking chronological aging in vitro [159].

9. Concluding Remarks

Caffeine, one of the most consumed and widely accepted neurostimulants, is also a powerful agent used in life science research. Due to its pleiotropic effects [163], caffeine is an active modulator of different enzymes and their regulatory pathways, which include important molecular players such as TOR kinases or DNA damage checkpoint kinases. Many of the studies reviewed here, which made use of the interaction between caffeine and *S. cerevisiae*, contributed to elucidating molecular mechanisms involved in biologic processes of general concern, such as DNA repair mechanisms, cancer, or aging. Using various approaches and setting multiple targets, the studies on caffeine–*S. cerevisiae* interaction generated outputs which could be extrapolated to higher organisms. In spite of the pleiotropic effects of caffeine, there is one mechanism universally accepted, i.e., the inhibitory effect on PI3 kinases, including the core kinases from the TOR complexes. However, since many of the puzzle pieces are still missing, it is no doubt that the duo caffeine–*S. cerevisiae* has not yet reached its full potential in opening doors to new knowledge.

Author Contributions: Conceptualization, L.L.R. and I.C.F.; resources, L.L.R. and I.C.F.; data curation, L.L.R. and I.C.F; writing—original draft preparation, L.L.R; writing—review and editing, I.C.F.; visualization, L.L.R. and I.C.F.; supervision, L.L.R. and I.C.F.; project administration, L.L.R. and I.C.F.; funding acquisition, L.L.R. and I.C.F. All authors have read and agreed to the published version of the manuscript.

Funding: This research received no external funding.

Conflicts of Interest: The authors declare no conflicts of interest.

References

1. Cappelletti, S.; Piacentino, D.; Sani, G.; Aromatario, M. Caffeine: Cognitive and physical performance enhancer or psychoactive drug? *Curr. Neuropharmacol.* **2015**, *13*, 71–88. [CrossRef] [PubMed]
2. Dewick, P.M. *Medicinal Natural Products: A Biosynthetic Approach*, 3rd ed.; John Wiley & Sons: West Sussex, UK, 2009; pp. 413–416.
3. Kaufmann, W.K.; Heffernan, T.P.; Beaulieu, L.M.; Doherty, S.; Frank, A.R.; Zhou, Y.; Bryant, M.F.; Zhou, T.; Luche, D.D.; Nikolaishvili-Feinberg, N.; et al. Caffeine and human DNA metabolism: The magic and the mystery. *Mutat. Res.* **2003**, *532*, 85–102. [CrossRef] [PubMed]
4. Karathia, H.; Vilaprinyo, E.; Sorribas, A.; Alves, R. *Saccharomyces cerevisiae* as a model organism: A comparative study. *PLoS ONE* **2011**, *6*, e16015. [CrossRef] [PubMed]
5. Duina, A.A.; Miller, M.E.; Keeney, J.B. Budding yeast for budding geneticists: A primer on the *Saccharomyces cerevisiae* model system. *Genetics* **2014**, *197*, 33–48. [CrossRef]
6. Goffeau, A.; Barrell, B.G.; Bussey, H.; Davis, R.W.; Dujon, B.; Feldmann, H.; Galibert, F.; Hoheisel, J.D.; Jacq, C.; Johnston, M.; et al. Life with 6000 genes. *Science* **1996**, *274*, 546–567. [CrossRef]
7. Castrillo, J.I.; Oliver, S. Yeast as a touchstone in post-genomic research: Strategies for integrative analysis in functional genomics. *J. Biochem. Mol. Biol.* **2004**, *37*, 93–106. [CrossRef]

8. Matuo, R.; Sousa, F.G.; Soares, D.G.; Bonatto, D.; Saffi, J.; Escargueil, A.E.; Larsen, A.K.; Henriques, J.A. *Saccharomyces cerevisiae* as a model system to study the response to anticancer agents. *Cancer Chemother. Pharmacol.* **2012**, *70*, 491–502. [CrossRef]
9. Dos Santos, S.C.; Sá-Correia, I. Yeast toxicogenomics: Lessons from a eukaryotic cell model and cell factory. *Curr. Opin. Biotechnol.* **2015**, *33*, 183–191. [CrossRef]
10. Lian, J.; Mishra, S.; Zhao, H. Recent advances in metabolic engineering of *Saccharomyces cerevisiae*: New tools and their applications. *Metab. Eng.* **2018**, *50*, 85–108. [CrossRef]
11. Nielsen, J. Yeast systems biology: Model organism and cell factory. *Biotechnol. J.* **2019**, *14*, e1800421. [CrossRef]
12. Coronas-Serna, J.M.; Valenti, M.; Del Val, E.; Fernández-Acero, T.; Rodríguez-Escudero, I.; Mingo, J.; Luna, S.; Torices, L.; Pulido, R.; Molina, M.; et al. Modeling human disease in yeast: Recreating the PI3K-PTEN-Akt signaling pathway in *Saccharomyces cerevisiae*. *Int. Microbiol.* **2020**, *23*, 75–87. [CrossRef] [PubMed]
13. Kuranda, K.; Leberre, V.; Sokol, S.; Palamarczyk, G.; François, J. Investigating the caffeine effects in the yeast *Saccharomyces cerevisiae* brings new insights into the connection between TOR, PKC and Ras/cAMP signalling pathways. *Mol. Microbiol.* **2006**, *61*, 1147–1166. [CrossRef] [PubMed]
14. Weber, E.; Rodriguez, C.; Chevallier, M.R.; Jund, R. The purine-cytosine permease gene of *Saccharomyces cerevisiae*: Primary structure and deduced protein sequence of the *FCY2* gene product. *Mol. Microbiol.* **1990**, *4*, 585–596. [CrossRef] [PubMed]
15. Qi, Z.; Xiong, L. Characterization of a purine permease family gene OsPUP7 involved in growth and development control in rice. *J. Integr. Plant. Biol.* **2013**, *55*, 1119–1135. [CrossRef]
16. Wagner, R.; Straub, M.L.; Souciet, J.L.; Potier, S.; de Montigny, J. New plasmid system to select for *Saccharomyces cerevisiae* purine-cytosine permease affinity mutants. *J. Bacteriol.* **2001**, *183*, 4386–4388. [CrossRef]
17. Tsujimoto, Y.; Shimizu, Y.; Otake, K.; Nakamura, T.; Okada, R.; Miyazaki, T.; Watanabe, K. Multidrug resistance transporters Snq2p and Pdr5p mediate caffeine efflux in *Saccharomyces cerevisiae*. *Biosci. Biotechnol. Biochem.* **2015**, *79*, 1103–1110. [CrossRef]
18. Sürmeli, Y.; Holyavkin, C.; Topaloğlu, A.; Arslan, M.; Kısakesen, H.İ.; Çakar, Z.P. Evolutionary engineering and molecular characterization of a caffeine-resistant *Saccharomyces cerevisiae* strain. *World J. Microbiol. Biotechnol.* **2019**, *35*, 183. [CrossRef]
19. Wang, M.; Deng, W.W.; Zhang, Z.Z.; Yu, O. Engineering an ABC transporter for enhancing resistance to caffeine in *Saccharomyces cerevisiae*. *J. Agric. Food Chem.* **2016**, *64*, 7973–7978. [CrossRef]
20. Kot, M.; Daniel, W.A. Caffeine as a marker substrate for testing cytochrome P450 activity in human and rat. *Pharmacol. Rep.* **2008**, *60*, 789–797.
21. Cusinato, D.A.C.; Martinez, E.Z.; Cintra, M.T.C.; Filgueira, G.C.O.; Berretta, A.A.; Lanchote, V.L.; Coelho, E.B. Evaluation of potential herbal-drug interactions of a standardized propolis extract (EPP-AF®) using an in vivo cocktail approach. *J. Ethnopharmacol.* **2019**, *245*, 112174. [CrossRef]
22. Aronsen, L.; Orvoll, E.; Lysaa, R.; Ravna, A.W.; Sager, G. Modulation of high affinity ATP-dependent cyclic nucleotide transporters by specific and non-specific cyclic nucleotide phosphodiesterase inhibitors. *Eur. J. Pharmacol.* **2014**, *745*, 249–253. [CrossRef] [PubMed]
23. Ding, R.; Shi, J.; Pabon, K.; Scotto, K.W. Xanthines down-regulate the drug transporter ABCG2 and reverse multidrug resistance. *Mol. Pharmacol.* **2012**, *81*, 328–337. [CrossRef] [PubMed]
24. Fuhr, U.; Jetter, A.; Kirchheiner, J. Appropriate phenotyping procedures for drug metabolizing enzymes and transporters in humans and their simultaneous use in the "cocktail" approach. *Clin. Pharmacol. Ther.* **2007**, *81*, 270–283. [CrossRef] [PubMed]
25. Bilodeau, P.S.; Winistorfer, S.C.; Kearney, W.R.; Robertson, A.D.; Piper, R.C. Vps27-Hse1 and ESCRT-I complexes cooperate to increase efficiency of sorting ubiquitinated proteins at the endosome. *J. Cell Biol.* **2003**, *63*, 237–243. [CrossRef]
26. Samanta, M.P.; Liang, S. Predicting protein functions from redundancies in large-scale protein interaction networks. *Proc. Natl. Acad. Sci. USA* **2003**, *100*, 12579–12583. [CrossRef]
27. Goldar, M.M.; Nishie, T.; Ishikura, Y.; Fukuda, T.; Takegawa, K.; Kawamukai, M. Functional conservation between fission yeast *moc1/sds23* and its two orthologs, budding yeast *SDS23* and *SDS24*, and phenotypic differences in their disruptants. *Biosci. Biotechnol. Biochem.* **2005**, *69*, 1422–1426. [CrossRef]
28. Wiederkehr, A.; Meier, K.D.; Riezman, H. Identification and characterization of *Saccharomyces cerevisiae* mutants defective in fluid-phase endocytosis. *Yeast* **2001**, *18*, 759–773. [CrossRef]

29. Hood-DeGrenier, J.K. Identification of phosphatase 2A-like Sit4-mediated signalling and ubiquitin-dependent protein sorting as modulators of caffeine sensitivity in *S. cerevisiae*. *Yeast* **2011**, *28*, 189–204. [CrossRef]
30. Schmitt, M.; Schwanewilm, P.; Ludwig, J.; Lichtenberg-Fraté, H. Use of *PMA1* as a housekeeping biomarker for assessment of toxicant-induced stress in *Saccharomyces cerevisiae*. *Appl. Environ. Microbiol.* **2006**, *72*, 1515–1522. [CrossRef]
31. Sayyed, K.; Le Vée, M.; Chamieh, H.; Fardel, O.; Abdel-Razzak, Z. Cigarette smoke condensate alters *Saccharomyces cerevisiae* efflux transporter mRNA and activity and increases caffeine toxicity. *Toxicology* **2018**, *409*, 129–136. [CrossRef]
32. Candreva, E.C.; Keszenman, D.J.; Barrios, E.; Gelós, U.; Nunes, E. Mutagenicity induced by hyperthermia, hot mate infusion, and hot caffeine in *Saccharomyces cerevisiae*. *Cancer Res.* **1993**, *53*, 5750–5753. [PubMed]
33. Dubeau, H.; Chung, Y.S. Effect of caffeine on ozone-sensitivity in *Saccharomyces cerevisiae*. *Mol. Gen. Genet.* **1984**, *195*, 361–363. [CrossRef] [PubMed]
34. Ferguson, L.R. Mutagenic and recombinogenic consequences of DNA-repair inhibition during treatment with 1,3-bis(2-chloroethyl)-1-nitrosourea in *Saccharomyces cerevisiae*. *Mutat. Res.* **1990**, *241*, 369–377. [CrossRef]
35. Ferguson, L.R.; Turner, P.M.; Baguley, B.C. Induction of mitotic crossing-over by the topoisomerase II poison DACA (N-[2-dimethylamino)ethyl]acridine-4-carboxamide) in *Saccharomyces cerevisiae*. *Mutat. Res.* **1993**, *289*, 157–163. [CrossRef]
36. Fominov, G.V.; Ter-Avanesian, M.D. Caffeine sensitivity of the yeast *Saccharomyces cerevisiae MCD4* mutant is related to alteration of calcium homeostasis and degradation of misfolded proteins. *Mol. Biol. (Mosk)* **2005**, *39*, 464–476. [CrossRef]
37. Courchesne, W.E.; Ozturk, S. Amiodarone induces a caffeine-inhibited, *MID1*-depedent rise in free cytoplasmic calcium in *Saccharomyces cerevisiae*. *Mol. Microbiol.* **2003**, *47*, 223–234. [CrossRef]
38. Kihlman, B.A.; Sturelid, S.; Hartley-Asp, B.; Nilsson, K. The enhancement by caffeine of the frequencies of chromosomal aberrations induced in plant and animal cells by chemical and physical agents. *Mutat. Res.* **1974**, *26*, 105–122. [CrossRef]
39. Nunes, E.; Brum, G.; Candreva, E.C.; Schenberg Frascino, A.C. Common repair pathways acting upon U.V.- and X-ray induced damage in diploid cells of *Saccharomyces cerevisiae*. *Int. J. Radiat. Biol. Relat. Stud. Phys. Chem. Med.* **1984**, *45*, 593–606. [CrossRef]
40. Hannan, M.A.; Nasim, A. Caffeine enhancement of radiation killing in different strains of *Saccharomyces cerevisiae*. *Mol. Gen. Genet.* **1977**, *158*, 111–116. [CrossRef]
41. Siede, W.; Obermaier, S.; Eckardt, F. Influence of different inhibitors on the activity of the RAD54 dependent step of DNA repair in *Saccharomyces cerevisiae*. *Radiat. Environ. Biophys.* **1985**, *24*, 1–7. [CrossRef]
42. Haynes, R.H. DNA repair and the genetic control of radiation sensitivity in yeast. In *Molecular Mechanisms for Repair of DNA*; Part B; Hanawalt, P., Setlow, R.B., Eds.; Academic Press: New York, NY, USA, 1975; pp. 529–540.
43. Li, H.; Zeng, J.; Shen, K. PI3K/AKT/mTOR signaling pathway as a therapeutic target for ovarian cancer. *Arch. Gynecol. Obstet.* **2014**, *290*, 1067–1078. [CrossRef] [PubMed]
44. Zaborowska, D.; Zuk, J. The effect of DNA replication on mutation of the *Saccharomyces cerevisiae* CDC8 gene. *Curr. Genet.* **1990**, *17*, 275–280. [CrossRef] [PubMed]
45. Kori, M.; Aydin, B.; Arga, K. A comprehensive overview of signaling pathways and their crosstalk in human cancers. In *The Most Recent Studies in Science and Art*; Arapgirlioglu, H., Atik, A., Hızıroglu, S., Elliott, R.L., Tasxlıdere, E., Eds.; Gece Kitapligi: Ankara, Turkey, 2018; pp. 771–784.
46. Nemavarkar, P.S.; Chourasia, B.K.; Pasupathy, K. Detection of gamma-irradiation induced DNA damage and radioprotection of compounds in yeast using comet assay. *J. Radiat. Res.* **2004**, *45*, 169–174. [CrossRef] [PubMed]
47. Vaidya, P.J.; Pasupathy, K. Radioprotective action of caffeine: Use of *Saccharomyces cerevisiae* as a test system. *Indian J. Exp. Biol.* **2001**, *39*, 1254–1257.
48. Anjaria, K.B.; Rao, B.S. Effect of caffeine on the genotoxic effects of gamma radiation and 4-NQO in diploid yeast. *J. Environ. Pathol. Toxicol. Oncol.* **2001**, *20*, 39–45. [CrossRef]
49. Tsabar, M.; Eapen, V.V.; Mason, J.M.; Memisoglu, G.; Waterman, D.P.; Long, M.J.; Bishop, U.K.; Haber, S.N. Caffeine impairs resection during DNA break repair by reducing the levels of nucleases Sae2 and Dna2. *Nucleic Acids Res.* **2015**, *43*, 6889–6901. [CrossRef]

50. Ciccia, A.; Elledge, S.J. The DNA damage response: Making it safe to play with knives. *Mol. Cell* **2010**, *40*, 179–204. [CrossRef]
51. Hustedt, N.; Gasser, S.M.; Shimada, K. Replication checkpoint: Tuning and coordination of replication forks in s phase. *Genes (Basel)*. **2013**, *4*, 388–434. [CrossRef]
52. Cussiol, J.R.R.; Soares, B.L.; Oliveira, F.M.B. From yeast to humans: Understanding the biology of DNA Damage Response (DDR) kinases. *Genet. Mol. Biol.* **2019**, *43*, e20190071. [CrossRef]
53. Heffernan, T.P.; Simpson, D.A.; Frank, A.R.; Heinloth, A.N.; Paules, R.S.; Cordeiro-Stone, M.; Kaufmann, W.K. An ATR- and Chk1-dependent S checkpoint inhibits replicon initiation following UVC-induced DNA damage. *Mol. Cell Biol.* **2002**, *22*, 8552–8561. [CrossRef]
54. Barlow, J.H.; Rothstein, R. Rad52 recruitment is DNA replication independent and regulated by Cdc28 and the Mec1 kinase. *EMBO J.* **2009**, *28*, 1121–1130. [CrossRef] [PubMed]
55. Harrison, J.C.; Haber, J.E. Surviving the breakup: The DNA damage checkpoint. *Annu. Rev. Genet.* **2006**, *40*, 209–235. [CrossRef] [PubMed]
56. Sandell, L.L.; Zakian, V.A. Loss of a yeast telomere: Arrest, recovery, and chromosome loss. *Cell* **1993**, *75*, 729–739. [CrossRef]
57. Lee, S.E.; Moore, J.K.; Holmes, A.; Umezu, K.; Kolodner, R.D.; Haber, J.E. *Saccharomyces* Ku70, mre11/rad50 and RPA proteins regulate adaptation to G2/M arrest after DNA damage. *Cell* **1998**, *94*, 399–409. [CrossRef]
58. Vaze, M.B.; Pellicioli, A.; Lee, S.E.; Ira, G.; Liberi, G.; Arbel-Eden, A.; Foiani, M.; Haber, J.E. Recovery from checkpoint-mediated arrest after repair of a double-strand break requires Srs2 helicase. *Mol. Cell* **2002**, *10*, 373–385. [CrossRef]
59. Barton, A.B.; Davies, C.J.; Hutchison, C.A., 3rd; Kaback, D.B. Cloning of chromosome I DNA from *Saccharomycescerevisiae*: Analysis of the FUN52 gene, whose product has homology to protein kinases. *Gene* **1992**, *117*, 137–140. [CrossRef]
60. Schweitzer, B.; Philippsen, P. NPK1, a nonessential protein kinase gene *in Saccharomyces cerevisiae* with similarity to *Aspergillus nidulans* nimA. *Mol. Gen. Genet.* **1992**, *234*, 164–167. [CrossRef]
61. Löffler, H.; Bochtler, T.; Fritz, B.; Tews, B.; Ho, A.D.; Lukas, J.; Bartek, J.; Krämer, A. DNA damage-induced accumulation of centrosomal Chk1 contributes to its checkpoint function. *Cell Cycle* **2007**, *6*, 2541–2548. [CrossRef]
62. Moura, D.J.; Castilhos, B.; Immich, B.F.; Cañedo, A.D.; Henriques, J.A.P.; Lenz, G.; Saffi, J. Kin3 protein, a NIMA-related kinase of *Saccharomyces cerevisiae*, is involved in DNA adduct damage response. *Cell Cycle* **2010**, *9*, 2220–2229. [CrossRef]
63. Chakraverty, R.K.; Kearsey, J.M.; Oakley, T.J.; Grenon, M.; de la Torre Ruiz, M.A.; Lowndes, N.F.; Hickson, I.D. Topoisomerase III acts upstream of Rad53p in the S-phase DNA damage checkpoint. *Mol. Cell Biol.* **2001**, *21*, 7150–7162. [CrossRef]
64. Mankouri, H.W.; Hickson, I.D. Top3 processes recombination intermediates and modulates checkpoint activity after DNA damage. *Mol. Biol. Cell* **2006**, *17*, 4473–4483. [CrossRef] [PubMed]
65. Crouch, R.J. Ribonuclease H: From discovery to 3D structure. *New Biol.* **1990**, *2*, 771–777. [PubMed]
66. Hyjek, M.; Figiel, M.; Nowotny, M. RNases H: Structure and mechanism. *DNA Repair* **2019**, *84*, 102672. [CrossRef] [PubMed]
67. Arudchandran, A.; Cerritelli, S.; Narimatsu, S.; Itaya, M.; Shin, D.Y.; Shimada, Y.; Crouch, R.J. The absence of ribonuclease H1 or H2 alters the sensitivity of *Saccharomyces cerevisiae* to hydroxyurea, caffeine and ethyl methanesulphonate: Implications for roles of RNases H in DNA replication and repair. *Genes Cells* **2000**, *5*, 789–802. [CrossRef]
68. Beauchamp, E.M.; Platanias, L.C. The evolution of the TOR pathway and its role in cancer. *Oncogene* **2013**, *32*, 3923–3932. [CrossRef]
69. Saxton, R.A.; Sabatini, D.M. mTOR signaling in growth, metabolism, and disease. *Cell* **2017**, *169*, 361–371. [CrossRef]
70. Yang, J.; Nie, J.; Ma, X.; Wei, Y.; Peng, Y.; Wei, X. Targeting PI3K in cancer: Mechanisms and advances in clinical trials. *Mol. Cancer* **2019**, *18*, 26. [CrossRef]
71. Costa, R.L.B.; Han, H.S.; Gradishar, W.J. Targeting the PI3K/AKT/mTOR pathway in triple-negative breast cancer: A review. *Breast. Cancer Res. Treat.* **2018**, *169*, 397–406. [CrossRef]
72. Janku, F.; Yap, T.A.; Meric-Bernstam, F. Targeting the PI3K pathway in cancer: Are we making headway? *Nat. Rev. Clin. Oncol.* **2018**, *15*, 273–291. [CrossRef]

73. Wullschleger, S.; Loewith, R.; Hall, M.N. TOR signaling in growth and metabolism. *Cell* **2006**, *124*, 471–484. [CrossRef]
74. Mohler, K.; Mann, R.; Kyle, A.; Reynolds, N.; Ibba, M. Aminoacyl-tRNA quality control is required for efficient activation of the TOR pathway regulator Gln3p. *RNA Biol.* **2018**, *15*, 594–603. [CrossRef]
75. Corona Velazquez, A.F.; Jackson, W.T. So many roads: The multifaceted regulation of autophagy induction. *Mol. Cell Biol.* **2018**, *38*, e00303–e00318. [CrossRef] [PubMed]
76. He, C.; Zhou, C.; Kennedy, B.K. The yeast replicative aging model. *Biochim. Biophys. Acta Mol. Basis. Dis.* **2018**, *1864*, 2690–2696. [CrossRef] [PubMed]
77. Kumar, P.; Awasthi, A.; Nain, V.; Issac, B.; Puria, R. Novel insights into TOR signalling in *Saccharomyces cerevisiae* through Torin2. *Gene* **2018**, *669*, 15–27. [CrossRef] [PubMed]
78. Zhou, H.; Luo, Y.; Huang, S. Updates of mTOR inhibitors. *Anti-Cancer Agents Med. Chem.* **2010**, *10*, 571–581. [CrossRef] [PubMed]
79. Loewith, R.; Jacinto, E.; Wullschleger, S.; Lorberg, A.; Crespo, J.L.; Bonenfant, D.; Oppliger, W.; Jenoe, P.; Hall, M.N. Two TOR complexes, only one of which is rapamycin sensitive, have distinct roles in cell growth control. *Mol. Cell* **2002**, *10*, 457–468. [CrossRef]
80. Loewith, R.; Hall, M.N. Target of rapamycin (TOR) in nutrient signaling and growth control. *Genetics* **2011**, *189*, 1177–1201. [CrossRef]
81. Reinke, A.; Chen, J.C.; Aronova, S.; Powers, T. Caffeine targets TOR complex I and provides evidence for a regulatory link between the FRB and kinase domains of Tor1p. *J. Biol. Chem.* **2006**, *281*, 31616–31626. [CrossRef]
82. Dikicioglu, D.; Dereli, E.E.; Eraslan, S.; Oliver, S.G.; Kirdar, B. *Saccharomyces cerevisiae* adapted to grow in the presence of low-dose rapamycin exhibit altered amino acid metabolism. *Cell Commun. Signal.* **2018**, *16*, 85. [CrossRef]
83. Rallis, C.; Codlin, S.; Bähler, J. TORC1 signaling inhibition by rapamycin and caffeine affect lifespan, global gene expression, and cell proliferation of fission yeast. *Aging Cell* **2013**, *12*, 563–573. [CrossRef]
84. Scott, P.H.; Lawrence, J.C., Jr. Attenuation of mammalian target of rapamycin activity by increased cAMP in 3T3-L1 adipocytes. *J. Biol. Chem.* **1998**, *273*, 34496–34501. [CrossRef] [PubMed]
85. Lee, M.B.; Carr, D.T.; Kiflezghi, M.G.; Zhao, Y.T.; Kim, D.B.; Thon, S.; Moore, M.D.; Li, M.A.K.; Kaeberlein, M. A system to identify inhibitors of mTOR signaling using high-resolution growth analysis in *Saccharomyces cerevisiae*. *Geroscience* **2017**, *39*, 419–428. [CrossRef] [PubMed]
86. Evans, S.K.; Burgess, K.E.; Gray, J.V. Recovery from rapamycin: Drug-insensitive activity of yeast target of rapamycin complex 1 (TORC1) supports residual proliferation that dilutes rapamycin among progeny cells. *J. Biol. Chem.* **2014**, *289*, 26554–26565. [CrossRef] [PubMed]
87. Wanke, V.; Cameroni, E.; Uotila, A.; Piccolis, M.; Urban, J.; Loewith, R.; De Virgilio, C. Caffeine extends yeast lifespan by targeting TORC1. *Mol. MicroBiol.* **2008**, *69*, 277–285. [CrossRef]
88. Heitman, J.; Movva, N.R.; Hall, M.N. Targets for cell cycle arrest by the immunosuppressant rapamycin in yeast. *Science* **1991**, *253*, 905–909. [CrossRef]
89. Lorenz, M.C.; Heitman, J. TOR mutations confer rapamycin resistance by preventing interaction with FKBP12-rapamycin. *J. Biol. Chem.* **1995**, *270*, 27531–27537. [CrossRef]
90. Kingsbury, J.M.; Cardenas, M.E. Vesicular trafficking systems impact TORC1-controlled transcriptional programs in *Saccharomyces cerevisiae*. *G3 (Bethesda)* **2016**, *6*, 641–652. [CrossRef]
91. Shamji, A.F.; Kuruvilla, F.G.; Schreiber, S.L. Partitioning the transcriptional program induced by rapamycin among the effectors of the Tor proteins. *Curr. Biol.* **2000**, *10*, 1574–1581. [CrossRef]
92. Komeili, A.; Wedaman, K.P.; O'Shea, E.K.; Powers, T. Mechanism of metabolic control: Target of rapamycin signaling links nitrogen quality to the activity of the Rtg1 and Rtg3 transcription factors. *J. Cell Biol.* **2000**, *151*, 863–878. [CrossRef]
93. Cooper, T.G. Transmitting the signal of excess nitrogen in *Saccharomyces cerevisiae* from the Tor proteins to the GATA factors: Connecting the dots. *FEMS Microbiol. Rev.* **2002**, *26*, 223–238. [CrossRef]
94. Conrad, M.; Schothorst, J.; Kankipati, H.N.; Van Zeebroeck, G.; Rubio-Texeira, M.; Thevelein, J.M. Nutrient sensing and signaling in the yeast *Saccharomyces cerevisiae*. *FEMS Microbiol. Rev.* **2014**, *38*, 254–299. [CrossRef] [PubMed]

95. Numamoto, M.; Tagami, S.; Ueda, Y.; Imabeppu, Y.; Sasano, Y.; Sugiyama, M.; Maekawa, H.; Harashima, S. Nuclear localization domains of GATA activator Gln3 are required for transcription of target genes through dephosphorylation in *Saccharomyces cerevisiae*. *J. Biosci. Bioeng.* **2015**, *120*, 121–127. [CrossRef] [PubMed]
96. Narumiya, S.; Thumkeo, D. Rho signaling research: History, current status and future directions. *FEBS Lett.* **2018**, *592*, 1763–1776. [CrossRef] [PubMed]
97. Lawson, C.D.; Ridley, A.J. Rho GTPase signaling complexes in cell migration and invasion. *J. Cell Biol.* **2018**, *217*, 447–457. [CrossRef]
98. Guan, X.; Guan, X.; Dong, C.; Jiao, Z. Rho GTPases and related signaling complexes in cell migration and invasion. *Exp. Cell Res.* **2020**, *388*, 111824. [CrossRef]
99. Delley, P.A.; Hall, M.N. Cell wall stress depolarizes cell growth via hyperactivation of RHO1. *J. Cell Biol.* **1999**, *147*, 163–174. [CrossRef]
100. Yan, G.; Lai, Y.; Jiang, Y. The TOR complex 1 is a direct target of Rho1 GTPase. *Mol. Cell* **2012**, *45*, 743–753. [CrossRef]
101. Zhu, M.; Wang, X.Q. Regulation of mTORC1 by small GTPases in response to nutrients. *J. Nutr.* **2020**, *150*, 1004–1011. [CrossRef]
102. Schmitz, H.P.; Huppert, S.; Lorberg, A.; Heinisch, J.J. Rho5p downregulates the yeast cell integrity pathway. *J. Cell Sci.* **2002**, *115*, 3139–3148.
103. Philip, B.; Levin, D.E. Wsc1 and Mid2 are cell surface sensors for cell wall integrity signaling that act through Rom2, a guanine nucleotide exchange factor for Rho1. *Mol. Cell Biol.* **2001**, *21*, 271–280. [CrossRef]
104. Guo, S.; Shen, X.; Yan, G.; Ma, D.; Bai, X.; Li, S.; Jiang, Y. A MAP kinase dependent feedback mechanism controls Rho1 GTPase and actin distribution in yeast. *PLoS ONE* **2009**, *4*, e6089. [CrossRef]
105. Yan, G.; Lai, Y.; Jiang, Y. TOR under stress: Targeting TORC1 by Rho1 GTPase. *Cell Cycle* **2012**, *11*, 3384–3388. [CrossRef] [PubMed]
106. Hirasaki, M.; Horiguchi, M.; Numamoto, M.; Sugiyama, M.; Kaneko, Y.; Nogi, Y.; Harashima, S. *Saccharomyces cerevisiae* protein phosphatase Ppz1 and protein kinases Sat4 and Hal5 are involved in the control of subcellular localization of Gln3 by likely regulating its phosphorylation state. *J. Biosci. Bioeng.* **2011**, *111*, 249–254. [CrossRef] [PubMed]
107. Tzima, E. Role of small GTPases in endothelial cytoskeletal dynamics and the shear stress response. *Circ. Res.* **2006**, *98*, 176–185. [CrossRef] [PubMed]
108. Nakashima, N.; Noguchi, E.; Nishimoto, T. *Saccharomyces cerevisiae* putative G protein, Gtr1p, which forms complexes with itself and a novel protein designated as Gtr2p, negatively regulates the Ran/Gsp1p G protein cycle through Gtr2p. *Genetics* **1999**, *152*, 853–867.
109. Bourne, H.R.; Sanders, D.A.; McCormick, F. The GTPase superfamily: A conserved switch for diverse cell functions. *Nature* **1990**, *348*, 125–132. [CrossRef]
110. Wang, Y.; Kurihara, Y.; Sato, T.; Toh, H.; Kobayashi, H.; Sekiguchi, T. Gtr1p differentially associates with Gtr2p and Ego1p. *Gene* **2009**, *437*, 32–38. [CrossRef]
111. Huang, J.; Zhu, H.; Haggarty, S.J.; Spring, D.R.; Hwang, H.; Jin, F.; Snyder, M.; Schreiber, S.L. Finding new components of the target of rapamycin (TOR) signaling network through chemical genetics and proteome chips. *Proc. Natl. Acad. Sci. USA* **2004**, *101*, 16594–16599. [CrossRef]
112. Gao, M.; Kaiser, C.A. A conserved GTPase-containing complex is required for intracellular sorting of the general amino-acid permease in yeast. *Nat. Cell Biol.* **2006**, *8*, 657–667. [CrossRef]
113. Dereli, E.E.; Arga, K.Y.; Dikicioglu, D.; Eraslan, S.; Erkol, E.; Celik, A.; Kirdar, B.; Di Camillo, B. Identification of novel components of target-of-rapamycin signaling pathway by network-based multi-omics integrative analysis. *OMICS* **2019**, *23*, 274–284. [CrossRef]
114. González, A.; Ruiz, A.; Casamayor, A.; Ariño, J. Normal function of the yeast TOR pathway requires the type 2C protein phosphatase Ptc1. *Mol. Cell Biol.* **2009**, *29*, 2876–2888. [CrossRef] [PubMed]
115. Zaborske, J.M.; Wu, X.; Wek, R.C.; Pan, T. Selective control of amino acid metabolism by the GCN2 eIF2 kinase pathway in *Saccharomyces cerevisiae*. *BMC Biochem.* **2010**, *11*, 29. [CrossRef] [PubMed]
116. White, J.T.; Cato, T.; Deramchi, N.; Gabunilas, J.; Roy, K.R.; Wang, C.; Chanfreau, G.F.; Clarke, S.G. Protein methylation and translation: Role of lysine modification on the function of yeast elongation factor 1A. *Biochemistry* **2019**, *58*, 4997–5010. [CrossRef] [PubMed]
117. Martínez-Muñoz, G.A.; Kane, P. Vacuolar and plasma membrane proton pumps collaborate to achieve cytosolic pH homeostasis in yeast. *J. Biol. Chem.* **2008**, *283*, 20309–20319. [CrossRef] [PubMed]

118. Banuelos, M.G.; Moreno, D.E.; Olson, D.K.; Nguyen, Q.; Ricarte, F.; Aguilera-Sandoval, C.R.; Gharakhanian, E. Genomic analysis of severe hypersensitivity to hygromycin B reveals linkage to vacuolar defects and new vacuolar gene functions in *Saccharomyces cerevisiae*. *Curr. Genet.* **2010**, *56*, 121–137. [CrossRef] [PubMed]
119. Lum, P.Y.; Armour, C.D.; Stepaniants, S.B.; Cavet, G.; Wolf, M.K.; Butler, J.S.; Hinshaw, J.C.; Garnier, P.; Prestwich, G.D.; Leonardson, A.; et al. Discovering modes of action for therapeutic compounds using a genome-wide screen of yeast heterozygotes. *Cell* **2004**, *116*, 121–137. [CrossRef]
120. Moser, B.A.; Brondello, J.M.; Baber-Furnari, B.; Russell, P. Mechanism of caffeine-induced checkpoint override in fission yeast. *Mol. Cell Biol.* **2000**, *20*, 4288–4294. [CrossRef]
121. Cid, V.J.; Durán, A.; del Rey, F.; Snyder, M.P.; Nombela, C.; Sánchez, M. Molecular basis of cell integrity and morphogenesis in *Saccharomyces cerevisiae*. *Microbiol. Rev.* **1995**, *59*, 345–386. [CrossRef]
122. Vicente, M.F.; Basilio, A.; Cabello, A.; Peláez, F. Microbial natural products as a source of antifungals. *Clin. Microbiol. Infect.* **2003**, *9*, 15–32. [CrossRef]
123. Levin, D.E. Cell wall integrity signaling in *Saccharomyces cerevisiae*. *Microbiol. Mol. Biol. Rev.* **2005**, *69*, 262–291. [CrossRef]
124. Truman, A.W.; Kim, K.Y.; Levin, D.E. Mechanism of Mpk1 mitogen-activated protein kinase binding to the Swi4 transcription factor and its regulation by a novel caffeine-induced phosphorylation. *Mol. Cell Biol.* **2009**, *29*, 6449–6461. [CrossRef] [PubMed]
125. Wang, K.; Vavassori, S.; Schweizer, L.M.; Schweizer, M. Impaired PRPP-synthesizing capacity compromises cell integrity signalling in *Saccharomyces cerevisiae*. *Microbiology* **2004**, *150*, 3327–3339. [CrossRef] [PubMed]
126. Ugbogu, E.A.; Wippler, S.; Euston, M.; Kouwenhoven, E.N.; de Brouwer, A.P.M.; Schweizer, L.M.; Schweizer, M. The contribution of the nonhomologous region of Prs1 to the maintenance of cell wall integrity and cell viability. *FEMS Yeast Res.* **2013**, *13*, 291–301. [CrossRef]
127. Sipling, T.; Zhai, C.; Panaretou, B. Emw1p/YNL313cp is essential for maintenance of the cell wall in *Saccharomyces cerevisiae*. *Microbiology* **2011**, *157*, 1032–1041. [CrossRef]
128. Castrejon, F.; Gomez, A.; Sanz, M.; Duran, A.; Roncero, C. The RIM101 pathway contributes to yeast cell wall assembly and its function becomes essential in the absence of mitogen-activated protein kinase Slt2p. *Eukaryot. Cell* **2006**, *5*, 507–517. [CrossRef] [PubMed]
129. Zolnierowicz, S.; Bollen, M. Protein phosphorylation and protein phosphatases. *EMBO J.* **2000**, *19*, 483–488. [CrossRef]
130. Sakumoto, N.; Mukai, Y.; Uchida, K.; Kouchi, T.; Kuwajima, J.; Nakagawa, Y.; Sugioka, S.; Yamamoto, E.; Furuyama, T.; Mizubuchi, H.; et al. A series of protein phosphatase gene disruptants in *Saccharomyces cerevisiae*. *Yeast* **1999**, *15*, 1669–1679. [CrossRef]
131. Yenush, L.; Merchan, S.; Holmes, J.; Serrano, R. pH-Responsive, posttranslational regulation of the Trk1 potassium transporter by the type 1-related Ppz1 phosphatase. *Mol. Cell Biol.* **2005**, *25*, 8683–8692. [CrossRef]
132. Wharton, R.P.; Aggarwal, A.K. mRNA regulation by Puf domain proteins. *Sci. STKE* **2006**, *2006*, pe37. [CrossRef]
133. Traven, A.; Lo, T.L.; Lithgow, T.; Heierhorst, J. The yeast PUF protein Puf5 has Pop2-independent roles in response to DNA replication stress. *PLoS ONE* **2010**, *5*, e10651. [CrossRef]
134. Saiardi, A.; Caffrey, J.J.; Snyder, S.H.; Shears, S.B. The inositol hexakisphosphate kinase family. Catalytic flexibility and function in yeast vacuole biogenesis. *J. Biol. Chem.* **2000**, *275*, 24686–24692. [CrossRef] [PubMed]
135. Dubois, E.; Scherens, B.; Vierendeels, F.; Ho, M.M.; Messenguy, F.; Shears, S.B. In *Saccharomyces cerevisiae*, the inositol polyphosphate kinase activity of Kcs1p is required for resistance to salt stress, cell wall integrity, and vacuolar morphogenesis. *J. Biol. Chem.* **2002**, *277*, 23755–23763. [CrossRef] [PubMed]
136. Saiardi, A.; Bhandari, R.; Resnick, A.C.; Snowman, A.M.; Snyder, S.H. Phosphorylation of proteins by inositol pyrophosphates. *Science* **2004**, *306*, 2101–2105. [CrossRef] [PubMed]
137. Saiardi, A.; Resnick, A.C.; Snowman, A.M.; Wendland, B.; Snyder, S.H. Inositol pyrophosphates regulate cell death and telomere length through phosphoinositide 3-kinase-related protein kinases. *Proc. Natl. Acad. Sci. USA* **2005**, *102*, 1911–1914. [CrossRef]
138. Gallegos, S.; Pacheco, C.; Peters, C.; Opazo, C.M.; Aguayo, L.G. Features of alpha-synuclein that could explain the progression and irreversibility of Parkinson's disease. *Front. Neurosci.* **2015**, *9*, 59. [CrossRef]
139. Kardani, J.; Roy, I. Understanding caffeine's role in attenuating the toxicity of α-synuclein aggregates: Implications for risk of Parkinson's disease. *ACS Chem. Neurosci.* **2015**, *6*, 1613–1625. [CrossRef]

140. Hong, C.T.; Chan, L.; Bai, C.-H. The Effect of caffeine on the risk and progression of Parkinson's Disease: A meta-analysis. *Nutrients* **2020**, *12*, 1860. [CrossRef]
141. Tsuzuki, J.; Newburgh, R.W. Inhibition of 5′-nucleotidase in rat brain by methylxanthines. *J. Neurochem.* **1975**, *25*, 895–896. [CrossRef]
142. Liao, H.H.; Thorner, J. Adenosine 3′,5′-phosphate phosphodiesterase and pheromone response in the yeast *Saccharomyces cerevisiae*. *J. Bacteriol.* **1981**, *148*, 919–925. [CrossRef]
143. Tsuboi, M.; Yanagishima, N. Effect of cyclic AMP, theophylline and caffeine on the glucose repression of sporulation in *Saccharomyces cerevisiae*. *Arch. MikroBiol.* **1973**, *93*, 1–12. [CrossRef]
144. Tortora, P.; Burlini, N.; Hanozet, G.M.; Guerritore, A. Effect of caffeine on glucose-induced inactivation of gluconeogenetic enzymes in *Saccharomyces cerevisiae*. A possible role of cyclic AMP. *Eur. J. Biochem.* **1982**, *126*, 617–622. [CrossRef]
145. Sarinová, M.; Tichá, E.; Obernauerová, M.; Gbelská, Y. Impact of mitochondrial function on yeast susceptibility to antifungal compounds. *Folia Microbiol. (Praha)* **2007**, *52*, 223–229. [CrossRef] [PubMed]
146. Harrison, D.E.; Strong, R.; Sharp, Z.D.; Nelson, J.F.; Astle, C.M.; Flurkey, K.; Nadon, N.L.; Wilkinson, J.E.; Frenkel, K.; Carter, C.S.; et al. Rapamycin fed late in life extends lifespan in genetically heterogeneous mice. *Nature* **2009**, *460*, 392–395. [CrossRef] [PubMed]
147. Powers, R.W., 3rd; Kaeberlein, M.; Caldwell, S.D.; Kennedy, B.K.; Fields, S. Extension of chronological life span in yeast by decreased TOR pathway signaling. *Genes Dev.* **2006**, *20*, 174–184. [CrossRef] [PubMed]
148. Baiges, I.; Arola, L. COCOA (Theobroma cacao) Polyphenol-rich extract increases the chronological lifespan of *Saccharomyces cerevisiae*. *J. Frailty Aging* **2016**, *5*, 186–190. [PubMed]
149. Rockenfeller, P.; Madeo, F. Ageing and eating. *Biochim. Biophys. Acta* **2010**, *1803*, 499–506. [CrossRef]
150. Longo, V.D.; Shadel, G.S.; Kaeberlein, M.; Kennedy, B. Replicative and chronological aging in *Saccharomyces cerevisiae*. *Cell Metab.* **2012**, *16*, 18–31. [CrossRef]
151. Fabrizio, P.; Pozza, F.; Pletcher, S.D.; Gendron, C.M.; Longo, V.D. Regulation of longevity and stress resistance by Sch9 in yeast. *Science* **2001**, *292*, 288–290. [CrossRef]
152. Bridi, J.C.; Barros, A.G.; Sampaio, L.R.; Ferreira, J.C.; Antunes Soares, F.; Romano-Silva, M.A. Lifespan extension induced by caffeine in *Caenorhabditis elegans* is partially dependent on adenosine signaling. *Front. Aging Neurosci.* **2015**, *7*, 220. [CrossRef]
153. Sutphin, G.L.; Bishop, E.; Yanos, M.E.; Moller, R.M.; Kaeberlein, M. Caffeine extends life span, improves healthspan, and delays age-associated pathology in *Caenorhabditis elegans*. *Longev. Healthspan* **2012**, *1*, 9. [CrossRef]
154. Loftfield, E.; Freedman, N.D.; Graubard, B.I.; Guertin, K.A.; Black, A.; Huang, W.-Y.; Shebl, F.M.; Mayne, S.T.; Sinha, R. Association of coffee consumption with overall and cause-specific mortality in a large US prospective cohort study. *Am. J. Epidemiol.* **2015**, *182*, 1010–1022. [CrossRef] [PubMed]
155. Fortes, C.; Forastiere, F.; Farchi, S.; Rapiti, E.; Pastori, G.; Perucci, C.A. Diet and overall survival in a cohort of very elderly people. *Epidemiology* **2000**, *11*, 440–445. [CrossRef]
156. Paganini-Hill, A.; Kawas, C.H.; Corrada, M.M. Non-alcoholic beverage and caffeine consumption and mortality: The leisure world cohort study. *Prev. Med.* **2007**, *44*, 305–310. [CrossRef] [PubMed]
157. Choi, K.M.; Lee, H.L.; Kwon, Y.Y.; Kang, M.S.; Lee, S.K.; Lee, C.K. Enhancement of mitochondrial function correlates with the extension of lifespan by caloric restriction and caloric restriction mimetics in yeast. *Biochem. Biophys. Res. Commun.* **2013**, *441*, 236–242. [CrossRef]
158. Nagai, S. Stabilizing effect of caffeine on a respirationally unstable strain of yeast. *Exp. Cell Res.* **1962**, *26*, 253–259. [CrossRef]
159. Pongpanich, M.; Patchsung, M.; Mutirangura, A. Pathologic replication-independent endogenous DNA double-strand breaks repair defect in chronological aging yeast. *Front. Genet.* **2018**, *9*, 501. [CrossRef] [PubMed]
160. Thongsroy, J.; Patchsung, M.; Pongpanich, M.; Settayanon, S.; Mutirangura, A. Reduction in replication-independent endogenous DNA double-strand breaks promotes genomic instability during chronological aging in yeast. *FASEB J.* **2018**, fj201800218RR. [CrossRef] [PubMed]
161. Hoeijmakers, J.H. DNA damage, aging, and cancer. *N. Engl. J. Med.* **2009**, *361*, 1475–1485. [CrossRef]

162. Thongsroy, J.; Matangkasombut, O.; Thongnak, A.; Rattanatanyong, P.; Jirawatnotai, S.; Mutirangura, A. Replication-independent endogenous DNA double-strand breaks in *Saccharomyces cerevisiae* model. *PLoS ONE* **2013**, *8*, e72706. [CrossRef]
163. Kolb, H.; Kempf, K.; Martin, S. Health effects of eoffee: Mechanism unraveled? *Nutrients* **2020**, *12*, 1842. [CrossRef]

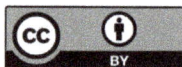

© 2020 by the authors. Licensee MDPI, Basel, Switzerland. This article is an open access article distributed under the terms and conditions of the Creative Commons Attribution (CC BY) license (http://creativecommons.org/licenses/by/4.0/).

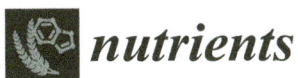

Review

Health Effects of Coffee: Mechanism Unraveled?

Hubert Kolb [1,2], Kerstin Kempf [2,*] and Stephan Martin [1,2]

1. Faculty of Medicine, University of Duesseldorf, Moorenstr. 5, 40225 Duesseldorf, Germany; hubert.kolb@hhu.de (H.K.); stephan.martin@uni-duesseldorf.de (S.M.)
2. West-German Centre of Diabetes and Health, Duesseldorf Catholic Hospital Group, Hohensandweg 37, 40591 Duesseldorf, Germany
* Correspondence: kerstin.kempf@wdgz.de; Tel.: +49-211-56-60-360-16

Received: 25 May 2020; Accepted: 18 June 2020; Published: 20 June 2020

Abstract: The association of habitual coffee consumption with a lower risk of diseases, like type 2 diabetes mellitus, chronic liver disease, certain cancer types, or with reduced all-cause mortality, has been confirmed in prospective cohort studies in many regions of the world. The molecular mechanism is still unresolved. The radical-scavenging and anti-inflammatory activity of coffee constituents is too weak to account for such effects. We argue here that coffee as a plant food has similar beneficial properties to many vegetables and fruits. Recent studies have identified a health promoting mechanism common to coffee, vegetables and fruits, i.e., the activation of an adaptive cellular response characterized by the upregulation of proteins involved in cell protection, notably antioxidant, detoxifying and repair enzymes. Key to this response is the activation of the Nrf2 (Nuclear factor erythroid 2-related factor-2) system by phenolic phytochemicals, which induces the expression of cell defense genes. Coffee plays a dominant role in that regard because it is the major dietary source of phenolic acids and polyphenols in the developed world. A possible supportive action may be the modulation of the gut microbiota by non-digested prebiotic constituents of coffee, but the available data are still scarce. We conclude that coffee employs similar pathways of promoting health as assumed for other vegetables and fruits. Coffee beans may be viewed as healthy vegetable food and a main supplier of dietary phenolic phytochemicals.

Keywords: coffee; phytochemicals; caffeine; diabetes; DNA damage; antioxidant; Nrf2; microbiota

1. Introduction

In recent years, numerous meta-analyses have come up with positive health outcomes associated with habitual coffee consumption in the general population, and this has changed the perception of coffee from that of a luxury stimulant drink to that of a health promoting beverage, if consumed within usual levels of intake. Positive health outcomes include lower incidences of type 2 diabetes mellitus, kidney stones, Parkinson's disease, gout, liver fibrosis, non-alcoholic fatty liver disease, liver cirrhosis, liver cancer and of chronic liver disease. This is the conclusion of an umbrella review of meta-analyses of multiple health outcomes, even after extensive correction for a large number of possible confounding factors [1], and also the result of the EPIC (European Prospective Investigation into Cancer and Nutrition Study) trial analyzing coffee consumption versus mortality [2]. Consumption of decaffeinated coffee was associated with similar beneficial outcomes, but only if data of large cohorts were available [3–5]. The molecular mechanism responsible for these putative health effects is still unresolved.

Epidemiological studies cannot prove causality, but it is remarkable that assumed health effects such as a lower risk of type 2 diabetes are seen at a global level, in different regions with different cultures and lifestyle. Moreover, a dose-response relationship between number of cups of coffee consumed per day and diabetes risk was observed, which is difficult to explain by an overlooked lifestyle factor [6].

However, it should not be ignored that heavy consumption of coffee may have a genetic basis, and that the latter accounts for better health outcomes. Drinking several cups of coffee per day would only be a marker of a favorable genetic background. Genome-wide association studies have identified an impact of several gene polymorphisms on caffeine or coffee intake [7–9]. Caffeine seems to be relevant for most genes identified, notably the gene CYP1A2 (cytochrome P450 isozyme 1A2) which is involved in the hepatic metabolism of caffeine. Carriers of the C variant at position 163 express less CYP1A2 and therefore metabolize caffeine more slowly than persons homozygous for the A allele [10]. Faster breakdown of caffeine is associated with more caffeine or coffee consumption.

Mendelian randomization studies made use of the finding that some genotypes are associated with increased coffee consumption. Nonetheless, there were no consistent associations of the genotype for faster caffeine metabolism (and more caffeine/coffee consumption) with positive health outcomes [11]. In spite of this, these findings do not invalidate the association of coffee consumption with health effects for several reasons. The difference between the high and low caffeine consumption genotypes of CYP1A2 is about 40 mg of caffeine, i.e., less than half a cup of coffee [7]. Habitual coffee consumption ranges from about 1 to more than 5 cups per day, which indicates that the daily dose is defined by something other than genetic reasons. Epidemiological studies find significant associations for cohorts that differ by consumption of 2 or more cups of coffee [1]. Among persons with the same CYP1A2 genotype, those drinking more coffee show better health outcomes, such as concerning Parkinson's disease or breast cancer [12,13]. Changes in coffee consumption were accompanied by a parallel change of health risk, i.e., type 2 diabetes. This argues against a major influence of genetic characteristics as well [14].

An epidemiological study of nearly 500,000 participants of the United Kingdom Biobank finds associations between the number of cups of coffee consumed per day and decreased all-cause mortality, regardless of genetic caffeine metabolism score, i.e., the circadian level of caffeine in circulation [15]. Caffeine also does not appear to account for the lower risk of type 2 diabetes with habitual coffee consumption, since this is also seen in association with drinking decaffeinated coffee. Impairment of glucose tolerance is observed after consumption of caffeinated, but not decaffeinated coffee, suggesting that other phytochemicals in coffee outweigh possible detrimental effects of caffeine. It has been suggested that polyphenols and other bioactives in decaffeinated coffee mediate these health effects [16].

We conclude that the possible mechanism of coffee-mediated health effects does not include a major role of caffeine actions (Figure 1). An important health promoting role of vitamins and minerals in the coffee brew seems improbable because, on average, there is no deficient intake in the developed world. Health effects therefore appear to be associated with other prominent constituents of the coffee brew. These include chlorogenic acids, trigonelline, N-methylpyridinium, the diterpenes kahweol and cafestol, polysaccharides, peptides and melanoidins. For several of these components, radical scavenging or anti-inflammatory activity has been postulated. We argue here that such hypotheses do not fit with the available data. Rather, beneficial effects of coffee probably employ the same pathway as recently suggested for "healthy" vegetables or fruits, i.e., the induction of a health promoting adaptive response of cells in the body. Additionally, non-digestible components of coffee may modulate the composition and function of the microbiota, as is known for other plant foods.

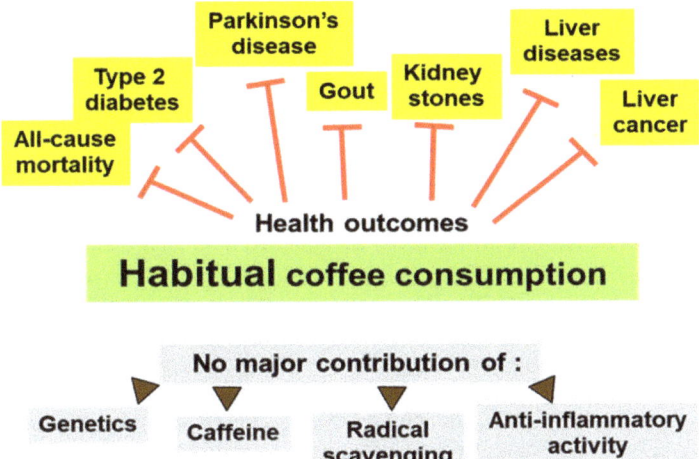

Figure 1. Health outcomes of coffee consumption. Prospective epidemiological studies consistently found a lower risk of several clinical outcomes and of all-cause mortality for habitual coffee consumption [1,2]. Most of these associations cannot be accounted for by genetic polymorphisms promoting coffee/caffeine consumption, by the caffeine content of coffee, or by its content of radical scavenging or anti-inflammatory constituents. Health effects of decaffeinated coffee could only be determined if sufficiently large cohorts were available for study. Otherwise, positive trends did not reach statistical significance, such as for Parkinson's disease.

2. Inefficient Radical Scavenging by Coffee Constituents

Several phenolic components of the coffee brew exhibit radical scavenging properties, which increase in quantity during roasting [17,18]. Although radical scavenging by ingested coffee components is still a quite common belief, there is ample evidence from animal and human studies showing that the concentrations of coffee constituents reached in plasma are too low for efficient radical scavenging. After consumption of coffee, peak plasma concentrations of phenolic metabolites range between 0.01 and 6 µmol/L, and caffeine concentrations may reach 30 µmol/L [19]. These values compare well with peak flavonoid concentrations seen in human plasma after consumption of 100 g of fruits and vegetables, which range between 0.03 µmol/L for apples and 5.9 µmol/L for cocoa [20]. Such concentrations are well below levels of endogenous antioxidant systems such as urate (160–450 µmol/L), ascorbate (30–150 µmol/L), α-tocopherol (15–40 µmol/L), glutamine (~500 µmol/L) or glutathione (>1 mmol/L in cells) [20–22]. In addition, the major coffee constituents caffeoylquinic acids, trigonelline and caffeine are weak antioxidants (one-electron reduction potential) in comparison to vitamins C or E, or glutathione (reviewed in Reference [23]), and thus cannot effectively reduce/regenerate oxidized forms of antioxidant vitamins or glutathione. Thus, radical scavenging by coffee components in vivo is limited and probably contributes little to the health effects of coffee (Figure 1). As discussed below, there is an antioxidative effect of coffee consumption because of the induction of endogenous radical scavenging enzymes.

3. Weak Anti-Inflammatory Action of Coffee

Cross-sectional studies of the level of circulating immune or inflammatory markers have reported small and not consistent variations in relation to habitual coffee consumption [24,25]. Randomized controlled trials of several weeks of coffee consumption in comparison to a water control were also performed and small reductions of some immune/inflammatory mediator concentrations were found, but the opposite was also reported [26–30]. Medium, but not dark roast coffee consumption increased the level of adiponectin [31]. A modulatory effect of habitual coffee consumption on the risk of an inflammatory disease, rheumatoid arthritis, was not observed [1,32]. Taken together, there may be a mild favorable anti-inflammatory response of the immune system to coffee consumption, but possible effects do not appear to reach clinical significance (Figure 1).

4. Phenolic Phytochemicals in Coffee May Account for Health Effects

Besides caffeine, major constituents of coffee are of a phenolic nature. These include roasting-induced degradation products of chlorogenic acids (caffeoylquinic acids), trigonelline and its roasting product, N-methylpyridinium. Melanoidins are also major components, these are roasting-dependent Maillard reaction products of carbohydrate residues with amino acids or protein side chains.

Coffee is entirely of plant origin. Thus, it is conceivable that its consumption causes similar health promoting responses in the human organism as described for many other plant foods. Virtually all plant-derived foods contain health promoting phytochemicals, and most of them are of a phenolic nature [33,34]. At present, there is no reason to assume that phenolic compounds of coffee are less "healthy" than comparable phytochemicals of tea, vegetables or fruits. However, coffee sticks out in one important regard: in habitual coffee drinkers, coffee is the primary dietary source of phytochemicals like phenolic acids and polyphenols, even in comparison to green tea in Japan [35–39]. At the level of populations, coffee provides around 40% of polyphenols and around 70% of phenolic acids consumed, followed by tea as the second major source.

We therefore propose that coffee employs similar molecular pathways for improving health as described for other plant foods such as broccoli, beetroot, berries, pomegranate, curcuma, cocoa and many others. Surprisingly, there seems to be one uniform response of cells when exposed to phenolic phytochemicals or their metabolites at concentrations observed in vivo after a meal, despite major differences in chemical structure of phenolic compounds. The cellular response is characterized by an increased expression of a large number of genes involved in antioxidative, detoxifying or repair mechanisms, this is also observed in vivo [40]. The molecular pathway involves the translocation of nuclear factor erythroid 2–related factor 2 (Nrf2) from cytosol to the nucleus, formation of heterodimers with small musculoaponeurotic fibrosarcoma (sMaf) proteins and binding to consensus DNA sequences, referred to as antioxidant response elements (ARE), electrophile response elements and more recently as cap'n'collar (CNC)-sMaf binding elements [41]. The response elements are present in the 5′-upstream region of several hundred cytoprotective genes, and binding of Nrf2/sMaf gives rise to increased gene expression of proteins involved in cell defense. These include antioxidant enzymes such as superoxide dismutase, catalase, glutathione peroxidase, glutamate-cysteine ligase and xenobiotic detoxifying enzymes, including nicotinamide adenine dinucleotide phosphate (NAD(P)H):quinone oxidoreductase-1, uridine 5′-diphospho (UDP)-glucuronosyltransferases or heme oxygenase-1 [42]. Decreased gene expression is seen for pro-inflammatory mediators like tumor necrosis factor-α or the NLRP3 (NOD-like receptor family, pyrin domain containing 3) inflammasome. Activation of Nrf2 is also required for the induction of mitochondrial biogenesis and antioxidant response. Furthermore, there is a regulation of substrate supply to mitochondria by Nrf2 [43–45] (Figure 2).

Under steady physiological conditions, the majority of newly synthesized Nrf2 is captured by the repressor protein Kelch-like ECH-associated protein 1 (Keap1) and channeled to proteasomal degradation via ubiquitylation by Cullin 3-based E3 ubiquitin ligase (Cul3). Keap1 is the main cellular sensor for stress molecules due to expression of 17 cysteine residues which are targets for modification by radical oxygen species (ROS), ROS-modified fatty acids or cyclic nucleotides, nitric oxide (NO) or other electrophiles [46]. Any modification suppresses the ability of Keap1 to transfer Nrf2 to proteasomes, which prevents Keap1 from capturing new Nrf2 molecules so that newly synthesized Nrf2 can translocate to the nucleus [47]. Phytochemicals may either directly target cysteines of Keap1, such as sulforaphane, or modify cell functions, resulting in oxidative stress and subsequent inactivation of Keap1. The interaction of different electrophiles with Keap1 leads to different patterns of modified cysteine residues, and to the activation of different patterns of cytoprotective genes, which may in part explain the different responses of cells to different phytochemicals [46].

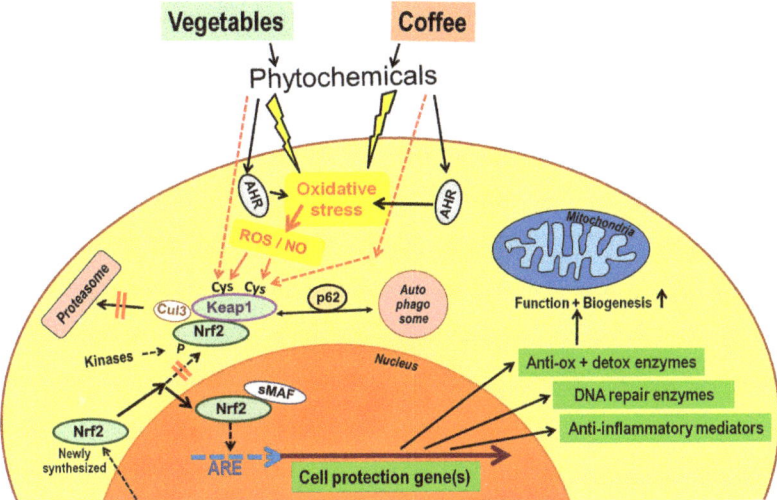

Figure 2. Phytochemicals activate the nuclear factor erythroid 2-related factor 2 (Nrf2) pathway. Exposure of cells to phenolics of vegetables or coffee leads to cell stress, including oxidative stress via mostly unknown pathways, except for some involvement of the aryl hydrocarbon receptor (AHR). Major sources of radical oxygen species (ROS) during oxidative stress are the mitochondrial respiratory chain and nicotinamide adenine dinucleotide phosphate (NADPH) oxidases of the NOX family. The nuclear factor Nrf2 is usually bound to Keap1 and the Cullin 3-based E3 ubiquitin ligase (Cul3), which is followed by transport to the proteasome for degradation. This process can be blocked by modification of one or more cysteine residues of Kelch-like ECH-associated protein 1 (Keap1) by ROS, ROS-modified fatty acids or cyclic nucleotides, by nitric oxide (NO), or by direct action of phytochemical electrophiles. The protein p62 blocks binding of Nrf2 to Keap1 and channels Keap1 to autophagic destruction. Several kinases, such as members of the Src family, can phosphorylate Nrf2 and may also interfere with routing to proteasomes. All these mechanisms prevent newly formed Nrf2 from being captured by Keap1, so that translocation to the nucleus is possible. In the nucleus, Nrf2 binds to small musculoaponeurotic fibrosarcoma (sMaf) protein, and the heterodimer interacts with the antioxidant response element (ARE) upstream of several hundred genes involved in cell defense mechanisms, resulting in enhanced transcription. The following points are not depicted in the scheme: AHR forms a complex with several other proteins including heat shock protein (hsp) 90. AHR activation by selective phytochemicals not only increases intracellular oxidative stress but also leads to translocation of the factor to the nucleus where it upregulates a set of genes involved in xenobiotic defense and immunoregulation. Some of the intranuclear Nrf2 molecules are phosphorylated. Nrf2 gene expression can be modified by affecting its transcription, such as by inhibitory microRNAs; additionally, Keap1 gene expression can also be modified.

Enhancement of Nrf2 activity may also result from blocking its binding to Keap1 by the autophagy adaptor protein p62, which channels Keap1 to degradation in autophagosomes. Proteasomal destruction of Nrf2 can also be inhibited via phosphorylation by several protein kinases, such as members of the Src family, by induction of transcription factors for the increased expression of Nrf2, or the downregulation of inhibitory microRNAs or of Keap1 expression [40,47,48] (Figure 2).

In order to prove that the adaptive response to plant phytochemicals indeed requires activation of the Nrf2 pathway, studies were performed with cells or animals with an inactivated or deleted Nrf2 gene. In the absence of Nrf2, all phytochemicals studied lost their cell protective activity. Phytochemicals included quercetin, epigallocatechin gallate (EGCG), resveratrol, isothiocyanates, allicin, curcumin and aspalathin [40,49–52]. The adaptive response to dietary phytochemicals often includes some anti-inflammatory activity, via suppression of nuclear factor kB (NFkB), which is the master regulator of inflammatory reactivity. This effect is either Nrf2-dependent or may be due to direct targeting of transcription factors NFkB or activator protein 1 by phytochemicals [40].

A second chemical sensor, engaged by phytochemicals as ligands, is the aryl hydrocarbon receptor (AHR), a transcription factor in the cytoplasm promoting the production of radical oxygen species and counterregulatory Nrf2 activity (Figure 2). Upon ligand binding, AHR is released from the complex with heat shock protein (hsp) 90 and is transported to the nucleus, where it dimerizes with the aryl hydrocarbon receptor nuclear translocator, followed by binding to AHR response elements upstream of a set of genes coding for detoxifying enzymes, such as the cytochrome P450 family 1 and immunoregulatory mediators [53–55] (not depicted in Figure 2).

5. Phenolic Constituents of Coffee Activate the Nrf2 Pathway

Exposure of cells or animals to coffee extracts has been observed to lead to increased expression of cytoprotective genes involved in the antioxidant defense, as well as in other chemoprotective or repair activities [56–62]. Decreased gene expression is seen for pro-inflammatory mediators like tumor necrosis factor-α or the NLRP3 inflammasome [60,63].

As seen for phytochemicals of other plants, these effects are mediated by the activation of the Nrf2 system and by inhibiting the pro-inflammatory NFkB pathway (Figure 2). The cytoprotective response seen in mice after consumption of coffee was suppressed after inactivation of the Nrf2 gene [64]. Many constituents of coffee can activate the Nrf2 pathway, with melanoidins of dark roast coffee contributing to these effects [56–58,60–62,65–68]. The diterpenes cafestol and kahweol present in coffee are known to elevate plasma low-density lipoprotein (LDL) and triacylglycerol concentration, while also exhibiting anti-inflammatory and antioxidant actions [69]. The latter cytoprotective action is also mediated by the Nrf2 system and is absent in Nrf2 gene knockout mice [64]. Several of the animal studies took care to apply doses of coffee extract comparable to the consumption of 2–5 cups of coffee in human adults [57,59–61].

Roasting of green coffee increases the ability to activate the Nrf2 pathway. In addition to this, dark roast coffee is more potent in that regard than light roast coffee, when analyzed in vivo [68,70,71]. The analysis of single coffee constituents has confirmed the differing activity of light versus dark roast coffee. Whereas N-methylpyridinium appears to be an activator of Nrf2 as potent as caffeoylquinic acids [56,66], trigonelline suppressed the activation of Nrf2. The lower content of trigonelline fits with the stronger activation of Nrf2 by dark roast coffee [56]. These effects in vitro were observed at physiologically relevant concentrations of 0.1 µmol/L [56]. Moreover, the studies of other constituents of coffee, such as chlorogenic acids, caffeic acid or kahweol, observed activation of Nrf2 at concentrations varying between 10 nmol/L and 3 µmol/L [56,62,65–67], which are in the range of peak concentrations in human plasma after coffee consumption.

Taken together, a large number of trials has shown that coffee or several of its isolated constituents are potent activators of antioxidant or cell-protective enzyme expression. Dark roast coffee appears to be more potent in that regard than light roast coffee. The available evidence indicates that the activation of Nrf2 pathways (to some extent via the aryl hydrocarbon receptor) is the major pathway involved.

Phenolic compounds are characterized in part by hydrophobic surface areas of the molecule. These regions tend to bind to hydrophobic pockets of accessible proteins in tissues and may cause their denaturation and aggregation, which can lead to cell stress, including oxidative stress, and activation of the Nrf2 system as a protective response. High doses of phenolic compounds can be cytotoxic [72–74], but these conditions are usually not reached after a meal of plant foods. For instance, an upper safe limit for the ingestion of green tea catechins has been defined and set as 800 mg epigallocatechin-3-gallate [75]. The phenomenon that tolerable doses of potential toxins induce increased resistance to the same or other chemical insults has been initially observed in toxicological research and defined as hormesis [76] and has been extended to the action of polyphenols [77]. Hormetic reaction schemes have been found or suggested to underlie many physiological processes [78–80].

Although the induction of a cytoprotective response in cells appears to be the dominant physiological reaction to coffee consumption, evidence for a cause–effect relationship with health outcomes is lacking, except for the beneficial effect of coffee intake on DNA integrity. Several randomized-controlled trials have observed that after a run-in period and 4–8 weeks of coffee or water consumption, values of spontaneous DNA strand breaks in blood lymphocytes were significantly lower in the coffee group, as determined by comet assay [81–83]. In one center, the initial trial [81] was repeated with a similar study protocol but the difference in favor of the coffee group was too small to be significant [84]. The level of spontaneous DNA strand breaks in blood lymphocytes is a relevant marker of general disease risk evaluated in epidemiological studies. A meta-analysis of 122 studies described significantly less disease risks for an 11–58% lower level of spontaneous DNA strand breaks, as determined by comet assay [85]. Coffee consumption (of a dark roast Arabica coffee blend shown to activate Nrf2), in three trials described above, resulted in 16–35% less spontaneous DNA strand breaks. These data indicate a cause–effect relationship between coffee consumption and a lower level of spontaneous DNA strand breaks, and that the effect is of physiologically relevant magnitude.

6. Other Possible Pathways of Coffee-Mediated Health Effects

Additional health promoting effects of coffee may occur in the gut, not requiring uptake and biochemical modification of coffee components. Indeed, a prebiotic effect of coffee consumption has been observed in animals and humans, including an increase of Bifidobacteria in humans and mice, and modulation of the Firmicutes to Bacteroidetes ratio in rats. In mice, feeding coffee led to higher levels of acetate, propionate and butyrate [86–88]. Candidate prebiotic constituents of coffee are soluble arabinogalactans and galactomannans, melanoidins and polyphenols [89–91]. However, in male Tsumura Suzuki obese diabetes mice, a mouse model of metabolic syndrome, daily coffee intake prevented nonalcoholic steatohepatitis but did not repair the altered levels of Gram-positive and Gram-negative bacteria and the increased abundance of Firmicutes, nor was there improvement of the disrupted short chain fatty acid profile [92]. Interestingly, feeding probiotic *Lactobacilli* caused the upregulation of Nrf2 in the liver, with concomitant resistance to oxidative injury [93].

To mediate long-term health effects, changes of the microbiota induced by coffee consumption needed to last for decades. A recent study observed that the initial substantial changes of the microbiota, seen after 3 months of introducing a specific diet, regressed thereafter to the original baseline state, which persisted despite continuation of the experimental diet for 12 months [94]. Similar trials of long-term coffee consumption have not been performed, thus the role of the gut microbiota in mediating health effects of coffee constituents remains unresolved.

7. Phytochemicals and Health—A Broader Perspective

One major function of phytochemicals, including those of *coffea* species, is to confer protection from environmental challenges such as exposure to UV radiation or toxins, and to prevent being eaten or damaged by pests or insects because of their noxious properties. At the relatively small doses ingested and taken up by humans, edible parts of plants are not toxic but induce a biological stress response [95]. Besides activation of the Nrf2 system, a number of other cellular responses have been noted, such as the stimulation of the sirtuin-forkhead box O pathway, of AMP-activated protein kinase, of mitogen-activated protein kinases, of the phosphatidylinositol-3-kinase (PI3K)—serine/threonine-specific protein kinase B (AKT) pathway, or modulation of the nuclear factor kB pathway [95–97]. Many outcomes of stress signaling are beneficial, such as the stimulation of antioxidant activity, of anti-inflammatory activity, of mitochondrial function, of DNA repair, of autophagy, of various metabolic parameters and of cell rejuvenation or apoptosis [98].

The many different signaling pathways involved in the cellular response to stress are interdependent and are part of a regulated network. Several studies have suggested a central role for the Nrf2 system.

For example, in the absence of Nrf2 gene activity, the mitochondria-dependent protection by broccoli extract or sulforaphane from pulmonary injury is almost abolished [49], as is the PI3K-AKT-dependent protection by Withania from liver injury [99], or the hemooxygenase-1-dependent protection by curcumin or phenethyl isothiocyanate from inflammatory stress [50]. The extracellular-signal-regulated kinase (ERK) forms a signaling pathway together with Nrf2 [100,101], as does AMPK with Nrf2 [102]. Sirtuin-1 and Nrf2 represent another joint pathway induced by phytochemicals [103].

It thus appears justified to consider the Nrf2 system as a central regulator of phytochemical-induced stress defenses. The type of cellular response may depend on chemical properties of the phytochemical studied, the cell type and developmental stage and further physiological factors.

8. Conclusions

Phytochemicals other than caffeine appear to account for most beneficial properties of coffee. As in vegetables or fruits, polyphenols and phenolic acids represent a major portion of phytochemicals in coffee beans. Phenolic phytochemicals of plant foods have one major pathway of health promoting effects in common, the induction of cell stress, which leads to the activation of an adaptive cell defense response, via activation of the Nrf2 system, translocation of Nrf2 to the nucleus and increased expression of Nrf2-dependent antioxidant and other cytoprotective genes. Furthermore, there is an improved biogenesis, antioxidant defense and substrate supply to mitochondria. Activation of the Nrf2 system and the subsequent cell defense response is also observed in response to exposure with coffee. Randomized controlled trials have found an improved preservation of DNA integrity after several weeks of coffee consumption, this outcome is also assumed to be mediated by the Nrf2 system. Polyphenols and other nondigestible constituents of coffee like polysaccharides and melanoidins share the ability to modify the composition and metabolic function of gut microbiota with similar components of other plant foods. Whether these effects contribute to the beneficial properties of coffee remains to be studied. Taken together, coffee employs similar pathways of beneficial physiological effects as were recently identified for vegetables or fruits. At the level of populations in the developed world, coffee provides more dietary phenolic phytochemicals than vegetables and fruits (Box 1).

Box 1. Key messages.

1. Habitual coffee consumption is associated with a lower risk of many chronic diseases and all-cause mortality.
2. The contribution of oxygen radical scavenging by coffee constituents to health effects is apparently small.
3. Coffee is a plant food and the majority of dietary phenolics consumed in the developed world come from coffee.
4. It is suggested that phenolic constituents of coffee exhibit similar health promoting effects as those from vegetables or fruits.
5. The main pathway of health effects of phenolic phytochemicals from plant food, as well as from coffee, is the activation of the Nrf2 system for an adaptive cytoprotective response.
6. Nrf2-dependent genes code for proteins with antioxidative, detoxifying, DNA repair or anti-inflammatory functions.

Author Contributions: H.K. developed the concept, drafted the manuscript and had primary responsibility for final content. K.K. and S.M. were responsible for discussion of the concept and critical revision of the manuscript. All authors have read and approved the final manuscript.

Funding: The authors report that no funding was received for this work.

Acknowledgments: We thank Christian Herder and Nanette Schloot, University of Düsseldorf, for critical reading, and Yasemin Kempf for proofreading the manuscript. This work was supported by the Freunde und Förderer der Heinrich-Heine-Universität Düsseldorf e.V.

Conflicts of Interest: H.K. received fees for providing consultant services to Tchibo GmbH. K.K. and S.M. reported no conflicts of interest.

Abbreviations

AHR	aryl hydrocarbon receptor
ARE	antioxidant response elements
CNC	cap'n'collar
Cul3	Cullin 3-based E3 ubiquitin ligase
CYP1A2	cytochrome P450 isozyme 1A2
DNA	desoxyribonucleic acid
EGCG	epigallocatechin gallate
EPIC	European Prospective Investigation into Cancer and Nutrition Study
HSP	heat shock protein
IRS	insulin receptor substrate
Keap1	Kelch-like ECH-associated protein 1
LDL	Low-density lipoprotein
NADPH	nicotinamide adenine dinucleotide phosphate
NFkB	nuclear factor kB
NLRP3	NOD-like receptor family, pyrin domain containing 3
NO	nitric oxide
Nrf2	Nuclear factor erythroid 2-related factor 2
ROS	radical oxygen species
sMaf	small musculoaponeurotic fibrosarcoma
UDP	uridine 5'-diphosphate

References

1. Poole, R.; Kennedy, O.J.; Roderick, P.; Fallowfield, J.A.; Hayes, P.C.; Parkes, J. Coffee consumption and health: Umbrella review of meta-analyses of multiple health outcomes. *BMJ* **2017**, *359*, 5024. [CrossRef]
2. Gunter, M.J.; Murphy, N.; Cross, A.J.; Dossus, L.; Dartois, L.; Fagherazzi, G.; Kaaks, R.; Kuhn, T.; Boeing, H.; Aleksandrova, K.; et al. Coffee drinking and mortality in 10 European countries: A multinational cohort study. *Ann. Intern. Med.* **2017**, *167*, 236–247. [CrossRef] [PubMed]
3. Carlstrom, M.; Larsson, S.C. Coffee consumption and reduced risk of developing type 2 diabetes: A systematic review with meta-analysis. *Nutr. Rev.* **2018**, *76*, 395–417. [CrossRef] [PubMed]
4. Je, Y.; Giovannucci, E. Coffee consumption and total mortality: A meta-analysis of twenty prospective cohort studies. *Br. J. Nutr.* **2014**, *111*, 1162–1173. [CrossRef] [PubMed]
5. Li, Q.; Liu, Y.; Sun, X.; Yin, Z.; Li, H.; Cheng, C.; Liu, L.; Zhang, R.; Liu, F.; Zhou, Q.; et al. Caffeinated and decaffeinated coffee consumption and risk of all-cause mortality: A dose-response meta-analysis of cohort studies. *J. Hum. Nutr. Diet* **2019**, *32*, 279–287. [CrossRef] [PubMed]
6. Cornelis, M.C. Coffee and type 2 diabetes: Time to consider alternative mechanisms? *Am. J. Clin. Nutr.* **2020**, *111*, 248–249. [CrossRef]
7. Cornelis, M.C.; Monda, K.L.; Yu, K.; Paynter, N.; Azzato, E.M.; Bennett, S.N.; Berndt, S.I.; Boerwinkle, E.; Chanock, S.; Chatterjee, N.; et al. Genome-wide meta-analysis identifies regions on 7p21 (AHR) and 15q24 (CYP1A2) as determinants of habitual caffeine consumption. *PLoS Genet.* **2011**, *7*, e1002033. [CrossRef]
8. Amin, N.; Byrne, E.; Johnson, J.; Chenevix-Trench, G.; Walter, S.; Nolte, I.M.; Vink, J.M.; Rawal, R.; Mangino, M.; Teumer, A.; et al. Genome-wide association analysis of coffee drinking suggests association with CYP1A1/CYP1A2 and NRCAM. *Mol. Psychiatry* **2012**, *17*, 1116–1129. [CrossRef]
9. Cornelis, M.C.; Byrne, E.M.; Esko, T.; Nalls, M.A.; Ganna, A.; Paynter, N.; Monda, K.L.; Amin, N.; Fischer, K.; Renstrom, F.; et al. Genome-wide meta-analysis identifies six novel loci associated with habitual coffee consumption. *Mol. Psychiatry* **2015**, *20*, 647–656. [CrossRef]
10. Nehlig, A. Interindividual differences in caffeine metabolism and factors driving caffeine consumption. *Pharmacol. Rev.* **2018**, *70*, 384–411. [CrossRef]
11. Cornelis, M.C.; Munafo, M.R. Mendelian randomization studies of coffee and caffeine consumption. *Nutrients* **2018**, *10*, 1343. [CrossRef] [PubMed]

12. Popat, R.A.; Van Den Eeden, S.K.; Tanner, C.M.; Kamel, F.; Umbach, D.M.; Marder, K.; Mayeux, R.; Ritz, B.; Ross, G.W.; Petrovitch, H.; et al. Coffee, ADORA2A, and CYP1A2: The caffeine connection in Parkinson's disease. *Eur. J. Neurol.* **2011**, *18*, 756–765. [CrossRef] [PubMed]
13. Kotsopoulos, J.; Ghadirian, P.; El Sohemy, A.; Lynch, H.T.; Snyder, C.; Daly, M.; Domchek, S.; Randall, S.; Karlan, B.; Zhang, P.; et al. The CYP1A2 genotype modifies the association between coffee consumption and breast cancer risk among BRCA1 mutation carriers. *Cancer Epidemiol. Biomarkers Prev.* **2007**, *16*, 912–916. [CrossRef]
14. Bhupathiraju, S.N.; Pan, A.; Manson, J.E.; Willett, W.C.; Van Dam, R.M.; Hu, F.B. Changes in coffee intake and subsequent risk of type 2 diabetes: Three large cohorts of US men and women. *Diabetologia* **2014**, *57*, 1346–1354. [CrossRef]
15. Loftfield, E.; Cornelis, M.C.; Caporaso, N.; Yu, K.; Sinha, R.; Freedman, N. Association of coffee drinking with mortality by genetic variation in caffeine metabolism: Findings from the UK Biobank. *JAMA Intern. Med.* **2018**, *178*, 1086–1097. [CrossRef] [PubMed]
16. Palatini, P. Coffee consumption and risk of type 2 diabetes. *Diabetologia* **2015**, *58*, 199–200. [CrossRef]
17. Opitz, S.E.; Goodman, B.A.; Keller, M.; Smrke, S.; Wellinger, M.; Schenker, S.; Yeretzian, C. Understanding the effects of roasting on antioxidant components of coffee brews by coupling on-line ABTS assay to high performance size exclusion chromatography. *Phytochem. Anal.* **2017**, *28*, 106–114. [CrossRef]
18. Kamiyama, M.; Moon, J.K.; Jang, H.W.; Shibamoto, T. Role of degradation products of chlorogenic acid in the antioxidant activity of roasted coffee. *J. Agric. Food Chem.* **2015**, *63*, 1996–2005. [CrossRef]
19. Lang, R.; Dieminger, N.; Beusch, A.; Lee, Y.M.; Dunkel, A.; Suess, B.; Skurk, T.; Wahl, A.; Hauner, H.; Hofmann, T. Bioappearance and pharmacokinetics of bioactives upon coffee consumption. *Anal. Bioanal. Chem.* **2013**, *405*, 8487–8503. [CrossRef]
20. Lotito, S.B.; Frei, B. Consumption of flavonoid-rich foods and increased plasma antioxidant capacity in humans: Cause, consequence, or epiphenomenon? *Free Radic. Biol. Med.* **2006**, *41*, 1727–1746. [CrossRef]
21. Lee, Y.H. Coffee consumption and gout: A Mendelian randomisation study. *Ann. Rheum. Dis.* **2019**, *78*, e130. [CrossRef] [PubMed]
22. Giustarini, D.; Colombo, G.; Garavaglia, M.L.; Astori, E.; Portinaro, N.M.; Reggiani, F.; Badalamenti, S.; Aloisi, A.M.; Santucci, A.; Rossi, R.; et al. Assessment of glutathione/glutathione disulphide ratio and S-glutathionylated proteins in human blood, solid tissues, and cultured cells. *Free Radic. Biol. Med.* **2017**, *112*, 360–375. [CrossRef] [PubMed]
23. Ludwig, I.A.; Clifford, M.N.; Lean, M.E.; Ashihara, H.; Crozier, A. Coffee: Biochemistry and potential impact on health. *Food Funct.* **2014**, *5*, 1695–1717. [CrossRef]
24. Calder, P.C.; Ahluwalia, N.; Brouns, F.; Buetler, T.; Clement, K.; Cunningham, K.; Esposito, K.; Jonsson, L.S.; Kolb, H.; Lansink, M.; et al. Dietary factors and low-grade inflammation in relation to overweight and obesity. *Br. J. Nutr.* **2011**, *106*, S5–S78. [CrossRef]
25. Hang, D.; Kvaerner, A.S.; Ma, W.; Hu, Y.; Tabung, F.K.; Nan, H.; Hu, Z.; Shen, H.; Mucci, L.A.; Chan, A.T.; et al. Coffee consumption and plasma biomarkers of metabolic and inflammatory pathways in US health professionals. *Am. J. Clin. Nutr.* **2019**, *109*, 635–647. [CrossRef]
26. Kempf, K.; Herder, C.; Erlund, I.; Kolb, H.; Martin, S.; Carstensen, M.; Koenig, W.; Sundvall, J.; Bidel, S.; Kuha, S.; et al. Effects of coffee consumption on subclinical inflammation and other risk factors for type 2 diabetes: A clinical trial. *Am. J. Clin. Nutr.* **2010**, *91*, 950–957. [CrossRef] [PubMed]
27. Loftfield, E.; Shiels, M.S.; Graubard, B.I.; Katki, H.A.; Chaturvedi, A.K.; Trabert, B.; Pinto, L.A.; Kemp, T.J.; Shebl, F.M.; Mayne, S.T.; et al. Associations of coffee drinking with systemic immune and inflammatory markers. *Cancer Epidemiol. Biomark. Prev.* **2015**, *24*, 1052–1060. [CrossRef]
28. Nieman, D.C.; Goodman, C.L.; Capps, C.R.; Shue, Z.L.; Arnot, R. Influence of 2-weeks ingestion of high chlorogenic acid coffee on mood state, performance, and postexercise inflammation and oxidative stress: A randomized, placebo-controlled trial. *Int. J. Sport Nutr. Exerc. Metab.* **2018**, *28*, 55–65. [CrossRef]
29. Martinez-Lopez, S.; Sarria, B.; Mateos, R.; Bravo-Clemente, L. Moderate consumption of a soluble green/roasted coffee rich in caffeoylquinic acids reduces cardiovascular risk markers: Results from a randomized, cross-over, controlled trial in healthy and hypercholesterolemic subjects. *Eur. J. Nutr.* **2019**, *58*, 865–878. [CrossRef]

30. Correa, T.A.; Rogero, M.M.; Mioto, B.M.; Tarasoutchi, D.; Tuda, V.L.; Cesar, L.A.; Torres, E.A. Paper-filtered coffee increases cholesterol and inflammation biomarkers independent of roasting degree: A clinical trial. *Nutrition* **2013**, *29*, 977–981. [CrossRef]
31. Kempf, K.; Kolb, H.; Gartner, B.; Bytof, G.; Stiebitz, H.; Lantz, I.; Lang, R.; Hofmann, T.; Martin, S. Cardiometabolic effects of two coffee blends differing in content for major constituents in overweight adults: A randomized controlled trial. *Eur. J. Nutr.* **2015**, *54*, 845–854. [CrossRef] [PubMed]
32. Lamichhane, D.; Collins, C.; Constantinescu, F.; Walitt, B.; Pettinger, M.; Parks, C.; Howard, B.V. Coffee and tea consumption in relation to risk of rheumatoid arthritis in the women's health initiative observational cohort. *J. Clin. Rheumatol.* **2019**, *25*, 127–132. [CrossRef]
33. Del Rio, D.; Rodriguez-Mateos, A.; Spencer, J.P.; Tognolini, M.; Borges, G.; Crozier, A. Dietary (poly)phenolics in human health: Structures, bioavailability, and evidence of protective effects against chronic diseases. *Antioxid. Redox. Signal.* **2013**, *18*, 1818–1892. [CrossRef] [PubMed]
34. Fraga, C.G.; Croft, K.D.; Kennedy, D.O.; Tomas-Barberan, F.A. The effects of polyphenols and other bioactives on human health. *Food Funct.* **2019**, *10*, 514–528. [CrossRef]
35. Burkholder-Cooley, N.; Rajaram, S.; Haddad, E.; Fraser, G.E.; Jaceldo-Siegl, K. Comparison of polyphenol intakes according to distinct dietary patterns and food sources in the Adventist Health Study-2 cohort. *Br. J. Nutr.* **2016**, *115*, 2162–2169. [CrossRef] [PubMed]
36. Grosso, G.; Stepaniak, U.; Topor-Madry, R.; Szafraniec, K.; Pajak, A. Estimated dietary intake and major food sources of polyphenols in the Polish arm of the HAPIEE study. *Nutrition* **2014**, *30*, 1398–1403. [CrossRef] [PubMed]
37. Taguchi, C.; Fukushima, Y.; Kishimoto, Y.; Suzuki-Sugihara, N.; Saita, E.; Takahashi, Y.; Kondo, K. estimated dietary polyphenol intake and major food and beverage sources among elderly Japanese. *Nutrients* **2015**, *7*, 10269–10281. [CrossRef] [PubMed]
38. Zamora-Ros, R.; Rothwell, J.A.; Scalbert, A.; Knaze, V.; Romieu, I.; Slimani, N.; Fagherazzi, G.; Perquier, F.; Touillaud, M.; Molina-Montes, E.; et al. Dietary intakes and food sources of phenolic acids in the European Prospective Investigation into Cancer and Nutrition (EPIC) study. *Br. J. Nutr.* **2013**, *110*, 1500–1511. [CrossRef]
39. Zamora-Ros, R.; Knaze, V.; Rothwell, J.A.; Hemon, B.; Moskal, A.; Overvad, K.; Tjonneland, A.; Kyro, C.; Fagherazzi, G.; Boutron-Ruault, M.C.; et al. Dietary polyphenol intake in Europe: The European Prospective Investigation into Cancer and Nutrition (EPIC) study. *Eur. J. Nutr.* **2016**, *55*, 1359–1375. [CrossRef]
40. Qin, S.; Hou, D.X. Multiple regulations of Keap1/Nrf2 system by dietary phytochemicals. *Mol. Nutr. Food Res.* **2016**, *60*, 1731–1755. [CrossRef]
41. Otsuki, A.; Yamamoto, M. Cis-element architecture of Nrf2-sMaf heterodimer binding sites and its relation to diseases. *Arch. Pharm. Res.* **2020**, *43*, 275–285. [CrossRef]
42. Tebay, L.E.; Robertson, H.; Durant, S.T.; Vitale, S.R.; Penning, T.M.; Dinkova-Kostova, A.T.; Hayes, J.D. Mechanisms of activation of the transcription factor Nrf2 by redox stressors, nutrient cues, and energy status and the pathways through which it attenuates degenerative disease. *Free Radic. Biol. Med.* **2015**, *88*, 108–146. [CrossRef] [PubMed]
43. Merry, T.L.; Ristow, M. Nuclear factor erythroid-derived 2-like 2 (NFE2L2, Nrf2) mediates exercise-induced mitochondrial biogenesis and the anti-oxidant response in mice. *J. Physiol.* **2016**, *594*, 5195–5207. [CrossRef] [PubMed]
44. Coleman, V.; Sa-Nguanmoo, P.; Koenig, J.; Schulz, T.J.; Grune, T.; Klaus, S.; Kipp, A.P.; Ost, M. Partial involvement of Nrf2 in skeletal muscle mitohormesis as an adaptive response to mitochondrial uncoupling. *Sci. Rep.* **2018**, *8*, 2446. [CrossRef] [PubMed]
45. Tsushima, M.; Liu, J.; Hirao, W.; Yamazaki, H.; Tomita, H.; Itoh, K. Emerging evidence for crosstalk between Nrf2 and mitochondria in physiological homeostasis and in heart disease. *Arch. Pharm. Res.* **2020**, *43*, 286–296. [CrossRef] [PubMed]
46. Unoki, T.; Akiyama, M.; Kumagai, Y. Nrf2 activation and its coordination with the protective defense systems in response to electrophilic stress. *Int. J. Mol. Sci.* **2020**, *21*, 545. [CrossRef]
47. Baird, L.; Yamamoto, M. The molecular mechanisms regulating the KEAP1-NRF2 pathway. *Mol. Cell. Biol.* **2020**, *40*, e00099-20. [CrossRef]
48. Shin, W.H.; Park, J.H.; Chung, K.C. The central regulator p62 between ubiquitin proteasome system and autophagy and its role in the mitophagy and Parkinson's disease. *BMB Rep.* **2020**, *53*, 56–63. [CrossRef]

49. Cho, H.Y.; Miller-DeGraff, L.; Blankenship-Paris, T.; Wang, X.; Bell, D.A.; Lih, F.; Deterding, L.; Panduri, V.; Morgan, D.L.; Yamamoto, M.; et al. Sulforaphane enriched transcriptome of lung mitochondrial energy metabolism and provided pulmonary injury protection via Nrf2 in mice. *Toxicol. Appl. Pharmacol.* **2019**, *364*, 29–44. [CrossRef]
50. Boyanapalli, S.S.; Paredes-Gonzalez, X.; Fuentes, F.; Zhang, C.; Guo, Y.; Pung, D.; Saw, C.L.; Kong, A.N. Nrf2 knockout attenuates the anti-inflammatory effects of phenethyl isothiocyanate and curcumin. *Chem. Res. Toxicol.* **2014**, *27*, 2036–2043. [CrossRef]
51. Ungvari, Z.; Bagi, Z.; Feher, A.; Recchia, F.A.; Sonntag, W.E.; Pearson, K.; De Cabo, R.; Csiszar, A. Resveratrol confers endothelial protection via activation of the antioxidant transcription factor Nrf2. *Am. J. Physiol. Heart Circ. Physiol.* **2010**, *299*, H18–H24. [CrossRef] [PubMed]
52. Dludla, P.V.; Muller, C.J.; Joubert, E.; Louw, J.; Essop, M.F.; Gabuza, K.B.; Ghoor, S.; Huisamen, B.; Johnson, R. Aspalathin protects the heart against hyperglycemia-induced oxidative damage by up-regulating Nrf2 expression. *Molecules* **2017**, *22*, 129. [CrossRef] [PubMed]
53. Furue, M.; Uchi, H.; Mitoma, C.; Hashimoto-Hachiya, A.; Chiba, T.; Ito, T.; Nakahara, T.; Tsuji, G. Antioxidants for healthy skin: The emerging role of aryl hydrocarbon receptors and nuclear factor-erythroid 2-related factor-2. *Nutrients* **2017**, *9*, 223. [CrossRef] [PubMed]
54. Neavin, D.R.; Liu, D.; Ray, B.; Weinshilboum, R.M. The role of the Aryl Hydrocarbon Receptor (AHR) in immune and inflammatory diseases. *Int. J. Mol. Sci.* **2018**, *19*, 3851. [CrossRef] [PubMed]
55. Rothhammer, V.; Quintana, F.J. The aryl hydrocarbon receptor: An environmental sensor integrating immune responses in health and disease. *Nat. Rev. Immunol.* **2019**, *19*, 184–197. [CrossRef]
56. Boettler, U.; Sommerfeld, K.; Volz, N.; Pahlke, G.; Teller, N.; Somoza, V.; Lang, R.; Hofmann, T.; Marko, D. Coffee constituents as modulators of Nrf2 nuclear translocation and ARE (EpRE)-dependent gene expression. *J. Nutr. Biochem.* **2011**, *22*, 426–440. [CrossRef]
57. Cavin, C.; Marin-Kuan, M.; Langouet, S.; Bezencon, C.; Guignard, G.; Verguet, C.; Piguet, D.; Holzhauser, D.; Cornaz, R.; Schilter, B. Induction of Nrf2-mediated cellular defenses and alteration of phase I activities as mechanisms of chemoprotective effects of coffee in the liver. *Food Chem. Toxicol.* **2008**, *46*, 1239–1248. [CrossRef]
58. Kalthoff, S.; Ehmer, U.; Freiberg, N.; Manns, M.P.; Strassburg, C.P. Coffee induces expression of glucuronosyltransferases by the aryl hydrocarbon receptor and Nrf2 in liver and stomach. *Gastroenterology* **2010**, *139*, 1699–1710. [CrossRef]
59. Salomone, F.; Li, V.G.; Vitaglione, P.; Morisco, F.; Fogliano, V.; Zappala, A.; Palmigiano, A.; Garozzo, D.; Caporaso, N.; D'Argenio, G.; et al. Coffee enhances the expression of chaperones and antioxidant proteins in rats with nonalcoholic fatty liver disease. *Transl. Res.* **2014**, *163*, 593–602. [CrossRef]
60. Shi, A.; Shi, H.; Wang, Y.; Liu, X.; Cheng, Y.; Li, H.; Zhao, H.; Wang, S.; Dong, L. Activation of Nrf2 pathway and inhibition of NLRP3 inflammasome activation contribute to the protective effect of chlorogenic acid on acute liver injury. *Int. Immunopharmacol.* **2018**, *54*, 125–130. [CrossRef]
61. Vicente, S.J.; Ishimoto, E.Y.; Torres, E.A. Coffee modulates transcription factor Nrf2 and highly increases the activity of antioxidant enzymes in rats. *J. Agric. Food Chem.* **2014**, *62*, 116–122. [CrossRef] [PubMed]
62. Volz, N.; Boettler, U.; Winkler, S.; Teller, N.; Schwarz, C.; Bakuradze, T.; Eisenbrand, G.; Haupt, L.; Griffiths, L.R.; Stiebitz, H.; et al. Effect of coffee combining green coffee bean constituents with typical roasting products on the Nrf2/ARE pathway in vitro and in vivo. *J. Agric. Food Chem.* **2012**, *60*, 9631–9641. [CrossRef] [PubMed]
63. Jung, K.A.; Kwak, M.K. The Nrf2 system as a potential target for the development of indirect antioxidants. *Molecules* **2010**, *15*, 7266–7291. [CrossRef] [PubMed]
64. Higgins, L.G.; Cavin, C.; Itoh, K.; Yamamoto, M.; Hayes, J.D. Induction of cancer chemopreventive enzymes by coffee is mediated by transcription factor Nrf2. Evidence that the coffee-specific diterpenes cafestol and kahweol confer protection against acrolein. *Toxicol. Appl. Pharmacol.* **2008**, *226*, 328–337. [CrossRef]
65. Balstad, T.R.; Carlsen, H.; Myhrstad, M.C.; Kolberg, M.; Reiersen, H.; Gilen, L.; Ebihara, K.; Paur, I.; Blomhoff, R. Coffee, broccoli and spices are strong inducers of electrophile response element-dependent transcription in vitro and in vivo—studies in electrophile response element transgenic mice. *Mol. Nutr. Food Res.* **2011**, *55*, 185–197. [CrossRef] [PubMed]

66. Boettler, U.; Volz, N.; Pahlke, G.; Teller, N.; Kotyczka, C.; Somoza, V.; Stiebitz, H.; Bytof, G.; Lantz, I.; Lang, R.; et al. Coffees rich in chlorogenic acid or N-methylpyridinium induce chemopreventive phase II-enzymes via the Nrf2/ARE pathway in vitro and in vivo. *Mol. Nutr. Food Res.* **2011**, *55*, 798–802. [CrossRef]
67. Fratantonio, D.; Speciale, A.; Canali, R.; Natarelli, L.; Ferrari, D.; Saija, A.; Virgili, F.; Cimino, F. Low nanomolar caffeic acid attenuates high glucose-induced endothelial dysfunction in primary human umbilical-vein endothelial cells by affecting NF-kappaB and Nrf2 pathways. *Biofactors* **2017**, *43*, 54–62. [CrossRef]
68. Priftis, A.; Mitsiou, D.; Halabalaki, M.; Ntasi, G.; Stagos, D.; Skaltsounis, L.A.; Kouretas, D. Roasting has a distinct effect on the antimutagenic activity of coffee varieties. *Mutat. Res. Genet. Toxicol. Environ. Mutagen.* **2018**, *829–830*, 33–42. [CrossRef]
69. Ren, Y.; Wang, C.; Xu, J.; Wang, S. Cafestol and Kahweol: A Review on their bioactivities and pharmacological properties. *Int. J. Mol. Sci.* **2019**, *20*, 4238. [CrossRef]
70. Paur, I.; Balstad, T.R.; Blomhoff, R. Degree of roasting is the main determinant of the effects of coffee on NF-kappaB and EpRE. *Free Radic. Biol. Med.* **2010**, *48*, 1218–1227. [CrossRef]
71. Sauer, T.; Raithel, M.; Kressel, J.; Munch, G.; Pischetsrieder, M. Activation of the transcription factor Nrf2 in macrophages, Caco-2 cells and intact human gut tissue by Maillard reaction products and coffee. *Amino Acids* **2013**, *44*, 1427–1439. [CrossRef] [PubMed]
72. Murakami, A. Dose-dependent functionality and toxicity of green tea polyphenols in experimental rodents. *Arch. Biochem. Biophys.* **2014**, *557*, 3–10. [CrossRef] [PubMed]
73. Karadas, O.; Mese, G.; Ozcivici, E. Cytotoxic tolerance of healthy and cancerous bone cells to anti-microbial phenolic compounds depend on culture conditions. *Appl. Biochem. Biotechnol.* **2019**, *188*, 514–526. [CrossRef] [PubMed]
74. Wu, H.; Chen, L.; Zhu, F.; Han, X.; Sun, L.; Chen, K. The cytotoxicity effect of resveratrol: Cell cycle arrest and induced apoptosis of breast cancer 4T1 Cells. *Toxins (Basel)* **2019**, *11*, 731. [CrossRef]
75. EFSA ANS Panel. Scientific opinion on the safety of green tea catechins. *EFSA J.* **2018**, *16*, 5239.
76. Calabrese, E.J. Hormesis is central to toxicology, pharmacology and risk assessment. *Hum. Exp. Toxicol.* **2010**, *29*, 249–261. [CrossRef]
77. Leri, M.; Scuto, M.; Ontario, M.L.; Calabrese, V.; Calabrese, E.J.; Bucciantini, M.; Stefani, M. Healthy effects of plant polyphenols: Molecular mechanisms. *Int. J. Mol. Sci.* **2020**, *21*, 1250. [CrossRef]
78. Miller, V.J.; Villamena, F.A.; Volek, J.S. Nutritional ketosis and mitohormesis: Potential implications for mitochondrial function and human health. *J. Nutr. Metab.* **2018**, *2018*, 5157645. [CrossRef]
79. Kolb, H.; Eizirik, D.L. Resistance to type 2 diabetes mellitus: A matter of hormesis? *Nat. Rev. Endocrinol.* **2011**, *8*, 183–192. [CrossRef]
80. Calabrese, E.J.; Mattson, M.P. How does hormesis impact biology, toxicology, and medicine? *NPJ Aging Mech. Dis.* **2017**, *3*, 13. [CrossRef]
81. Bakuradze, T.; Lang, R.; Hofmann, T.; Eisenbrand, G.; Schipp, D.; Galan, J.; Richling, E. Consumption of a dark roast coffee decreases the level of spontaneous DNA strand breaks: A randomized controlled trial. *Eur. J. Nutr.* **2015**, *54*, 149–156. [CrossRef] [PubMed]
82. Schipp, D.; Tulinska, J.; Sustrova, M.; Liskova, A.; Spustova, V.; Lehotska, M.M.; Krivosikova, Z.; Rausova, K.; Collins, A.; Vebraite, V.; et al. Consumption of a dark roast coffee blend reduces DNA damage in humans: Results from a 4-week randomised controlled study. *Eur. J. Nutr.* **2019**, *58*, 3199–3206. [CrossRef] [PubMed]
83. Pahlke, G.; Attapah, E.; Aichinger, G.; Ahlberg, K.; Hochkogler, C.; Schipp, D.; Somoza, V.; Marko, D. Dark coffee consumption protects human blood cells from spontaneous DNA damage. *J. Funct. Foods* **2019**, *55*, 285–295. [CrossRef]
84. EFSA Panel on NDA. Scientifc opinion on Coffee C21 and protection of DNA from strand breaks. *EFSA J.* **2020**, *18*, 6055.
85. Valverde, M.; Rojas, E. Environmental and occupational biomonitoring using the Comet assay. *Mutat. Res.* **2009**, *681*, 93–109. [CrossRef] [PubMed]
86. Jaquet, M.; Rochat, I.; Moulin, J.; Cavin, C.; Bibiloni, R. Impact of coffee consumption on the gut microbiota: A human volunteer study. *Int. J. Food Microbiol.* **2009**, *130*, 117–121. [CrossRef]
87. Cowan, T.E.; Palmnas, M.S.; Yang, J.; Bomhof, M.R.; Ardell, K.L.; Reimer, R.A.; Vogel, H.J.; Shearer, J. Chronic coffee consumption in the diet-induced obese rat: Impact on gut microbiota and serum metabolomics. *J. Nutr. Biochem.* **2014**, *25*, 489–495. [CrossRef]

88. Nakayama, T.; Oishi, K. Influence of coffee (*Coffea arabica*) and galacto-oligosaccharide consumption on intestinal microbiota and the host responses. *FEMS Microbiol. Lett.* **2013**, *343*, 161–168. [CrossRef]
89. Gniechwitz, D.; Brueckel, B.; Reichardt, N.; Blaut, M.; Steinhart, H.; Bunzel, M. Coffee dietary fiber contents and structural characteristics as influenced by coffee type and technological and brewing procedures. *J. Agric. Food Chem.* **2007**, *55*, 11027–11034. [CrossRef]
90. Williamson, G. The role of polyphenols in modern nutrition. *Nutr. Bull.* **2017**, *42*, 226–235. [CrossRef]
91. Perez-Burillo, S.; Rajakaruna, S.; Pastoriza, S.; Paliy, O.; Rufian-Henares, J.A. Bioactivity of food melanoidins is mediated by gut microbiota. *Food Chem.* **2020**, *316*, 126309. [CrossRef] [PubMed]
92. Nishitsuji, K.; Watanabe, S.; Xiao, J.; Nagatomo, R.; Ogawa, H.; Tsunematsu, T.; Umemoto, H.; Morimoto, Y.; Akatsu, H.; Inoue, K.; et al. Effect of coffee or coffee components on gut microbiome and short-chain fatty acids in a mouse model of metabolic syndrome. *Sci. Rep.* **2018**, *8*, 16173. [CrossRef] [PubMed]
93. Saeedi, B.J.; Liu, K.H.; Owens, J.A.; Hunter-Chang, S.; Camacho, M.C.; Eboka, R.U.; Chandrasekharan, B.; Baker, N.F.; Darby, T.M.; Robinson, B.S.; et al. Gut-resident lactobacilli activate hepatic Nrf2 and protect against oxidative liver injury. *Cell Metab.* **2020**, *31*, 956–968. [CrossRef] [PubMed]
94. Fragiadakis, G.K.; Wastyk, H.C.; Robinson, J.L.; Sonnenburg, E.D.; Sonnenburg, J.L.; Gardner, C.D. Long-term dietary intervention reveals resilience of the gut microbiota despite changes in diet and weight. *Am. J. Clin. Nutr.* **2020**, *111*, 1127–1136. [CrossRef]
95. Son, T.G.; Camandola, S.; Mattson, M.P. Hormetic dietary phytochemicals. *Neuromolecular Med.* **2008**, *10*, 236–246. [CrossRef]
96. Martel, J.; Ojcius, D.M.; Ko, Y.F.; Ke, P.Y.; Wu, C.Y.; Peng, H.H.; Young, J.D. Hormetic effects of phytochemicals on health and longevity. *Trends Endocrinol. Metab.* **2019**, *30*, 335–346. [CrossRef]
97. Yahfoufi, N.; Alsadi, N.; Jambi, M.; Matar, C. The immunomodulatory and anti-inflammatory role of polyphenols. *Nutrients* **2018**, *10*, 1618. [CrossRef]
98. Liu, K.; Luo, M.; Wei, S. The bioprotective effects of polyphenols on metabolic syndrome against oxidative stress: Evidences and perspectives. *Oxid. Med. Cell Longev.* **2019**, *2019*, 6713194. [CrossRef]
99. Palliyaguru, D.L.; Chartoumpekis, D.V.; Wakabayashi, N.; Skoko, J.J.; Yagishita, Y.; Singh, S.V.; Kensler, T.W. Withaferin A induces Nrf2-dependent protection against liver injury: Role of Keap1-independent mechanisms. *Free Radic. Biol. Med.* **2016**, *101*, 116–128. [CrossRef]
100. Hao, Q.; Wang, M.; Sun, N.X.; Zhu, C.; Lin, Y.M.; Li, C.; Liu, F.; Zhu, W.W. Sulforaphane suppresses carcinogenesis of colorectal cancer through the ERK/Nrf2UDP glucuronosyltransferase 1A metabolic axis activation. *Oncol. Rep.* **2020**, *43*, 1067–1080.
101. Zhao, S.J.; Liu, H.; Chen, J.; Qian, D.F.; Kong, F.Q.; Jie, J.; Yin, G.Y.; Li, Q.Q.; Fan, J. Macrophage GIT1 contributes to bone regeneration by regulating inflammatory responses in an ERK/NRF2-dependent way. *J. Bone Miner. Res.* **2020**. [CrossRef] [PubMed]
102. Lei, L.; Chai, Y.; Lin, H.; Chen, C.; Zhao, M.; Xiong, W.; Zhuang, J.; Fan, X. Dihydroquercetin activates AMPK/Nrf2/HO-1 signaling in macrophages and attenuates inflammation in LPS-induced endotoxemic mice. *Front. Pharmacol.* **2020**, *11*, 662. [CrossRef] [PubMed]
103. Lu, J.; Huang, Q.; Zhang, D.; Lan, T.; Zhang, Y.; Tang, X.; Xu, P.; Zhao, D.; Cong, D.; Zhao, D.; et al. The protective effect of DiDang Tang against AlCl3-Induced oxidative stress and apoptosis in PC12 cells through the activation of SIRT1-mediated Akt/Nrf2/HO-1 pathway. *Front. Pharmacol.* **2020**, *11*, 466. [CrossRef] [PubMed]

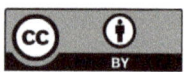

© 2020 by the authors. Licensee MDPI, Basel, Switzerland. This article is an open access article distributed under the terms and conditions of the Creative Commons Attribution (CC BY) license (http://creativecommons.org/licenses/by/4.0/).

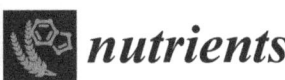

Review

Effects of Coffee and Its Components on the Gastrointestinal Tract and the Brain–Gut Axis

Amaia Iriondo-DeHond [1], José Antonio Uranga [2], Maria Dolores del Castillo [1] and Raquel Abalo [2,3,*]

[1] Food Bioscience Group, Department of Bioactivity and Food Analysis, Instituto de Investigación en Ciencias de la Alimentación (CIAL) (CSIC-UAM), Calle Nicolás Cabrera, 9, 28049 Madrid, Spain; amaia.iriondo@csic.es (A.I.-D.); mdolores.delcastillo@csic.es (M.D.d.C.)

[2] High Performance Research Group in Physiopathology and Pharmacology of the Digestive System NeuGut-URJC, Department of Basic Health Sciences, Faculty of Health Sciences, Campus de Alcorcón, Universidad Rey Juan Carlos (URJC), Avda. de Atenas s/n, 28022 Madrid, Spain; jose.uranga@urjc.es

[3] Associated Unit to Institute of Medicinal Chemistry (Unidad Asociada I+D+i del Instituto de Química Médica, IQM), Spanish National Research Council (Consejo Superior de Investigaciones Científicas, CSIC), 28006 Madrid, Spain

* Correspondence: raquel.abalo@urjc.es; Tel.: +34-914-888854

Abstract: Coffee is one of the most popular beverages consumed worldwide. Roasted coffee is a complex mixture of thousands of bioactive compounds, and some of them have numerous potential health-promoting properties that have been extensively studied in the cardiovascular and central nervous systems, with relatively much less attention given to other body systems, such as the gastrointestinal tract and its particular connection with the brain, known as the brain–gut axis. This narrative review provides an overview of the effect of coffee brew; its by-products; and its components on the gastrointestinal mucosa (mainly involved in permeability, secretion, and proliferation), the neural and non-neural components of the gut wall responsible for its motor function, and the brain–gut axis. Despite in vitro, in vivo, and epidemiological studies having shown that coffee may exert multiple effects on the digestive tract, including antioxidant, anti-inflammatory, and antiproliferative effects on the mucosa, and pro-motility effects on the external muscle layers, much is still surprisingly unknown. Further studies are needed to understand the mechanisms of action of certain health-promoting properties of coffee on the gastrointestinal tract and to transfer this knowledge to the industry to develop functional foods to improve the gastrointestinal and brain–gut axis health.

Keywords: brain–gut axis; caffeine; coffee; coffee by-products; dietary fiber; enteric; gastrointestinal; melanoidins; mucosa; myenteric

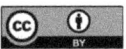

1. Introduction

In the past years, coffee has gone from being the villain in the movie to the paradoxical hero. In 1991, the International Agency for Research on Cancer (IARC), the specialized cancer agency of the World Health Organization (WHO), classified coffee as "possibly carcinogenic to humans" (Group 2B). This assessment was made on the basis of limited evidence on the association of urinary bladder cancer and coffee consumption. In 2016, after a re-evaluation based on more than 1000 observational and experimental studies, 23 scientists from 10 different countries concluded that the extensive scientific literature does not show evidence of an association between coffee consumption and cancer [1]. Therefore, coffee was moved from Group 2B ("possibly carcinogenic to humans") to Group 3 ("not classifiable as to carcinogenicity"). In addition, the IARC found that there is evidence that coffee consumption may actually help reduce occurrence of certain cancers (colon, prostate, endometrial, melanoma, and liver) [1,2].

The "coffee paradox" consists of the fact that caffeine raises blood pressure, but drinking coffee is associated with a lower risk of hypertension [3]. In fact, daily coffee consumption is associated with a decrease in the prevalence of heart attack, despite the tendency to smoke in coffee drinkers [4]. In addition, moderate consumption of 3–4 cups of coffee a day is associated with greater longevity and lower risk of all-cause mortality [5]. Coffee consumption has also evidence-based beneficial associations with metabolic diseases (type 2 diabetes, metabolic syndrome, renal stones, and different liver conditions) and neurodegenerative diseases (Parkinson's and Alzheimer's disease) [2]. Therefore, coffee consumption is recommended as part of a healthy diet [6,7], since it contains several bioactive compounds with therapeutic properties [8].

Table 1 shows the chemical composition of green, roasted, and brewed coffee. The composition of the green coffee bean is severely affected by the roasting process, during which, among others, the Maillard reaction occurs. This reaction reduces the amount of free chlorogenic acids (CGAs), but other antioxidant compounds are formed, such as melanoidins that incorporate CGA to their backbone (Table 1) [9]. These compounds, among others formed during processing, are responsible for the brown color of roasted coffee beans and contribute to the antioxidant capacity of coffee [10]. On the other hand, the Maillard reaction produces newly formed contaminants, such as acrylamide. The European Commission indicates that levels of acrylamide in coffee can be lowered by the following mitigation approaches: controlling roasting conditions or treating with asparaginase [11]. Roasted coffee is a complex mixture of thousands of bioactive compounds, and some of them have potential health-promoting properties such as antioxidant, anti-inflammatory, antifibrotic, or antiproliferative effects [5].

Table 1. Chemical composition of Arabica green, roasted, filtered, and cold brew coffee.

Constituent	Green Coffee Beans (100 g)	Roasted Coffee Beans (100 g)	Filtered Coffee Brew (330 mL)	Cold Brew Coffee (330 mL)
Carbohydrates	9–12.5 g	38 g	0 g	0.1 g
Fiber	46–53 g	31–38 g	1.2 g	0 g
Lipids	15–18 g	17 g	0.1 g	0 g
Proteins	8.5–12 g	7.5–10 g	0.1 g	0.1 g
Free amino acids	0.2–0.8 g	ND	NR	NR
Tryptophan	0.14 g	NR	0.028 g	NR
GABA	0.11 g	NR	NR	NR
Caffeine	0.8–1.4 g	1.3 g	0.244 g	0.412 g
Melatonin	0.7 mg	0.9 mg	0.026 mg	NR
Serotonin	1.3 mg	0.9 mg	0.048 mg	NR
Trigonelline	0.6–2.0 g	1 g	0.026 g	NR
Chlorogenic acids	4.1–9.2 g	1.9–2.7 g	0.009 g	13.2 g
Melanoidins	0 g	23 g	0.6 g	NR
Acrylamide	0 µg	24.4 µg	0.6–8.5 µg	1.4–1.8 µg
Ash	3–5.4 g	4.5 g	0.1 g	0 g
References	[9,12–16]	[9,12,14,17]	[12,13,17–26]	[19,21,27–29]

GABA, γ-aminobutyric acid; ND, not detected; NR, not reported.

The brewing procedure will also have an influence on the biochemical composition of the final coffee cup (Table 1) [30]. Coffee brewing is a solid–liquid extraction that involves water absorption by ground roasted coffee, solubilization of ground coffee in hot water, and separation of the water extract from spent coffee grounds. Many variables will affect the composition of the coffee cup, such as coffee particle size, time of extraction, pressure, type of filter, and water temperature, among others [31]. In the last years, consumers have shown great interest in "cold brew", a coffee beverage prepared with cold water (room temperature or refrigerated water) for up to 24 h [32]. Recent studies indicate that hot and cold brew coffees have small but important differences, particularly in the total antioxidant capacity of the resulting coffee [21]. Although melanoidins have not been characterized in cold brew coffee (Table 1) [33], water extraction temperature causes differential solubility of these molecules [34]. Therefore, further studies are needed to complete the chemical characterization of this popular beverage.

Whatever the brewing method, coffee and its components exert profound effects on the body, and some have already been mentioned above. As for any other food or beverage, the gastrointestinal tract is the first body system that gets in contact with coffee, and local effects do occur. Of course, other gastrointestinal effects occur after absorption of the different coffee components, with these also worth mentioning. Thus, the first part of this review focuses on the effects that coffee, its by-products and its components have been demonstrated to produce in the gastrointestinal tract. These may affect the function of different components of the gut wall (namely, mucosa, muscle, and intrinsic innervation), along the different organs of the gastrointestinal tract (Figure 1), and therefore their effects related with gastrointestinal cancer, inflammation, and mucosa functions (permeability, secretion) as well as in motor function will be discussed.

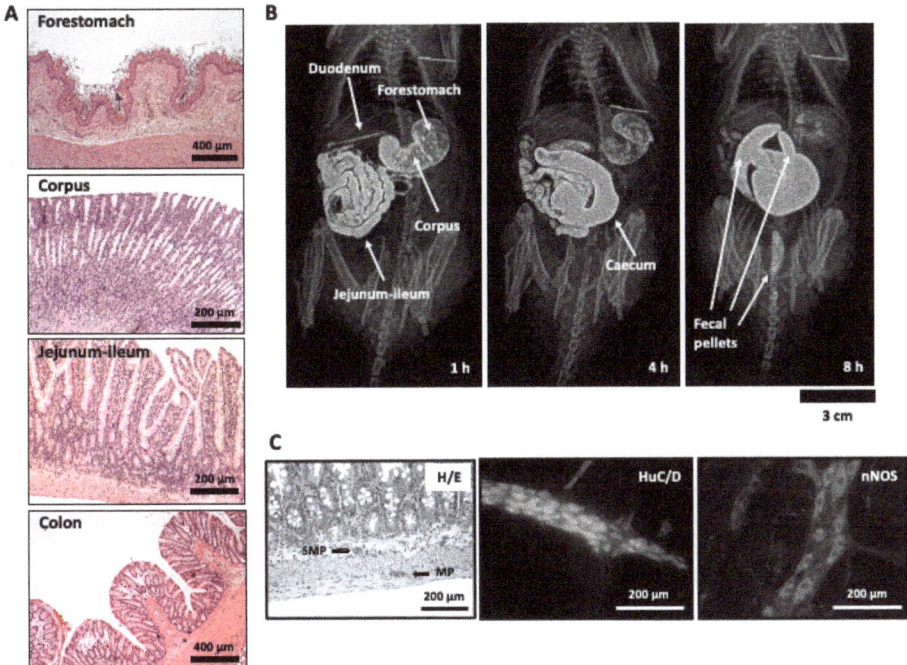

Figure 1. (**A**) Histological appearance of the wall of forestomach, corpus, jejunum-ileum (the longest part of the small intestine), and colon. (**B**) Organs of the rat gastrointestinal tract visualized by radiographic methods at different time points after intragastric barium administration in a conscious rat. Since rats do not vomit, barium can only progress towards the anus: 1 h after contrast, the two parts of the rat stomach (forestomach and corpus) can be distinguished, as well as the duodenum and the jejunum-ileum; 4 h after contrast, the stomach and small intestine can still be partially seen but now the cecum is filled with contrast; 8 h after contrast, the stomach and small intestine are barely seen, but the cecum is well filled with contrast and some fecal pellets are present within the colon. (**C**) Microscopic images showing the appearance of the enteric nervous system: left, location of the submucous (SMP) and the myenteric plexuses (MP) within the rat ileal wall in histological sections, stained with hematoxylin/eosin (H/E); middle and right, whole-mount or "sheet-like" preparations (from guinea pig ileum), obtained after dissecting away mucosa, submucosa, and circular muscle, leaving behind only the longitudinal muscle layer with the myenteric plexus attached; whole-mount preparations were processed immunohistochemically to show all the neurons with the pan-neuronal marker HuC/D (middle), or the specific subpopulation of neurons immunoreactive to neuronal nitric oxide synthase (nNOS), for which both somata and nerve fibers, but not nuclei, can be distinguished (right).

Furthermore, the gastrointestinal tract is functionally connected with the brain, through the so-called brain–gut axis (or gut–brain axis) [35]. Whereas the effects of coffee and its components on the brain have been deeply studied, those on the brain–gut axis have received comparatively little attention. However, a large amount of evidence has accumulated on the association between psychological factors and gut sensory, motor, and immune functioning [36]. Accordingly, it is now recognized that a healthy brain–gut axis is key for emotional and affective stability, adequate responses to stress, and visceral pain modulation [37]. In fact, the increased awareness about the importance of the brain–gut interaction in gastrointestinal disorders has even given rise to the field of psychogastroenterology [38,39]. Thus, this review also briefly describes the effects that coffee, its by-products and its components have on the brain–gut axis and their possible role in this area.

2. Coffee and the Gastrointestinal Tract: Focus on the Mucosa

The effects of coffee on the gastrointestinal tract have been studied for years in order to understand its hypothetical stimulating or inhibiting properties and its mechanisms of action. This problem has been addressed through numerous epidemiological studies. These works have been mainly focused on neoplastic diseases, with conflicting results, although there is evidence suggesting that coffee may be associated with lower risk of some cancers. Indeed, systematic reviews have found a protective effect of coffee on liver, hepatocellular, and breast cancers. However, coffee seems to increase the risk for lung cancer development, whereas the association of coffee with other cancers such as those of the pancreas, bladder, ovaries, and prostate is controversial [40,41]. Regarding cancers of the digestive tract, most meta-analyses have revealed a modest or dose–response-inverse association between coffee and the risk of colorectal cancer (CRC) [42–48]. In particular, coffee consumption has been found to be inversely associated with risk of CRC in a dose-dependent manner in the northern regions of Israel [49] or among Japanese women [50]. Furthermore, a recent prospective observational study including 1171 patients, most of them with metastatic CRC, showed an increase in survival up to 8 months for those who consumed daily four or more cups of coffee [51]. Differences related with race or sex seem to be important when assessing results that can sometimes be conflicting. Thus, a meta-analysis by Micek et al. (2019) [52] did not find any evidence for the association between coffee intake and CRC risk but, when using pooled groups, coffee consumption was related with a decreased risk of colon cancer in never-smokers and in Asian countries, and with an increased risk of rectal cancer in the general population, not considering women, never-smokers, and European countries. Similarly, a systematic review and meta-analysis of 24 prospective studies on CRC showed that coffee exerts a protective effect in men and women combined and in men alone. Regarding ethnicity, a significant protective association was noted in European men and in Asian women. Decaffeinated coffee exhibited a protective effect in both men and women [53]. On the contrary, other researchers have found no protective evidence for coffee. It is worth mentioning the EPIC cohort study by Dik et al. (2014) [54] that involved more than 400,000 Europeans and showed no association between coffee consumption and CRC. Park et al. (2018) [55] also found no relationship between CRC and coffee consumption in a large prospective multiethnic cohort study involving 4096 patients. Similarly, prospective studies among Swedish women did not find any relationship between CRC and the intake of four or more cups of coffee per day [56]. The same type of study among the British population also found no relationship between coffee and stomach, small bowel, or colorectal cancers [57]. In this respect, the results of gastric cancer are difficult to evaluate. Some meta-analyses affirm that coffee diminishes the risk of gastric cancer [58] but in other cases the results are conflicting, depending directly on the sex of the patients [59,60] or on the part of the stomach studied, with a direct relationship being found between coffee intake and gastric cardia cancer but not other cancers affecting the stomach [61]. Similarly, the association with esophageal cancer does not seem clear since there are systematic reviews that affirm that the relationship between coffee consumption and the incidence of this cancer either does not exist [61,62] or is attributable to the temperature of the beverage [63]. On the contrary, a meta-analysis comparing coffee and tea found a significant correlation between coffee and esophageal cancer [64].

Results of epidemiologic studies on non-neoplastic pathologies are also controversial. Some meta-analyses have shown that overall coffee did not seem to be a causal factor for chronic gastroesophageal reflux disease (GERD) [65], whereas an Italian study found an adverse effect of coffee among Barrett's esophagus (BE) patients [66]. On the contrary, a survey in the United States did not find any association between coffee intake and the risk of BE [67].

The variability described above may be due to many causes, including sex, ethnicity, lifestyles, and the numerous bioactive compounds present in coffee. In fact, it soon became evident that caffeine, considered the main component of coffee, was not really the only bioactive compound in coffee. In particular, the discovery during the second half of the last century, that even decaffeinated coffee causes an increase in gastric acid secretion and a reduction in the competence of the lower esophageal sphincter [68,69], led to an investigation of the physiological effect of the other coffee derived-compounds. As mentioned above, coffee composition depends on many factors such as coffee origin, method of preparation (water steam temperature, roasting, etc), resulting in variable effects on physiology and microbiome [41,70–73].

Thus, studies conducted in vivo with animal models or volunteers, or in vitro with isolated cells to separately evaluate the effects of the various compounds present in coffee, are much less numerous than the epidemiological reports. The interspecific differences in metabolism or the different doses tested have a great impact on the results obtained. However, although still incomplete and somehow leading to contradictory results, the efforts to investigate the mechanisms by which coffee manifests its effects and the specific compounds responsible for them have already shed some light on the subject, as shown next.

2.1. In Vitro Studies

2.1.1. Coffee

Since the decade of 1980, several studies have investigated whether coffee or its derivatives have carcinogenic effects. These studies identified potentially harmful compounds such as hydrogen peroxide (H_2O_2) in various coffee preparations. However, these studies were carried out in bacterial models that lacked the enzymes of peroxisomes, and thus this supposed carcinogenic effect could not apply to humans. The compounds in coffee that are responsible for the generation of these potential harmful effects were not identified either [74,75].

Similarly, the anti-inflammatory properties have been investigated in coffee preparations such as coffee "charcoal", a herbal preparation produced by roasting green dried coffee and milling to powder. In this case, the intestinal cells increased their barrier function, and inflammatory mediators such as interleukin (IL) IL-6, IL-8, tumor necrosis factor (TNF), methyl-accepting chemotaxis protein-1 (MCP-1), and prostaglandin (PG) E2 were inhibited [76]. However, this preparation also preserves most of the compounds in coffee and it is difficult to identify a specific molecule responsible for these effects.

In line, the incubation of CaCo2 cells (a human colorectal adenocarcinoma cell line), with regular, filtered, decaffeinated, or instant coffee resulted in an induction of the transcription of uridine diphosphate (UDP) glucuronosyltransferases (UGT1A), proteins with indirect antioxidant properties. The responsible molecule for this upregulation remained elusive also in this case [77].

2.1.2. Caffeine

The alkaloid caffeine is amongst the most studied coffee components [41]. Caffeine has been considered to possess antioxidant properties, although very high doses were needed to demonstrate them [78]. On the contrary, when physiological concentrations were used, caffeine did not show any antioxidant activity measured by oxygen-radical absorbing capacity. However, the antioxidant activity was significant when using 1-methylxanthine and 1-methyluric acid, the main metabolites of caffeine in humans. The antioxidant effects of these compounds are equivalent to those produced by ascorbic acid and uric acid, respectively [79]. This does not rule out, however, the involvement of other mechanisms.

Colonic cell lines have also been used to assess the anti-inflammatory activity of caffeine. Co-cultures of human colorectal adenocarcinoma cell line CaCo2 and 3T3-L1 adipocytes in the presence of caffeine have shown that caffeine inhibits the secretion of inflammatory cytokines interleukin (IL) IL-8 and plasminogen activator inhibitor-1 (PAI-1) and decreases lipid accumulation in adipocytes, whereas it has no effect on 3T3-L1 cells alone [80]. Related to this, CaCo2, goblet, and macrophage cell lines have also been co-cultured to study the effects on mechanisms relevant for inflammatory bowel disease (IBD).

In fact, more recent studies focused on caffeine tend to show the opposite. Moreover, caffeine has also been shown to increase sensitivity to radiotherapy of RKO cells in the transition from G1 to G2 phases in the cell cycle [81]. Caffeine may also act synergistically with the suppressor gene phosphatase and tensin homolog (PTEN), suppressing cell growth and inducing apoptosis in several human CRC cell lines but not in fibroblasts. This effect was induced through downregulation of the serine/threonine kinase (AKT) kinase pathway, and modulation of the p44/42MAPK pathway even in the absence of p53 [82]. Additionally, caffeine inhibits hypoxia-inducible factor-1 (HIF-1) in HT29 CRC cells cultured in hypoxic conditions. It also reduces vascular endothelial growth factor (VEGF) promoter activity and IL-8 expression, essential factors involved in tumor angiogenesis. The inhibition of kinases such as extracellular signal-regulated kinase (ERK1/2), *p38*, and AKT through blockade of their phosphorylation might also be the mechanism elicited by caffeine in this case. Additionally, it also inhibited cell migration stimulated by the adenosine A3 receptor [83]. These effects of caffeine may be different in cells of different origin or when it is administered synergically with other molecules. Thus, caffeine cannot inhibit ERK phosphorylation and the consequent epidermal growth factor (EGF)- and H-Ras-induced neoplastic transformation in the JB6 P epithelial cell line [84]. Similarly, caffeine activates the ERK signaling pathway in the Colo-205 CRC cell line, resulting in an increase of the anti-apoptotic protein myeloid cell leukemia 1 (Mcl-1) and a higher resistance to paclitaxel [85]. This effect was not observed with the HT-29 cell line, although in this case incubation with caffeine lasted only 20 h [86]. These differences can be explained considering particularities in cell lines, exposure time, and/or concentration of caffeine assayed. It is also important to consider that in vitro research may not fully reflect the complex relationships in multicellular organisms nor the dosage finally reaching the different tissues in vivo. Regarding this, Guertin et al. (2015) [87] studied a large number of serum metabolites present in coffee drinkers and found that some caffeine-related metabolites were inversely associated with CRC. Experimental in vivo studies are needed to understand the mechanisms underlying the exact caffeine–cancer association.

2.1.3. Polyphenols

Polyphenols are other important compounds present in coffee. They include different concentrations of CGAs, composed of quinic acid with trans-cinnamic acids, with the caffeoylquinic acids (CQAs), especially the 5-O-caffeoylquinic acid (5-CQA) and one of the metabolites of CGA, caffeic acid (CA), as the most studied [70,73]. Polyphenols have strong antioxidant properties both in decaffeinated and regular coffee and may also reduce the activation of proinflammatory factors such as nuclear factor-kβ (NF-kβ) in cultured myoblasts proportionally to CGA concentration, with regular coffee being twice as potent as decaffeinated coffee [88]. Similarly, Zhao et al. (2008) [89] demonstrated that the secretion of IL-8 induced by H_2O_2 or by tumor necrosis factor-receptor (TNF-R) activation may be blocked by 5-CQA in a dose-dependent manner in human intestinal epithelial CaCo2 cells. These effects are interesting since over-expression of pro-inflammatory elements and increased amounts of reactive oxygen species (ROS) are closely associated with DNA damage and multiple cell-signaling pathways involved in pathogenesis of important diseases such as cancer [41,90]. Moreover, 5-CQA and especially CA inhibit cell growth in the transition from G1 to G2/M phases of the cell cycle in the HT-29 CRC cell line [91]. In relation to this, it has been demonstrated that CA affects cyclin D1 expression in the same cell line. Cyclin D1 is required for G1/S transition in the cell cycle and over-expressed in many cancers. The levels of this protein are downregulated through the over-expression of the signal transducer and activator of transcription 5 (STAT5) protein and a decrease in activating transcription factor 2 (ATF-2) protein expression [92]. Overexpression of STAT5 may result in increased apoptosis, and decreased ATF-2 expression may have an anticancer action [73]. As with caffeine, a direct effect of CA has been shown on the inhibition of ERK phosphorylation, with the result of the downregulation of the neoplastic transformation of JB6 P1 cells [84]. CA also induces apoptosis and reduces invasiveness of other colorectal cell lines such as the murine CT26 cell line and in cell lines from different origin such as leukemia or endothelial cells [73]. On the contrary, Choi et al. (2015) [86] did not find any antiproliferative effect of CA or CGA on the same HT-29 cell line. However, in this case, shorter periods of incubation were assayed (20 h in [86] vs. 48–96 h in [91]).

Another important element that influences protein expression are epigenetic marks. One key factor of such regulation is the addition of methyl groups to DNA. 5-CQA and CA have resulted as strong inhibitors of DNA methylation in vitro. A DNA methyltransferase inhibition of up to 80% of normal values was achieved when the higher concentration was tested [93]. The meaning of this effect is yet to be determined.

Finally, polyphenols may also exhibit some effect on epithelial permeability. T84 CRC cells mounted in Ussing-type chambers and incubated in the presence of physiological concentrations of hydroxycinnamic acids and flavonoids showed that some of them, such as ferulic and isoferulic acids, significantly increase the expression of proteins of the tight junction complexes (zonulin 1 (ZO-1) and claudin-4) but reduce others such as occludin. In contrast, CA had no effects on the transcription of either ZO-1 or occludin [94].

2.1.4. Diterpenes

Diterpenes are fatty acyl esters that have also attracted attention as coffee bioactive compounds. They are present at variable quantities in coffee beans and unfiltered coffee but in small amounts in filtered and soluble coffee [41,73]. The most studied is kahweol, which has been shown to behave as a potent inhibitor of in vitro cell viability. HT-29 CRC cells decrease their viability after exposure to kahweol at smaller concentrations than those of caffeine, CA, or CGA. This effect is mediated by an increase in the pro-apoptotic caspase-3 and a decrease in the expression of anti-apoptotic Bcl-2 and phosphorylated AKT in a dose-dependent manner [86]. The apoptotic action of kahweol has also been observed with other colorectal carcinoma cell lines (HCT116, SW480, and LoVo). In these cell lines, in addition to the HT-29 line, kahweol stimulates the activating transcription factor 3 (ATF-3), a factor known to act as a tumor suppressor in CRC that downregulates cyclin D1 and enhances p53 protein. Inhibition of ERK1/2 and glycogen synthase kinase 3 beta (GSK3β) kinases blocked kahweol-mediated ATF-3 expression [95]. Accordingly, the same authors found that kahweol decreases cyclin D1 concentration without affecting its mRNA levels. Degradation in proteasomes might be the cause of this reduction since proteasome inhibitors blocked the decrease of cyclin D1 protein levels. In accordance with this, kahweol induces the activation of ERK1/2, c-Jun N-terminal kinase (JNK), and GSK3β kinases, resulting in phosphorylation of cyclin D1, which leads to proteasomal degradation. The antiproliferative action of kahweol was not observed in the normal colon cell line CCD-18-Co [95]. In addition, kahweol may significantly attenuate the expression of the heat shock protein 70 (HSP70), causing a cytotoxic effect that is increased when cells are incubated with the chaperone inhibitor triptolide [86]. NF-kβ is another key regulatory factor implicated in inflammation and immune response that is overexpressed in many cancers [96]. Kahweol blocks NF-kβ activation through inhibiting the IkB kinase (IKK) activity. Similarly, both kahweol and cafestol, another diterpene, significantly suppress the pro-inflammatory cyclooxygenase-2 (COX-2) protein and its mRNA expression in a dose-dependent manner [97]. Anti-oxidant properties of kahweol and cafestol have also been demonstrated in non-digestive cell types such as hepatocytes, neurons, or fibroblasts, where they have been shown to be highly protective against H_2O_2-induced oxidative DNA damage and the generation of superoxide radicals via different mechanisms, such as the induction of cytoprotective enzymes such as the heme oxygenase-1 (HO-1) [98–100].

2.1.5. Maillard Reaction Products: Melanoidins

Finally, melanoidins formed during the roasting process present interesting health-promoting properties. Indeed, several biological activities, such as antioxidant, antimicrobial, anticariogenic, anti-inflammatory, antihypertensive, and antiglycative activities, have been attributed to coffee melanoidins [10]. It is considered that the amount of melanoidins with antioxidant properties depend on the roasting conditions [15]. These antioxidant properties may be higher than in other sources, as shown by their ability to inhibit lipid peroxidation in an in vitro model of simulated gastric digestion [101] or in other non-digestive systems [41,102]. However, the exact mechanisms involved in such functions remain to be studied in detail.

2.2. In Vivo Studies

2.2.1. Coffee

The potentially protective effect of coffee appeared to be supported by the first studies carried out in animals. Indeed, it was demonstrated that the chronic feeding of rodents with coffee did not increase but decreased in some cases (as in the stomach) the incidence of spontaneous tumors [103,104]. Similarly, coffee protected rats against the effects of carcinogens such as 1,2-dimethylhydrazine in the colon, although not in the small intestine [105], and it also elicited a 14-fold induction of the antioxidant and cytoprotective transferases UGT1A in the stomach of transgenic mice [77]. However, its mechanisms of action have not yet been fully elucidated. In this way, coffee consumption of over 1 cup of coffee daily in colon cancer patients has been associated with a significant attenuation of ERK, a kinase directly involved in the development of colon cancer [84]. On the other hand, differences in coffee consumers and non-consumers have been found with regard to DNA methylation levels of genes related with coffee-associated effects. The potential epigenetic action of coffee may also be mediated by sex hormones and cell type since it was only observed in women who never used hormone therapy and in mononuclear cells from blood but not from saliva [106].

Coffee has also been related with a transient damage of gastric mucosa since it increases permeability to sucrose in healthy volunteers [107].

Lastly, coffee consumption has been shown to have an impact on gut microbiota both in experimental animals and humans, even with only 3 cups a day. Decreased amounts of *Escherichia coli*, *Enterococcus* spp., *Clostridium* spp., and *Bacteroides* spp. have been reported, together with an upregulation of *Lactobacillus* spp. and *Bifidobacterium* spp. populations. In any case, the exact implications of these changes induced by coffee on the microbiota need to be determined [108–110].

2.2.2. Caffeine

With regards to specific compounds such as caffeine, their concentration, as already mentioned, changes strongly according to coffee brand and method of preparation, which makes it very difficult to assess caffeine intake on a population basis [41].

Caffeine is rapidly absorbed in the stomach and small intestine and has been proposed to reduce cancer risk by altering the metabolism of carcinogens such as 2-amino-1-methyl-6-phenylimidazo (4,5-*b*) pyridine (PhIP), as shown in rats. PhIP is an amine to which humans are strongly exposed from cooked meat and fish and, accordingly, it has been implicated in CRC. Regarding this, coffee has been shown to increase the expression of enzymes involved in the detoxification of PhIP, such as glutathione *S*-transferase (GST) [111]. As a result, caffeine decreased the number of PhIP-induced colonic aberrant crypt foci (ACF) preneoplastic lesions [112]. Interestingly, a study with human healthy volunteers showed that unfiltered coffee elicited an increase in the detoxification capability and anti-mutagenic properties of the colorectal mucosa through an increase in glutathione concentration [113]. However, it is important to note that when the carcinogenic effect of PhIP was combined with a fatty diet, cell proliferation increased without caffeine being able to prevent it, which is a factor to be considered when interpreting epidemiological studies [114]. Likewise, in a rat CRC model induced by N-methyl-N-nitro-N-nitrosoguanidine (MNNG), coffee decreased the development of dysplastic crypts in a caffeine-independent way, although both decaffeinated coffee and caffeine decreased inflammatory stress and DNA damage [115]. On the contrary, previous studies with a model of stomach carcinogenesis induced in rats by MNNG and NaCl showed that lipid peroxidation in the glandular stomach mucosa was inhibited by caffeine treatment, resulting in less gastric tumors [116]. Differences in caffeine dosage and administration and method of tumor induction might explain these contradictory results.

2.2.3. Polyphenols

Regarding polyphenols, studying ileostomy subjects, Olthof et al. (2001) [117] determined that about one-third of CGA is absorbed in the small intestine. The rest of the polyphenols reach the colon, where simpler molecules are produced by breakdown due to microbial activity and, thus, very few of the absorbed molecules retain the structure of the parent CQAs present in coffee. Therefore, microbial action is necessary for absorption of phenols but also the individual microbiome itself is modulated by them [70,72,118]. As a result, the CQA derivatives that are ultimately absorbed are very varied. It is not clear then whether they prevent or induce cell damage, and their overall effect in the body is far from being understood since the number of studies regarding CGA effects in vivo is very limited [41,73]. In any case, CA might be implicated in the decrease of cancer metabolism. Kang et al. (2011) [84] showed that lung metastasis induced in mice by infusion of CT-26 colon cancer cells are inhibited after CA administration. CA strongly suppresses the activity of mitogen-activated MAPK/ERK kinase (MEK1), a protein kinase whose constitutive activation results in cell transformation, and TOPK, a serine/threonine kinase expressed in high levels in CRC and an activator of ERKs. CA binds directly to either MEK1 or lymphokine-activated killer t-cell-originated protein kinase-like protein (TOPK) in an ATP-noncompetitive manner.

2.2.4. Diterpenes

A third group of bioactive compounds assayed in vivo are the diterpenes cafestol and kahweol. These compounds act in rats as chemoprotectants against PhIP. In this case, PhIP–DNA adduct formation in the colon was reduced up to 54% compared to controls. Similarly, these diterpenes reduced buccal carcinogenesis in hamster after dimethylbenz (a) anthracene (DMBA) treatment [119]. The effects of kahweol and cafestol seem dependent on the continuous presence of these compounds in the diet since they are reversible following their removal. These detoxicant effects might be mediated by the ability of kahweol and cafestol to induce GST and other metabolic enzymes such as UGT1A. In this way, it has been shown that diterpene ingestion results in 2.5-fold induction of GST and a dose-dependent increase in UGT1A in rats [99,120]. In mice, kahweol seems to be a more potent inductor of GST than cafestol [121]. A chemoprotective role of kahweol and cafestol by the direct prevention of carcinogen–DNA binding should also not be discarded [99].

The studies on the effects of these diterpenes in humans are scarce but an increase in total cholesterol in serum has been reported [122]. However, the variability in the concentration of cafestol and kahweol in commercial coffee makes it difficult to answer the question as to whether the beneficial effects observed in animals may occur in humans consuming moderate amounts of coffee without inducing hypercholesterolemia. This question remains open, although considering the difference between the dose needed for hypercholesterolemia and for enzyme induction in model animals, beneficial effects in humans might also be expected without an increase in blood cholesterol [99].

2.2.5. Maillard Reaction Products: Melanoidins and Acrylamide

Maillard reaction is a main chemical event taking place during coffee roasting. Melanoidins are produced during coffee roasting due to the Maillard reaction. As mentioned above, melanoidins display a wide range of beneficial properties. In a mouse model of IBD induced by dextran sodium sulfate (DSS), a correlation between the exposure to melanoidins and the attenuation of inflammation has been shown, although the precise mechanisms involved remain to be elucidated [123]. It would be interesting to investigate if their antioxidant and metal chelating activity, antimicrobial activity, and the ability to modulate colonic microflora, as well as antihypertensive activities described in vitro (see above), are reproducible in model animals.

Finally, it is worth mentioning that melanoidins behave in vivo as dietary fiber, being largely indigestible by humans and fermented in the gut [41,102]. Melanoidins might be relevant contributors to colonic health since their intake may reach up to 20% of the recommended daily intake of dietary fiber [15]. This will be more deeply discussed in the following section, focused on the effects of coffee and its components on gastrointestinal motility.

Acrylamide is also produced during roasting of coffee due to the high temperatures employed in this step of the food processing. After absorption, a significant fraction of acrylamide is converted metabolically to the chemically reactive and genotoxic glycidamide. Acrylamide is a very soluble carcinogen that has been shown to cause tumors in experimental animals at multiple organ sites, but not in digestive organs [124]. Interestingly, epidemiological studies have failed thus far to provide evidence of an increased risk of most types of cancer after exposure to acrylamide in humans [124,125].

However, acrylamide is not without effects on the gastrointestinal epithelium, as some reports in experimental animals (rats) have shown vascular congestion, mucosal erosions, and depletion of the protective surface mucus together with widespread inflammatory infiltration in gastric samples after 4-week oral administration of acrylamide at 30 mg/kg, due to severe oxidative stress manifested as a significant increase in lipid peroxidation and depletion of antioxidant enzymes in gastric tissue, as well as, likely, high nitric oxide (NO) production after inducible nitric oxide synthase (iNOS) induction [126].

3. Coffee and the Gastrointestinal Tract: Focus on Motor Function

Gastrointestinal motility is a complex process involving different elements. The element more directly responsible of motor function is the smooth muscle, of which two layers are found in all gastrointestinal organs: the circular (inner and thicker) and the longitudinal (outer and thinner) layers (their names refer to the orientation of their smooth muscle cells, around or along the longitudinal axis of the gastrointestinal tract; the stomach has an additional, oblique smooth muscle layer).

Between the inner and the outer muscle layers lie the myenteric plexus, the part of the enteric nervous system (ENS, intrinsic innervation of the gastrointestinal tract) directly responsible of gastrointestinal motor function [127]. In the myenteric plexus, different subpopulations of myenteric neurons participate in the generation of the different motor patterns, such as the peristaltic reflex, i.e., the basic motor pattern that allows the luminal contents to progress distally thanks to the oral contraction and aboral relaxation of the circular muscle, together with coordinated changes in the length of the longitudinal muscle. The enteric glial cells (which were previously considered simply as supportive cells for neurons, but now are recognized to exert important signaling functions) also collaborate to coordinate motility [128]. In addition, the interstitial cells of Cajal (ICC), located at different levels within the muscle layers and myenteric plexus, play a pacemaker role and generate stereotyped activity patterns (i.e., slow waves [129]).

Moreover, extrinsic innervation from the autonomic nervous system (vagal and pelvic nerves belonging to its parasympathetic branch, and splanchnic nerves belonging to the sympathetic branch) as well as hormones secreted within the gut wall (from enterochromaffin cells (ECs), L cells, etc.) or reaching the gut wall via the blood stream from different extrinsic endocrine glands, are classically recognized as important modulators of gastrointestinal tract motor function.

Finally, immune cells (mast cells in particular [127,130]) and microbiota may produce and release mediators and metabolites, respectively, that may remarkably alter motility and either contribute to maintain a healthy gut or facilitate the development of gut disorders.

The effects of coffee and its components on gastrointestinal tract motor function in general and the specific mechanisms involved have been relatively scarcely evaluated.

3.1. Effects of Coffee Brew on Gastrointestinal Motility

Despite the popular use of coffee around the world, the effects of this beverage on gastrointestinal motor function have surprisingly been evaluated only scarcely, especially when compared with those on other systems such as the cardiovascular and the central nervous systems. It was soon demonstrated that coffee reduces lower esophageal sphincter pressure [131] and stimulates secretion from the stomach [69]. Both effects may cause or aggravate heartburn, the most frequent effect attributed to coffee. This might be caused by direct irritation of the esophageal mucosa or by promoting GERD [132], which may favor the development of Barrett's esophagus (BE) (see above).

Using a barostat, coffee was found to prolong the adaptive relaxation of the proximal stomach, compared with an isotonic control solution, suggesting that it might slow gastric emptying [132]. However, other studies, using scintigraphy or applied potential tomography, indicate a lack of effect in stomach motor function, or even accelerated gastric emptying, in a portion of individuals [132–135]. These conflicting results may have been due to methodological differences, including the selection of participants (healthy or dyspeptic) or the type of coffee drink used for the studies [132]. Despite early associations of coffee drinking and functional dyspepsia [136], these were later attributed to study bias related with characteristics of patients (higher adiposity [137], more attentive to their symptoms [138]). Indeed, despite the relaxing effects of the proximal stomach, coffee did not modify gastric wall compliance, wall tension, or sensory function [139]. No association has been confirmed to occur either with peptic ulcer disease [132].

Caffeine-containing beverages (75–300 mg) were shown to induce a dose-related secretion from the small intestine [140], although coffee by itself had no significant effect on sodium and water transport, maybe due to compensatory effects by other coffee components [141]. Despite the common believe that coffee favors diarrhea, the effects on jejunal and ileal fluid secretion were not associated with changes in small bowel transit [140]. Orocecal transit studies did not find any significant effect of coffee compared with control solutions either [135]. However, these results could be due to the use of lactulose as a substrate for assessing transit, since this compound by itself accelerates transit and may have masked the possible effects of coffee [132,142].

In an early study, using radiographic techniques, it was shown that coffee, drunk together with a low-fat breakfast, induced a contraction of the gallbladder that was similar for regular and caffeinated coffee [143]. Years after, this was also demonstrated for regular coffee using ultrasonography, although no control drink was used as a comparator [144]. Further research, using a better controlled experimental design, confirmed that caffeinated and decaffeinated coffee induces cholecystokinin release and gallbladder contraction [145], which may explain why patients with symptomatic gallstones often avoid drinking coffee.

Regarding colonic motility, it was soon found that coffee, either caffeinated or not, promotes the desire to defecate at least in one-third of the population, predominantly women, and that this was associated with an increase in rectosigmoid motor activity. Furthermore, it was found that this increase occurred as soon as 4 min after drinking the coffee, caffeinated or not, but not after drinking hot water. Since (unsweetened) coffee contains no calories, and its effects on the gastrointestinal tract cannot be justified by its volume load, acidity, or osmolality, it was soon recognized that it must have pharmacological effects [132]. Thus, these findings were interpreted as mediated indirectly by a component of coffee other than caffeine, which, by acting on epithelial receptors in the stomach or small bowel, would trigger a gastrocolonic response, speculated at that time to be due to the release of cholecystokinin or another hormone [146].

Interestingly, these results were further supported using ambulatory colonic manometry [147]. In a study with 12 healthy volunteers, a probe was placed up to the mid-transverse colon and the following day the effects of four different drinks were evaluated: unsweetened black coffee, unsweetened decaffeinated coffee, a 1000 kcal meal, and water. Caffeinated coffee significantly increased colonic motor activity, including both propagated and simultaneous contractions, which were 60% and 23% greater than those of water and decaffeinated coffee, respectively, and similar to the effect of the meal. Both the caffeinated coffee and the meal (but not the decaffeinated coffee) produced a strong gastrocolonic response, but no significant effect of gender was detected in this case. Compared to water, coffee increased propagating contractions by 50%, suggesting that this drink may induce propulsive motor activity, and this was accompanied by a higher incidence of abdominal cramps, flatulence, and urination, leading to confirmation of the popular belief that coffee stimulates colonic motor activity. The effect of caffeinated coffee was similar to that of the meal during the first 30 min, although it was of shorter duration (1–1.5 h vs. 2–2.5 h). Decaffeinated coffee seemed to also enhance colonic motor activity but was less potent than caffeinated coffee and seemed to exert this effect only at the more proximal colonic sites recorded. The short latency of the effect of coffee (of either kind) after its ingestion was again interpreted as due to the involvement of an indirect mechanism, probably a neurohumoral response mediated by the small bowel, since gastric emptying of coffee occurs as soon as 15–20 min [148]. The authors acknowledged that the specific molecule involved was not yet known but mentioned different possibilities, such as cholecystokinin, exorphins (opioid-like molecules present in coffee), gastrin, or motilin, as well as the fact that other active ingredients contained in coffee could add their own direct effects on gut smooth muscle. Importantly, the authors suggested that the effect demonstrated for coffee could be beneficial for patients with colonic disorders such as slow transit constipation but might be detrimental to patients with diarrhea or fecal incontinence [147].

In these regards, Gkegkes et al. recently published a systematic review and meta-analysis in which they evaluated the evidence suggesting a potential role of coffee to prevent postoperative ileus [149]. Postoperative ileus is a significant complication of surgery, and management is not yet optimal. The underlying cause of this clinically relevant problem is multiple, including surgical manipulation itself, opioid analgesics, inflammation, electrolyte fluctuations, and imbalances in the autonomic function and gastrointestinal hormonal system [150,151]. Although frequently self-resolving, postoperative ileus represents an important clinical and economic burden, particularly hospital expenses, due to delayed discharge [152]. In addition to other measures, prokinetic agents (alvimopam, ghrelin agonists, neostigmine and serotonin receptor antagonists), chewing gum, gastrograffin, and coffee are used for management. The authors focused on coffee and found four randomized controlled trials as eligible for their study, with three of them referring to colorectal procedures [153–155] and only one to gynecological surgery [150], with a total of 341 patients (the sample size in each study was 58–114 patients). Coffee was administered postoperatively to 156 patients. The most remarkable results were (1) coffee did not significantly increase complications compared with the control group; (2) coffee significantly decreased the time period until the first bowel movement, as well as the time to tolerance of solid food, the first flatus, and the first defecation; (3) no significant effects were found regarding the length of hospital stay. Decaffeinated coffee was proved to reduce time to initiation of bowel movement [155], suggesting that caffeine is not necessary for coffee effect, and it was suggested that maybe CGAs and melanoidins could have a role [15]. Both display antioxidant effects, whereas melanoidins may contribute a fiber effect to coffee anti-ileus properties (see below). Moreover, the authors proposed that other chemically active agents might be formed during decaffeination [149]. Other mechanisms that may contribute to the positive effects of coffee are related with the anti-inflammatory effects of some of its compounds. In these regards, C-reactive protein (CRP) levels, used as a marker of postoperative complications, were found to be significantly lower in patients given coffee after removal of the nasogastric tube on the first postoperative day compared with the group of patients that were not given coffee. Furthermore, in that study, lower CRP levels were associated with reduced time to initiation of bowel movements, as well as reduced rates of postsurgical complications and hospitalization time, particularly in patients with a right colon tumor [155]. Another important conclusion of this meta-analysis is that, compared with alvimopam (a peripheral opioid antagonist), which also showed good results to reduce the constipating impact of opioid use associated with surgery [156,157], coffee may be a much cheaper therapeutic strategy to achieve comparable results [149]. As in other studies using coffee, the limitations highlighted by the authors include the differences in quality and quantity of administered coffee, together with low number of participants and heterogeneity of patients and operations.

In general, it can be said that studies performed thus far evaluating the effects of coffee in humans are relatively scarce, with relatively low numbers of participants and mainly healthy (other than those participating in the studies related with postoperative ileus), with high heterogeneity in the kind of coffee used and not too high methodological quality. In addition, no animal study could be found using coffee itself to test motility-related parameters, in contrast with studies of the effects of particular coffee components, as will be discussed next.

3.2. Caffeine

In vitro studies have mainly tested the effects of caffeine, whose pharmacology is quite complex. Thus, caffeine is a non-selective adenosinergic antagonist. In addition, in many cell types, caffeine releases calcium (Ca^{2+}) from internal stores through ryanodine receptors (RyR) and also increases the content of cyclic adenosine monophosphate (cAMP) by inhibiting the activity of phosphodiesterases [158].

Interestingly, caffeine has been used as a tool to investigate the contractile and/or electrical properties of the different components of the gut wall involved in motor function along the gastrointestinal tract [159], including the myenteric plexus (both neurons and glial cells), the smooth muscle cells, and ICCs, as well as their dependency on intracellular calcium dynamics.

The effects exerted in vitro by caffeine in the gastrointestinal smooth muscle have been tested using different techniques, including the recording of contractile activity of smooth muscle strips (which contain also myenteric plexus and ICCs) in organ baths, and the electrophysiological recording of cultured single smooth muscle cells. In these experiments, the effects of caffeine were shown to be dose-dependent, with low doses (0.1–0.3 mM) relaxing and high doses (>0.3 mM) producing a transient contraction followed by relaxation [160].

Moreover, caffeine at relatively high doses (1–10 mM) inhibits slow waves (generated by ICCs) in different gastrointestinal tissues from different species [161], including the human jejunum [162]. In addition, despite early reports of no effects of caffeine on glial cells [163], more recent studies have shown that caffeine at 0.01 mM produced an immediate and sustained Ca^{2+} response in all myenteric glial cells from mouse colon, confirming that they have ryanodine-sensitive Ca^{2+} stores [164]. Thus, caffeine might modulate glial cell function at relatively low doses, and this, in turn, may have an impact on gastrointestinal motor activity through coordinated responses with the myenteric neurons.

The effect of caffeine on the myenteric neurons has been studied using cultured isolated neurons/ganglia or whole-mount preparations (see Figures 1 and 2). In cultured myenteric neurons, caffeine was shown to concentration-dependently stimulate Ca^{2+} release, in a quantal and saturable manner, from intracellular Ca^{2+} stores that are refilled via depolarization-induced Ca^{2+} increases. This effect was shown to be sensitive to the RyR antagonists ryanodine, dantrolene, and procaine, but did not involve the participation of cAMP phosphodiesterase inhibition [163]. However, caffeine-releasable ryanodine-sensitive calcium stores are not the only subset of cytosolic Ca^{2+} storage and the calcium ionophore ionomycin applied after maximal caffeine effect in Fura-2-loaded myenteric neurons achieved further increases in intracellular free Ca^{2+} ($[Ca^{2+}]i$) [163]. An important drawback of these studies in cultured myenteric neurons/ganglia is that it is difficult to identify the functional subpopulations of myenteric neurons, although heterogeneity of the responses to caffeine (as well as to other drugs) is clearly observed, suggesting that it might affect different neuronal subtypes [163].

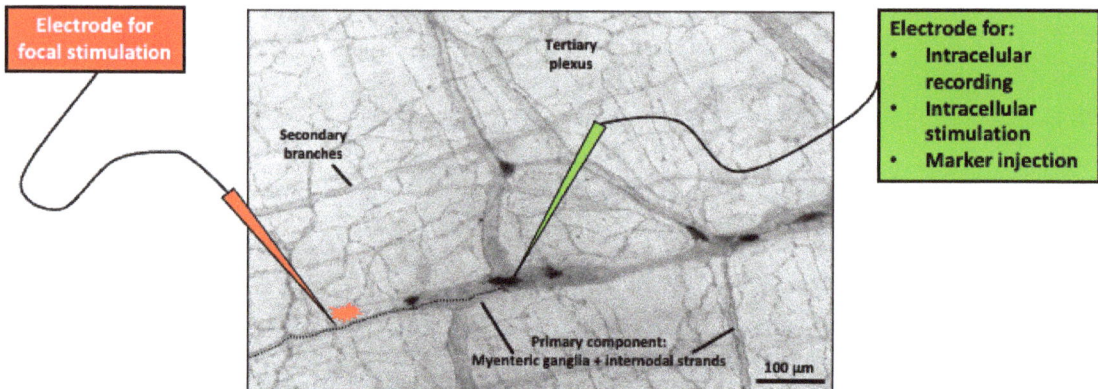

Figure 2. Intracellular recording from myenteric neurons. A fixed whole-mount preparation, processed immunohistochemically to show calretinin positive neurons, is used to illustrate how electrical activity of myenteric neurons would be recorded using current clamp electrophysiological modality. Calretinin immunoreactivity in guinea pig ileum whole-mount preparations allows one to distinguish the different components of the myenteric plexus: the primary component, which includes the myenteric ganglia and the internodal strands; the secondary branches that run circumferentially; and the tertiary plexus, a web of fine nerves that correspond to axons derived from excitatory longitudinal muscle motor neurons [165]. The intracellular recording electrode is represented in green (right)—this electrode allows for the recording of neuronal electrical activity, as well as direct intracellular stimulation of the cell with depolarizing or hyperpolarizing continuous or pulsed current, and marker injection to allow the impaled neuron to be visualized after immunohistochemical processing. The electrode for focal, extracellular stimulation is represented in red (left); this is placed on top of a circumferential internodal nerve strand. If the strand carries an axon (represented as a dotted line) that synapses on the impaled neuron, then focal stimuli (represented as a red blast symbol) will cause neurotransmitter release from the axon terminal and a postsynaptic potential on the impaled neuron (see Figure 3 for morphological and electrophysiological classifications of myenteric neurons).

In order to evaluate the effects of drugs on specific subpopulations of myenteric neurons, the use of whole-mount preparations is a better option. Whole-mount preparations are "sheets" of longitudinal muscle with the myenteric plexus attached. The other gut wall layers, i.e., mucosa, submucosa, and circular muscle, are dissected away to facilitate intracellular recording of myenteric neuron electrical activity. In addition, these experiments allow for the definition of the morphology of the impaled neuron through intracellular injection of a marker during recording, as well as its chemical code, by use of immunohistochemistry after fixation (Figure 2).

In these experiments, ryanodin-sensitive calcium stores were demonstrated to play a particularly important role in a specific subpopulation of myenteric neurons whose electrophysiological features (in whole-mount preparations) highly depend on $[Ca^{2+}]i$, the so-called AH/type II neurons (Figure 3), which are identified as intrinsic primary afferent neurons [166]. Morphologically, these are multipolar neurons with a smooth soma and projections to the mucosa and other myenteric neurons. Electrophysiologically, these neurons are characterized by relatively broad action potentials (APs) (i.e., the falling phase of their

APs display a "hump"), followed by two afterhyperpolarizations (AHPs); an early, short (ms) AHP; and a late, long-lasting (4–20 s) AHP [166]. Similar to cardiomyocytes, the broad AP is due to the influx of both sodium and calcium through voltage-gated channels. Importantly, Ca^{2+} entry during the AP is associated with a transient increase in $[Ca^{2+}]i$, released from RyR-sensitive stores, which amplifies calcium influx. This calcium-induced calcium release (CICR), in turn, leads to potassium efflux through calcium-operated potassium channels, which underlies the characteristic slow AHP of these neurons. Thus, activity-dependent CICR has been suggested to be a mechanism to grade the output of AH neurons according to the intensity of sensory input. Furthermore, AH neurons display relatively high resting levels of $[Ca^{2+}]i$, which, through the same indirect mechanism involving potassium efflux, maintain low their resting potential and reduce their excitability [167].

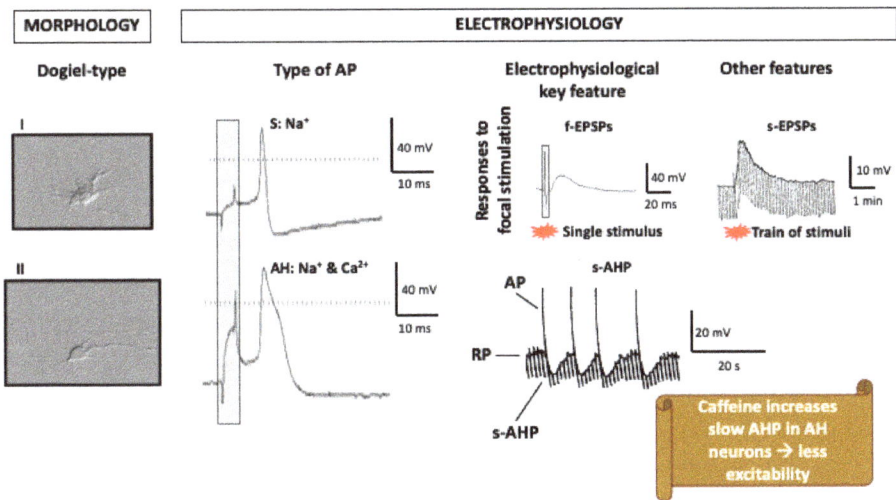

Figure 3. Morphological and electrophysiologic features of myenteric neurons and effect of caffeine on AH/II neurons. By use of intracellular recording methods illustrated in Figure 2, two main classes of myenteric neurons can be distinguished. According to morphology (left), neurons are classified as Dogiel type I (top) or Dogiel type II (bottom). These neurons broadly correspond to electrophysiological types S and AH, respectively. S neurons display short sodium-dependent APs, whereas APs of AH neurons are wider and depend on the entry of both Na^+ and Ca^{2+}, displaying a "hump" during the falling phase of the AP, due to Ca^{2+} entry. S neurons respond to single focal electrical stimuli with fast excitatory postsynaptic potentials (f-EPSPs), which are not seen in AH neurons, although both classes may respond to trains of focal stimulation with slow excitatory postsynaptic potentials (s-EPSPs). Finally, AH neurons display a s-AHP, due to K^+ efflux dependent on the increase in intracellular free Ca^{2+} ($[Ca^{2+}]i$) released from ryanodine-dependent stores. This s-AHP is increased and prolonged by caffeine, making these neurons, which are intrinsic peripheral nerve afferents, less excitable. Abbreviations: AP, action potential; f-EPSP, fast excitatory postsynaptic potential; RP, resting potential; s-AHP, slow after hyperpolarization; s-EPSP, slow excitatory postsynaptic potentials. Light grey blocks with dotted border, artifact of the stimulus; red blast symbol, focal stimulus.

Interestingly, activation of AH myenteric neurons by caffeine turns into a reduction of their excitability due to the increase in $[Ca^{2+}]i$ released from ryanodine-dependent stores and the consequent potassium-mediated hyperpolarization [167,168]. How this translates into in vivo effects is not clear, but it is important to remember that AH/type II myenteric neurons extend projections to the mucosa where caffeine might activate them directly, leading to the indirect inhibitory effect suggested by these in vitro studies.

3.3. Polyphenols

Wood and collaborators used intracellular recording of enteric neurons and CA as a tool to understand the mechanisms underlying pathophysiology of secretory diarrhea associated with food allergies [169]. Antigen-evoked mast cell degranulation in the small and large intestine starts an immediate (type I) hypersensitivity reaction characterized by mucosal hypersecretion [170] and strong contractions of the musculature [171], which are sensitive to tetrodotoxin and atropine, meaning that these reactions implicate the participation of the ENS. Exposure to an antigen, then, triggers a coordinated immunoneural defense program response aimed at getting rid of the antigenic threat, which translates into watery diarrhea, fecal urgency, and abdominal pain [172]. In the study by Wood et al., CA, which is a 5-lipoxygenase inhibitor [173], was able to partially suppress the hyperexcitability of submucous neurons induced by β-lactoglobulin in the small intestine of guinea pigs, which was used as a model of anaphylactic responses associated with food allergies [169]. Thus, this study demonstrated the involvement of leukotrienes in the secretory response of submucous neurons to food antigens. However, to our knowledge, the in vitro effects of CA on the myenteric neurons in the context of food allergy has not been tested thus far.

Of note, CA and CGA may exert an important neuroprotective role in the context of Parkinson's disease (PD), including on the ENS, which is discussed in Section 4. However, to our knowledge, the potential impact of these polyphenols on gastrointestinal motility altered in preclinical models of PD or in patients, has not been specifically evaluated.

3.4. Dietary Fiber

Dietary fiber is also present in coffee. Our group evaluated the effect of two coffee-derived by-products proposed as natural sources of dietary fiber on in vivo rat gastrointestinal motility using radiographic methods after intragastric administration of barium as contrast (Figure 1B illustrates this procedure). In one of them, different experiments were performed to evaluate the properties of instant spent coffee grounds (SCGs) [174]. The gastrointestinal motility study was performed after the 1st, 14th, and 28th intragastric administration of SCGs. The product accelerated transit in both the small intestine (since the cecum of the rats was reached significantly more quickly than that of control rats), and the colon (since formation of fecal pellets occurred also much more quickly in SCGs-exposed than in vehicle-treated animals). However, this effect was restricted to the first radiographic session, after the first SCG dose, whereas it was not apparent after the 14th or the 28th doses. Thus, the dietary fiber effect acutely produced by SCG administration seemed to be followed by tolerance development, although no sign of impaired motility was found in any animal. The acute pro-motility effects of SCG demonstrated in that study could be influenced by short chain fatty acids (SCFAs), which have been shown to be released during SCGs fermentation by colon microbiota from medium and dark roasted coffee beans at concentrations higher than 10 mM [175], and SCFAs (10–200 mM) stimulate colonic motility [176]. Interestingly, an aqueous extract of coffee silverskin, another coffee by-product, may also display dietary fiber effect since total SCFAs derived from coffee silverskin extract fermentation were higher in feces of rats treated with the extract for 28 days [177]. Although its precise in vivo effects on gastrointestinal motility still needs to be determined, it might be related with the presence of melanoidins in it (see Section 3.5).

3.5. Maillard Reaction Products: Melanoidins and Acrylamide

The other radiographic study of gastrointestinal motility performed by our group evaluated the effect of melanoidins from the previously mentioned aqueous extract of coffee silverskin [178]. Coffee silverskin is the tegument of the outer layer of the coffee bean, representing approximately 4.2% (w/w) of the coffee cherry and is the only by-product produced during coffee roasting [179]. Coffee silverskin has been proposed as a sustainable natural source of prebiotics, antioxidants, and dietary fiber [180]. The antioxidant properties of coffee silverskin extract are due to the presence of CGA [181], but also to the melanoidins generated during the roasting process [182]. Melanoidins are high molecular weight brown polymeric compounds generated during the last stage of the Maillard reaction [183], and those derived from coffee are described as "Maillardized dietary fiber" [184]. Thus, the fiber effect was studied in vivo, in healthy male Wistar rats, at a dose of 1 g/kg in drinking water. After 4 weeks, the rats received barium sulphate by gavage and radiographs were taken 0–8 h afterwards. In addition, the colonic bead expulsion test was performed to specifically determine the possible effects on colonic propulsion. In line with the previous study with SCGs, melanoidins accelerated transit in small intestine (since the caecum was reached significantly more quickly in melanoidin-exposed rats than in control animals) and tended to accelerate fecal pellet formation, although this effect was not significant. Interestingly, fecal pellets from the melanoidin group tended to be slightly larger, which might have been a result of the higher fiber intake in this group, making the fecal pellets slightly more effective to mechanically stimulate the colon. Moreover, melanoidins did not significantly alter the latency of expulsion of a bead inserted 3 cm into the colorectum, suggesting that the motor agents (intrinsic and extrinsic innervation, smooth muscle, and ICCs) involved in the colonic propulsion at this level were not altered by dietary exposure to coffee silverskin-derived melanoidins and that these may have potential to be used as a functional food ingredient [178]. Interestingly, Argirova et al. (2010) [185] showed that melanoidins act upon muscle tone and might facilitate Ca^{2+} influx into the cells of isolated gastric muscle layers. Thus, these compounds might exert their pro-motility action not only through a fiber effect, but also through the direct activation of gastrointestinal smooth muscle cells, which needs to be confirmed to occur also using isolated intestinal muscle tissue.

As mentioned above, acrylamide is formed as a result of Maillard reaction between amino acids and sugars during heating [186], which occurs also during coffee roasting. Although the dietary intake of acrylamide in humans is difficult to assess, the estimated dietary exposure for the general population ranges from 0.3 to 0.8 µg/kg of body weight per day [187]. This is due to the exposure, not only to coffee, but also to other foods (chips, cereals) and industrial products (those related with polymer, glues and paper, water treatment, and cosmetic industries [126]) that may also contain acrylamide in relevant concentrations to impact human health. Despite the fact that the digestive tract is one of the main routes of acrylamide absorption, and the fact that intake of acrylamide-containing foods, including coffee, is still growing, its effect on the ENS neurons has scarcely been assessed, yet this is important because acrylamide is a peripheral nervous system toxin.

Acrylamide effects were studied in a coculture model of intestinal myenteric neurons, smooth muscle cells, and glia [188]. In this study, acrylamide was added to the cocultures in doses ranging from 0.01 mM to 12 mM, followed by incubation for 24, 96, or 144 h. In contrast with botulinum toxin A, which was also tested in the same system and only altered neuronal function, acrylamide damaged enteric neuron structure when used at 0.5–2 mM. At these doses, the damage was selective for the axonal structures, without affecting survival, whereas at higher doses, neuronal survival was significantly reduced. Axonal loss was accompanied by reduced acetylcholine release, which was negligible at 4 mM. The mechanism involved synaptic vesicle synthesis and function, but not choline uptake. Neuronal loss at high doses involved mainly a necrotic mechanism, although a low frequency of noncaspase-3-mediated apoptotic death was also demonstrated. Interestingly, it was also shown that after low-dose acrylamide challenge, axon regeneration was possible. In fact, axon growth occurred more rapidly than in control cultures over the 24–96 h period after low-dose challenge, suggesting the involvement of compensatory mechanisms after the initial damaging insult. However, neurotransmitter release was found to lag behind axonal regrowth by at least several days. Interestingly, all the changes described were selective to neurons (irrespective of the underlying phenotype), with enteric glial cells apparently not being affected [188].

Acrylamide has also been shown to produce neurotoxic effects on the ENS after oral administration to experimental animals. Early studies showed changes in the ENS in acrylamide-treated rats resembling those of streptozotocin-induced diabetic animals, with alterations of the catecholaminergic content, a decrease in the amount of calcitonin gene-related peptide (CGRP), and a corresponding increase in the levels of vasoactive intestinal peptide (VIP) [189]. However, those studies did not evaluate whether these changes were associated with neuronal loss, axonal degeneration, or altered function. More recently, the effects of acrylamide administration have been studied in pig models. The results suggest that even low doses of acrylamide affect the structure and function of the gastrointestinal tract and cause a significant response of ENS neurons. For example, the expression of cocaine- and amphetamine-regulated transcript (CART), which exerts a crucial role in neuronal response to stress stimuli and neuroprotection, was increased, particularly in the myenteric plexus of the small intestine in immature female pigs receiving a low or a high dose of acrylamide by the oral route for 28 days, which was interpreted to occur as part of the neuronal protection/recovery processes within the gastrointestinal tract in response to this pathological stimulus [190]. Galanin is another peptide with neuroprotective properties that mediates survival or regeneration after neural injury and exerts anti-inflammatory activities [191,192]. Thus, in the same porcine model, the population of galanin-like immunoreactive neurons was found to be increased in both the submucous and myenteric plexuses of the stomach, even at low doses. Moreover, the submucous and myenteric neuronal populations of cells immunoreactive to galanin and simultaneously immunoreactive to VIP, nNOS, or CART were increased. These findings were, again, interpreted by the authors as a neurotrophic/neuroprotective role of galanin (in possible co-operation with VIP, nNOS, and CART) in the recovery processes in the gastric ENS after acrylamide intoxication [193]. One more paper of this series was published in the year 2019 and found similar results in the pig duodenum. As before, acrylamide was used at a low (0.5 µg/kg) daily dose considered tolerable, or at a 10-fold dose (5 µg/kg), by the oral route for 4 weeks. Both treatments led to significant increases in the percentage of neurons immunoreactive to substance P (SP), CGRP, galanin, nNOS, and vesicular acetylcholine transporter (VACHT), although the high dose exerted more intense changes. In this case too, the interpretation given by the authors is that all these changes may be compensatory plastic effects in an attempt to protect neurons from damage and restore enteric neuronal homeostasis [194]. Of note, although acrylamide activates microglial cells both in vivo and in vitro, leading to the release of proinflammatory cytokines, and consequently contributing to neuronal damage [195], the involvement of enteric glial cells in enteric neuronal alterations induced by acrylamide has not been specifically evaluated yet, except for the above-mentioned study that used cocultures of intestinal myenteric neurons, smooth muscle cells, and glia, and did not show any acrylamide-induced alterations in this last cell type [188].

4. Coffee and the Brain–Gut Axis

As already mentioned, coffee is a natural source of compounds (Figure 4) able to exert crucial effects in the brain–gut axis [196].

Interestingly, when "brain–gut axis" and "coffee" are combined as keywords in Pubmed, only three papers are retrieved (as of 29th November 2020), and two of them lead with the relationship of coffee with PD (see below) [197,198]. The other one is a recent study by Papakonstantinou et al. [199], who performed a randomized, double blind, crossover clinical trial (ClinicalTrials.gov ID: NCT02253628) with 40 healthy young (20–55 years of age) individuals of both sexes to study the effect of 200 mL coffee beverages containing 160 mg caffeine (hot and cold instant coffee, cold espresso, hot filtered coffee) on (1) self-reported gastrointestinal symptoms, (2) salivary gastrin, (3) stress indices (salivary cortisol and α-amylase) and psychometric measures, and (4) blood pressure. Importantly, the participants were daily coffee consumers, and the study was performed in non-stressful conditions. There was no effect of coffee on self-reported anxiety levels. Furthermore, the participants reported a very low score (1 out of 10) for all the questions pertaining to negative gastrointestinal symptoms (i.e., abdominal discomfort, bloating, dyspepsia, and heartburn), chronic stress, and negative feelings, whereas the score was high (9 out of

10) for all the questions pertaining to positive feelings. Coffee consumption significantly increased salivary α-amylase activity, with significant differences only between cold instant and filtered coffee at 15 and 30 min after intake. Irrespective of coffee type, salivary gastrin was temporarily increased, whereas salivary cortisol or self-reported anxiety levels were not affected. However, at the end of the experimental periods, blood pressure was significantly increased (but within the healthy physiological levels), independently of coffee type/temperature. Although many studies have addressed the cardiovascular and central effects of coffee and caffeine, the report by Papakonstantinou et al. seems to be the only study specifically evaluating their effects on the brain–gut axis as a whole, in the same individuals and under the same conditions. Thus, it was demonstrated that acute coffee consumption in non-stressful conditions was not associated with gastrointestinal symptoms but activated the sympathetic nervous system, associated with increases in salivary α-amylase and blood pressure but not salivary cortisol, which was interpreted as due to a possible anti-stress effect of coffee [199], possibly contributed by a coffee compound other than caffeine. Thus, it is important to study the effects not only of coffee, but also of its components, on the brain–gut axis.

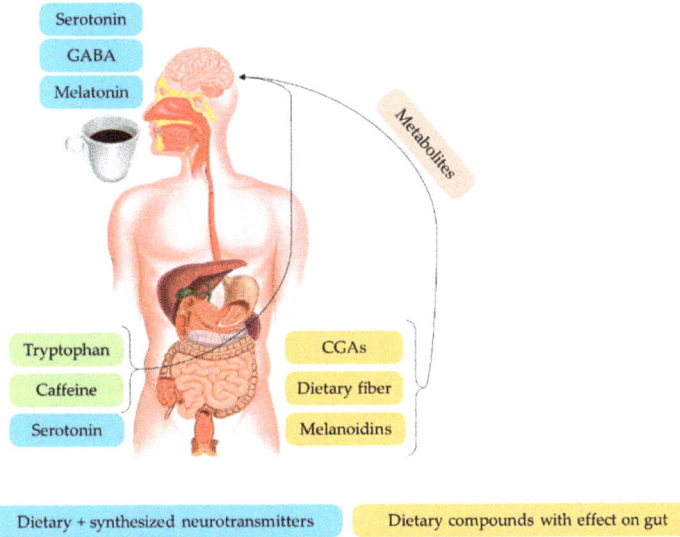

Figure 4. Effect of coffee compounds on the brain–gut axis. Abbreviations: CGAs, chlorogenic acids; GABA, γ-amino butyric acid.

4.1. Caffeine

Caffeine is the main psychoactive compound found in coffee (Table 1). It is consumed from the diet and absorbed into the blood, stimulates the sympathetic nervous system activity, and easily crosses the blood–brain barrier (BBB) with stimulatory effects also on the central nervous system (CNS) [196,200]. Caffeine has an effect on the CNS by modulating different neuronal pathways.

Thus, both in animal and human studies, changes in dopaminergic systems have been observed after caffeine exposure [201]. Different studies suggest that caffeine increases extracellular dopamine concentrations [202], as well as the expression of dopaminergic receptors [203] and transporters, which leads to an improvement of cognitive dysfunction and attention [204]. In addition, it has been reported that caffeine is able to combat the loss of dopaminergic neurons, inducing neuroprotection and attenuating neurological diseases in animal models [205], which may be particularly useful in the context of PD (see below). However, dopaminergic activity is increased in schizophrenia and addictions. Therefore, the effects of coffee and caffeine must be considered also in these patients. Importantly, people with schizophrenia have relatively high intakes of coffee and caffeine, due to different reasons, including the willingness to relieve boredom and apathy or the side effects of antipsychotic medication, such as sedation or dry mouth [206]. In general, it is recommended that these patients reduce coffee consumption [207].

On the other hand, it has been reported that there is a possible interaction between caffeine and glutamatergic signaling. Chronic caffeine consumption can attenuate blast-induced memory deficit in adult male C57BL/6 mice, which is correlated with neuroprotective effects against glutamate excitotoxicity, inflammation, astrogliosis, and neuronal loss at different stages of injury [208]. Moreover, caffeine consumption could also reduce the loss of glutamatergic nerve terminals in the hippocampus, restoring diabetes-induced memory dysfunction in mice [209].

Additionally, caffeine has been found to decrease the activity of the γ-aminobutyric acid (GABA) ergic system and modulate GABA receptors, leading to neurobehavioral effects [201]. Chronic caffeine intake may be related to long-term decrease in GABA [210].

Finally, a recent review by Jee et al. (2020) has indicated that caffeine consumption has different neurological and psychiatric effects in men and women [211], highlighting the importance of evaluating the influence of gender on the effects of coffee and its components on the brain–gut axis. Specifically, the authors showed that caffeine consumption reduces the risk of stroke, dementia, and depression in women and of PD in men. However, caffeine has a negative effect of increasing sleep disorders and anxiety in both male and female adolescents [211].

4.2. Polyphenols

Coffee is also a source of CGA (Table 1), a hydroxycinnamic acid with health-promoting properties such as antioxidant, antibacterial, and anti-inflammatory activities, among others [212]. The majority of ingested CGA is hydrolyzed to CA and quinic acid, and further metabolized by gut microbiota into various aromatic acid metabolites [213]. There is controversial information regarding the ability of CGA and its metabolites to cross the BBB [214,215]. However, neuroprotective effects due to its antioxidant and anti-inflammatory properties have been previously described [215].

As mentioned for caffeine, CA and CGA are coffee components with antioxidant properties and neuroprotective effects against dopaminergic neurotoxicity [216,217] that have been suggested to underlie the decrease in PD risk associated with coffee consumption [218,219]. Interestingly, one of the cardinal symptoms of PD is constipation, and this seems to occur already 10–20 years prior to the presentation of PD motor symptoms [220], with lower bowel movement frequencies predicting the future PD crisis [221]. Moreover, neurodegeneration occurs in PD patients and animal models, and robust evidence suggests that PD could start in the ENS and spread from there to the CNS via the vagal nerve [222,223]. In a recent report, CA or CGA were tested in a rotenone-induced PD mouse model [224]. In this model, mice were subcutaneously implanted an osmotic mini pump, allowing the administration of rotenone at 2.5 mg/kg/day (corresponding to environmental exposure levels of rotenone via pesticides) for 4 weeks. CA (30 mg/kg/day) or CGA (50 g/kg/day) were administered 5 days a week, starting 1 week before rotenone exposure, up to its end. The effects of treatments on central dopaminergic and enteric neurons were evaluated after sacrifice and performed 1 day after rotenone treatment ended. In addition, cultures of rat enteric neurons and glial cells were exposed to rotenone (1–5 nM) with or without exposure to CA (10 or 25 μM) or CGA (25 μM). Remarkably, besides beneficial effects on central structures and cells relevant to PD (namely, nigral dopaminergic neurons and astrocytes), it was demonstrated that administration of CA or CGA at least partially prevented the changes induced by rotenone, which affected both neurons and enteric glial cells in the intestinal myenteric plexus of treated mice. Importantly, all these effects were reproduced in vitro. The precise mechanism was not clarified but it was proposed that CA or CGA pretreatment may enhance the reactivity of glial cells to produce antioxidative molecules in response to rotenone exposure. Although the CA and CGA doses used were probably 2–5 times higher than those consumed daily by coffee drinkers, the results are clearly promising. In fact, the authors suggested that it may be possible to use a food-based promising therapeutic strategy of neuroprotection to improve not only motor but also non-motor symptoms of PD, such as constipation, although the effects of CA and CGA on gastrointestinal motility were not specifically evaluated in this report [224].

During the last stage of preparation of this manuscript, a report by the group of Rogulja [225] was published showing that there is a key connection between beneficial effects of sleep and gut health. They demonstrated that severe sleep loss causes accumulation of ROS in the gut (but not the brain) of both flies and mice, which was associated with death of the flies (the short cycle of sleep restriction did not allow for it to be demonstrated also in mice). Importantly, all these effects could be prevented by oral administration of antioxidant compounds or through gut-targeted transgenic expression of antioxidant enzymes. Many people use caffeinated coffee to keep awake, and while caffeine may favor insomnia [211], the antioxidant components of coffee (like melatonin, one of the antioxidant compounds used in the mentioned study by Rogulja and collaborators, [225]) may prevent accumulation of ROS in the gut and avoid the deleterious effect of voluntary sleep restriction.

4.3. Aminoacids and Their Derived Hormones

One of the compounds found naturally in coffee is tryptophan (Trp), an essential amino acid that must be supplied in the diet. Tryptophan is absorbed using the sodium-dependent neutral amino acid transporter, sodium-dependent neutral amino acid transporter (B^0AT-1), which needs to be stabilized through interaction with the angiotensin-converting enzyme 2 (ACE2) [226]. Tryptophan absorption results in the secretion of α-defensins, cysteine-rich cationic peptides with antibiotic activity against a wide range of bacteria and other microbes, making dietary Trp essential for gut microbiota homeostasis [227,228]. Importantly, the aberrant absorption of Trp (which may occur due to cell surface downregulation of ACE2 during chronic stress, [229], or infection by the severe acute respiratory syndrome coronavirus 2 (SARS-CoV-2) [230]) leads to manifestations of colitis, such as diarrhea [231]. This amino acid is also essential for vitamin B_3 (niacin) synthesis, and the deficit of this vitamin causes pellagra, a disease characterized by diarrhea, inflammation, and protein malnutrition, with skin and CNS manifestations [232]. Importantly, recent studies also revealed that niacin deficiency might be associated with Alzheimer's, Parkinson's, and Huntington's diseases; cognitive impairment; or schizophrenia [232].

Once Trp is consumed and absorbed from the gut, it is made available in the circulation (the majority bound to albumin) and crosses the BBB to be involved in serotonin synthesis in the CNS [233,234]. Serotonin is a neurotransmitter that regulates different physiological aspects, such as behavior, learning, appetite, and glucose homeostasis [235]. Five percent of total body serotonin is brain-derived [235], whereas the majority of serotonin (95%) is produced from Trp in the ECs of the gastrointestinal tract [233]. ECs act as a sensory transduction component in the gastrointestinal mucosa. Serotonin is released by ECs after food intake, intraluminal distension, or efferent vagal stimulation, and its primary targets are the mucosal projections of primary afferent neurons including the vagal nerve [236]. Dietary and peripheral serotonin do not cross the BBB, implying that peripheral serotonin exerts different functions compared to brain-derived serotonin [235]. Peripheral serotonin is involved in the regulation of glucose and lipid homeostasis by acting on pancreatic β-cells, on hepatic cells, and on white adipocytes [235]. Serotonin is also involved in the regulation of visceral pain, secretion, and initiation of the peristaltic reflex, and altered levels of this hormone are also detected in many different psychiatric disorders. Symptoms of some gastrointestinal functional disorders may be due to deregulation of CNS activity, dysregulation at the peripheral level (intestine), or a combination of both (brain–gut axis) by means of neuro-endocrine-immune stimuli. In addition, several studies have demonstrated the profibrogenic role of serotonin in the liver, showing that it works synergistically with platelet-derived growth factor in stimulating hepatic stellate cell proliferation [237].

Another neurotransmitter synthesized from Trp in the brain is melatonin [238]. Melatonin has a crucial role in the control of the circadian cycle and it is also a powerful free radical scavenger and antioxidant [239]. Coffee is a source of melatonin, but the bioavailability of this compound in humans is low (around 3%) [240] and caffeine reduces endogenous nocturnal melatonin levels [238], with a significant impact on duration and quality of sleep [211].

GABA is a major inhibitory neurotransmitter of the CNS and is normally present in high concentrations in many brain regions. It is also found in green coffee beans (Table 1). Although the ability of GABA to cross the BBB is still unclear [241], its analgesic, anti-anxiety and hypotensive properties may be due to a local effect on gastrointestinal receptors, to circulating GABA, or to certain amount of GABA that might cross the BBB [196,242].

4.4. Maillard Reaction Products: Melanoidins

Dietary fiber and melanoidins, the latter also known as Maillardized dietary fiber [184], are likewise present in coffee (Table 1) and have health-promoting properties in the gut and possibly in the brain. Dietary melanoidins, similarly to fiber, escape gastrointestinal digestion, reach the colon, and become substrates for the gut microbiota [243]. In the gut, dietary fiber increases fecal bulk, contributes to normal bowel function and to accelerated intestinal transit [244]. Non-digestible carbohydrates are fermented by the microbiota into SCFAs, and these metabolites have been attributed several health effects [196]. Curiously, studies carried out in male Tsumura Suzuki obese diabetes (TSOD) mice, an accepted mouse model of metabolic syndrome, showed that caffeine and CGA improved plasma SCFA profile after 16 weeks of daily consumption of these compounds. However, in this study coffee had no effects probably because dietary fiber content in coffee composition differs by brand [245]. SCFAs influence gastrointestinal epithelial cell integrity, glucose homeostasis, lipid metabolism, appetite regulation, and immune function and are able to cross the BBB [246]. Interestingly, human studies have reported that dietary fiber can be isolated from SCGs and have chronobiotic effects [247], in addition to promoting short-term appetite and reducing energy consumption [248]. Moreover, a very recent randomized, crossover study of 14 healthy subjects reported that coffee melanoidins consumed at breakfast reduce daily energy intake and modulate postprandial glycemia and other biomarkers [249].

5. Conclusions

Coffee is a complex variable mixture of many compounds whose effects may vary according to their origin, processing, bioavailability, and possible synergistic and/or antagonistic effects.

Epidemiological studies have suggested that coffee brew may exert multiple effects on the digestive tract, including antioxidant, anti-inflammatory, and antiproliferative effects on the mucosa, and pro-motility effects on the muscle layers. However, in high contrast with what is known for other body systems and functions (i.e., cardiovascular system, CNS), the knowledge accumulated thus far regarding the effects of coffee and specific coffee-derived compounds on the gastrointestinal tract as a whole or on their different organs, as well as the specific mechanisms of action exerted on the different cell types present in the gut wall along the whole system, is strikingly scarce, despite the fact that the gastrointestinal tract is the first body system that comes in contact with ingested coffee. Furthermore, the impact of coffee and its derivatives on brain–gut axis health (from emotions to neurodegeneration) has only recently been addressed.

Coffee is recognized as one of the most popular beverages and largest traded produces worldwide, with millions of people consuming it on a daily basis [250]. Furthermore, the coffee plant *Coffee* sp. offers much more than the traditional beverage, and its by-products, including coffee flowers, leaves, pulp, husk, parchment, green coffee, silver skin, and SCGs, have become an attractive potential source of ingredients for new functional foods [251].

Hopefully, the currently huge interest in coffee and coffee by-products will help obtain robust scientific evidence clarifying their impact and mechanisms of action underlying their health-promoting properties in the gastrointestinal tract. Moreover, it is possible that targeted functional foods will soon be developed to specifically protect or improve gastrointestinal and brain–gut axis health.

Author Contributions: Conceptualization, R.A.; writing—original draft preparation, A.I.-D., J.A.U., M.D.d.C., R.A.; writing—review and editing, R.A. and M.D.d.C.; funding acquisition, R.A. and M.D.d.C. All authors have read and agreed to the published version of the manuscript.

Funding: The project "Nuevos conocimientos para la sostenibilidad del sector cafetero" was funded by Consejo Superior de Investigaciones Científicas (CSIC) (201970E117); "Generación de nuevos ingredientes y alimentos beneficiosos dirigidos a condiciones de riesgo y al bienestar global de personas con cáncer colorrectal (TERÁTROFO, IDI-20190960)" and "Novel coffee by-product beverages for an optimal health of the brain-gut axis (COFFEE4BGA)" were funded by the Ministerio de Ciencia e Innovación (PID2019-111510RB-I00).

Institutional Review Board Statement: Not applicable.

Informed Consent Statement: Not applicable.

Data Availability Statement: Data sharing not applicable.

Acknowledgments: We thank Yolanda López-Tofiño and Gema Vera for their technical assistance in recording of X-ray and whole-mount images, respectively.

Conflicts of Interest: The authors declare no conflict of interest.

Abbreviations

$[Ca^{2+}]i$	intracellular free Ca^{2+}
5-CQA	5-O-caffeoylquinic acid
ACF	aberrant crypt foci
ACE2	angiotensin-converting enzyme 2
AHP	afterhyperpolarization
AKT	serine/threonine kinase Akt
AP	action potential
PKB	protein kinase B
ATF-2	activating transcription factor 2
ATF-3	activating transcription factor 3
B^0AT-1	sodium-dependent neutral amino acid transporter
BBB	blood–brain-barrier
BE	Barrett's esophagus
CA	caffeic acid
Ca^{2+}	calcium
cAMP	cyclic adenosine monophosphate
CART	cocaine- and amphetamine-regulated transcript
CGA	chlorogenic acid
CGRP	calcitonin gene-related peptide
CICR	calcium-induced calcium release
CNS	central nervous system
COX-2	cyclooxygenase-2
CQA	caffeoylquinic acid
CRC	colorectal cancer
CRP	C-reactive protein
DMBA	dimethylbenz(a)anthracene
DSS	dextran sodium sulfate
EC	enterochromaffin cell
EGF	epidermal growth factor
ENS	enteric nervous system

ERK	extracellular signal-regulated kinase
f-EPSP	fast excitatory postsynaptic potential
GABA	γ-aminobutyric acid
GERD	gastroesophageal reflux disease
GSK3β	glycogen synthase kinase 3 beta
GST	glutathione S-transferase
HE	hematoxylin/eosin
HIF-1	hypoxia-inducible factor-1
HO-1	heme oxygenase-1
HSP 70	heat shock protein 70
IARC	International Agency for Research on Cancer
IBD	inflammatory bowel disease
ICC	interstitial cells of Cajal
IKK	IkB kinase
IL-	interleukin-
iNOS	inducible nitric oxide synthase
JNK	c-Jun N-terminal kinase
MAPK	mitogen-activated protein kinase
Mcl-1	myeloid cell leukemia 1
MCP-1	methyl-accepting chemotaxis protein-1
SAPK	stress-activated protein kinase
MEK	MAPK/ERK kinase
MNNG	N-methyl-N-nitro-N-nitrosoguanidine
MP	myenteric plexus
ND	not detected
NF-kβ	nuclear factor-kβ
nNOS	nitric oxide synthase
NO	nitric oxide
NR	not reported
PAI-1	plasminogen activator inhibitor-1
PD	Parkinsons's disease
PTEN	phosphatase and tensin homolog
PG	prostaglandin
PhIP	2-amino-1-methyl-6-phenylimidazo[4,5-b]pyridine
ROS	reactive oxygen species
RP	resting potential
RyR	ryanodine receptors
s-AHP	slow afterhyperpolarization
SARS-CoV-2	severe acute respiratory syndrome coronavirus 2
SCFA	short chain fatty acid
SCG	spent coffee grounds
s-EPSP	slow excitatory postsynaptic potential
SMP	submucous plexus
SP	substance P
spp.	species
STAT5	signal transducer and activator of transcription 5
TNF-R	tumor necrosis factor-receptor
TNF	tumor necrosis factor
TOPK	lymphokine-activated killer t-cell-originated protein kinase-like protein
Trp	tryptophan
UDP	uridine diphosphate
UGT1A	UDP glucuronosyltransferases
VACHT	vesicular acetylcholine transporter
VEGF	vascular endothelial growth factor
VIP	vasoactive intestinal peptide
WHO	World Health Organization
ZO-1	zonulin-1

References

1. Loomis, D.; Guyton, K.Z.; Grosse, Y.; Lauby-Secretan, B.; El Ghissassi, F.; Bouvard, V.; Benbrahim-Tallaa, L.; Guha, N.; Mattock, H.; Straif, K. Carcinogenicity of Drinking Coffee, Mate, and Very Hot Beverages. *Lancet Oncol.* **2016**, *17*, 877–878. [CrossRef]
2. Grosso, G.; Godos, J.; Galvano, F.; Giovannucci, E.L. Coffee, Caffeine, and Health Outcomes: An Umbrella Review. *Annu. Rev. Nutr.* **2017**, *37*, 131–156. [CrossRef] [PubMed]
3. Grosso, G.; Stepaniak, U.; Polak, M.; Micek, A.; Topor, R.; Stefler, D.; Szafraniec, K.; Pajak, A. Europe PMC Funders Group Coffee Consumption and Risk of Hypertension in the Polish Arm of the HAPIEE Cohort Study. *Eur. J. Clin. Nutr.* **2016**, *70*, 109–115. [CrossRef] [PubMed]
4. Liebeskind, D.S.; Sanossian, N.; Fu, K.A.; Wang, H.-J.; Arab, L. The Coffee Paradox in Stroke: Increased Consumption Linked with Fewer Strokes. *Nutr. Neurosci.* **2016**, *19*, 406–413. [CrossRef] [PubMed]
5. Poole, R.; Kennedy, O.J.; Roderick, P.; Fallowfield, J.A.; Hayes, P.C.; Parkes, J. Coffee Consumption and Health: Umbrella Review of Meta-Analyses of Multiple Health Outcomes. *BMJ* **2017**, *359*, j5024. [CrossRef]
6. Guallar, E.; Blasco-Colmenares, E.; Arking, D.E.; Zhao, D. Moderate Coffee Intake Can Be Part of a Healthy Diet. *Ann. Intern. Med.* **2017**, *167*, 283–284. [CrossRef]
7. Del Castillo, M.D.; Iriondo-Dehond, A.; Iriondo-Dehond, M.; Gonzalez, I.; Medrano, A.; Filip, R.; Uribarri, J. Healthy Eating Recommendations: Good for Reducing Dietary Contribution to the Body's Advanced Glycation/Lipoxidation End Products Pool? *Nutr. Res. Rev.* **2020**, 1–57. [CrossRef]
8. Del Castillo, M.D.; Iriondo-DeHond, A.; Fernandez-Gomez, B.; Martinez-Saez, N.; Rebollo-Hernanz, M.; Martín-Cabrejas, M.A.; Farah, A. *Coffee Antioxidants in Chronic Diseases*; The Royal Society of Chemistry: London, UK, 2019; ISBN 9781788015028.
9. Farah, A. Coffee Constituents. *Coffee Emerg. Health Eff. Dis. Prev.* **2012**, *1*, 21–58.
10. Moreira, A.S.P.; Nunes, F.M.; Domingues, M.R.; Coimbra, M.A. Coffee Melanoidins: Structures, Mechanisms of Formation and Potential Health Impacts. *Food Funct.* **2012**, *3*, 903–915. [CrossRef]
11. Juncker, J. European Commission COMMISSION REGULATION (EU) 2017/2158 of 20 November 2017 Establishing Mitigation Measures and Benchmark Levels for the Reduction of the Presence of Acrylamide in Food. *Off. J. Eur. Union* **2017**, *204*, 24–44.
12. Belitz, H.-D.; Grosch, W.; Schieberle, P. Coffee, tea, cocoa. In *Food Chemistry*, 4th ed.; Belitz, H.-D., Grosch, W., Schieberle, P., Eds.; Springer: Leipzig, Germany, 2009; pp. 938–951.
13. Martins, A.C.C.L.; Gloria, M.B.A. Changes on the Levels of Serotonin Precursors—Tryptophan and 5-Hydroxytryptophan—during Roasting of Arabica and Robusta Coffee. *Food Chem.* **2010**, *118*, 529–533. [CrossRef]
14. Ramakrishna, A.; Giridhar, P.; Sankar, K.U.; Ravishankar, G.A. Melatonin and Serotonin Profiles in Beans of Coffea Species. *J. Pineal Res.* **2012**, *52*, 470–476. [CrossRef] [PubMed]
15. Vitaglione, P.; Fogliano, V.; Pellegrini, N. Coffee, Colon Function and Colorectal Cancer. *Food Funct.* **2012**, *3*, 916. [CrossRef] [PubMed]
16. Kim, Y.; Jhon, D.-Y. Changes of the Chlorogenic Acid, Caffeine, Gama-Aminobutyric Acid (GABA) and Antioxdant Activities during Germination of Coffee Bean (Coffea Arabica). *Emir. J. Food Agric.* **2018**, *30*, 675. [CrossRef]
17. EFSA CONTAM Panel (EFSA Panel on Contaminants in the Food Chain). Scientific Opinion on Acrylamide in Food. *EFSA J.* **2015**, *13*, 4104.
18. Gniechwitz, D.; Brueckel, B.; Reichardt, N.; Blaut, M.; Steinhart, H.; Bunzel, M. Coffee Dietary Fiber Contents and Structural Characteristics as Influenced by Coffee Type and Technological and Brewing Procedures. *J. Agric. Food Chem.* **2007**, *55*, 11027–11034. [CrossRef]
19. Angeloni, G.; Guerrini, L.; Masella, P.; Innocenti, M.; Bellumori, M.; Parenti, A. Characterization and Comparison of Cold Brew and Cold Drip Coffee Extraction Methods. *J. Sci. Food Agric.* **2019**, *99*, 391–399. [CrossRef]
20. Jeszka-Skowron, M.; Frankowski, R.; Zgoła-Grześkowiak, A. Comparison of Methylxantines, Trigonelline, Nicotinic Acid and Nicotinamide Contents in Brews of Green and Processed Arabica and Robusta Coffee Beans—Influence of Steaming, Decaffeination and Roasting Processes on Coffee Beans. *LWT* **2020**, *125*, 109344. [CrossRef]
21. Rao, N.; Fuller, M.; Grim, M. Physiochemical Characteristics of Hot and Cold Brew Coffee Chemistry: The Effects of Roast Level and Brewing Temperature on Compound Extraction. *Foods* **2020**, *9*, 902. [CrossRef]
22. Fogliano, V.; Morales, F.J. Estimation of Dietary Intake of Melanoidins from Coffee and Bread. *Food Funct.* **2011**, *2*, 117–123. [CrossRef]
23. Galuch, M.B.; Magon, T.F.S.; Silveira, R.; Nicácio, A.E.; Pizzo, J.S.; Bonafe, E.G.; Maldaner, L.; Santos, O.O.; Visentainer, J.V. Determination of Acrylamide in Brewed Coffee by Dispersive Liquid–Liquid Microextraction (DLLME) and Ultra-Performance Liquid Chromatography Tandem Mass Spectrometry (UPLC-MS/MS). *Food Chem.* **2019**, *282*, 120–126. [CrossRef] [PubMed]
24. Doello, K.; Ortiz, R.; Alvarez, P.J.; Melguizo, C.; Cabeza, L.; Prados, J. Latest in Vitro and in Vivo Assay, Clinical Trials and Patents in Cancer Treatment Using Curcumin: A Literature Review. *Nutr. Cancer* **2018**, *70*, 569–578. [CrossRef]
25. Mesías, M.; Morales, F.J. Acrylamide in Coffee: Estimation of Exposure from Vending Machines. *J. Food Compos. Anal.* **2016**, *48*, 8–12. [CrossRef]
26. Starbucks Blonde Roast. Available online: https://www.starbucks.com/menu/product/873068625/hot?parent=%2Fdrinks%2Fhot-coffees%2Fbrewed-coffees (accessed on 3 September 2020).
27. Starbucks Coffee España Sociedad Limitada. *Información Nutricional*; Starbucks Coffee España Sociedad Limitada: Madrid, Spain, 2020.
28. Kang, D.; Lee, H.U.; Davaatseren, M.; Chung, M.S. Comparison of Acrylamide and Furan Concentrations, Antioxidant Activities, and Volatile Profiles in Cold or Hot Brew Coffees. *Food Sci. Biotechnol.* **2020**, *29*, 141–148. [CrossRef]

29. Starbucks Starbucks®Cold Brew Coffee. Available online: https://www.starbucks.com/menu/product/2121255/iced?parent=%2Fdrinks%2Fcold-coffees%2Fcold-brews (accessed on 3 September 2020).
30. Gloess, A.N.; Schönbächler, B.; Klopprogge, B.; D'Ambrosio, L.; Chatelain, K.; Bongartz, A.; Strittmatter, A.; Rast, M.; Yeretzian, C. Comparison of Nine Common Coffee Extraction Methods: Instrumental and Sensory Analysis. *Eur. Food Res. Technol.* **2013**, *236*, 607–627. [CrossRef]
31. Angeloni, G.; Guerrini, L.; Masella, P.; Bellumori, M.; Daluiso, S.; Parenti, A.; Innocenti, M. What Kind of Coffee Do You Drink? An Investigation on Effects of Eight Different Extraction Methods. *Food Res. Int.* **2019**, *116*, 1327–1335. [CrossRef]
32. Lane, S.; Palmer, J.; Christie, B.; Ehlting, J.; Le, C. Can Cold Brew Coffee Be Convenient? A Pilot Study For Caffeine Content in Cold Brew Coffee Concentrate Using High Performance Liquid Chromatography. *Arbutus Rev.* **2017**, *8*, 15–23. [CrossRef]
33. Rao, N.Z.; Fuller, M. Acidity and Antioxidant Activity of Cold Brew Coffee. *Sci. Rep.* **2018**, *8*, 1–9. [CrossRef] [PubMed]
34. Nunes, F.M.; Coimbra, M.A. Melanoidins from Coffee Infusions. Fractionation, Chemical Characterization, and Effect of the Degree of Roast. *J. Agric. Food Chem.* **2007**, *55*, 3967–3977. [CrossRef] [PubMed]
35. Carabotti, M.; Scirocco, A.; Maselli, M.A.; Severi, C. The Gut-Brain Axis: Interactions between Enteric Microbiota, Central and Enteric Nervous Systems. *Ann. Gastroenterol.* **2015**, *28*, 203–209.
36. Koloski, N.; Holtmann, G.; Talley, N.J. Is There a Causal Link between Psychological Disorders and Functional Gastrointestinal Disorders? *Expert Rev. Gastroenterol. Hepatol.* **2020**, *14*, 1047–1059. [CrossRef] [PubMed]
37. Labanski, A.; Langhorst, J.; Engler, H.; Elsenbruch, S. Stress and the Brain-Gut Axis in Functional and Chronic-Inflammatory Gastrointestinal Diseases: A Transdisciplinary Challenge. *Psychoneuroendocrinology* **2020**, *111*, 104501. [CrossRef] [PubMed]
38. Keefer, L.; Palsson, O.S.; Pandolfino, J.E. Best Practice Update: Incorporating Psychogastroenterology Into Management of Digestive Disorders. *Gastroenterology* **2018**, *154*, 1249–1257. [CrossRef] [PubMed]
39. Van Tilburg, M.A.L. Psychogastroenterology: A Cure, Band-Aid, or Prevention? *Children* **2020**, *7*, 121. [CrossRef] [PubMed]
40. Wierzejska, R. Coffee Consumption vs. Cancer Risk—A Review of Scientific Data. *Rocz. Państwowego Zakładu Hig.* **2015**, *66*, 293–298.
41. Ludwig, I.A.; Clifford, M.N.; Lean, M.E.J.; Ashihara, H.; Crozier, A. Coffee: Biochemistry and Potential Impact on Health. *Food Funct.* **2014**, *5*, 695–1717. [CrossRef] [PubMed]
42. Lukic, M.; Licaj, I.; Lund, E.; Skeie, G.; Weiderpass, E.; Braaten, T. Coffee Consumption and the Risk of Cancer in the Norwegian Women and Cancer (NOWAC) Study. *Eur. J. Epidemiol.* **2016**, *31*, 905–916. [CrossRef]
43. Li, G.; Ma, D.; Zhang, Y.; Zheng, W.; Wang, P. Coffee Consumption and Risk of Colorectal Cancer: A Meta-Analysis of Observational Studies. *Public Health Nutr.* **2013**, *16*, 346–357. [CrossRef]
44. Tian, C.; Wang, W.; Hong, Z.; Zhang, X. Coffee Consumption and Risk of Colorectal Cancer: A Dose-Response Analysis of Observational Studies. *Cancer Causes Control* **2013**, *24*, 1265–1268. [CrossRef]
45. Galeone, C.; Turati, F.; La Vecchia, C.; Tavani, A. Coffee Consumption and Risk of Colorectal Cancer: A Meta-Analysis of Case-Control Studies. *Cancer Causes Control* **2010**, *21*, 1949–1959. [CrossRef]
46. Hu, Y.; Ding, M.; Yuan, C.; Wu, K.; Smith-Warner, S.A.; Hu, F.B.; Chan, A.T.; Meyerhardt, J.A.; Ogino, S.; Fuchs, C.S.; et al. Association Between Coffee Intake After Diagnosis of Colorectal Cancer and Reduced Mortality. *Gastroenterology* **2018**, *154*, 916–926.e9. [CrossRef] [PubMed]
47. Inoue, M.; Tajima, K.; Hirose, K.; Hamajima, N.; Takezaki, T.; Kuroishi, T.; Tominaga, S. Tea and Coffee Consumption and the Risk of Digestive Tract Cancers: Data from a Comparative Case-Referent Study in Japan. *Cancer Causes Control* **1998**, *9*, 209–216. [CrossRef] [PubMed]
48. Giovannucci, E. Meta-Analysis of Coffee Consumption and Risk of Colorectal Cancer. *Am. J. Epidemiol.* **1998**, *147*, 1043–1052. [CrossRef] [PubMed]
49. Schmit, S.L.; Rennert, H.S.; Rennert, G.; Gruber, S.B. Coffee Consumption and the Risk of Colorectal Cancer. *Cancer Epidemiol. Biomark. Prev.* **2016**, *25*, 634–639. [CrossRef]
50. Je, Y.; Liu, W.; Giovannucci, E. Coffee Consumption and Risk of Colorectal Cancer: A Systematic Review and Meta-Analysis of Prospective Cohort Studies. *Int. J. Cancer* **2009**, *124*, 1662–1668. [CrossRef]
51. Mackintosh, C.; Yuan, C.; Ou, F.-S.; Zhang, S.; Niedzwiecki, D.; Chang, I.-W.; O'Neil, B.H.; Mullen, B.C.; Lenz, H.-J.; Blanke, C.D.; et al. Association of Coffee Intake with Survival in Patients With Advanced or Metastatic Colorectal Cancer. *JAMA Oncol.* **2020**, *6*, 1713. [CrossRef]
52. Micek, A.; Gniadek, A.; Kawalec, P.; Brzostek, T. Coffee Consumption and Colorectal Cancer Risk: A Dose-Response Meta-Analysis on Prospective Cohort Studies. *Int. J. Food Sci. Nutr.* **2019**, *70*, 986–1006. [CrossRef]
53. Sartini, M.; Bragazzi, N.L.; Spagnolo, A.M.; Schinca, E.; Ottria, G.; Dupont, C.; Cristina, M.L. Coffee Consumption and Risk of Colorectal Cancer: A Systematic Review and Meta-Analysis of Prospective Studies. *Nutrients* **2019**, *11*, 694. [CrossRef]
54. Dik, V.K.; Bueno-De-Mesquita, H.B.; Van Oijen, M.G.H.; Siersema, P.D.; Uiterwaal, C.S.P.M.; Van Gils, C.H.; Van Duijnhoven, F.J.B.; Cauchi, S.; Yengo, L.; Froguel, P.; et al. Coffee and Tea Consumption, Genotype-Based CYP1A2 and NAT2 Activity and Colorectal Cancer Risk—Results from the EPIC Cohort Study. *Int. J. Cancer* **2014**, *135*, 401–412. [CrossRef]
55. Park, S.Y.; Freedman, N.D.; Haiman, C.A.; Le Marchand, L.; Wilkens, L.R.; Setiawan, V.W. Prospective Study of Coffee Consumption and Cancer Incidence in Non-White Populations. *Cancer Epidemiol. Biomark. Prev.* **2018**, *27*, 928–935. [CrossRef]
56. Terry, P.; Bergkvist, L.; Holmberg, L.; Wolk, A. Coffee Consumption and Risk of Colorectal Cancer in a Population Based Prospective Cohort of Swedish Women. *Gut* **2001**, *49*, 87–90. [CrossRef] [PubMed]

57. Tran, K.T.; Coleman, H.G.; McMenamin, Ú.C.; Cardwell, C.R. Coffee Consumption by Type and Risk of Digestive Cancer: A Large Prospective Cohort Study. *Br. J. Cancer* **2019**, *120*, 1059–1066. [CrossRef] [PubMed]
58. Xie, Y.; Huang, S.; He, T.; Su, Y. Coffee Consumption and Risk of Gastric Cancer: An Updated Meta-Analysis. *Asia Pac. J. Clin. Nutr.* **2016**, *25*, 578–588. [PubMed]
59. Bidel, S.; Hu, G.; Jousilahti, P.; Pukkala, E.; Hakulinen, T.; Tuomilehto, J. Coffee Consumption and Risk of Gastric and Pancreatic Cancer—A Prospective Cohort Study. *Int. J. Cancer* **2013**, *132*, 1651–1659. [CrossRef] [PubMed]
60. Larsson, S.C.; Giovannucci, E.; Wolk, A. Coffee Consumption and Stomach Cancer Risk in a Cohort of Swedish Women. *Int. J. Cancer* **2006**, *119*, 2186–2189. [CrossRef] [PubMed]
61. Ren, J.S.; Freedman, N.D.; Kamangar, F.; Dawsey, S.M.; Hollenbeck, A.R.; Schatzkin, A.; Abnet, C.C. Tea, Coffee, Carbonated Soft Drinks and Upper Gastrointestinal Tract Cancer Risk in a Large United States Prospective Cohort Study. *Eur. J. Cancer* **2010**, *46*, 1873–1881. [CrossRef] [PubMed]
62. Turati, F.; Galeone, C.; La Vecchia, C.; Garavello, W.; Tavani, A. Coffee and Cancers of the Upper Digestive and Respiratory Tracts: Meta-Analyses of Observational Studies. *Ann. Oncol.* **2011**, *22*, 536–544. [CrossRef]
63. Islami, F.; Boffetta, P.; Ren, J.S.; Pedoeim, L.; Khatib, D.; Kamangar, F. High-Temperature Beverages and Foods and Esophageal Cancer Risk—A Systematic Review. *Int. J. Cancer* **2009**, *125*, 491–524. [CrossRef]
64. Zheng, J.-S.; Yang, J.; Fu, Y.-Q.; Huang, T.; Huang, Y.-J.; Li, D. Effects of Green Tea, Black Tea, and Coffee Consumption on the Risk of Esophageal Cancer: A Systematic Review and Meta-Analysis of Observational Studies. *Nutr. Cancer* **2013**, *65*, 1–16. [CrossRef]
65. Kim, J.; Oh, S.W.; Myung, S.K.; Kwon, H.; Lee, C.; Yun, J.M.; Lee, H.K. Association between Coffee Intake and Gastroesophageal Reflux Disease: A Meta-Analysis. *Dis. Esophagus* **2014**, *27*, 311–317. [CrossRef]
66. Filiberti, R.A.; Fontana, V.; De Ceglie, A.; Blanchi, S.; Grossi, E.; Della Casa, D.; Lacchin, T.; De Matthaeis, M.; Ignomirelli, O.; Cappiello, R.; et al. Association between Coffee or Tea Drinking and Barrett's Esophagus or Esophagitis: An Italian Study. *Eur. J. Clin. Nutr.* **2017**, *71*, 980–986. [CrossRef] [PubMed]
67. Sajja, K.C.; El-Serag, H.B.; Thrift, A.P. Coffee or Tea, Hot or Cold, Are Not Associated With Risk of Barrett's Esophagus. *Clin. Gastroenterol. Hepatol.* **2016**, *14*, 769–772. [CrossRef] [PubMed]
68. Marotta, R.B.; Floch, M.H. Diet and Nutrition in Ulcer Disease. *Med. Clin. N. Am.* **1991**, *75*, 967–979. [CrossRef]
69. Cohen, S.; Booth, G.H. Gastric Acid Secretion and Lower-Esophageal-Sphincter Pressure in Response to Coffee and Caffeine. *N. Engl. J. Med.* **1975**, *293*, 897–899. [CrossRef]
70. Moco, S.; Martin, F.P.J.; Rezzi, S. Metabolomics View on Gut Microbiome Modulation by Polyphenol-Rich Foods. *J. Proteome Res.* **2012**, *11*, 4781–4790. [CrossRef]
71. Rubach, M.; Lang, R.; Skupin, C.; Hofmann, T.; Somoza, V. Activity-Guided Fractionation to Characterize a Coffee Beverage That Effectively down-Regulates Mechanisms of Gastric Acid Secretion as Compared to Regular Coffee. *J. Agric. Food Chem.* **2010**, *58*, 4153–4161. [CrossRef]
72. Selma, M.V.; Espín, J.C.; Tomás-Barberán, F.A. Interaction between Phenolics and Gut Microbiota: Role in Human Health. *J. Agric. Food Chem.* **2009**, *57*, 6485–6501. [CrossRef]
73. Bułdak, R.J.; Hejmo, T.; Osowski, M.; Bułdak, Ł.; Kukla, M.; Polaniak, R.; Birkner, E. The Impact of Coffee and Its Selected Bioactive Compounds on the Development and Progression of Colorectal Cancer In Vivo and In Vitro. *Molecules* **2018**, *23*, 3309. [CrossRef]
74. Dorado, G.; Barbancho, M.; Pueyo, C. Coffee Is Highly Mutagenic in the L-Arabinose Resistance Test InSalmonella Typhimurium. *Environ. Mutagen.* **1987**, *9*, 251–260. [CrossRef]
75. Nagao, M.; Fujita, Y.; Wakabayashi, K. Mutagens in Coffee and Other Beverages. *Environ. Health Perspect.* **1986**, *67*, 89–91. [CrossRef]
76. Weber, L.; Kuck, K.; Jürgenliemk, G.; Heilmann, J.; Lipowicz, B.; Vissiennon, C. Anti-Inflammatory and Barrier-Stabilising Effects of Myrrh, Coffee Charcoal and Chamomile Flower Extract in a Co-Culture Cell Model of the Intestinal Mucosa. *Biomolecules* **2020**, *10*, 1033. [CrossRef] [PubMed]
77. Kalthoff, S.; Ehmer, U.; Freiberg, N.; Manns, M.P.; Strassburg, C.P. Coffee Induces Expression of Glucuronosyltransferases by the Aryl Hydrocarbon Receptor and Nrf2 in Liver and Stomach. *Gastroenterology* **2010**, *139*, 1699–1710.e2. [CrossRef] [PubMed]
78. Devasagayam, T.P.A.; Kamat, J.P.; Mohan, H.; Kesavan, P.C. Caffeine as an Antioxidant: Inhibition of Lipid Peroxidation Induced by Reactive Oxygen Species. *Biochim. Biophys. Actan Biomembr.* **1996**, *1282*, 63–70. [CrossRef]
79. Lee, C. Antioxidant Ability of Caffeine and Its Metabolites Based on the Study of Oxygen Radical Absorbing Capacity and Inhibition of LDL Peroxidation. *Clin. Chim. Acta* **2000**, *295*, 141–154. [CrossRef]
80. Mitani, T.; Nagano, T.; Harada, K.; Yamashita, Y.; Ashida, H. Caffeine-Stimulated Intestinal Epithelial Cells Suppress Lipid Accumulation in Adipocytes. *J. Nutr. Sci. Vitaminol. (Tokyo)* **2017**, *63*, 331–338. [CrossRef] [PubMed]
81. Choi, E.K.; Ji, I.M.; Lee, S.R.; Kook, Y.H.; Griffin, R.J.; Lim, B.U.; Kim, J.-S.; Lee, D.S.; Song, C.W.; Park, H.J. Radiosensitization of Tumor Cells by Modulation of ATM Kinase. *Int. J. Radiat. Biol.* **2006**, *82*, 277–283. [CrossRef]
82. Saito, Y.; Gopalan, B.; Mhashilkar, A.M.; Roth, J.A.; Chada, S.; Zumstein, L.; Ramesh, R. Adenovirus-Mediated PTEN Treatment Combined with Caffeine Produces a Synergistic Therapeutic Effect in Colorectal Cancer Cells. *Cancer Gene Ther.* **2003**, *10*, 803–813. [CrossRef]
83. Merighi, S.; Benini, A.; Mirandola, P.; Gessi, S.; Varani, K.; Simioni, C.; Leung, E.; Maclennan, S.; Baraldi, P.G.; Borea, P.A. Caffeine Inhibits Adenosine-Induced Accumulation of Hypoxia-Inducible Factor-1α, Vascular Endothelial Growth Factor, and Interleukin-8 Expression in Hypoxic Human Colon Cancer Cells. *Mol. Pharmacol.* **2007**, *72*, 395–406. [CrossRef]

84. Kang, N.J.; Lee, K.W.; Kim, B.H.; Bode, A.M.; Lee, H.-J.; Heo, Y.-S.; Boardman, L.; Limburg, P.; Lee, H.J.; Dong, Z. Coffee Phenolic Phytochemicals Suppress Colon Cancer Metastasis by Targeting MEK and TOPK. *Carcinogenesis* **2011**, *32*, 921–928. [CrossRef]
85. Mhaidat, N.M.; Alzoubi, K.H.; Al-Azzam, S.I.; Alsaad, A.A. Caffeine Inhibits Paclitaxel-Induced Apoptosis in Colorectal Cancer Cells through the Upregulation of Mcl-1 Levels. *Mol. Med. Rep.* **2014**, *9*, 243–248. [CrossRef]
86. Choi, D.W.; Lim, M.S.; Lee, J.W.; Chun, W.; Lee, S.H.; Nam, Y.H.; Park, J.M.; Choi, D.H.; Kang, C.D.; Lee, S.J.; et al. The Cytotoxicity of Kahweol in HT-29 Human Colorectal Cancer Cells Is Mediated by Apoptosis and Suppression of Heat Shock Protein 70 Expression. *Biomol. Ther. (Seoul)* **2015**, *23*, 128–133. [CrossRef] [PubMed]
87. Guertin, K.A.; Loftfield, E.; Boca, S.M.; Sampson, J.N.; Moore, S.C.; Xiao, Q.; Huang, W.-Y.; Xiong, X.; Freedman, N.D.; Cross, A.J.; et al. Serum Biomarkers of Habitual Coffee Consumption May Provide Insight into the Mechanism Underlying the Association between Coffee Consumption and Colorectal Cancer. *Am. J. Clin. Nutr.* **2015**, *101*, 1000–1011. [CrossRef] [PubMed]
88. Chu, Y.-F.; Chen, Y.; Black, R.M.; Brown, P.H.; Lyle, B.J.; Liu, R.H.; Ou, B. Type 2 Diabetes-Related Bioactivities of Coffee: Assessment of Antioxidant Activity, NF-KB Inhibition, and Stimulation of Glucose Uptake. *Food Chem.* **2011**, *124*, 914–920. [CrossRef]
89. Zhao, Z.; Shin, H.S.; Satsu, H.; Totsuka, M.; Shimizu, M. 5-Caffeoylquinic Acid and Caffeic Acid Down-Regulate the Oxidative Stress- and TNF-α-Induced Secretion of Interleukin-8 from Caco-2 Cells. *J. Agric. Food Chem.* **2008**, *56*, 3863–3868. [CrossRef] [PubMed]
90. Bøhn, S.K.; Blomhoff, R.; Paur, I. Coffee and Cancer Risk, Epidemiological Evidence, and Molecular Mechanisms. *Mol. Nutr. Food Res.* **2014**, *58*, 915–930. [CrossRef]
91. Murad, L.D.; da Soares, N.C.P.; Brand, C.; Monteiro, M.C.; Teodoro, A.J. Effects of Caffeic and 5-Caffeoylquinic Acids on Cell Viability and Cellular Uptake in Human Colon Adenocarcinoma Cells. *Nutr. Cancer* **2015**, *67*, 532–542. [CrossRef]
92. Oleaga, C.; Ciudad, C.J.; Noé, V.; Izquierdo-Pulido, M. Coffee Polyphenols Change the Expression of STAT5B and ATF-2 Modifying Cyclin D1 Levels in Cancer Cells. *Oxid. Med. Cell. Longev.* **2012**, *2012*, 1–17. [CrossRef]
93. Lee, W.J.; Zhu, B.T. Inhibition of DNA Methylation by Caffeic Acid and Chlorogenic Acid, Two Common Catechol-Containing Coffee Polyphenols. *Carcinogenesis* **2006**, *27*, 269–277. [CrossRef]
94. Bergmann, H.; Rogoll, D.; Scheppach, W.; Melcher, R.; Richling, E. The Ussing Type Chamber Model to Study the Intestinal Transport and Modulation of Specific Tight-Junction Genes Using a Colonic Cell Line. *Mol. Nutr. Food Res.* **2009**, *53*, 1211–1225. [CrossRef]
95. Park, G.H.; Song, H.M.; Jeong, J.B. The Coffee Diterpene Kahweol Suppresses the Cell Proliferation by Inducing Cyclin D1 Proteasomal Degradation via ERK1/2, JNK and GKS3β-Dependent Threonine-286 Phosphorylation in Human Colorectal Cancer Cells. *Food Chem. Toxicol.* **2016**, *95*, 142–148. [CrossRef]
96. Karin, M.; Greten, F.R. NF-KB: Linking Inflammation and Immunity to Cancer Development and Progression. *Nat. Rev. Immunol.* **2005**, *5*, 749–759. [CrossRef] [PubMed]
97. Kim, J.Y.; Jung, K.S.; Jeong, H.G. Suppressive Effects of the Kahweol and Cafestol on Cyclooxygenase-2 Expression in Macrophages. *FEBS Lett.* **2004**, *569*, 321–326. [CrossRef] [PubMed]
98. Lee, K.J.; Jeong, H.G. Protective Effects of Kahweol and Cafestol against Hydrogen Peroxide-Induced Oxidative Stress and DNA Damage. *Toxicol. Lett.* **2007**, *173*, 80–87. [CrossRef] [PubMed]
99. Cavin, C.; Holzhaeuser, D.; Scharf, G.; Constable, A.; Huber, W.; Schilter, B. Cafestol and Kahweol, Two Coffee Specific Diterpenes with Anticarcinogenic Activity. *Food Chem. Toxicol.* **2002**, *40*, 1155–1163. [CrossRef]
100. Hwang, Y.P.; Jeong, H.G. The Coffee Diterpene Kahweol Induces Heme Oxygenase-1 via the PI3K and P38/Nrf2 Pathway to Protect Human Dopaminergic Neurons from 6-Hydroxydopamine-Derived Oxidative Stress. *FEBS Lett.* **2008**, *582*, 2655–2662. [CrossRef]
101. Tagliazucchi, D.; Verzelloni, E.; Conte, A. Effect of Dietary Melanoidins on Lipid Peroxidation during Simulated Gastric Digestion: Their Possible Role in the Prevention of Oxidative Damage. *J. Agric. Food Chem.* **2010**, *58*, 2513–2519. [CrossRef]
102. Faist, V.; Erbersdobler, H.F. Metabolic Transit and in Vivo Effects of Melanoidins and Precursor Compounds Deriving from the Maillard Reaction. *Ann. Nutr. Metab.* **2001**, *45*, 1–12. [CrossRef]
103. Würzner, H.-P.; Lindström, E.; Vuataz, L.; Luginbühl, H. A 2-Year Feeding Study of Instant. Coffees in Rats. II. Incidence and Types of Neoplasms. *Food Cosmet. Toxicol.* **1977**, *15*, 289–296. [CrossRef]
104. Stalder, R.; Bexter, A.; Würzner, H.P.; Luginbühl, H. A Carcinogenicity Study of Instant Coffee in Swiss Mice. *Food Chem. Toxicol.* **1990**, *28*, 829–837. [CrossRef]
105. Gershbein, L.L. Action of Dietary Trypsin, Pressed Coffee Oil, Silymarin and Iron Salt on 1,2-Dimethylhydrazine Tumorigenesis by Gavage. *Anticancer Res.* **1994**, *14*, 1113–1116.
106. Chuang, Y.-H.; Quach, A.; Absher, D.; Assimes, T.; Horvath, S.; Ritz, B. Coffee Consumption Is Associated with DNA Methylation Levels of Human Blood. *Eur. J. Hum. Genet.* **2017**, *25*, 608–616. [CrossRef] [PubMed]
107. Cibicková, E.; Cibicek, N.; Zd'ánský, P.; Kohout, P. The Impairment of Gastroduodenal Mucosal Barrier by Coffee. *Acta Medica Hradec. Kral.* **2004**, *47*, 273–275. [CrossRef]
108. Cuervo, A.; Hevia, A.; López, P.; Suárez, A.; Diaz, C.; Sánchez, B.; Margolles, A.; González, S. Phenolic Compounds from Red Wine and Coffee Are Associated with Specific Intestinal Microorganisms in Allergic Subjects. *Food Funct.* **2016**, *7*, 104–109. [CrossRef]
109. Nakayama, T.; Oishi, K. Influence of Coffee (Coffea Arabica) and Galacto-Oligosaccharide Consumption on Intestinal Microbiota and the Host Responses. *FEMS Microbiol. Lett.* **2013**, *343*, 161–168. [CrossRef] [PubMed]
110. Jaquet, M.; Rochat, I.; Moulin, J.; Cavin, C.; Bibiloni, R. Impact of Coffee Consumption on the Gut Microbiota: A Human Volunteer Study. *Int. J. Food Microbiol.* **2009**, *130*, 117–121. [CrossRef] [PubMed]

111. Turesky, R.J.; Richoz, J.; Constable, A.; Curtis, K.D.; Dingley, K.H.; Turteltaub, K.W. The Effects of Coffee on Enzymes Involved in Metabolism of the Dietary Carcinogen 2-Amino-1-Methyl-6-Phenylimidazo[4,5-b]Pyridine in Rats. *Chem. Biol. Interact.* **2003**, *145*, 251–265. [CrossRef]
112. Carter, O.; Wang, R.; Dashwood, W.M.; Orner, G.A.; Fischer, K.A.; Löhr, C.V.; Pereira, C.B.; Bailey, G.S.; Williams, D.E.; Dashwood, R.H. Comparison of White Tea, Green Tea, Epigallocatechin-3-Gallate, and Caffeine as Inhibitors of PhIP-Induced Colonic Aberrant Crypts. *Nutr. Cancer* **2007**, *58*, 60–65. [CrossRef]
113. Den Braak, V.; Jong, D.; Rijt, V.; Ruijter, D.; Katan, P. Nagengast The Effect of Unfiltered Coffee on Potential Biomarkers for Colonic Cancer Risk in Healthy Volunteers: A Randomized Trial. *Aliment. Pharmacol. Ther.* **2000**, *14*, 1181–1190.
114. Wang, R.; Dashwood, W.M.; Löhr, C.V.; Fischer, K.A.; Pereira, C.B.; Louderback, M.; Nakagama, H.; Bailey, G.S.; Williams, D.E.; Dashwood, R.H. Protective versus Promotional Effects of White Tea and Caffeine on PhIP-Induced Tumorigenesis and β-Catenin Expression in the Rat. *Carcinogenesis* **2008**, *29*, 834–839. [CrossRef]
115. Soares, P.V.; Kannen, V.; Junior, A.A.J.; Garcia, S.B. Coffee, but Neither Decaffeinated Coffee nor Caffeine, Elicits Chemoprotection Against a Direct Carcinogen in the Colon of Wistar Rats. *Nutr. Cancer* **2019**, *71*, 615–623. [CrossRef]
116. Nishikawa, A.; Furukawa, F.; Imazawa, T.; Ikezaki, S.; Hasegawa, T.; Takahashi, M. Effects of Caffeine on Glandular Stomach Carcinogenesis Induced in Rats by N-Methyl-N′-Nitro-N-Nitrosoguanidine and Sodium Chloride. *Food Chem. Toxicol.* **1995**, *33*, 21–26. [CrossRef]
117. Olthof, M.R.; Hollman, P.C.H.; Katan, M.B. Chlorogenic Acid and Caffeic Acid Are Absorbed in Humans. *J. Nutr.* **2001**, *131*, 66–71. [CrossRef] [PubMed]
118. Olthof, M.R.; Hollman, P.C.H.; Buijsman, M.N.C.P.; van Amelsvoort, J.M.M.; Katan, M.B. Chlorogenic Acid, Quercetin-3-Rutinoside and Black Tea Phenols Are Extensively Metabolized in Humans. *J. Nutr.* **2003**, *133*, 1806–1814. [CrossRef] [PubMed]
119. Miller, E.G.; McWhorter, K.; Rivera-Hidalgo, F.; Wright, J.M.; Hirsbrunner, P.; Sunahara, G.I. Kahweol and Cafestol: Inhibitors of Hamster Buccal Pouch Carcinogenesis. *Nutr. Cancer* **1991**, *15*, 41–46. [CrossRef]
120. Huber, W.W.; McDaniel, L.P.; Kaderlik, K.R.; Teitel, C.H.; Lang, N.P.; Kadlubar, F.F. Chemoprotection against the Formation of Colon DNA Adducts from the Food-Borne Carcinogen 2-Amino-1-Methyl-6-Phenylimidazo[4,5-b]Pyridine (PhIP) in the Rat. *Mutat. Res. Mol. Mech. Mutagen.* **1997**, *376*, 115–122. [CrossRef]
121. Lam, L.K.; Sparnins, V.L.; Wattenberg, L.W. Isolation and Identification of Kahweol Palmitate and Cafestol Palmitate as Active Constituents of Green Coffee Beans That Enhance Glutathione S-Transferase Activity in the Mouse. *Cancer Res.* **1982**, *42*, 1193–1198.
122. De Roos, B.; Sawyer, J.K.; Katan, M.B.; Rudel, L.L. Validity of Animal Models for the Cholesterol-Raising Effects of Coffee Diterpenes in Human Subjects. *Proc. Nutr. Soc.* **1999**, *58*, 551–557. [CrossRef]
123. Anton, P.M.; Craus, A.; Niquet-Léridon, C.; Tessier, F.J. Highly Heated Food Rich in Maillard Reaction Products Limit an Experimental Colitis in Mice. *Food Funct.* **2012**, *3*, 941. [CrossRef]
124. Rice, J.M. The Carcinogenicity of Acrylamide. *Mutat. Res. Toxicol. Environ. Mutagen.* **2005**, *580*, 3–20. [CrossRef] [PubMed]
125. Pelucchi, C.; La Vecchia, C.; Bosetti, C.; Boyle, P.; Boffetta, P. Exposure to Acrylamide and Human Cancer—A Review and Meta-Analysis of Epidemiologic Studies. *Ann. Oncol.* **2011**, *22*, 1487–1499. [CrossRef]
126. El-Mehi, A.E.; El-Sherif, N.M. Influence of Acrylamide on the Gastric Mucosa of Adult Albino Rats and the Possible Protective Role of Rosemary. *Tissue Cell* **2015**, *47*, 273–283. [CrossRef] [PubMed]
127. Furness, J.B. *The Enteric Nervous System*; Blackwell Publishing: Oxford, UK, 2006.
128. Grundmann, D.; Loris, E.; Maas-Omlor, S.; Huang, W.; Scheller, A.; Kirchhoff, F.; Schäfer, K. Enteric Glia: S100, GFAP, and Beyond. *Anat. Rec.* **2019**, *302*, 1333–1344. [CrossRef] [PubMed]
129. Takaki, M. Gut Pacemaker Cells: The Interstitial Cells of Cajal (ICC). *J. Smooth Muscle Res.* **2003**, *39*, 137–161. [CrossRef] [PubMed]
130. Uranga, J.A.; Martínez, V.; Abalo, R. Mast Cell Regulation and Irritable Bowel Syndrome: Effects of Food Components with Potential Nutraceutical Use. *Molecules* **2020**, *25*, 4314. [CrossRef]
131. Thomas, F.B.; Steinbaugh, J.T.; Fromkes, J.J.; Mekhjian, H.S.; Caldwell, J.H. Inhibitory Effect of Coffee on Lower Esophageal Sphincter Pressure. *Gastroenterology* **1980**, *79*, 1262–1266. [CrossRef]
132. Boekema, P.J.; Samsom, M.; van Henegouwen, G.P.B.; Smout, A.J. Coffee and Gastrointestinal Function: Facts and Fiction: A Review. *Scand. J. Gastroenterol.* **1999**, *34*, 35–39.
133. Chang, L.M.; Chen, G.H.; Chang, C.S.; Lien, H.C.; Kao, C.H. Effect of Coffee on Solid-Phase Gastric Emptying in Patients with Non-Ulcer Dyspepsia. *Gaoxiong Yi Xue Ke Xue Za Zhi* **1995**, *11*, 425–429.
134. Lien, H.-C.; Chen, G.-H.; Chang, C.-S.; Kao, C.-H.; Wang, S.-J. The Effect of Coffee on Gastric Emptying. *Nucl. Med. Commun.* **1995**, *16*, 923–926. [CrossRef]
135. Boekema, P.J.; Lo, B.; Samsom, M.; Akkermans, L.M.A.; Smout, A.J.P.M.; Lo, B.; Samsom, M.; Akkermans, L.; Smout, A. The Effect of Coffee on Gastric Emptying and Oro-Caecal Transit Time. *Eur. J. Clin. Investig.* **2000**, *30*, 129–134. [CrossRef]
136. Elta, G.H.; Behler, E.M.; Colturi, T.J. Comparison of Coffee Intake and Coffee-Induced Symptoms in Patients with Duodenal Ulcer, Nonulcer Dyspepsia, and Normal Controls. *Am. J. Gastroenterol.* **1990**, *85*, 1339–1342.
137. Shirlow, M.J.; Mathers, C.D. A Study of Caffeine Consumption and Symptoms: Indigestion, Palpitations, Tremor, Headache and Insomnia. *Int. J. Epidemiol.* **1985**, *14*, 239–248. [CrossRef] [PubMed]
138. Talley, N.J. Coffee and Nonulcer Dyspepsia. *Am. J. Gastroenterol.* **1993**, *88*, 966. [PubMed]
139. Boekema, P.J.; Samsom, M.; Roelofs, J.M.; Smout, A.J. Effect of Coffee on Motor and Sensory Function of Proximal Stomach. *Dig. Dis. Sci.* **2001**, *46*, 945–951. [CrossRef] [PubMed]

140. Wald, A.; Back, C.; Bayless, T.M. Effect of Caffeine on the Human Small Intestine. *Gastroenterology* **1976**, *71*, 738–742. [CrossRef]
141. Wagner, S.M.; Mekhjian, H.S.; Caldwell, J.H.; Thomas, F.B. Effects of Caffeine and Coffee on Fluid Transport in the Small Intestine. *Gastroenterology* **1978**, *75*, 379–381. [CrossRef]
142. Brettholz, E.; Meshkinpour, H. The Effect of Coffee on Mouth To-Cecum Transit Time. *Gastroenterology* **1985**, *88*, 1335.
143. Glatzel, H.; Hackenberg, K. Wirkungen von Koffeinhaltigem Und Koffeinfreiem Kaffee Auf Die Verdauungsfunktion. *Med. Klin.* **1967**, *62*, 625–628.
144. Matzkies, F.; Perisoara, A. Ultrasound Study of the Effects of Coffee on the Motoric Function of the Gallbladder. *Fortschr. Med.* **1985**, *103*, 713–714.
145. Douglas, B.R.; Jansen, J.B.; Tham, R.T.; Lamers, C.B. Coffee Stimulation of Cholecystokinin Release and Gallbladder Contraction in Humans. *Am. J. Clin. Nutr.* **1990**, *52*, 553–556. [CrossRef]
146. Brown, S.R.; Cann, P.A.; Read, N.W. Effect of Coffee on Distal Colon Function. *Gut* **1990**, *31*, 450–453. [CrossRef]
147. Rao, S.S.C.; Welcher, K.; Zimmerman, B.; Stumbo, P. Is Coffee a Colonic Stimulant? *Eur. J. Gastroenterol. Hepatol.* **1998**, *10*, 113–118. [CrossRef] [PubMed]
148. Chvasta, T.E.; Cooke, A.R. Emptying and Absorption of Caffeine from the Human Stomach. *Gastroenterology* **1971**, *61*, 838–843. [CrossRef]
149. Gkegkes, I.D.; Minis, E.E.; Iavazzo, C. Effect of Caffeine Intake on Postoperative Ileus: A Systematic Review and Meta-Analysis. *Dig. Surg.* **2020**, *37*, 22–31. [CrossRef] [PubMed]
150. Güngördük, K.; Özdemir, İ.A.; Güngördük, Ö.; Gülseren, V.; Gokçü, M.; Sancı, M. Effects of Coffee Consumption on Gut Recovery after Surgery of Gynecological Cancer Patients: A Randomized Controlled Trial. *Am. J. Obstet. Gynecol.* **2017**, *216*, e1–e145. [CrossRef]
151. Vather, R.; O'Grady, G.; Bissett, I.P.; Dinning, P.G. Postoperative Ileus: Mechanisms and Future Directions for Research. *Clin. Exp. Pharmacol. Physiol.* **2014**, *41*, 358–370. [CrossRef]
152. Sarawate, C.A.; Lin, S.-J.; Walton, S.M.; Crawford, S.Y.; Goldstein, J.L. Economic Burden of Postoperative Ileus (POI) in Abdominal Surgical Procedures. *Gastroenterology* **2003**, *124*, A828. [CrossRef]
153. Müller, S.A.; Rahbari, N.N.; Schneider, F.; Warschkow, R.; Simon, T.; von Frankenberg, M.; Bork, U.; Weitz, J.; Schmied, B.M.; Büchler, M.W. Randomized Clinical Trial on the Effect of Coffee on Postoperative Ileus Following Elective Colectomy. *Br. J. Surg.* **2012**, *99*, 1530–1538. [CrossRef]
154. Dulskas, A.; Klimovskij, M.; Vitkauskiene, M.; Samalavicius, N.E. Effect of Coffee on the Length of Postoperative Ileus After Elective Laparoscopic Left-Sided Colectomy. *Dis. Colon Rectum* **2015**, *58*, 1064–1069. [CrossRef]
155. Piric, M.; Pasic, F.; Rifatbegovic, Z.; Konjic, F. The Effects of Drinking Coffee While Recovering from Colon and Rectal Resection Surgery. *Med. Arch.* **2015**, *69*, 357. [CrossRef]
156. Büchler, M.W.; Seiler, C.M.; Monson, J.R.T.; Flamant, Y.; Thompson-Fawcett, M.W.; Byrne, M.M.; Mortensen, E.R.; Altman, J.F.B.; Williamson, R. Clinical Trial: Alvimopan for the Management of Post-Operative Ileus after Abdominal Surgery: Results of an International Randomized, Double-Blind, Multicentre, Placebo-Controlled Clinical Study. *Aliment. Pharmacol. Ther.* **2008**, *28*, 312–325. [CrossRef]
157. Bell, T.J.; Poston, S.A.; Kraft, M.D.; Senagore, A.J.; Delaney, C.P.; Techner, L. Economic Analysis of Alvimopan in North American Phase III Efficacy Trials. *Am. J. Health Pharm.* **2009**, *66*, 1362–1368. [CrossRef] [PubMed]
158. Institute of Medicine (US). Committee on Military Nutrition Research Pharmacology of Caffeine. In *Caffeine for the Sustainment of Mental Task Performance: Formulations for Military Operations*; National Academies Press (US): Washington, DC, USA, 2001.
159. Ito, Y.; Osa, T.; Kuriyama, H. Topical Differences of Caffeine Action on the Smooth Muscle Cells of the Guinea Pig Alimentary Canal. *Jpn. J. Physiol.* **1974**, *24*, 217–232. [CrossRef] [PubMed]
160. Tokutomi, Y.; Tokutomi, N.; Nishi, K. The Properties of Ryanodine-Sensitive Ca 2+ Release in Mouse Gastric Smooth Muscle Cells. *Br. J. Pharmacol.* **2001**, *133*, 125–137. [CrossRef]
161. Domae, K.; Hashitani, H.; Suzuki, H. Regional Differences in the Frequency of Slow Waves in Smooth Muscle of the Guinea-Pig Stomach. *J. Smooth Muscle Res.* **2008**, *44*, 231–248. [CrossRef] [PubMed]
162. Lee, H.; Hennig, G.W.; Fleming, N.W.; Keef, K.D.; Spencer, N.J.; Ward, S.M.; Sanders, K.M.; Smith, T.K. The Mechanism and Spread of Pacemaker Activity Through Myenteric Interstitial Cells of Cajal in Human Small Intestine. *Gastroenterology* **2007**, *132*, 1852–1865. [CrossRef] [PubMed]
163. Kimball, B.C.; Yule, D.I.; Mulholland, M.W. Caffeine- and Ryanodine-Sensitive Ca2+ Stores in Cultured Guinea Pig Myenteric Neurons. *Am. J. Physiol. Liver Physiol.* **1996**, *270*, G594–G603. [CrossRef]
164. Broadhead, M.J.; Bayguinov, P.O.; Okamoto, T.; Heredia, D.J.; Smith, T.K. Ca2+ Transients in Myenteric Glial Cells during the Colonic Migrating Motor Complex in the Isolated Murine Large Intestine. *J. Physiol.* **2012**, *590*, 335–350. [CrossRef]
165. Brookes, S.J.H. Classes of Enteric Nerve Cells in the Guinea-Pig Small Intestine. *Anat. Rec.* **2001**, *262*, 58–70. [CrossRef]
166. Furness, J. Intrinsic Primary Afferent Neuronsof the Intestine. *Prog. Neurobiol.* **1998**, *54*, 1–18. [CrossRef]
167. Hillsley, K.; Kenyon, J.L.; Smith, T.K. Ryanodine-Sensitive Stores Regulate the Excitability of AH Neurons in the Myenteric Plexus of Guinea-Pig Ileum. *J. Neurophysiol.* **2000**, *84*, 2777–2785. [CrossRef]
168. Rugiero, F.; Gola, M.; Kunze, W.A.A.; Reynaud, J.; Furness, J.B.; Clerc, N. Analysis of Whole-cell Currents by Patch Clamp of Guinea-pig Myenteric Neurones in Intact Ganglia. *J. Physiol.* **2002**, *538*, 447–463. [CrossRef] [PubMed]
169. Liu, S.; Hu, H.-Z.; Gao, N.; Gao, C.; Wang, G.; Wang, X.; Peck, O.C.; Kim, G.; Gao, X.; Xia, Y.; et al. Neuroimmune Interactions in Guinea Pig Stomach and Small Intestine. *Am. J. Physiol. Liver Physiol.* **2003**, *284*, G154–G164. [CrossRef] [PubMed]

170. Baird, A.W.; Cuthbert, A.W. Neuronal Involvement in Type 1 Hypersensitivity Reactions in Gut Epithelia. *Br. J. Pharmacol.* **1987**, *92*, 647–655. [CrossRef] [PubMed]
171. Barnette, M.S.; Grous, M. Characterization of the Antigen-Induced Contraction of Colonic Smooth Muscle from Sensitized Guinea Pigs. *Am. J. Physiol. Liver Physiol.* **1992**, *262*, G144–G149. [CrossRef]
172. Wood, J. Allergies and the Brain-in-the-Gut. *Clin. Perspect Gastroenterol.* **2000**, *4*, 343–348.
173. Koshihara, Y.; Neichi, T.; Murota, S.; Lao, A.; Fujimoto, Y.; Tatsuno, T. Caffeic Acid Is a Selective Inhibitor for Leukotriene Biosynthesis. *Biochim. Biophys. Acta* **1984**, *792*, 92–97.
174. Iriondo-DeHond, A.; Cornejo, F.S.; Fernandez-Gomez, B.; Vera, G.; Guisantes-Batan, E.; Alonso, S.G.; Andres, M.I.S.; Sanchez-Fortun, S.; Lopez-Gomez, L.; Uranga, J.A.; et al. Bioaccesibility, Metabolism, and Excretion of Lipids Composing Spent Coffee Grounds. *Nutrients* **2019**, *11*, 1411. [CrossRef]
175. López-Barrera, D.M.; Vázquez-Sánchez, K.; Loarca-Piña, M.G.F.; Campos-Vega, R. Spent Coffee Grounds, an Innovative Source of Colonic Fermentable Compounds, Inhibit Inflammatory Mediators in Vitro. *Food Chem.* **2016**, *212*, 282–290. [CrossRef]
176. Fukumoto, S.; Tatewaki, M.; Yamada, T.; Fujimiya, M.; Mantyh, C.; Voss, M.; Eubanks, S.; Harris, M.; Pappas, T.N.; Takahashi, T. Short-Chain Fatty Acids Stimulate Colonic Transit via Intraluminal 5-HT Release in Rats. *Am. J. Physiol. Integr. Comp. Physiol.* **2003**, *284*, R1269–R1276. [CrossRef]
177. Iriondo-DeHond, A.; Rios, M.B.; Herrera, T.; Rodriguez-Bertos, A.; Nuñez, F.; San Andres, M.I.; Sanchez-Fortun, S.; del Castillo, M.D. Coffee Silverskin Extract: Nutritional Value, Safety and Effect on Key Biological Functions. *Nutrients* **2019**, *11*, 2693. [CrossRef]
178. De la Cruz, S.T.; Iriondo-DeHond, A.; Herrera, T.; Lopez-Tofiño, Y.; Galvez-Robleño, C.; Prodanov, M.; Velazquez-Escobar, F.; Abalo, R.; Castillo, M.D. del An Assessment of the Bioactivity of Coffee Silverskin Melanoidins. *Foods* **2019**, *8*, 68. [CrossRef] [PubMed]
179. Iriondo-DeHond, A.; Aparicio García, N.; Velazquez Escobar, F.; San Andres, M.I.; Sanchez-Fortun, S.; Blanch, G.P.; Fernandez-Gomez, B.; Guisantes Batan, E.; del Castillo, M.D. Validation of Coffee By-Products as Novel Food Ingredients. *Innov. Food Sci. Emerg. Technol.* **2019**, *51*, 194–204. [CrossRef]
180. Del Castillo, M.D.; Martinez-Saez, N.; Amigo-Benavent, M.; Silvan, J.M. Phytochemomics and Other Omics for Permitting Health Claims Made on Foods. *Food Res. Int.* **2013**, *54*, 1237–1249. [CrossRef]
181. Murthy, P.S.; Naidu, M.M.; Srinivas, P. Production of α-Amylase under Solid-State Fermentation Utilizing Coffee Waste. *J. Chem. Technol. Biotechnol.* **2009**, *84*, 1246–1249. [CrossRef]
182. Esquivel, P.; Jiménez, V.M. Functional Properties of Coffee and Coffee By-Products. *Food Res. Int.* **2012**, *46*, 488–495. [CrossRef]
183. Mesías, M.; Delgado-Andrade, C. Melanoidins as a Potential Functional Food Ingredient. *Curr. Opin. Food Sci.* **2017**, *14*, 37–42. [CrossRef]
184. Silván, J.M.; Morales, F.J.; Saura-Calixto, F. Conceptual Study on Maillardized Dietary Fiber in Coffee. *J. Agric. Food Chem.* **2010**, *58*, 12244–12249. [CrossRef]
185. Argirova, M.D.; Stefanova, I.D.; Krustev, A.D.; Turiiski, V.I. Testing Biological Activity of Model Maillard Reaction Products: Studies on Gastric Smooth Muscle Tissues. *Amino Acids* **2010**, *38*, 797–803. [CrossRef]
186. Stadler, R.H.; Blank, I.; Varga, N.; Robert, F.; Hau, J.; Guy, P.A.; Robert, M.-C.; Riediker, S. Acrylamide from Maillard Reaction Products. *Nature* **2002**, *419*, 449–450. [CrossRef]
187. World Health Organization (WHO). Health Implications of Acrylamide in Food. Available online: http://apps.who.int/iris/handle/10665/4256 (accessed on 10 November 2020).
188. Lourenssen, S.; Miller, K.G.; Blennerhassett, M.G. Discrete Responses of Myenteric Neurons to Structural and Functional Damage by Neurotoxins in Vitro. *Am. J. Physiol. Liver Physiol.* **2009**, *297*, G228–G239. [CrossRef]
189. Belai, A.; Burnstock, G. Acrylamide-Induced Neuropathic Changes in Rat Enteric Nerves: Similarities with Effects of Streptozotocin-Diabetes. *J. Auton. Nerv. Syst.* **1996**, *58*, 56–62. [CrossRef]
190. Palus, K.; Makowska, K.; Całka, J. Acrylamide-Induced Alterations in the Cocaine- and Amphetamine-Regulated Peptide Transcript (CART)-like Immunoreactivity within the Enteric Nervous System of the Porcine Small Intestines. *Ann. Anat. Anat. Anzeiger* **2018**, *219*, 94–101. [CrossRef] [PubMed]
191. Liu, H.-X.; Hökfelt, T. The Participation of Galanin in Pain Processing at the Spinal Level. *Trends Pharmacol. Sci.* **2002**, *23*, 468–474. [CrossRef]
192. Locker, F.; Lang, A.A.; Koller, A.; Lang, R.; Bianchini, R.; Kofler, B. Galanin Modulates Human and Murine Neutrophil Activation in Vitro. *Acta Physiol.* **2015**, *213*, 595–602. [CrossRef]
193. Palus, K.; Makowska, K.; Całka, J. Alterations in Galanin-Like Immunoreactivity in the Enteric Nervous System of the Porcine Stomach Following Acrylamide Supplementation. *Int. J. Mol. Sci.* **2019**, *20*, 3345. [CrossRef]
194. Palus, K.; Całka, J. Influence of Acrylamide Administration on the Neurochemical Characteristics of Enteric Nervous System (ENS) Neurons in the Porcine Duodenum. *Int. J. Mol. Sci.* **2019**, *21*, 15. [CrossRef]
195. Zong, C.; Hasegawa, R.; Urushitani, M.; Zhang, L.; Nagashima, D.; Sakurai, T.; Ichihara, S.; Ohsako, S.; Ichihara, G. Role of Microglial Activation and Neuroinflammation in Neurotoxicity of Acrylamide in Vivo and in Vitro. *Arch. Toxicol.* **2019**, *93*, 2007–2019. [CrossRef]
196. Lyte, J.M. Eating for 3.8 × 10^{13}: Examining the Impact of Diet and Nutrition on the Microbiota-Gut-Brain Axis through the Lens of Microbial Endocrinology. *Front. Endocrinol. (Lausanne)* **2019**, *10*, 1–14. [CrossRef]
197. Mulak, A. Brain-Gut-Microbiota Axis in Parkinson's Disease. *World J. Gastroenterol.* **2015**, *21*, 10609. [CrossRef]
198. Scheperjans, F.; Pekkonen, E.; Kaakkola, S.; Auvinen, P. Linking Smoking, Coffee, Urate, and Parkinson's Disease—A Role for Gut Microbiota? *J. Parkinsons. Dis.* **2015**, *5*, 255–262. [CrossRef]

199. Papakonstantinou, E.; Kechribari, I.; Sotirakoglou, K.; Tarantilis, P.; Gourdomichali, T.; Michas, G.; Kravvariti, V.; Voumvourakis, K.; Zampelas, A. Acute Effects of Coffee Consumption on Self-Reported Gastrointestinal Symptoms, Blood Pressure and Stress Indices in Healthy Individuals. *Nutr. J.* **2015**, *15*, 26. [CrossRef] [PubMed]
200. European Food Safety Authority (EFSA). Scientific Opinion on the Safety of Caffeine. *EFSA J.* **2015**, *13*, 1–21.
201. Alasmari, F. Caffeine Induces Neurobehavioral Effects through Modulating Neurotransmitters. *Saudi Pharm. J.* **2020**, *28*, 445–451. [CrossRef] [PubMed]
202. Solinas, M.; Ferré, S.; You, Z.-B.; Karcz-Kubicha, M.; Popoli, P.; Goldberg, S.R. Caffeine Induces Dopamine and Glutamate Release in the Shell of the Nucleus Accumbens. *J. Neurosci.* **2002**, *22*, 6321–6324. [CrossRef]
203. Volkow, N.D.; Wang, G.-J.; Logan, J.; Alexoff, D.; Fowler, J.S.; Thanos, P.K.; Wong, C.; Casado, V.; Ferre, S.; Tomasi, D. Caffeine Increases Striatal Dopamine D2/D3 Receptor Availability in the Human Brain. *Transl. Psychiatry* **2015**, *5*, e549. [CrossRef]
204. Pandolfo, P.; Machado, N.J.; Köfalvi, A.; Takahashi, R.N.; Cunha, R.A. Caffeine Regulates Frontocorticostriatal Dopamine Transporter Density and Improves Attention and Cognitive Deficits in an Animal Model of Attention Deficit Hyperactivity Disorder. *Eur. Neuropsychopharmacol.* **2013**, *23*, 317–328. [CrossRef]
205. Manalo, R.V.M.; Medina, P.M.B. Caffeine Protects Dopaminergic Neurons From Dopamine-Induced Neurodegeneration via Synergistic Adenosine-Dopamine D2-Like Receptor Interactions in Transgenic Caenorhabditis Elegans. *Front. Neurosci.* **2018**, *12*, 137. [CrossRef]
206. Hughes, J.R.; McHugh, P.; Holtzman, S. Alcohol & Drug Abuse: Caffeine and Schizophrenia. *Psychiatr. Serv.* **1998**, *49*, 1415–1417.
207. Winston, A.P.; Hardwick, E.; Jaberi, N. Neuropsychiatric Effects of Caffeine. *Adv. Psychiatr. Treat.* **2005**, *11*, 432–439. [CrossRef]
208. Ning, Y.-L.; Yang, N.; Chen, X.; Zhao, Z.-A.; Zhang, X.-Z.; Chen, X.-Y.; Li, P.; Zhao, Y.; Zhou, Y.-G. Chronic Caffeine Exposure Attenuates Blast-Induced Memory Deficit in Mice. *Chin. J. Traumatol.* **2015**, *18*, 204–211. [CrossRef]
209. Duarte, J.M.N.; Agostinho, P.M.; Carvalho, R.A.; Cunha, R.A. Caffeine Consumption Prevents Diabetes-Induced Memory Impairment and Synaptotoxicity in the Hippocampus of NONcZNO10/LTJ Mice. *PLoS ONE* **2012**, *7*, e21899. [CrossRef] [PubMed]
210. Hahn, S.; Kim, Y.H.; Seo, H.S. Immediate Decrease in γ-AminoButyric Acid after Caffeine Intake in Adolescents: A Preliminary MRS Study. *Investig. Magn. Reson. Imaging* **2017**, *21*, 102–105. [CrossRef]
211. Jee, H.J.J.; Lee, S.G.G.; Bormate, K.J.J.; Jung, Y.-S.S. Effect of Caffeine Consumption on the Risk for Neurological and Psychiatric Disorders: Sex Differences in Human. *Nutrients* **2020**, *12*, 3080. [CrossRef] [PubMed]
212. Farah, A.; Monteiro, M.; Donangelo, C.M.; Lafay, S. Chlorogenic Acids from Green Coffee Extract Are Highly Bioavailable in Humans. *J. Nutr.* **2008**, *138*, 2309–2315. [CrossRef]
213. Fernandez-Gomez, B.; Lezama, A.; Amigo-Benavent, M.; Ullate, M.; Herrero, M.; Martín, M.Á.; Mesa, M.D.; del Castillo, M.D. Insights on the Health Benefits of the Bioactive Compounds of Coffee Silverskin Extract. *J. Funct. Foods* **2016**, *25*, 197–207. [CrossRef]
214. Lardeau, A.; Poquet, L. Phenolic Acid Metabolites Derived from Coffee Consumption Are Unlikely to Cross the Blood-Brain Barrier. *J. Pharm. Biomed. Anal.* **2013**, *76*, 134–138. [CrossRef]
215. Nabavi, S.F.; Tejada, S.; Setzer, W.N.; Gortzi, O.; Sureda, A.; Braidy, N.; Daglia, M.; Manayi, A.; Nabavi, S.M. Chlorogenic Acid and Mental Diseases: From Chemistry to Medicine. *Curr. Neuropharmacol.* **2016**, *15*, 471–479. [CrossRef]
216. Barros Silva, R.; Santos, N.A.G.; Martins, N.M.; Ferreira, D.A.S.; Barbosa, F.; Oliveira Souza, V.C.; Kinoshita, Â.; Baffa, O.; Del-Bel, E.; Santos, A.C. Caffeic Acid Phenethyl Ester Protects against the Dopaminergic Neuronal Loss Induced by 6-Hydroxydopamine in Rats. *Neuroscience* **2013**, *233*, 86–94. [CrossRef]
217. Singh, S.S.; Rai, S.N.; Birla, H.; Zahra, W.; Kumar, G.; Gedda, M.R.; Tiwari, N.; Patnaik, R.; Singh, R.K.; Singh, S.P. Effect of Chlorogenic Acid Supplementation in MPTP-Intoxicated Mouse. *Front. Pharmacol.* **2018**, *9*, 757. [CrossRef]
218. Ascherio, A.; Zhang, S.M.; Hernán, M.A.; Kawachi, I.; Colditz, G.A.; Speizer, F.E.; Willett, W.C. Prospective Study of Caffeine Consumption and Risk of Parkinson's Disease in Men and Women. *Ann. Neurol.* **2001**, *50*, 56–63. [CrossRef]
219. Hong, C.T.; Chan, L.; Bai, C.-H. The Effect of Caffeine on the Risk and Progression of Parkinson's Disease: A Meta-Analysis. *Nutrients* **2020**, *12*, 1860. [CrossRef] [PubMed]
220. Fasano, A.; Visanji, N.P.; Liu, L.W.C.; Lang, A.E.; Pfeiffer, R.F. Gastrointestinal Dysfunction in Parkinson's Disease. *Lancet Neurol.* **2015**, *14*, 625–639. [CrossRef]
221. Abbott, R.D.; Petrovitch, H.; White, L.R.; Masaki, K.H.; Tanner, C.M.; Curb, J.D.; Grandinetti, A.; Blanchette, P.L.; Popper, J.S.; Ross, G.W. Frequency of Bowel Movements and the Future Risk of Parkinson's Disease. *Neurology* **2001**, *57*, 456–462. [CrossRef] [PubMed]
222. Braak, H.; Tredici, K.; Del Rüb, U.; de Vos, R.A.; Steur, E.N.J.; Braak, E. Staging of Brain Pathology Related to Sporadic Parkinson's Disease. *Neurobiol. Aging* **2003**, *24*, 197–211. [CrossRef]
223. Perez-Pardo, P.; Kliest, T.; Dodiya, H.B.; Broersen, L.M.; Garssen, J.; Keshavarzian, A.; Kraneveld, A.D. The Gut-Brain Axis in Parkinson's Disease: Possibilities for Food-Based Therapies. *Eur. J. Pharmacol.* **2017**, *817*, 86–95. [CrossRef] [PubMed]
224. Miyazaki, I.; Isooka, N.; Wada, K.; Kikuoka, R.; Kitamura, Y.; Asanuma, M. Effects of Enteric Environmental Modification by Coffee Components on Neurodegeneration in Rotenone-Treated Mice. *Cells* **2019**, *8*, 221. [CrossRef] [PubMed]
225. Vaccaro, A.; Kaplan Dor, Y.; Nambara, K.; Pollina, E.A.; Lin, C.; Greenberg, M.E.; Rogulja, D. Sleep Loss Can Cause Death through Accumulation of Reactive Oxygen Species in the Gut. *Cell* **2020**, *181*, 1307–1328.e15. [CrossRef]
226. Singer, D.; Camargo, S.M.R. Collectrin and ACE2 in Renal and Intestinal Amino Acid Transport. *Channels* **2011**, *5*, 410–423. [CrossRef]
227. Bevins, C.L. Events at the Host-Microbial Interface of the Gastrointestinal Tract. V. Paneth Cell α-Defensins in Intestinal Host Defense. *Am. J. Physiol. Gastrointest. Liver Physiol.* **2005**, *289*, 173–176. [CrossRef]

228. Hashimoto, T.; Perlot, T.; Rehman, A.; Trichereau, J.; Ishiguro, H.; Paolino, M.; Sigl, V.; Hanada, T.; Hanada, R.; Lipinski, S.; et al. ACE2 Links Amino Acid Malnutrition to Microbial Ecology and Intestinal Inflammation. *Nature* **2012**, *487*, 477–481. [CrossRef]
229. Yisireyili, M.; Uchida, Y.; Yamamoto, K.; Nakayama, T.; Cheng, X.W.; Matsushita, T.; Nakamura, S.; Murohara, T.; Takeshita, K. Angiotensin Receptor Blocker Irbesartan Reduces Stress-Induced Intestinal Inflammation via AT1a Signaling and ACE2-Dependent Mechanism in Mice. *Brain Behav. Immun.* **2018**, *69*, 167–179. [CrossRef] [PubMed]
230. Garg, M.; Christensen, B.; Lubel, J.S. Letter: Gastrointestinal ACE2, COVID-19 and IBD—Opportunity in the Face of Tragedy? *Gastroenterology* **2020**. [CrossRef]
231. Camargo, S.M.R.; Vuille-dit-Bille, R.N.; Meier, C.F.; Verrey, F. ACE2 and Gut Amino Acid Transport. *Clin. Sci.* **2020**, *134*, 2823–2833. [CrossRef] [PubMed]
232. Mousa, T.Y.; Mousa, O.Y. *Nicotinic Acid Deficiency*; StatPearls Publishing: Treasure Island, FL, USA, 2020.
233. O'Mahony, S.M.; Clarke, G.; Borre, Y.E.; Dinan, T.G.; Cryan, J.F. Serotonin, Tryptophan Metabolism and the Brain-Gut-Microbiome Axis. *Behav. Brain Res.* **2015**, *277*, 32–48. [CrossRef] [PubMed]
234. Paredes, S.D.; Barriga, C.; Reiter, R.J.; Rodríguez, A.B. Assessment of the Potential Role of Tryptophan as the Precursor of Serotonin and Melatonin for the Aged Sleep-Wake Cycle and Immune Function: Streptopelia Risoria as a Model. *Int. J. Tryptophan Res.* **2009**, *2*, 23–36. [CrossRef] [PubMed]
235. El-Merahbi, R.; Löffler, M.; Mayer, A.; Sumara, G. The Roles of Peripheral Serotonin in Metabolic Homeostasis. *FEBS Lett.* **2015**, *589*, 1728–1734. [CrossRef]
236. Voigt, J.P.; Fink, H. Serotonin Controlling Feeding and Satiety. *Behav. Brain Res.* **2015**, *277*, 14–31. [CrossRef]
237. Stasi, C.; Sadalla, S.; Milani, S. The Relationship Between the Serotonin Metabolism, Gut-Microbiota and the Gut-Brain Axis. *Curr. Drug Metab.* **2019**, *20*, 646–655. [CrossRef]
238. Peuhkuri, K.; Sihvola, N.; Korpela, R. Dietary Factors and Fluctuating Levels of Melatonin. *Food Nutr. Res.* **2012**, *56*, 17252. [CrossRef]
239. Johns, J. Estimation of Melatonin Blood Brain Barrier Permeability. *J. Bioanal. Biomed.* **2011**, *3*, 64–69. [CrossRef]
240. Andersen, L.P.H.; Werner, M.U.; Rosenkilde, M.M.; Harpsøe, N.G.; Fuglsang, H.; Rosenberg, J.; Gögenur, I. Pharmacokinetics of Oral and Intravenous Melatonin in Healthy Volunteers. *BMC Pharmacol. Toxicol.* **2016**, *17*, 1–5. [CrossRef] [PubMed]
241. Boonstra, E.; de Kleijn, R.; Colzato, L.S.; Alkemade, A.; Forstmann, B.U.; Nieuwenhuis, S. Neurotransmitters as Food Supplements: The Effects of GABA on Brain and Behavior. *Front. Psychol.* **2015**, *6*, 6–11. [CrossRef] [PubMed]
242. Briguglio, M.; Dell'Osso, B.; Panzica, G.; Malgaroli, A.; Banfi, G.; Dina, C.Z.; Galentino, R.; Porta, M. Dietary Neurotransmitters: A Narrative Review on Current Knowledge. *Nutrients* **2018**, *10*, 591. [CrossRef] [PubMed]
243. Pérez-Burillo, S.; Rajakaruna, S.; Pastoriza, S.; Paliy, O.; Rufián-Henares, J.Á. Bioactivity of Food Melanoidins Is Mediated by Gut Microbiota. *Food Chem.* **2020**, *316*, 126309. [CrossRef]
244. Barroso, J.M. Commission Regulation (EU) No 432/2012. *Off. J. Eur. Union* **2012**, *13*, 9.
245. Nishitsuji, K.; Watanabe, S.; Xiao, J.; Nagatomo, R.; Ogawa, H.; Tsunematsu, T.; Umemoto, H.; Morimoto, Y.; Akatsu, H.; Inoue, K.; et al. Effect of Coffee or Coffee Components on Gut Microbiome and Short-Chain Fatty Acids in a Mouse Model of Metabolic Syndrome. *Sci. Rep.* **2018**, *8*, 16173. [CrossRef]
246. Holscher, H.D. Dietary Fiber and Prebiotics and the Gastrointestinal Microbiota. *Gut Microbes* **2017**, *8*, 172–184. [CrossRef]
247. Oseguera-Castro, K.Y.; Madrid, J.A.; Martínez Madrid, M.J.; García, O.P.; Del Castillo, M.D.; Campos-Vega, R. Antioxidant Dietary Fiber Isolated from Spent Coffee (*Coffea Arabica* L.) Grounds Improves Chronotype and Circadian Locomotor Activity in Young Adults. *Food Funct.* **2019**, *10*, 4546–4556. [CrossRef]
248. Campos-Vega, R.; Arreguín-Campos, A.; Cruz-Medrano, M.A.; del Castillo, B.M.D. Spent Coffee (*Coffea Arabica* L.) Grounds Promote Satiety and Attenuate Energy Intake: A Pilot Study. *J. Food Biochem.* **2020**, e13204. [CrossRef]
249. Walker, J.M.; Mennella, I.; Ferracane, R.; Tagliamonte, S.; Holik, A.K.; Hölz, K.; Somoza, M.M.; Somoza, V.; Fogliano, V.; Vitaglione, P. Melanoidins from Coffee and Bread Differently Influence Energy Intake: A Randomized Controlled Trial of Food Intake and Gut-Brain Axis Response. *J. Funct. Foods* **2020**, *72*, 104063. [CrossRef]
250. International Coffee Organization. *Crop Year Production by Country*; International Coffee Organization: London, UK, 2020.
251. Klingel, T.; Kremer, J.I.; Gottstein, V.; Rajcic de Rezende, T.; Schwarz, S.; Lachenmeier, D.W. A Review of Coffee By-Products Including Leaf, Flower, Cherry, Husk, Silver Skin, and Spent Grounds as Novel Foods within the European Union. *Foods* **2020**, *9*, 665. [CrossRef] [PubMed]

MDPI
St. Alban-Anlage 66
4052 Basel
Switzerland
Tel. +41 61 683 77 34
Fax +41 61 302 89 18
www.mdpi.com

Nutrients Editorial Office
E-mail: nutrients@mdpi.com
www.mdpi.com/journal/nutrients

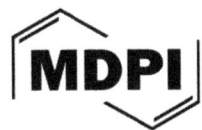

www.ingramcontent.com/pod-product-compliance
Lightning Source LLC
LaVergne TN
LVHW070052120526
838202LV00102B/2127